Diagnosing and Treating Common Problems in Paediatrics

THE ESSENTIAL EVIDENCE-BASED STUDY GUIDE

DR MICHAEL B O'NEILL

Consultant Paediatrician
Mayo General Hospital, Co. Mayo, Ireland

DR MICHELLE MARY MCEVOY

Consultant General Paediatrician
Great Ormond Street Hospital, London, United Kingdom

PROFESSOR ALF J NICHOLSON

Consultant Paediatrician
Children's University Hospital, Dublin, Ireland

Foreword by
TERENCE STEPHENSON

Nuffield Professor of Child Health, Institute of Child Health, UCL
Honorary Consultant Paediatrician, University College
and Great Ormond Street Hospitals
Chair, UK Academy of Medical Royal Colleges
Past President, Royal College of Paediatrics and Child Health

Radiology section compiled by
DR STEPHANIE RYAN

Consultant Radiologist
Children's University Hospital, Dublin, Ireland

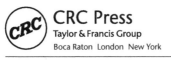

CRC Press
Taylor & Francis Group
Boca Raton London New York

CRC Press is an imprint of the
Taylor & Francis Group, an **informa** business

CRC Press
Taylor & Francis Group
6000 Broken Sound Parkway NW, Suite 300
Boca Raton, FL 33487-2742

No claim to original U.S. Government works

Printed on acid-free paper
Version Date: 20151016

ISBN-13: 978-1-908911-90-2 (pbk)
ISBN-13: 978-1-315379-43-2 (ebk)

Visit the Taylor & Francis Web site at
http://www.taylorandfrancis.com

and the CRC Press Web site at
http://www.crcpress.com

CONTENTS

Foreword   v

Preface   vi

About the authors   viii

How to use the CD for learning   ix

Acknowledgements   x

1 Evidence-based medicine: the basics   1

2 Communication   9

3 First response   16

4 The child with a fever   43

5 The child with recurrent infections   75

6 The afebrile infant with excessive crying   94

7 Common problems with infant feeding   114

8 Food allergy in children   133

9 The child with vomiting   152

10 The child with abdominal pain   175

11 The child with diarrhoea   201

12 Constipation in children   220

13 Failure to thrive (inclusive of eating disorders) 237

14 Nocturnal enuresis   259

15 Daytime wetting   276

16 Cough in children   293

17 The child with wheeze   313

18 The child with suspected congenital heart disease   334

19 Recurrent headaches in children   358

20 Seizures   380

21 Sleep problems in children   402

22 The child with developmental delay   421

23 The child with Down's syndrome   450

24 The child with a limp   466

25 The pale child   486

26 Short stature   507

27 The child with a pubertal development disorder   521

28 The child with diabetes mellitus   537

29 Childhood and adolescent obesity   556

30 The child with an acute rash   572

31 The child with a chronic rash   594

32 Attention deficit hyperactivity disorder in children   620

Index   639

FOREWORD

This book stands out because it is written from such a pragmatic and helpful viewpoint.

No child comes to the doctor with a big sticker on his or her forehead saying 'I have meningitis' or 'I have pneumonia'. Children see paediatricians because they are ill, they have a headache, they have a cough, they are vomiting. It falls to the paediatrician, community or hospital, to sort the wheat from the chaff, to triage those who need urgent investigation and treatment, those for whom it can wait, and those where doing nothing and simply counselling the child and their carers is the right course.

Emma Lazarus wrote in 1883:

> *Give me your tired, your poor,*
> *Your huddled masses yearning to breathe free,*
> *The wretched refuse of your teeming shore.*
> *Send these, the homeless, tempest-tossed to me,*
> *I lift my lamp beside the golden door.*

The paediatrician's role is to be the lamp which shines a light on a child's problem, and this book will help every paediatrician to do just that.

When I teach undergraduates or postgraduates, I try to persuade them to think exactly the way this book approaches children's illnesses. All of medicine is applied problem solving – the patient presents with a problem and the doctor's role is to bring their expertise to bear in helping solve that problem. This book will help the clinician, whether practitioner or student of paediatrics, to take a history (what we are told), examine the child (what we find), frame a list of differential diagnoses, undertake sensible tests, and offer a management plan.

In addition, it is all backed up with crisp examples illustrating how an evidence-based medicine approach to published articles can inform our practice and there are multiple choice questions to 'test yourself' on what you have learned.

Professor Terence Stephenson
BSc, BM, BCh, DM, FRCP, FRCPCH, FRACP, FRCPI, FHKAP
Nuffield Professor of Child Health,
Institute of Child Health, University College London
Honorary Consultant Paediatrician,
University College and Great Ormond Street Hospitals
Chair, UK Academy of Medical Royal Colleges
Past President, Royal College of Paediatrics and Child Health
March 2014

PREFACE

We are what we repeatedly do.
We are the sum of all our experiences, both positive and negative.

I am reminded of these two phrases when dealing with children and their parents. Our interactions with families will frame how those families view their experiences. It is with this in mind that this book has been written. While it is different from the usual textbook, its primary aims are to impart practical knowledge to the reader and an evidence-based strategy for treatment, in an attempt to make the reader smarter and, as a consequence, to enhance the care they provide to both children and parents. Currently, medical information is widely available, and as a consequence doctors need to be adept at managing and providing accurate information, because this is what the customer (patient) wants and also it is what doctors would want for themselves. Which of the following two answers is more suitable for you?

1. *The treatment for condition X, which I am suggesting for you, is more effective than standard treatment in one in eight patients.*
2. *This treatment works reasonably well in patients with your condition.*

If you chose answer 1 read on; if not, close this book.

THE BOOK'S STRUCTURE

Each chapter is devoted to a symptom. The chapter commences with the learning objectives, followed by relevant background material that is essential for the reader to know in depth. History and examination sections then follow, complete with 'red flags' to look out for. Questions are posed and answered as to which investigations are relevant.

The management section outlines clarifying and pitfall avoidance strategies. This section addresses the parent perspective first, and the reader is guided through this perspective, which must be addressed if the consultation is to be viewed as satisfactory by the parents. Pitfall avoidance for the doctor is also offered (to avoid rookie mistakes) to ensure that the symptom is correctly interpreted. The management of specific conditions is outlined. In this management section, specific questions are posed and evidence-based answers are offered. In most cases evidence from randomised controlled trials is offered. This element of the book is unique. A question is posed and answered, but it is done in a structured fashion. The quality of the evidence is weighted (Jadad score), the setting is outlined, relevant data on the participants, intervention, outcomes, results (inclusive of numbers needed to treat) and conclusion are provided. A commentary is then provided to explain the results in a clinical context. The use of this format generates accurate information for the parent. Parents want effective treatment but are also anxious to avoid harm to their child; therefore, discussing the effectiveness of treatment in terms of number needed to treat is very useful, i.e. in children with acute otitis media, with adequate analgesia, one child in every 12 treated with antibiotics benefits from the treatment (*see* Chapter 4: The Child With a Fever, Evidence 4). This type of information is of practical use in clinical practice.

Suggestions for follow-up and when to refer are also offered as a guide to primary care physicians. Clarification statements are offered for parental misconceptions. These misconceptions may influence parental treatment strategies or their adherence to treatment and should be addressed in the initial consultation, prior to recommending a treatment strategy. It is prudent to remember that what we might consider to be universally acceptable in fact may not be accepted by parents, e.g. children should be immunised unless there is a medical contraindication.

Each chapter ends with a series of multiple-choice questions. A review of these questions indicates your level of knowledge – on average, 90% indicates a good base of knowledge of the symptom.

Three chapters are different from the others in structure. These are Chapter 1: Evidence-Based Medicine: The Basics; Chapter 2: Communication; and Chapter 3: First Response, which deals with emergencies in paediatrics.

The CD component of this book has an extensive clinical slide and X-ray collection. The clinical slides are a useful adjunct for the reader to recognise clinical conditions that are described in this book, where their clinical features are provided in a table to aid recognition. The X-ray section is a stand alone component which comprises 66 cases. Each case commences with a clinical caveat and the reader is asked to identify the anomalies, which are outlined in subsequent text and indicated on the radiological image.

Michael B O'Neill
Mayo General Hospital, County Mayo, Ireland
March 2014

ABOUT THE AUTHORS

Dr O'Neill qualified as a graduate of University College Cork, Ireland. He received his paediatric training in Ireland and Canada, where he trained at Queens University, Kingston, Ontario, and at the Hospital for Sick Children, Toronto, Ontario. He was awarded his FRCPC in 1986 and was awarded a master's in health service administration from Dalhousie University, Halifax, Nova Scotia, in 1992. He was appointed Head of the Division of General Paediatrics and Associate Professor of Paediatrics at McMaster University in Hamilton in 1992. He returned to Ireland in 1996 to his current position as Consultant Paediatrician at Mayo General Hospital, Castlebar, County Mayo, Ireland. In 1999 he was appointed as one of the two National Specialty Directors for the Higher Specialist Training Programme in Paediatrics, a post he held until 2007.

Dr McEvoy is a graduate of the Royal College of Surgeons of Ireland. She trained in Ireland and was awarded her MRCPI in 2007 and completed her Higher Specialist Training in Paediatrics in 2012. She completed her master's in medical education at Queen's University Belfast, Ireland, in 2011. In 2013 she took up her current appointment as Consultant Paediatrician at Great Ormond Street Hospital, London, in general paediatrics.

Professor Nicholson is a graduate of University College Dublin. He received his paediatric training in Ireland and England at Saint Mary's Hospital, Manchester, and in Australia at the Royal Children's Hospital in Melbourne. He was awarded his MRCP (London) in 1987. He returned to Ireland in 1990 as a Consultant Paediatrician at the Longford Westmeath Regional Hospital in Mullingar and was subsequently appointed as Professor of Paediatrics for the Royal College of Surgeons in Ireland and Consultant Paediatrician at the Children's University Hospital, Temple Street, Dublin, in 2008. In 1999 he was appointed as one of the two National Specialty Directors for the Higher Specialist Training Programme in Paediatrics, a post he held until 2006. He has been the Irish representative to the European Academy of Paediatrics and is currently the National Clinical Lead for Paediatrics in Ireland.

HOW TO USE THE CD FOR LEARNING

The CD that accompanies this book contains clinical slides and radiological cases. At the end of select chapters there is a list of slides that relate to the symptoms discussed within the chapter. Prior to reading the chapter, users are recommended to review the appropriate clinical slides. This will help reinforce the material contained in each chapter. The slides have the abnormalities listed in text at the bottom of the slide. Frequently reviewing the slides will aid recognition of the clinical entities they reflect. Remember the maxim: 'a picture is worth a thousand words'.

The radiology section of the CD consists of 66 cases with 156 images. There are eight sections:

1. Respiratory (14 cases; 19 images)
2. Cardiac and vascular (6 cases; 23 images)
3. ENT (3 cases; 14 images)
4. Abdomen (not renal) (10 cases; 19 images)
5. Renal (8 cases; 25 images)
6. Bones (8 cases; 19 images)
7. Neurology (14 cases; 25 images)
8. Spine (3 cases; 12 images).

Each case commences with a short clinical scenario and a radiological investigation is shown. The reader should review the scenario and the radiological investigation, and answer the following questions:

1. What is the most likely diagnosis from a clinical perspective?
2. What are the likely radiological features that should be sought?

The abnormal findings are subsequently outlined. To aid learning the reader should consider the scenario, list a short differential diagnosis and list the expected radiological features.

CD materials can be found at http://resourcecentre.routledge.com/books/9781908911902

ACKNOWLEDGEMENTS

The authors would like to thank Ms Julia Reynolds and the staff of the Medical Library at Mayo General Hospital for their assistance in retrieving articles that are cited in this book.

Professor Nicholson wishes to thank both his secretary Norma Mc Eneaney and Tommy Nolan for his work in relation to the clinical photographs.

I would like to thank my parents Michael and Kathleen for opportunities provided and my wife Janet and our four children Kate, Sarah, Rachel and Eoghan for their love and support.   MBO'N

I would like to acknowledge the support of my parents, Charlie (now sadly deceased) and Breda (now in her eighties), my wife Helen and our four wonderful children (Katie, Mark, Marie Louise and Alfie). Thanking them for all their support and love.   AJN

Chapter One

EVIDENCE-BASED MEDICINE:
THE BASICS

This chapter will answer five questions on evidence-based medicine (EBM).

QUESTION 1: WHAT IS THE DEFINITION OF EVIDENCE-BASED MEDICINE?

EBM is the conscientious, explicit and judicious use of current best evidence in making decisions about the care of individual patients. This is the definition offered by Dr David Sackett (one of the pioneers of EBM) in 1996.[1] The patient is at the centre of this quest and the doctor's task is to provide the information to facilitate the patient's choice.

QUESTION 2: WHAT IS THE ORIGIN OF EVIDENCE-BASED MEDICINE?

The development of EBM has been a process. In the 1940s controlled clinical trials were commencing, but it wasn't until the 1970s that Professor Archie Cochrane enunciated the principles that were later to form the basis of EBM. However, developing these concepts into a practical methodology and employing them in everyday clinical practice was initially achieved by Dr David Eddy (Duke University, North Carolina) and by Dr David Sackett and Dr Gordon Guyatt at McMaster University in Hamilton, Ontario, in the late 1980s. The essentials of EBM were incorporated into the book *Users' Guides to the Medical Literature: A Manual for Evidence-Based Clinical Practice*, written by the Evidence-Based Medicine Working Group and edited by Gordon Guyatt and Drummond Rennie.[2]

QUESTION 3: HOW DO I BEGIN TO PRACTISE EVIDENCE-BASED MEDICINE?

Evidence-based practice involves asking and answering questions, e.g. will a 3-year-old with no risk factors for asthma but with acute viral wheeze benefit from oral steroids or will a 4-year-old with acute otitis media benefit from antibiotic treatment? These questions have similar elements: first, the population (children with otitis media or asthma); second, there is an intervention (antibiotic or steroid therapy); third, a comparison (analgesia or bronchodilator treatment); and fourth, a clinical outcome (avoidance of antibiotic treatment and steroid treatment with associated side effects). This gives rise to the structured clinical question PICO format, where P refers to patient or problem, I refers to the intervention, C refers to the comparison and O refers to the outcome.

QUESTION 4: WHERE DO I GET INFORMATION ON EVIDENCE-BASED MEDICINE?

The following websites provide evidence-based summaries:

- The Cochrane Library – www.thecochranelibrary.com
- Trip – www.tripdatabase.com
- PubMed Clinical Queries – www.ncbi.nlm.nih.gov/pubmed/clinical
- DynaMed – https://dynamed.ebscohost.com
- Embase – www.embase.com
- UpToDate – www.uptodate.com

Specific sites that publish evidence-based guidelines include the National Institute for Health and Care Excellence and the Scottish Intercollegiate Guidelines Network.

Many people search PubMed and get perhaps thousands of citations per search. This is not useful, as no one has time to trawl through each citation and review the abstract for relevance; it is more appropriate to have 10 relevant citations. Prior to using PubMed it is essential to be familiar with search strategies. The online tutorials provided by PubMed ultimately save time. If you are unable to answer the following questions you need to do these tutorials: What is the PMID number? What are clinical queries? What does MeSH mean? Where do the words 'related citations' appear on the screen?

QUESTION 5: WHAT DO I NEED TO KNOW ABOUT RANDOMISED CONTROLLED TRIALS IN RELATION TO EVIDENCE-BASED MEDICINE?

Randomised controlled trials (RCTs) are being used increasingly in medicine to define therapy effectiveness. The core concept of RCTs is that study groups are very similar, with the only variable within the study being the intervention, and therefore the resulting outcome is attributed to the intervention. The word 'randomised' refers to distributing measured characteristics, e.g. age or disease severity, equally in each group. An advantage of the randomisation process is that unmeasured variables are likely to be equally distributed among the groups. A useful way to analyse RCTs is outlined as follows.

Aim of study

The aim should state why the study is being undertaken. For example, in adolescents with acute migraine headaches, how effective in the treatment of pain is strategy A as compared with strategy B? The question asked is explicit and clearly defined.

Methods

- **Participants**. The eligibility of the study population needs to be understood. What are the criteria for entry into the study and what features result in exclusion from the study? The reader should be aware of the recruitment process – were participants recruited from hospital clinics or general practitioners' practices or were advertisements used in the paper? The description of the population allows the physician to relate the studied population to his or her own practice. Recruitment of patients from a tertiary care centre asthma clinic is likely to result in patients with severe disease being recruited into the study and the results may not be applicable to a doctor working in a primary care setting.
- **Intervention**. What is the intervention in the study? This needs to be stated clearly, e.g. patients will be randomised to receive treatment A or placebo.
- **Outcomes**. What are the primary outcomes? Primary outcomes need to be relevant and measurable, e.g. in an adolescent with migraine, as defined by the International Headache Society criteria for migraine, what is the impact of treatment X versus treatment Y, on the presence of pain at 2 hours? The primary outcome is defined (pain-free at 2 hours) and a method for measurement (e.g. visual analogue scale) must be outlined. Secondary outcome must be stated prior to the study commencing.
- **Sample size and its calculation**. In determining the sample size the following need to be evaluated: (a) an estimate of an important outcome difference that would be clinically relevant, (b) the alpha level (type I error), (c) the statistical power (type II error) and (d) for continuous outcomes, the standard deviation of the mean. The size effect is inversely related to the sample size. Traditionally the alpha level is set at $P < 0.05$, i.e. a 1 in 20 chance that the results are incorrect. Type II errors indicate there is no difference, when in fact there is.
- **Randomisation**. Once the group of eligible participants has been determined, there is a need to separate them into two groups, with the proviso that each participant has an equal chance of being assigned into either group. This is the basis of correct randomisation. In effect, when this is done correctly important characteristics of the patients will be equally divided into the two groups. The best way to randomise is to utilise a central computer-based randomisation. This has the added advantage of being remote from the investigators and patients, which makes it difficult to predict which patient will be assigned to the intervention or the control group. Utilising sealed, opaque envelopes sounds like a good idea, but if there is a way of influencing the group to which the patient is assigned, then this randomisation process is flawed and should not be used. Some older studies used

date of birth (odd versus even days) or days of the week on which the participant attended, to define the group to which he or she is assigned; this is not randomisation, as participants do not have an equal chance of being assigned to either group. The process is referred to as 'pseudo-randomisation'. This concept of 'not knowing' or being unable to predict the group to which the next patient will be assigned is called allocation concealment and is employed to reduce bias.

- **Blinding** refers to withholding information that relates to the intervention from persons who may be influenced by this knowledge, especially if the outcomes are subjective. The term 'double-blind' indicates that both patients and investigators are unaware of the treatment allocation – this reduces bias. Double-blinding is not possible if a surgical intervention is being evaluated against a medical treatment. If the primary outcome is objective, e.g. death, then blinding is not a concern, because the measurement of the outcome cannot be influenced. On the contrary, where the measurement can be influenced the blinding of the assessor is crucial. In reviewing an RCT, it is essential to know who the assessor of the outcome is, and that they are unaware of which particpant received which intervention. This needs to be ensured (if possible).

- **Statistical methods** refer to the analysis of the data to determine magnitude of the treatment effect.

Results

- The presence of a **flow diagram** is very useful. This diagram indicates (a) the number of patients who were eligible, (b) those who participated, (c) those who received the intended treatment and (d) those who were analysed in respect to the primary outcome. When reviewing the flow diagram, certain observations should be made: (a) of those eligible, how many agreed to participate and what were explanations offered for non-participation? (b) of those who were randomised to the intended treatment, what percentage was not analysed in determining the results of the study?

- **Baseline data**. If the randomisation was undertaken correctly, then the groups should be similar for baseline characteristics, as each person's assigned group was determine by chance. If baseline characteristics are similar between groups then the reader is reassured that the randomisation has been done correctly.

- **Numbers analysed**. The numbers analysed are important, because if the difference between those who commenced the intervention and those for whom data are available is significantly different, the results are not valid. If 100 patients are assigned to the intervention arm, loss of five patients will not have a great bearing on the results; however, if the number is 20, then the reader should be concerned and look for an explanation of same (this is the basis of the '5 and 20' rule: 5 or less is acceptable, 20 or greater is very concerning). The concept of intention-to-treat analysis is that patients are analysed in the group to which they were assigned, and if data are not available then an assumption is made that they have experienced a poor outcome. For example, in a study of a medical and surgical intervention, 100 patients are assigned to each group. In the medical group all 100 patients receive the intervention and 40 get better. However, in the surgical group of the 100 patients assigned, only 70 have the procedure and 35 get better. Which treatment should I recommend? The percentage success of the medical treatment is 40/100 (40%) and the surgical treatment is 35/70 (50%). The surgical treatment offers the better outcome, but the 30 patients who did not receive the surgical treatment must be taken into account and analysed in the group to which they were assigned; as no data are available we must assume a negative outcome and therefore the surgical success rate was 35/100 (35%). The medical treatment is preferred. Intention-to-treat analysis is an important concept to bear in mind if there is a significant dropout rate. The reader can often do the analysis him- or herself if it is not provided by the authors.

- **Primary outcomes with confidence intervals**. The primary outcome of the study is the result, which the reader wishes to know. For binary results the relative risk and the absolute risk need to be reported. The absolute risk is useful for the clinician, but it must be applied to a similar population from which it was derived. If in a study on migraine therapy 75% of patients receiving treatment A achieve the primary outcome in comparison with 50% of patients receiving treatment B, then the absolute risk difference is 25%. This is called the absolute risk reduction (ARR) and 1/ARR equals the number needed to treat (NNT). In the example given, the NNT = 1/25% (1/0.25), or 4, which means that one in four persons who received treatment A had a better outcome that those who received treatment B.

- If the study is repeated on multiple occasions the results will vary, and the range of these variations are the **confidence intervals** (CIs), which provide the reader with the range of effect sizes. If the CIs are narrow the reader is reassured that the results are valid; however, if the CIs are wide or cross the line of no effect, the reader should view the results with caution.

- **Secondary outcomes**. The secondary outcomes of the study must be predefined; if not, then the results should be interpreted with caution, e.g. in a study on asthma treatment if the primary outcome is achieved in 60% of 5- to 7-year-olds and in 75% of 10- to 12-year-olds, are the results clinically relevant? If this finding was assessed from incidental analysis of the data it reflects 'data dredging'. The impact of age must have been stated as part of the outcomes before the study was begun and the necessary age stratification undertaken.

- **Harms**. Studies must report harms or adverse events that accrue to patients. In deciding whether to accept or reject a treatment option, parents are influenced by the negative impact of treatment. It is an 'opportunity cost': if this treatment is pursued the chance of a positive impact is x but this has to be balanced against potential harms y. This can be usefully expressed as the number needed to harm (NNH). For example, if a treatment has a serious side effect occurring in 1% of children, the NNH equals 1/1% (1/0.01), or 1 in 100.

Discussion

The discussion component of the paper should ideally contain the following: (a) the principle results and their limitations, (b) the mechanism or biological plausibility of the results, (c) the results in context of the published literature and (d) the generalisability of the results. The concept of generalisability is crucial, as the clinician, on reading the paper, will ponder the answer to the question: Are the patients who received the study treatment similar to the patients I treat? If they are, then use of the treatment is likely to produce the expected results; however, if the population is different, the results may not translate and a clinical judgement needs to be used.

Recommendation

Having defined the benefit in context of the risk, the doctor is able to make a recommendation to the patient – or in the case of a young patient, the parents – and it is up to the patient to decide whether he or she will follow it or not.

ASSESSING QUALITY OF RANDOMISED CONTROLLED TRIALS

The quality of an RCT is important if treatment decisions are to be based on the results. This book uses the Jadad scale as a measure of quality because it is easily applied and it gives a numerical value. The Jadad score consists of the following items, for which a score of 1 is awarded if present or 0 if absent.

- Was the study described as randomised?
- Was the method used to generate the sequence of randomisation described and appropriate?
- Was the study described as double-blind?
- Was the method of double-blinding described and appropriate, e.g. identical placebo?
- Was there a description of withdrawals and dropouts?

For the following items, 1 or 0 is deducted (–1 if present, 0 if absent).

- The method used to generate the sequence of randomisation was described but was inappropriate, e.g. patients allocated by year of birth.
- The study was described as double-blind but the method of blinding was inappropriate, e.g. tablets versus injection with no double placebo.

CLARIFYING AND PITFALL AVOIDANCE IN RANDOMISED CONTROLLED TRIALS

- Asking a person to join a study. **Rationale and Pitfall**: avoidance of bias is an important tenet in RCTs that must be present throughout. Therefore the concept of 'equipoise' is important. When recruiting potential participants the conversation should be devoid of statements like 'this is a good treatment and you should agree to participate' but rather, 'no one knows' and that is why the study is being done.

- Flow diagram. **Pitfall**: the flow diagram should prompt specific questions, especially if there was major difficulty in recruiting patients, very high refusal rates or significant loss to follow-up (>20%). If the treatment was effective but associated with high dropout rates or high failure-to-recruit rates then the reasons for these occurrences should be sought.
- Secondary outcomes. **Pitfall**: Were they predefined? Are they biologically plausible? The finding of potentially important results, e.g. different outcomes at different ages, is interesting; however, such results must be interpreted with caution if they were not predefined secondary outcomes. Often researchers will register their protocol online prior to the commencement of the study, and therefore outcomes are predefined. Interesting findings that are noted need to be tested prospectively in another study to determine if they are valid.
- NNT and CI. **Rationale**: the CI of NNT can be calculated with the following formula.

$$NNT = \pm\ 1.96\ \sqrt{\ \frac{CER \times (1\text{-}CER)}{\text{Number of control patients}} + \frac{EER \times (1\text{-}EER)}{\text{Number of experimental patients}}}$$

CER = control event rate
EER = experimental event rate
$\sqrt{\ }$ = square root

- Generalisability of results. **Rationale**: a central concept of EBM is applying the intervention or treatment to the individual patient; therefore, the study population should reflect the population encountered by the doctor.
- 'Not significant' does not mean 'no effect'. **Pitfall**: small studies will often report non-significant results, even when this is not the case. If larger studies are undertaken, clinically important results become evident.
- 'Statistically significant' does not necessarily mean 'clinically important'. **Rationale**: statistical significance means that 1 in 20 results will be incorrect. It is the magnitude of the treatment effect that matters.
- Bias and its impact. **Pitfall**: clinical effects can be overestimated if the study is performed incorrectly. Non-randomised studies can overestimate the treatment by 40%, non-double-blind studies by 17% and small trials by 30%. The use of the Jadad score in assessing clinical trials enhances the reader's awareness of this pitfall.
- Interim analysis. **Rationale**: an interim analysis is performed prior to the completion of a study, especially if there are concerns relating to potential adverse effects accruing. When prophylaxis with penicillin in sickle-cell disease was being assessed, the interim analysis indicated a higher death rate in those not receiving the penicillin; this prompted the termination of the study and the recommendation for prophylaxis.
- Hierarchy of evidence. **Rationale**: the correct analysis of RCTs results in formation

of systematic review, which is at the apex of the quality pyramid, followed by the RCT. Other study types are of lesser quality.

- Time for searching. **Pitfall**: learn how to search correctly. This is analogous to learning to type; sure you can use one or two fingers, but if you were to use all your fingers, in the long run a lot of time is saved.

References

1. Sackett DL, Rosenberg WM, Gray JA, *et al.* Evidence Based Medicine: what it is and what it isn't. *BMJ* 1996; **312**: 71–72.
2. Guyatt G, Rennie D, Meade MO, *et al.* (eds). The Evidence-Based Working Group. *Users' Guides to the Medical Literature: essentials of evidence-based clinical practice.* 2nd ed. New York, London: McGraw-Hill Medical; 2008.

Chapter Two

COMMUNICATION

While communication is central to effective interaction with patients, three areas are worthy of special mention:
1. breaking bad news
2. motivational interviewing (MI)
3. dealing with difficult parents.

BREAKING BAD NEWS

For parents the moment when bad news is broken to them by a doctor is never forgotten. Breaking bad news does occur in paediatric practice but not with the frequency that it occurs in adult medicine. For many trainees their first experience may relate to newborn infants who are born with Down's syndrome or have complications of prematurity. It may occur unexpectedly in a child who presents with a common symptom but the aetiology is sinister, e.g. the child with bruising who is diagnosed with leukaemia. Breaking bad news is a skill that must be learnt by all doctors and it must be done after a period of reflection.

The following strategies are helpful in breaking bad news.
- Gather the information that you will need, and anticipate the likely questions and what answers you will offer. Communication is a complex process and what a doctor says to a parent is not necessarily what a parent hears.
- Decide on the environment in which the news is delivered. It should ideally be in a private room with seating for all. Those present should include both parents and the baby if possible, doctors (consultant and some team members) and members of the nursing staff. After the news is broken the parents will have much more contact with the nursing staff than the medical staff on the ward. All should be seated so that eye contact can be maintained. All mobile phones and pagers must be turned off. The time to be given to the process must be adequate.
- Make an assessment of the parents' state. Are they able to listen? Are they distraught because they are fearful for their child? Most parents will know that something is amiss and will want to know what is wrong.
- If the news pertains to a newborn, congratulate them on the birth of their child. This is an important event for them and needs to be recognised and celebrated.

Explain in clear and simple language what the medical concerns are and what conclusions you have drawn. Explain to them the likelihood of your diagnosis being correct. Try to be as honest as is possible. For example, if the child has presented to a general hospital with bruising and the blood films shows blast cells, indicate that this suggests a diagnosis of leukaemia but that further tests are required and these will be completed in a specialist unit. Avoid using jargon language, avoid excessive bluntness and do not remove hope from the parents in the initial discussion. Check for parental understanding of what they have heard.

- Be empathetic to the emotional response. This is probably the most difficult news they will ever receive. Parental emotional responses vary. Some parents become quiet, unable to think, others commence to cry or become angry. There is no correct emotional response when receiving bad news; however, it is beneficial if the doctor tries to name the response that the parents are exhibiting and reassure them that it is normal. There needs to be time for the emotional response to be expressed.

- Parents will want to know what the plan is for their child. The 'broad strokes' should be outlined, but often another meeting will be required. Allow time for parents' questions to be answered. Offer honest answers and if you don't know the answer, say so, or indicate that you will seek out the answer and report back to them. Prior to completing the interview made a time for a follow-up meeting.

- Ensure one person in the meeting has documented what was said and has recorded the agreed-upon actions. Ensure that these are done and indicate to the parents the time frame that will be required. The record of the communication should be placed in the patient's chart to allow for a consistent message to be given.

- Parents who have received bad news may want to talk to someone who has gone through a similar experience and this should be facilitated.

MOTIVATIONAL INTERVIEWING (MI)

Scenario 1: an 11-year-old boy is referred to your clinic because he is overweight (currently on the 85th centile). Both his mother and father are overweight. His father is a lorry driver who eats at roadside restaurants while working. His sister, currently 19 years of age, was overweight but since starting college a year ago she has lost significant weight, which she attributes to improved exercise and a change in eating habits.

Scenario 2: a 5-year-old boy has had four admissions to hospital for uncontrolled asthma in the past year. On each occasion he responds well to treatment and is medically ready for discharge within 24 hours. The parents both continue to smoke in the home and are reluctant to give their child inhaled steroids, lest he develop side effects.

In these two scenarios change needs to occur to ensure health gain for the child. Change is characteristically described as occurring in five stages. The first is **pre-contemplation**, where a person has no intention of changing, often because the person does not view his or her behaviour as problematic or does not recognise that there is a problem. These individuals may be referred to as 'being in denial' or resistant. The second stage is **contemplation**, where the person is aware that a problem exists and seriously considers action but has not made a commitment to action. The third stage is **preparation**, where the person is intent upon taking action but may still be weighing up the pros and cons of action. The fourth stage is **action**, where awareness exists, commitment is clear and effort is expended to achieve a desired outcome. The fifth stage is **maintenance**, where the new behaviour has replaced the old behaviour and the risk of relapse becomes less.

MI can be used to enhance the change process. The four principles of MI are (1) empathy, seeing the world through patients' or parents' eyes; (2) development of discrepancy, assessing how things are versus how they would like them to be; (3) rolling with resistance, not challenging the parents' view but rolling with it, as arguing will only entrench their viewpoint; and (4) supporting self-efficacy, recognising that the parents have the ability to make effective changes.

How to operationalise MI? There are four stages:

1. asking open-ended questions
2. reflective listening
3. affirmation
4. providing summary statements.

Prior to commencing MI, the doctor should ask the parents: 'Do you mind if we talk about . . .?' In the scenarios illustrated here it may be the repeated readmissions for asthma or the child who is overweight. This shows respect for the parent and can aid engagement. This can be followed by the open-ended questions: What would you like to be different? What things need to change for things to be different? What will happen if things do not change?

Reflective listening is paraphrasing what the parent is saying back to him or her. Such sentences can begin 'it sounds like', 'what I hear you saying is', 'I get the sense that'.

In conjunction with these statements there may be a need to point out discrepancies, e.g. 'I hear you say that you enjoy smoking and that you don't want your child to have asthma attacks. Why do you think the asthma attacks are occurring so frequently?'

Affirmations are statements that are made to reflect the parents' strengths, past successes and desire to change, e.g. 'I notice that you are showing a lot of insight as to why your child is being hospitalised so frequently.' These affirmations acknowledge what the parents and child have achieved, and validation of their efforts is required.

Summaries are used to bring together what the parents have said. It is important to reflect back accurately what a parent has said, so careful listening is required.

MI is a useful skill to develop and with practice the doctor becomes more skilful (*see* Evidence 1). Not all parents will be receptive, as is their choice, but it facilitates a change process for families.

DEALING WITH DIFFICULT PARENTS

Clinical encounters in paediatrics differ from adult medicine, as the paediatrician has to address the needs of the child or adolescent and his or her parents. For many children, their illnesses are self-limiting and the child recovers, much to the delight of his or her parents; unfortunately, however, this is not always the case, and for the doctor there are some encounters that are difficult and challenging.

What contributes to difficult encounters? The factors may be parent, physician or system related.

Parent-related issues include:
- increased stress levels that are illness related
- worry related to the diagnosis
- previous negative experience of healthcare system
- impact of the illness on working lives of parents
- child may have chronic disease and the parents are adjusting to the diagnosis and the impact it has on family life.

Physician-related issues include:
- doctor's personality (poor listening skills)
- doctor's attitude to the illness (physician may consider it mild, e.g. bronchiolitis, but for parents, with no medical experience, this may be anxiety provoking)
- limited experience of the doctor (may be uncertain about diagnosis, limited knowledge of paediatric conditions), or cultural differences (may not understand expectations of the parents, including their expectations regarding the style of communication).

Systems-related issues include:
- creating an environment that will enhance dissatisfaction, e.g. overbooking clinics
- rushing the clinic visit for the patient because of time constraints will create unhappiness
- utilising an inappropriate communication environment, e.g. having lack of privacy when talking to the parents may cause intense irritation, especially if they wish to keep their child's health difficulties private.

Difficult encounters can be reduced if the following advice is adhered to.
- Establish boundaries early. Let the parents know what your role is in the care of their child. This is particularly important if they are attending several specialists.
- If the child or adolescent is presenting with a condition that has a psychological

component to it, mention this to the parents early in the consultation process when you are discussing potential aetiologies and aggravating factors.

- Avoid over-investigating patients or agreeing to 'one more test to reassure the parents'. Put the child's interest first and explain this to the parents.
- Adopt a positive listening style. Pay attention to cues that the parents are unhappy or annoyed by assessing their body language, and seek clarification from them by using statements such as 'I notice that . . .'. Avoid using 'you statements', e.g. 'you are angry', as this is likely to aggravate the parents.
- Acknowledge environmental issues, e.g. the lack of privacy, the overbooked clinic. This indicates an awareness of the situation on your part, which most parents will appreciate.

Dealing with the difficult encounter

There are clinical encounters that are both difficult and challenging. When you are experiencing a difficult encounter the following strategies are helpful.

- Recognise that the encounter is difficult. Clarify with the parent your observation by saying, 'I notice that . . .. Am I correct in this assumption?' Once the parent responds, ask: 'What do you think the cause is?'
- Always pause and wait for the parent to reflect – he or she may not notice that the situation is tense or difficult.
- If the parents are overtly critical, often they will use 'you statements', e.g. 'You are not listening to what we are saying'. Before responding, ask yourself, are they correct?
- Exercise caution in how you respond. Focus on the primary goal of addressing the healthcare needs of their child.
- Attempt to assess what is the driver of this difficult encounter by reviewing parent, physician and environment factors.
- If you are experiencing a difficult encounter beyond your comfort zone, withdraw from it and seek advice from a more experienced colleague, especially if you have limited experience in paediatrics.
- Difficult encounters can be reduced if the following are adhered to:
  - introduce yourself to the parents and child if old enough
  - recognise potential negative occurrences that can irritate parents (e.g. excessive waiting without explanation or apology, unsatisfactory environment, a doctor who is not attentive to their concerns)
  - be engaged in the consultation process as it is occurring.

Strategies to deal with demanding families who have ongoing clinical care requirements for their child

- Ask yourself why you find them demanding. There are multiple reasons why this may be the case:
  - the parents may be unfriendly and threatening – it is how they are

- they may wish to drive their own investigation and treatment strategies, thereby being in control of the situation
- they may make excessive demands on time and resources that are inappropriate because they feel that that is what their child requires
- they may be hostile to the doctor and other healthcare professionals for unknown reasons.

- Learn about the family. Find out their background and what may be the triggers for their demanding behaviour. Look for parent, physician and environmental factors. Check for negative experiences that may have moulded their current response. Find out how they deal with stressful situations. Assess if any harm has occurred to their child while receiving medical care. These actions are going to take time, but if they are to become less demanding the physician will need to understand what the main drivers for their behaviour are.
- Clearly explain your role in their child's care, especially the specifics of what you can and cannot do. This boundary setting will need to be explained on several occasions.
- Attempt to be proactive: plan elective care provision in a timely fashion and ensure that it occurs. If they miss a clinic visit, telephone to find out why. Reschedule the visit in a timely fashion.
- Explain how acute medical care is usually provided to children with similar conditions to their child and adhere to the same process for them. Making an exception to the general rule can become the new rule and will be an expectation of the family.
- If the parents continue to be demanding then weigh up and consider the benefits of sharing the child's care with another doctor, or ask the parents if that is their wish.
- For doctors involved with difficult families on an ongoing basis there is a clear need for them to address how they deal with the stress that these families can induce. Discussion with colleagues can help but more defined stress reduction strategies are required.

EVALUATING THE EVIDENCE

Evidence 1	
Theme E1	**Teaching motivational interviewing**
Question	Can motivational interviewing be effectively taught to doctors in training?
Design	RCT
Level of evidence	Jadad 3
Setting	Department of paediatrics, academic medical centre, the United States
Participants	Paediatric trainees in from years 1 to 4 in a residency training program
Intervention	Participants were randomised to a behaviour change programme (the Collaborative Management in Paediatrics programme) or a wait-list control group. The Collaborative Management in Paediatrics programme is a 9-hour behavioural change curriculum based on brief MI plus written feedback on communication skills (based on a 3-month objective structured clinical examination).
Outcomes	The primary outcome was the percentage change in MI-consistent behaviour (%MICO) at baseline and at 7 months using objective structured clinical examinations with standardised patients who portrayed parents of asthmatic children in three stages of change (not ready, unsure and ready).
Main results	Of 84 paediatric trainees, 29 were eligible, of whom 11 (38%) declined to participate. Of the eight allocated to the intervention group, all eight (100%) completed the study, and of the ten allocated to the control group, eight (80%) completed the study. The percentage improvement (%MICO) was 16% for patients ready for intervention and patients ready for change, 20% for those who were unsure and 18% for those who were not ready.
Conclusion	Paediatric trainee skills in behavioural change counselling improved following the combination of training in brief MI and written feedback.
Commentary	Quality improvement is a central theme in healthcare currently. This study, through MI, sought to enhance outcome for patients through MI. This is an important skill that all doctors require, although the resources employed were significant (in terms of video reviews and written feedback) and may not be available to all institutions. The lack of engagement of 38% of trainees is a concern, but if this skill is included in the medical curriculum that difficulty will be overcome. The need to recertify in MI, like many other aspects of medicine, would seem sensible.
Reference	Lozano P, McPhilips HA, Hartzler B, *et al*. Randomized trial of teaching brief motivational interviewing to pediatric trainees to promote healthy behaviors in families. *Arch Pediatr Adolesc Med.* 2010; **164**(6): 561–6.

Chapter Three

FIRST RESPONSE

This chapter looks at clinical symptoms that require prompt attention from the doctor. Common symptoms discussed include acute stridor, acute wheeze, transient loss of consciousness, anaphylaxis and coma, which incorporates treatment of shock, sepsis, diabetic ketoacidosis, bacterial meningitis and status epilepticus. Each symptom is described, the potential differential diagnosis is provided, potentially useful assessment tools outlined and management steps indicated. A key element in dealing with emergencies is ensuring treatments are given in a timely fashion; therefore, keep an eye on the clock, the patient is depending on you.

ACUTE STRIDOR

Clinical condition	Clinical feature	Differentiating features
Croup	Stridor	Cough resembling the bark of a seal, hoarseness
Foreign body aspiration	Stridor	History of choking 80%, absence of cough that resembles bark of a seal
Epiglottitis	Stridor	High fever, sitting erect (sniffing position), drooling, dysphagia, absence of barky cough
Bacterial tracheitis	Stridor	High fever, looks toxic, failure of stridor to resolve with nebulised adrenaline, usually does not drool, as can swallow secretions, does *not* choose sniffing position as preferred comfort position
Peritonsillar abscess	Stridor (not prominent)	Severe sore throat, difficulty in swallowing
Retropharyngeal abscess	Stridor	Fever, drooling, neck swelling with lymphadenopathy
Anaphylaxis	Stridor (as part of oral syndrome)	History of trigger event, Swelling of lips and oral mucosa
Laryngomalacia	Stridor (intermittent) position dependent	

Croup

Assessment tool

Croup score (modified Westley clinical scoring system)

Indicators of disease severity	Score
Inspiratory stridor	
none	0
only with agitation or activity	1
at rest	2
Intercostal retractions	
none	0
mild	1
moderate	2
severe	3
Air entry	
normal	0
mildly decreased	1
severely decreased	2
Cyanosis	
none	0
with agitation or activity	4
at rest	5
Level of consciousness	
normal	0
altered	5

Note: possible score 0–17; <4 = mild croup; 4–6 = moderate croup; >6 = severe croup.

Severity classification: follow croup score classification to guide therapy and management

Score	Severity	Management	Treatment considerations
<4	Mild	Outpatient	Supportive Consider corticosteroids
4–6	Moderate	Inpatient or observation	Corticosteroids Oxygen (for hypoxia) Epinephrine
>6	Severe	Inpatient, consider intensive care unit	Corticosteroids Oxygen (for hypoxia) Epinephrine Consider helium oxygen Consider intubation

---

CLINICAL SEVERITY REASSESSMENT SCHEDULE
- *Mild*: reassess every 4 hours, consider discharge
- *Moderate*: reassess every 2 hours, consider admission
- *Severe*: reassess every 1 hour, consider intensive care unit admission

---

The best indicator of croup severity is the respiratory rate. This is not included in the scoring systems, as it is an age-dependent variable. The scoring systems, in general, do not have strong evidence; however, for the trainee they offer a strategy to assess the child and determine the impact of treatment.

Pitfall avoidance
- Reduce patient anxiety (blow bubbles in front of the patient).
- Do not cannulate the patient, as crying will aggravate the stridor.
- Avoid X-rays – croup is a clinical diagnosis. If chest X-ray is performed, evaluate for the 'steeple sign'.

Investigations
- None usually required

Treatment strategies
- Nebulise budesonide (*see* Evidence 1)
- Oral dexamethasone (*see* Evidence 1)
- Nebulised adrenaline (*see* Evidence 2, 3)

Foreign body aspiration
Pitfall avoidance
- A history of choking will be absent in 20%.
- Stridor will predominate without the characteristic croupy cough.
- Treatment with dexamethasone and nebulised adrenaline will be ineffective.

Investigation
- Chest X-ray is useful if the item swallowed is radio-opaque. A normal chest X-ray does not imply an absence of a foreign body.

Treatment strategy
- Refer for bronchoscopy to remove the foreign body.

Epiglottitis

Pitfall avoidance

- With immunisation this condition is becoming infrequent but should be considered with the characteristic history.
- Do *not* examine the throat.
- If the child fails to respond to nebulised adrenaline, epiglottitis should be considered.
- If the child is being intubated, the normal anatomy will be distorted and to aid the anaesthetist gently compress the rib cage to expel air from the trachea and a bubble will form. This reflects the entrance to the trachea and the tube should be aimed toward the bubble to facilitate intubation.

Investigations

- A chest X-ray should *not* be undertaken. Getting a patient with epiglottitis to lie recumbent can lead to airway obstruction.

Treatment strategy

- Endotracheal intubation (*see* earlier Pitfall Avoidance section)
- Antibiotic treatment
- Intravenous cefotaxime

Bacterial tracheitis

Pitfall avoidance

- Failure to consider the diagnosis in a child with upper airway obstruction who fails to respond to nebulised adrenaline.
- Not recognising that a child who looks toxic with stridor but does assume the sniffing position and is not drooling has bacterial tracheitis.
- If the trachea is tender and the child is reluctant to cough, think of bacterial tracheitis.

Treatment strategy

- Intravenous antibiotics: first-line treatment is cefotaxime and flucloxacillin, as the common organisms are *Staphylococcus aureus*, *Moraxella catarrhalis*, *Streptococcus pneumoniae* and *Haemophilus influenzae*.
- Endotracheal intubation is required.

ACUTE WHEEZE

Clinical condition	Clinical feature	Differentiating features
Asthma	Acute wheeze	Specific trigger, upper respiratory tract infection, allergen, family history of asthma, eczema, smoking
Bronchiolitis	Wheeze	<9 months, upper respiratory tract infection, wet cough characteristic, hyperinflated, crackles and wheeze
Foreign body aspiration	Recurrent wheeze	History of choking (maybe forgotten), recurrent wheeze with a wet cough Appears to be a poorly controlled asthma patient May have unilateral wheeze
Congenital airway anomaly	Noisy breathing from birth	History of a wet cough
Recurrent aspiration	Recurrent wheeze	Acute onset of dyspnoea, tachypnoea, risk group cerebral palsy, gastro-oesophageal reflux disease
Mycoplasma infections	Wheeze	Cough, fever, wheeze

Assessment tools

Methods of calculating the asthma score and the severity of asthma*

Variable	Asthma scoring		
	1 Point	2 Points	3 Points
Respiratory rate (breaths/minute)			
2–3 years	≤34	35–39	≥40
4–5 years	≤30	31–35	≥36
6–12 years	≤26	27–30	≥31
>12 years	≤23	24–27	≥28
Oxygen saturation (%)	>95 with room air	90–95 with room air	<90 with room air or supplemental oxygen
Auscultation	Normal breathing or end-expiratory wheezing	Expiratory wheezing	Inspiratory and expiratory wheezing, diminished breath sounds or both
Retractions	None or intercostal	Intercostal and substernal	Intercostal, substernal and supraclavicular
Dyspnoea	Speaks in sentences or coos and babbles	Speaks in partial sentences or utters short cries	Speaks in single words or short phrases or grunts

(continued)

Severity of Asthma			
	Mild	*Moderate*	*Severe*
Peak expiratory flow rate (best of 5 attempts, scored as a percentage of predicted value)	>70%	50–70%	<50%
Asthma score	5–7	8–11	12–15

Note: *the overall asthma score (range: 5–15 points) is calculated by adding the scores for each of the five variables: respiratory rate, oxygen saturation, auscultation, retractions and dyspnoea. The overall asthma score is then used to stratify children according to the severity of disease. When the peak expiratory flow rate is known and reliable, it, rather than the asthma score, should be used to stratify the children according to severity.

For the trainees this scoring system provides a practical approach to assess if the treatment strategy is working in a child with acute asthma. Children who are not used to performing pulmonary function tests may be uncooperative, if they are distressed and thus peak expiratory flow rates may not be reliable.

The 12-Point Preschool Respiratory Assessment Measure

Sign	0	1	2	3
Suprasternal retractions	Absent		Present	
Scalene muscle contraction	Absent		Present	
Air entry*	Normal	Decreased at bases	Widespread decrease	Absent/Minimal
Wheezing*	Absent	Expiratory only	Inspiratory and expiratory	Audible without stethoscope/silent chest with minimal air entry
Oxygen saturation	≥95%	92%–94%	<92%	

Note: *if asymmetric findings between the right and left lungs, the most severe side is rated.

The Preschool Respiratory Assessment Measure (PRAM) is an indicator of asthma severity. It is useful for the preschool population and a change in score of 3 is clinically relevant. Pulmonary function tests are not routinely available for assessment in children under 5 years of age; therefore, clinical assessment scores such as the PRAM are useful.

Acute asthma

Pitfall avoidance

- Failure to assess severity
- Failure to use oxygen with bronchodilator treatment
- Not ensuring early use of steroids
- Being guided by the oxygen saturation ONLY and ignoring the clinical features of the child
- Failing to intensify treatment if clinical response is suboptimal
- Failing to give the parents a written action plan on discharge
- Failure to define the asthma trigger especially if history of food allergy

Treatment strategy

- Oxygen
- Bronchodilator treatment (for mild to moderate asthma metered-dose inhaler with spacer delivery is equivalent to nebulised treatment; however, in status asthmaticus nebulised treatment is preferred, which is addressed here):
  - nebulised salbutamol, dose 0.1 mg/kg of 5 mg/mL solution ×3
  - ipratropium bromide, administer with salbutamol, dose 250 mg (*see* Evidence 4)
- Steroids: prednisolone 1–2 mg/kg (*see* Evidence 4)
- If patient fails to show improvement, consider magnesium sulphate 25–50 mg/ kg over 20 minutes (*see* Evidence 6). Contact your consultant if there is failure to improve

Bronchiolitis

Treatment strategy

- Utilise oxygen via soft nasal prongs, at a flow rate of 2 L/min (higher flows may cause distress to the infant).
- Place a nasogastric feeds if the infant is unable to feed.
- Utilise hypertonic saline 3% in children with bronchiolitis (*see* Evidence 7 in Chapter 17: The Child With Wheeze).
- Bronchodilator treatment is not proven to be effective (may give short-term relief).
- Ipratropium bromide is not proven to be effective (may give short term relief).
- Nebulised or inhaled steroids are of no benefit.

ACUTE SYNCOPE

Syncope is the sudden loss of consciousness and postural tone and complete recovery in a short period of time. Presyncope is the feeling that one is about to lose conscious-ness but it does not occur, although there is a transient loss of tone.

Features

Clinical condition	Clinical feature	Differentiating features
Syncope (vasodepressor syncope)	Loss of consciousness (from erect to supine position)	Presyncope symptoms Full recall (no retrograde amnesia)
Orthostatic syncope	Syncope on position change (supine to erect)	Clear trigger
Postural orthostatic tachycardia syndrome	Erect position	
Cardiac syncope (2%–6% of cases)		
prolonged QT interval	Syncope	No presyncope symptoms Genetic syndromes with prolonged QT interval include Romano–Ward's syndrome, Jervell and Lange–Nielsen's syndrome (with congenital deafness) Check for medication use: tricyclic antidepressants, macrolide antibiotics, anti-fungal agents
supraventricular tachycardia; Wolff–Parkinson–White's syndrome	Syncope	Tachycardia noted by patient, electrocardiogram (ECG) evaluate for delta wave for Wolff–Parkinson–White's syndrome Patients may induce vagal manoeuvres, e.g. vomiting to terminate the supraventricular tachycardia
structural cardiac disease; critical aortic stenosis; anomalous left coronary artery; hypertrophic obstructive cardiomyopathy	Syncope on exercise (sudden event) Ask if clasp hand to chest prior to loss of consciousness	Presyncopal symptoms of chest pain, dizziness, shortness of breath on exercise
Central nervous system causes		
seizure	Syncope in supine position	No prodromal presyncope symptoms, seizure before loss of consciousness, typical associated seizure symptoms, tongue biting, frothing at mouth, no recall post event, post-ictal sleep
migraine (vertebrobasilar)	Loss of consciousness	Occipital headache, visual change (unilateral), vomiting, and rotational movements (vertigo) and vomiting
hyperventilation syndrome	Loss of consciousness	Presyncopal symptoms include feeling of apprehension, fast shallow breathing, tingling around the lips, difficulty breathing in (not out) Full recall of events
breath-holding spells (*see* Chapter 20: Seizures)	Loss of consciousness	Transient, direct trigger evident

Pitfall avoidance

- Syncope is rare under 6 years of age.
- 'Red flag' recognition: exercise-induced syncope (mid-stride syncope), chest pain, congenital heart disease, family history of sudden death, hypertrophic obstructive cardiomyopathy, and pacemaker placement.

Investigations

- Evaluate pre-hospital vital signs inclusive of heart rate and blood pressure.
- ECG – check for the following:
  - supraventricular tachycardia – heart rate >220 beats/minute
  - Wolff–Parkinson–White's syndrome – ECG findings include short PR interval, delta wave and a wide QRS complex
  - long QT interval – ECG findings include QTc >0.45 seconds
  - hypertrophic obstructive cardiomyopathy – ECG features may indicate hyper-trophy but cardiac echocardiogram required to confirm diagnosis and clinical severity.
- Electroencephalogram if any of the following: prolonged loss of consciousness, post syncope lethargy, failure to recall presyncope event (these symptoms suggest that the event was not a simple syncope event).

Treatment strategies

- Vasodepressor syncope: (a) reassurance, (b) with presyncope symptoms encour-age to cross legs, (c) encourage fluids – avoid dehydration, (d) if simple measures are inadequate and symptoms persist, fludrocortisone is used, although data on effectiveness are limited, (e) most parents will wish for cardiology consultation if symptoms persist.
- Orthostatic syncope: (a) reassure that condition is benign, (b) advise transitioning from the lying to the standing position to allow for blood pressure adaptation, (c) if standing, ensure movement of leg muscle to prevent pooling of blood.
- Postural orthostatic tachycardia syndrome (for cardiology consultation).
- Prolonged QT interval for cardiology consultation.
- Supraventricular tachycardia: (a) attempt vagal manoeuvres, (b) use adenosine at a dose of 0.1 mg/kg (maximum first dose, 6 mg) by rapid infusion – use vein in right arm in antecubital fossa if possible, (c) may double first dose if no response (maximum dose is 12 mg), (d) if non-responsive, obtain cardiology opinion.
- Wolff–Parkinson–White's syndrome: obtain cardiology consultation, propranolol frequently used to control rhythm disturbance.
- Hypertrophic obstructive cardiomyopathy: (a) obtain cardiology opinion, (b) activ-ity restriction may be necessary, (c) beta blockers effective for symptom control, (d) severe cases may require surgery.
- Critical aortic stenosis: obtain cardiology consultation.
- Anomalous coronary syndrome: obtain cardiology consultation.

ANAPHYLAXIS IN CHILDREN AND ADOLESCENTS

(*See* Evidence 4 in Chapter 8: Food Allergy in Children)

Anaphylaxis has been defined as a 'severe, life-threatening generalised or systemic hypersensitivity reaction'. Anaphylaxis is highly likely to be present when *any one of the following three criteria are met.*

1. Acute onset of an illness (minutes to hours) with involvement of the skin, mucosa or both, with generalised hives (urticaria), pruritus or flushing swollen lips or tongue and **at least one of the following**:
   - ○ respiratory compromise characterised by stridor, bronchospasm, dyspnoea or hypoxia
   - ○ cardiovascular compromise characterised by hypotension and/or collapse.
2. **Two or more** of the following that occur rapidly after exposure to a likely allergen for that patient (minutes to hours):
   - ○ involvement of the skin and mucosal tissue characterised by generalised hives (urticaria), itch, flushing and swelling
   - ○ respiratory compromise characterised by stridor, bronchospasm, dyspnoea or hypoxia
   - ○ cardiovascular compromise characterised by hypotension and/or collapse
   - ○ persistent gastrointestinal symptoms characterised by crampy abdominal pain and vomiting.
3. **Hypotension** after exposure to known allergen for that patient (minutes to hours):
   - ○ hypotension for children is defined as systolic blood pressure <70 mmHg from 1 month to 1 year; <70 mmHg + (age × 2) from 1 to 10 years; and ≤90 mmHg from 11 to 17 years.

Pitfall avoidance

- Recognise that the major aetiologies for anaphylaxis in children (from an Australian study) are foods (56%), drugs (5%), insects (5%) and unknown (34%).
- Remember that a history of *asthma* is a major risk factor; therefore, good asthma control is essential.
- Poor adherence to treatment plans or poor symptom perception leads to poorer outcome (patients who do not carry antihistamines with them or who do not use intramuscular adrenaline at the onset of anaphylaxis).

Principles of treatment

Principles of treatment are to manage the acute episode and to prevent recurrence.

Assess severity of anaphylaxis

Grade	1: Mild	2: Moderate	3: Severe
Skin	Sudden itching of eyes and nose, generalised pruritus, flushing, urticaria, angioedema	Any of the previous	Any of the previous
GI tract	Oral pruritus, oral 'tingling', mild lip swelling, nausea or emesis, mild abdominal pain	Any of the previous plus crampy abdominal pain, diarrhoea, recurrent vomiting	Any of the previous plus loss of bowel control
Respiratory	Nasal congestion and/or sneezing, rhinorrhoea, throat pruritus, throat tightness, mild wheezing	Any of the previous plus hoarseness, 'barky' cough, difficulty swallowing, stridor, dyspnoea, moderate wheezing	Any of the previous plus cyanosis or saturation <92%, respiratory arrest
Cardiovascular	Tachycardia (increase >15 beats/minute)	Any of the previous	Hypotension* and/or collapse, dysrhythmia, severe bradycardia and/or cardiac arrest
Neurological	Change in activity level plus anxiety	'Light-headedness' feeling of 'pending doom'	Confusion, loss of consciousness

Note: *hypotension defined as systolic blood pressure: 1 month to 1 year <70 mmHg; 1–10 years < [70 mmHg + (2 × age)]; 11–17 years <90 mmHg. The severity score should be based on the organ system most affected. Bold face symptoms and signs are mandatory indication for the use of adrenaline. This table allows the doctor to characterise the severity of the reaction; however, anaphylaxis is an emergency and active treatment is required.

Action plan

- *Evaluate airway, breathing, circulation*
- *Assess severity of anaphylaxis* (*see* Assess Severity of Anaphylaxis table above)
- If respiratory distress, hypotension or collapses, *administer intramuscular adrenaline* into the vastus lateralis muscle (lateral aspect of the thigh); *this is the most important initial treatment*:
  - dose of adrenaline 0.01 mL/kg: adrenaline 1:1000 OR
  - <10 kg: 1:1000 adrenaline 0.01 mL/kg
  - 10–30 kg: self-injectable device (0.15 mg)
  - ≥30 kg: self-injectable device (0.3 mg)
- If *hypotension* or *collapse* administer:
  - high-flow oxygen
  - normal saline 20 mL/kg intravenously or intraosseously
  - corticosteroid
  - antihistamine
  - if no responses in 5 minutes repeat the intramuscular adrenaline and repeat fluid bolus

- If *stridor* present:
  - high-flow oxygen
  - nebulised adrenaline
  - if respiratory distress persists or no response in 5 minutes, administer IM adrenaline, nebulised corticosteroid and obtain IV access
  - if no response in 5–10 minutes, repeat nebulised adrenaline and consider further intramuscular adrenaline
  - intravenous corticosteroid
  - intravenous antihistamine
- If *wheeze* present:
  - high-flow oxygen
  - nebulised beta-2 agonist
  - if respiratory distress or no response within 5–10 minutes, administer intramuscular adrenaline
  - obtain intravenous access
  - if no response in 5–10 minutes, repeat nebulised beta-2 agonist
  - consider intramuscular adrenaline and consider intravenous beta-2 agonists
  - intravenous corticosteroid
  - intravenous antihistamine
- *Angioedema only* or *urticaria only*:
  - antihistamine
  - if known to be asthmatic, give beta-2 agonist and oral prednisolone
  - observe for 4 hours, as this may be early stage of anaphylaxis
  - PLUS persisting vomiting and/or abdominal pain consider intramuscular adrenaline

Discharge plan

- Ensure that the child or parents have self-injectable adrenaline with them
- Evaluate the written treatment plan (especially if adherence was suboptimal)
- Medications on discharge to include antihistamines and prednisolone (1–2 mg/kg for 3 days)
- Communicate with primary care physician
- If necessary, consider referral to allergist or consultant with a specific expertise in allergy

COMA (PROGRESSIVE LOSS OF CONSCIOUSNESS)

The aetiology of coma is extensive; however, the mnemonic TIPS AEIOU is useful (*see* outline provided). When presented with a child or adolescent in coma, the doctor needs to have a methodical approach to assessment and investigation to define the aetiology of the coma.

Trauma	Seizures, stroke, shunt malfunction	Infection
Insulin (hypoglycaemia), inborn errors of metabolism, intussusception	Alcohol misuse	Overdose
Psychiatric conditions	Electrolyte abnormalities, encephalopathy, diabetic ketoacidosis	Uraemia

Clinical condition	Clinical features	Differentiating features
Shock	Reduced level of consciousness	Capillary refill >2 seconds, cool or mottled peripheries, blood pressure <5th centile for age, urine output <1 mL/kg/hour
Sepsis	Reduced level of consciousness	Elevated or reduced temperature, increased heart rate, increased respiratory rate, increased or decreased white blood cell count or a non-blanching rash
Bacterial meningitis	Reduced level of consciousness	Fever, vomiting, irritability of movement, stiff neck (>18 months, usually), bulging fontanelle, purpuric rash that is progressive
Status epilepticus	Reduced level of consciousness	Seizure duration >30 minutes
Diabetic ketoacidosis	Reduced level of consciousness	Symptoms depend on timed elapse before clinical presentation, polydipsia, polyuria, thirst, weight loss, Kussmaul's breathing
Inborn errors of metabolism, elevated ammonia levels	Reduced level of consciousness	Trigger may be related to upper respiratory tract infection

While the differential diagnosis is extensive, the initial response should be to consider the following conditions are outlined: shock, sepsis, bacterial meningitis, status epilepticus, diabetic ketoacidosis and inborn errors of metabolism. The initial assessment should always include the ABCs: Airway, Breathing and Circulation.

The ongoing assessment of the child with reduced level of consciousness, in the emergency department, using the Glasgow Coma Scale, is essential. Reducing levels of consciousness indicate either that (a) the primary aetiology has not been discerned or (b) that the treatment being provided is inadequate. Having a practical approach to the assessment of coma is essential. There will be a percentage of cases however where the aetiology will not be determined (*see* Evidence 9).

Glasgow Coma Scale with modification for children

Best eye response

1	No eye opening
2	Eye opening to pain
3	Eye opening to verbal command
4	Eyes open spontaneously

Best verbal response (use one of the following)

	Adult version (Age 5+)	Children's modification	Grimace response for preverbal or intubated patients
1	No verbal response	No vocal response	No response to pain
2	Incomprehensible sounds	Occasionally whimpers and/or moans	Mild grimace to pain
3	Inappropriate words	Cries inappropriately	Vigorous grimace to pain
4	Confused	Less than usual ability and/or spontaneous irritable cry	Less than usual spontaneous ability or only response to touch stimuli
5	Oriented	Alert, babbles, coos, words or sentences to usual ability	Spontaneous normal facial/oromotor activity

Best motor response

1	No motor response to pain
2	Abnormal extension to pain
3	Abnormal flexion to pain
4	Withdrawal to painful stimuli
5	Localises to painful stimuli or withdraws to touch
6	Obeys commands or performs normal spontaneous movements

AVPU SCALE

Record the condition that best describes the patient:

Alert
responds to **V**oice
responds to **P**ain
Unresponsive

Shock

Pitfall avoidance

- Define the aetiology of shock; do not assume hypovolaemic shock only – consider cardiac failure, sepsis, and anaphylaxis.

- Consider ileus in children with gastroenteritis who do not respond to fluid boluses, especially if there is also reduced urine output.
- Ensure adequate access for fluids, move to intraosseous access early rather than delaying treatment.

Investigations
- Full blood count, urea, electrolytes, creatinine, blood gases, lactate

Treatment
- Fluid bolus 20 mL/kg 0.9% sodium chloride
- Check the response as indicated by reduction in heart rate and increase in blood pressure
- Further fluid boluses guided by physiological responses to a maximum of 60 mL/kg
- If 40 mL/kg of fluid administered and patient is still non-responsive, administer dopamine intravenously (ensure senior decision-maker is supporting these decisions)

Sepsis
Pitfall avoidance
- Failure to recognise the early symptoms and signs of sepsis
- Use the Glasgow meningococcal score (*see* Chapter 25: The Pale Child)
- Refractory hypotension is an indicator of a poor prognosis (as is deteriorating levels of consciousness

Investigations
- Full blood count, blood culture, C-reactive protein, chest X-ray, urine culture, polymerase chain reaction tests for meningococcus and pneumococcus, lumbar puncture if no contraindication, joint aspiration if clinically indicated

Treatment
- Intravenous antibiotics administration immediately after cultures are obtained. Cefotaxime is an appropriate initial choice.
- Intravenous fluids (as for shock)
- Oxygen
- Blood pressure support if necessary (as for shock)
- Consider where care is best administered, either high dependency unit or intensive care unit
- Early consultation with clinical microbiologist or infectious disease consultant if uncertainty regarding antibiotic coverage

Bacterial meningitis

Pitfall avoidance

- Do not perform a lumbar puncture in a child with a decreasing level of consciousness
- Provide chemoprophylaxis for close contacts

Investigations

- Obtain polymerase chain reaction tests for pneumococcus and meningococcus
- Full blood count, urea and electrolytes, blood gases, coagulation profile if petechiae present

Treatment

- Immediate antibiotics at general practice clinic if child presents there
- Establish intravenous access and correct hypotension
- Immediate intravenous antibiotics administration using cefotaxime and clindamycin (for suspected pneumococcus)
- Move to a high dependency unit or intensive care unit
- The mortality rate for meningococcal septicaemia can be as high as 10% and pneumococcal meningitis morbidity can be as high as 70%; consequently, good communication is required with parents

Status epilepticus

Pitfall avoidance

- Check blood glucose level
- If under 18 months or on isoniazid, consider pyridoxine
- If suspected cocaine, use phenobarbitone
- Phenytoin is first treatment in head injury
- The maximal rate of phenytoin infusion is 1 mg/kg/min and ECG monitoring is required

Investigation

- Glucose
- If on anticonvulsants, check levels
- Serum calcium, magnesium, electrolytes and blood gases
- Neuroimaging: computed tomography of the brain
- Electroencephalogram

Treatment

(*See* Evidence 7, 8)

- First-line treatment if no intravenous access:
  - buccal or rectal lorazepam 0.1 mg/kg (maximum, 4 mg)
  - or buccal midazolam 0.5 mg (maximum, 10 mg)

- o or rectal diazepam 0.5 mg/kg (maximum, 20 mg)
- If intravenous access established:
  - o intravenous lorazepam 0.1 mg/kg
  - o or intravenous midazolam 0.1 mg/kg (maximum, 10 mg)
  - o or intravenous diazepam 0.3 mg/kg (maximum, 5 mg if <5 years; maximum, 10 mg if >5 years)
- If no response after 5 minutes, repeat first-line treatment
- Second-line treatment: intravenous phenytoin 20 mg/kg in normal saline over 20 minutes; if <18 months, consider phenobarbitone
- Further treatment requires consultant input

Diabetic ketoacidosis

Pitfall avoidance
- Carefully document fluid intake and output.
- Do not rehydrate the younger child with DKA aggressively (avoid large bolus rapid rehydration).
- The presence of epigastric pain may reflect hypovolaemia.
- Elevated white blood cell count does not automatically reflect infection.

Investigation
- Full blood count, urea, electrolytes, creatinine, blood gases, serum ketones, urinalysis for glucose and ketones

Treatment
- Fluid management:

  Requirements = Maintenance + deficit − fluid administered

- Give requirements over 48 hours:

  Hourly rate = (48-hour maintenance + deficit − resuscitation fluid) divided by 48

- Give potassium after resuscitation fluid has been administered unless anuria is present; administer 20 mmol/500 mL of fluid
- Continuous low-dose insulin is preferred; administer at 0.1 units/kg/hour
- Use the ISPAD guideline[1] for specific detail and contact the paediatrician on call

EVALUATING THE EVIDENCE

Evidence 1	
Theme E1	*Steroid therapy for croup*
Question	Which is more effective in croup: nebulised budesonide or oral dexamethasone?
Study design	Randomised controlled trial
Level of evidence	Jadad 5
Setting	Emergency department in two children's hospitals, Canada
Participants	Children aged 3–5 years, with a croup syndrome characterised by hoarseness, barky cough, inspiratory stridor and a Westley croup score of 2 or greater after 15 minutes of mist therapy and whose parents were available for telephone contact 1 week after their attendance at the emergency department, were eligible to participate.
Intervention	Three interventions were compared: (1) nebulised budesonide 2 mg with an oral dexamethasone placebo, (2) budesonide placebo with oral dexamethasone 0.6 mg/kg and (3) budesonide 2 mg and oral dexamethasone 0.6 mg/kg. Participants were observed until the croup score reached 1, or until they were discharged or received epinephrine (adrenaline) or until 4 hours had elapsed, whichever was shortest.
Outcome	The primary outcome was a reduction in Westley croup score of 2 points, indicating a clinical response to the intervention.
Main results	Two hundred and thirty-five children were eligible for enrolment, but 36 were not randomised: 26 parents refused and 10 did not contact the study team. Of the 199, 65 children were randomised to the budesonide-only group, 69 to the dexamethasone-only group and 64 to the budesonide and dexamethasone group. The mean croup scores for budesonide only was 3.5, with a response rate of 74%; for dexamethasone only it was 3.6, with a response rate of 83%; and for budesonide and dexamethasone it was 3.8, with a response rate of 72%. The response to dexamethasone alone was best (absolute risk reduction = 9%; number needed to treat = 12). Only one patient was hospitalised.
Conclusion	Outcomes in all three groups were similar, but oral dexamethasone has the advantage of ease of administration, ready availability and cost.
Commentary	In this study 20% of patients had a previous episode of croup and one-third had a positive family history of asthma. Two patients (3%) in each group required epinephrine (adrenaline) as rescue therapy, 19 (10%) required additional steroid treatment, one-third visited their family doctor post discharge from the emergency department and 20 (10%) had croup symptoms at 1 week on telephone contact. These facts are relevant to the practising clinician and are useful to parents when outlining the natural history of croup. While the dose of dexamethasone used in this study was 0.6 mg/kg, doses at 0.15 mg/kg are effective. The use of nebulised saline (mist responders) is a strategy to remove children with mild croup from studies.
Reference	Klassen TP, Craig WR, Moher D, *et al*. Nebulized budesonide and oral dexamethasone for treatment of croup: a randomized controlled trial. *JAMA*. 1998; **279**(20): 1629–32.

Evidence 2	
Theme E2	***Adrenaline and acute stridor***
Question	How effective is racemic epinephrine by intermittent positive pressure breathing for the treatment of croup?
Study design	Randomised controlled trial
Level of evidence	Jadad 5
Setting	Intensive care setting, academic medical centre, the United States
Participants	Infants and children with inspiratory stridor at rest who had no evidence of epi-glottitis on direct visualisation of the epiglottis and whose stridor did not improve on exposure to mist for 15–30 minutes, in a specially designed room, were eligible for inclusion in the study. These children are considered at risk of developing more severe signs and symptoms of severe airway obstruction. Participants were assessed utilising the Westley croup scoring system.
Intervention	Subjects were randomised to receive nebulised racemic epinephrine (adrenaline) or nebulised saline (both solutions had the same distinctive odour), administered by intermittent positive pressure breathing.
Outcome	The primary outcome was the reduction in croup score at 10 and 30 minutes.
Main results	Forty-three patients were eligible for inclusion, 23 were randomised but three were withdrawn due to a technical fault in the administration of the treatment. There were 10 in each group, aged 4 months to 4 years. All 10 patients responded to the racemic epinephrine, with clinical improvement at 10 and 30 minutes and a reduction in croup scores from 3.9 to 1.7. The saline group did not display a clinical reduction in croup scores with pre-treatment scores of 4.1 and 3.7 at 10 minutes and 3.1 at 30 minutes (absolute risk reduction = 100%; number needed to treat = 1). The outcomes of the control group in terms of clinical deterioration and the requirement for intubation were not detailed in the results section. No adverse effects were reported after the administration of the racemic epinephrine.
Conclusion	Racemic epinephrine was effective in treating acute severe croup.
Commentary	This randomised, double-blind study was the first to demonstrate the effectiveness of adrenaline epinephrine in the treatment of severe croup. It took place in an era when epiglottitis was much more common than now. The Westley score was utilised to assess severity. This is a 17-point scoring system with five parameters: (1) level of consciousness (normal 0, disorientated 5); (2) cyanosis (none 0, cyanosed with agitation 4, cyanosed at rest 5); (3) stridor (none 0, when agitated 1, at rest 2); (4) air entry (normal 0, decreased 1, markedly decreased 2); and (5) retractions (none 0, mild 1, moderate 2, severe 3). Children with Westley croup scores of 4 in the emergency department give rise to clinical concern and a reduction to 2 post intervention would ease clinical concerns. Current practice is to minimise invasive interventions in children with croup. Distraction techniques can reduce the anxiety levels in children, e.g. blowing bubbles adjacent to them. Racemic epinephrine is no longer available and consequently the L form of epinephrine (adrenaline) is used.
Reference	Westley CR, Cotton EK, Brooks JG. Nebulised racemic epinephrine by IPPB for the treatment of croup: a double-blind study. *Am J Dis Child.* 1978; **132**(5): 484–7.

Evidence 3	
Theme E3	*Adrenaline in the treatment of croup*
Question	Which is more effective in moderate to severe croup: L-epinephrine (adrenaline) (LE) or racemic epinephrine (adrenaline)?
Study design	Randomised controlled trial
Level of evidence	Jadad 5
Setting	Emergency department, children's hospital, the United States
Participants	Children 6 months to 6 years with a diagnosis of croup defined as acute inspiratory stridor, dyspnoea, suprasternal or intercostal retractions with preceding coryzal symptoms. The Downes and Raphaely croup score was used post 20 minutes of mist therapy (nebulised saline). Children with spasmodic croup, defined as a sudden attack of stridor, usually during the night without antecedent fever or signs of an upper respiratory infection, were excluded.
Intervention	Identical vials were used containing 0.5 mL of 2.25% racemic epinephrine (RE) in 4.5 mL of normal saline or 5 mL of 1:1000 LE, which were administered by a nebulisers to children with croup score of 6 or greater. Participants with scores of 8 or greater were administered intramuscular dexamethasone at a dose of 0.6 mg/kg. Supplemental oxygen was administered to children with oxygen saturation <95%.
Outcome	The primary outcome was the reduction in croup score at 0, 15 and 30 minutes.
Main results	Thirty-one patients were enrolled, 16 in the RE group and 15 in the LE group. Two patients in the RE group were excluded, as during the treatment they required intubation, and one patient in the LE group was excluded because of a diagnosis of tracheal stenosis from a previous intubation. The median age in the RE group was 11.5 months and in the LE group it was 11 months. Each group improved after treatment with a reduction in croup scores of at least 2 points. One patient in each group required an additional aerosol treatment for their clinical condition and four RE patients and three LE patients were administered additional intramuscular dexamethasone. A total of three patients in the RE group were intubated and none in the LE group were.
Conclusion	Both forms of epinephrine (adrenaline) were effective in the treatment of croup. The L form is more readily available and cheaper and consequently should be utilised to treat moderate to severe croup.
Commentary	The patients in this study had moderate to severe croup, as assessed by the Downes and Raphaely scoring system. This croup scoring system utilises five parameters to grade severity: (1) inspiratory breath sounds (0 = normal; 1 = harsh with rhonchi; 2 = delayed); (2) stridor (0 = none; 1 = inspiratory; 2 = inspiratory and expiratory); (3) cough (0 = none; 1 = hoarse cry; 2 = bark); (4) retractions/nasal flaring (0 = none; 1 = suprasternal/present; 2 = suprasternal and intercostal/present); and (5) [cyanosis (but now use oxygen saturation levels to assess cyanosis)] <95% (0 = none; 1 = in room air; 2 = in 40% oxygen). An analysis of a score of 6 or greater suggests significant respiratory distress and the need to consider epinephrine (adrenaline). While this therapy improved the stridor, additional treatment aerosols were needed in 6% of patients and dexamethasone in 20%. Respiratory rate is an important indicator of croup severity and its reduction post treatment an indicator of improvement.

(*continued*)

Evidence 3	
Theme E3	***Adrenaline in the treatment of croup***
Commentary (*cont.*)	Respiratory rate is not included in this croup score, as it is an age-dependent variable.
Reference	Waisman Y, Klein BL, Boenning DA, *et al.* Prospective randomized double-blind study comparing L-epinephrine and racemic epinephrine aerosols in the treatment of laryngotracheitis (croup). *Pediatrics.* 1992; **89**(2): 302–6.

Evidence 4	
Theme E4	***The role of oral steroid therapy in acute asthma***
Question	How effective is oral prednisolone in the treatment of acute asthma?
Study design	Randomised controlled trial
Level of evidence	Jadad 5
Setting	Ward setting, children's hospital, England
Participants	Children 18 months or older with an acute asthma attack who required admission to hospital were eligible for enrolment.
Intervention	Subjects were randomised to receive prednisolone 2 mg/kg or placebo and then were randomised to receive nebulised salbutamol 5 mg every 1–4 hours as necessary or nebulised salbutamol 0.15 mg/kg (maximum dose 5 mg) every 30 minutes for 3 hours. Asthma severity was assessed utilising heart rate and respiratory rate, peak expiratory flow rate, oxygen saturation and a clinical severity score.
Outcome	The primary outcome measure was discharge rates at 4 hours post admission.
Main results	Of the 105 eligible patients, 12 were excluded due to recent oral steroid therapy, three had additional croupy symptoms and two parents refused consent. Ten children were excluded because their symptoms were mild. Seventy-eight children were enrolled but there were eight withdrawals: two with rapid improvement (one each from steroid and placebo group), two with vomiting (in the placebo group) and four with clinical deterioration (all in the placebo group). In the prednisolone group plus standard salbutamol of 19 patients, six (32%) were discharged, and in the low-dose salbutamol group of 18 patients, 11 (61%) were discharged. In the placebo group plus standard salbutamol of 18 patients, three (17%) were discharged, and in the low-dose salbutamol group of 15 patients, three (29%) were discharged. In the prednisolone group, 17 (46%) were discharged, as opposed to six (18%) in the placebo group (absolute risk reduction = 28%; number needed to treat = 4). Age of children ranged from 1.5 to 14.2 years with a mean age of 4.7.
Conclusion	Oral prednisolone in acute asthma is effective and facilitates early discharge from hospital.
Commentary	Oral steroids were effective in treating children with acute asthma. The children were aged from 18 months to 14 years and 50% were exposed to parental smoking. The dose of prednisolone at 2 mg/kg was not associated with significant side effects. The early use of oral prednisolone contributed to the early discharge of patients at 4 hours.
Reference	Connett GJ, Warde C, Wooler E, *et al.* Prednisolone and salbutamol in the hospital treatment of acute asthma. *Arch Dis Child.* 1994; **70**(3): 170–3.

Evidence 5

Theme E5	**Ipratropium in acute asthma**
Question	What is the effect of nebulised ipratropium on the hospitalisation rates of children?
Study design	Randomised controlled trial
Level of evidence	Jadad 5
Setting	Paediatric emergency department, academic medical centre, the United States
Participants	Children 2–18 years of age with acute exacerbation of asthma were eligible for inclusion. Asthma was classified as mild (peak expiratory flow rate (PEFR) was >70% of predicted or the asthma score was 5–7), moderate (PEFR was 50%–70% of predicted or the asthma score was 8–11), or severe (PEFR was <50% of predicted or the asthma score was 12–15).
Intervention	During the treatment of a moderate or severe asthma attack, all children received nebulised salbutamol (2.5 or 5 mg per dose, depending on body weight) every 20 minutes for three doses as needed. A corticosteroid (2 mg/kg) was given orally with their second dose of salbutamol. Children in the treatment group received 500 µg of ipratropium bromide with the second and third doses of salbutamol; the control group received normal saline (placebo).
Outcome	The primary outcome was the reduction in hospitalisation rates for children with moderate to severe asthma attacks.
Main results	Of the 480 children enrolled, 46 had rapid resolution of symptoms and 434 were randomised (215 to the treatment group and 219 to the control group). In the treatment group, asthma was moderate for 79 and severe for 136; in the control group, asthma was moderate in 84 and severe in 135. The overall hospitalisation rate was 27.4% in the ipratropium group and 36.5% in the placebo group (absolute risk reduction (ARR) = 8.9%; number needed to treat (NNT) = 12). For severe asthma the admission rate was 37.5% for ipratropium and 52.6% for placebo (ARR = 15.1%; NNT = 7).
Conclusion	Ipratropium when administered in moderate to severe asthma is effective in reducing hospital admission rates.
Commentary	This study indicates the effectiveness of ipratropium in the treatment of acute asthma and reinforces the importance of timeliness in the provision of care. The asthma score utilised in this study comprised five parameters:

1. dyspnoea (1 = speaks in sentences or coos or babbles; 2 = speaks in short sentences or utters short cries; 2 = speaks in single words or short phrases or grunts)
2. retractions (1 = none or intercostal; 2 = intercostal and substernal; 3 = intercostal, substernal and supraclavicular)
3. auscultation (1 = normal breathing or end-expiratory wheezing; 2 = expiratory wheezing; 3 = inspiratory and expiratory wheezing, diminished breath sounds or both)
4. oxygen saturation % (1 = >95% in room air; 2 = 90%–95% with room air; 3 = <90 with room air or supplemental oxygen)
5. respiratory rate (for children aged 2–3 years, 4–5 years, 6–12 years, >12 years children scored 1 for respiratory rates ≤34, ≤30, ≤26 and ≤23, respectively; scored 2 for respiratory rates 35–39, 31–35, 27–30 and 24–27, respectively; and scored 3 for respiratory rates ≥40, ≥36, ≥31 and ≥28, respectively).

(continued)

Evidence 5	
Theme E5	**Ipratropium in acute asthma**
Commentary (*cont.*)	This study utilised the hospitalisation rates for the primary outcome as opposed to length of stay in the emergency department, which is influenced by other factors that are independent of drug therapy, such as the availability of beds in the hospital or the time needed to arrange discharge medications or transportation.
Reference	Qureshi F, Pestian J, Davis P, *et al.* Effect of nebulized ipratropium on the hospitalization rates of children with asthma. *N Engl J Med.* 1998; **339**(15): 1030–5.

Evidence 6	
Theme E6	**Intravenous magnesium in asthma**
Question	What is the utilisation of magnesium sulphate in acute asthma management?
Study design	Retrospective medical record review
Level of evidence	
Setting	Emergency departments in six children's hospitals, Canada
Participants	Children were included if they received a discharge diagnosis of acute asthma. Children were aged 2–17. First-time wheezers were excluded.
Intervention	Chart review from September 2008 to March 2009 of acute asthma attendances.
Outcome	The primary outcome was the use of magnesium sulphate in a Canadian paediatric emergency department for previously healthy children aged 2–17 years of age requiring hospitalisation for acute asthma. A secondary outcome was investigation of the timely use of asthma treatments and admission rates to hospital.
Main results	One thousand, three hundred and fifty-eight visits were identified; however, only 1116 met the inclusion criteria. The mean age was 6.1 ± 3.8 years. One hundred and fifty-four (13.8%) were admitted, of whom 19 (12.3%) received intravenous magnesium; only two (0.02%) received intravenous magnesium in the emergency department and were discharged. Of the admitted patients, 45% did not receive frequent ipratropium, 27% did not receive corticosteroids within 1 hour and 53% did not receive frequent salbutamol with ipratropium and corticosteroids within 1 hour of triage. Forty-two (53%) of 90 hospitalised children were not given intensive asthma treatment in their initial presentation to the emergency department. Factors that determined use of intravenous magnesium included hospitalisation in the past year (odds ratio (OR): 3.8), Previous intensive care unit admission (OR: 11.2), Current use of oral steroids (OR: 4.0) and severe asthma (OR: 6.1).
Conclusion	Intravenous magnesium is infrequently used in the treatment of children with acute asthma and there was significant variability between centres. There is a need to adhere to the timelines in acute asthma care.
Commentary	Retrospective studies can give an insight into clinical practice, which aids the reflective process. In this study, 107 (70%) of the admitted patients did not have an intravenous cannula in place reflected a change in practice. The ability of the doctors to incorporate timelines in rendering care improves the outcome for the patient. In this study many patients received partial care despite the presence of guidelines.

(*continued*)

Evidence 6	
Theme E6	*Intravenous magnesium in asthma*
Commentary (*cont.*)	Contributing factors include the non-use of guidelines, creating one's own variation of the guideline, human factors inclusive of forgetfulness or implementation issues and resource limitation. When presented with a child with acute asthma, the doctor needs to know the treatment protocol but must also ensure the treatment is delivered in a timely fashion.
Reference	Schuh S, Zemek R, Plint A, *et al.* Magnesium use in asthma pharmacotherapy: a Pediatric Emergency Research Canada study. *Pediatrics.* 2012; **129**(5): 852–9.

Evidence 7	
Theme E7	*Drug treatment for status epilepticus*
Question	How effective is drug treatment for status epilepticus?
Study design	Retrospective cohort study
Level of evidence	
Setting	Eight emergency departments in Australia and New Zealand
Participants	The charts of patients presenting to the emergency department with convulsive status epilepticus (CSE) were reviewed. CSE was defined as seizure activity lasting 10 minutes, which is at variance with the commonly accepted time frame of 30 minutes.
Intervention	Patients were treated in a sequential manner with anti-epileptic drugs, depending on local protocols, which would have been adapted from recommendations of the Advanced Paediatric Life Support Group.
Outcome	The primary outcome was the strategy that resulted in termination of CSE and the timelines adopted in treatment.
Main results	Over a 5-year-period 542 episodes of convulsive status epilepticus (CSE) were identified. For 94%, the in-hospital seizure duration was greater than 30 minutes. Ages ranged from 18 days to 20 years, with a mean age of 3 years. Of the 542 episodes, 227 responded to benzodiazepines, 190 responded to a second-line anticonvulsant, 120 required rapid sequence intubation (RSI), two had hypoglycaemia and were treated with dextrose infusion, one spontaneously ceased seizing without treatment and two patients died. The aetiologies of CSE were epilepsy (35%), underlying neurological disease (24%), febrile convulsions (21%), no aetiology (14%), neurological infections (3%) and electrolyte disturbances including hypoglycaemia (1%).
Conclusion	CSE is an emergency, with many children having a prolonged pre-hospital and hospital seizure duration. There is a need to have a clear and specific strategy to treat these children to minimise morbidity. Adhering to published guidelines should aid this process.
Commentary	A previous Australian study revealed that 74% of paediatric seizures given pre-hospital treatment did not require further treatment beyond 10 minutes; consequently, restricting the study to patients with CSE may have selected out those likely to respond to benzodiazepines.

(continued)

Evidence 7	
Theme E7	*Drug treatment for status epilepticus*
Commentary (*cont.*)	The lessons from this study are: a) cumulative doses of benzodiazepines are in keeping with published recommendations but were frequently administered in multiple incremental doses rather than in one to two boluses b) the answer to when RSI should be used in the treatment of CSE needs to be considered. The authors were unable to define the relative contributions of respiratory depression and the presence of ongoing CSE. Standard guidelines suggest that RSI should be used after 40 minutes of CSE; however, the present study shows a reluctance to follow this advice, given that the median pre-hospital seizure duration was 45 minutes.
Reference	Lewena S, Pennington V, Acworth J, *et al.* Emergency management of pediatric convulsive status epilepticus: a multicenter study of 542 patients. *Pediatr Emerg Care.* 2009; **25**(2): 83–7.

Evidence 8	
Theme E8	*Non-intravenous drug therapy of seizures*
Question	Which is more effective in the treatment of seizures: buccal midazolam or rectal diazepam?
Study design	Randomised controlled trial
Level of evidence	Jadad 1
Setting	Emergency departments, four children's hospitals, England
Participants	Children, older than 6 months, presenting to the emergency department with generalised seizures who did not have intravenous access established, had not a diagnosis of chronic epilepsy or had received pre-hospital rescue treatment, were eligible for enrolment.
Intervention	Children received either buccal midazolam or rectal diazepam. The buccal midazolam was filtered through a needle or straw into the buccal cavity between the gum and the cheeks. The doses of midazolam and diazepam were 0.5 mg per/kg (2.5 mg for those aged 6–12 months; 5 mg for those 1–4 years, 7.5 mg for those 5–9 years and 10 mg for those 10 years or older).
Outcome	The primary outcome was cessation of the seizure within 10 minutes without respiratory depression and the lack of reoccurrence of the seizure within 1 hour. If seizure activity was present at 10 minutes then intravenous lorazepam was administered (100 µg/kg).
Main results	Consent was obtained for 219 separate episodes for 177 patients. Of the 42 patients recruited more than once, seven were recruited within a week, four within a month and the remainder within 2 months. For the 109 in the buccal midazolam group, 61 (56%) achieved the primary outcome, compared with 30 (27%) of the rectal diazepam group (absolute risk reduction = 29%; number needed to treat = 4). Respiratory depression occurred in five (5%) of the buccal midazolam group compared with six (7%) in the rectal diazepam group.

(*continued*)

Evidence 8	
Theme E8	***Non-intravenous drug therapy of seizures***
Conclusion	Buccal midazolam was more effective than rectal diazepam in the treatment of seizures in children and was not associated with increased respiratory depression.
Commentary	In reality, achieving intravenous access in a seizing child can be difficult. The use of alternate treatment options is required. The use of buccal midazolam is superior to rectal diazepam. Currently rectal diazepam is utilised by carers and paramedics in the pre-hospital treatment of seizures as was seen in approximately one-third of the patients in this study. While participants in this study had concerns with the use of buccal midazolam in the presence of acute seizure activity, they reported that it was easy to administer. This experience needs to be validated in the pre-hospital setting, but is likely to receive support from parents, especially if teaching videos are developed that demonstrate administration in the presence of an acute seizure event.
Reference	McIntyre J, Robertson S, Norris E, *et al*. Safety and efficacy of buccal midazolam versus rectal diazepam for emergency treatment of seizures in children: a randomised controlled trial. *Lancet*. 2005; **366**(9481): 205–10.

Evidence 9	
Theme E9	***The aetiology of coma***
Question	What is the aetiology and outcome from non-traumatic coma?
Study design	Prospective population-based study
Level of evidence	
Setting	Northern National Health Service region of England, department of child health, academic medical centre, England
Participants	Children and adolescents aged 1 month to 15 years and 11 months, with a significant depression of conscious level (defined as a Glasgow Coma Scale score of 12; for children younger than 5, the Saint James modification of the Glasgow Coma Scale was used), with a duration of at least 6 hours and not related to trauma, were eligible for inclusion.
Intervention	Children admitted to any hospital in the region with coma were identified and all deaths during the study period recorded by the Office for Population Census and Surveys were analysed.
Outcome	The primary outcomes were incidence of non-traumatic coma, aetiology and outcome of the affected population.
Main results	A total of 345 episodes of non-traumatic coma were identified, of which 283 met the inclusion criteria. Sixty-two were excluded, 37 because duration of unconsciousness was <6 hours, 19 had terminal malignant diseases, three did not meet the age criteria, two were trauma-related coma, one notified out of study period. Three children had more than one episode of coma; therefore, 278 were included in the final analysis. The incidence of coma was 30.8/100 000 children under the age of 16.

(continued)

Evidence 9	
Theme E9	*The aetiology of coma*
Main results (*cont.*)	The incidence in the first year of life was 130/100 000. The aetiologies were as follows for the 278 patients: infection, 107; intoxication, 29; epilepsy, 28; complications of congenital abnormalities, 22; accidents, 19 (seven had smoke inhalation, four were accidental strangulation, three had burns, three from drowning); metabolic, 15 (eight had diabetic ketoacidosis, three had medium chain acyl-CoA dehydrogenase deficiency (MCAD) and four had other inborn errors); and unknown, 41 and others, 17. Of the 278 participants, there were 59 pre-hospital deaths and 66 died in hospital, giving an overall mortality rate of 127 (45.6%). Late follow-up was available in 141 children, of whom 94 (66%) had no detectable impairment and 40 had cognitive or behavioural morbidity.
Conclusion	The aetiology of coma is diverse but it has a high mortality; therefore, the clinician needs to have a specific strategy when assessing and treating these children.
Commentary	Children under 1 year of age are at the highest risk of coma but the diagnosis may be further complicated by the non-specific nature of the symptoms and signs. The absence of a defined aetiology in 14% of patients (despite extensive investigations) is concerning; however, in 50% of these cases an infectious aetiology was suspected and in another quarter a metabolic cause was considered likely but unproven.
Reference	Wong CP, Forsyth RJ, Kelly TP, *et al*. Incidence, aetiology, and outcome of non-traumatic coma: a population based study. *Arch Dis Child*. 2001; **84**(3): 193–9.

Reference

1. Wolfsdorf J, Craig ME, Daneman D, *et al*. Diabetic ketoacidosis in children and adolescents with diabetes. *Pediatr Diabetes*. 2009; **10**(Suppl 12): 118–33.

SLIDES

1. Acute meningococcal sepsis
2. Meningococcal disease
3. Meningococcal disease (widespread purpura)

Chapter Four

THE CHILD WITH A FEVER

COMMON SCENARIO

'He's had a temperature all day. I've been giving him regular Calpol and Nurofen, and it brings it down, but an hour later, it's back up again.'

LEARNING OBJECTIVES

- Recognise 'red flags' in the history or examination that indicate serious bacterial infection (SBI)
- List the differential causes of acute, chronic and recurrent fever
- Develop a rationale approach to the initial investigations required in child presenting with fever
- Understand the management of common causes of fever in childhood
- Recognise when referral and hospital admission for further investigation and treatment is required
- Understand the treatment options available in treating the febrile child

BACKGROUND

Fever is by far the commonest presenting complaint in childhood and a cause of immense parental anxiety. For practitioners, it represents a diagnostic challenge. Practitioners need the ability to distinguish the acutely unwell child with a potential SBI from the well child with a common viral illness. SBIs include meningitis, sepsis, osteomyelitis, septic arthritis, cellulitis, urinary tract infections (UTIs), pneumonia and enteritis. Signs of underlying meningitis or septicaemia should be looked for in all febrile patients without an obvious source for fever. A history of fever in a child presenting afebrile is important. A fever than subsides with antipyretic treatment cannot be dismissed as secondary to a virus. In contrast, hypothermia in infants may indicate serious infection.

Fever of unknown origin is defined as an acute febrile illness in which aetiology is not apparent after a detailed history and examination. One in five acutely ill, non-toxic-appearing children have an unidentifiable source of fever.

Recurrent fevers are defined as three or more episodes of fever in a 6-month period, with no medical illness to explain the fevers and with an interval of at least 7 days between febrile episodes. Recurrent fevers with a regular pattern of onset should be distinguished from fevers with an irregular pattern of onset. Recurrent fevers can be due to infections, neoplastic or inflammatory disorders.

The gold standard for assessment of fever is a rectal temperature measurement. A parent's tactile assessment of the child's forehead identifies the presence of fever in approximately 50%–75% of cases. Fever is defined as a rectal temperature greater than 38°C. The accuracy of oral temperature measurement is dependent on the correct positioning of the thermometer under the tongue. Tympanic thermometers have reasonable accuracy and are in general the most practical means of recording temperature. For children at higher risk of sepsis, the threshold for fever tends to be lower.

Patients at high risk of SBI:
- infants under 2 months of age
- transplant recipients
- immunosuppressed children
- asplenic patients.

For infants under 2 months of age presenting with fever, the rate of SBI is higher. It is estimated to be 25% in infants less than 2 weeks of age, 13% in infants less than 4 weeks of age and 8% in infants between 4 and 8 weeks of age.

Neonates under 28 days of age are at increased risk of serious infections because of:
- immaturity of immune system
- risk of infection acquired during delivery
- clinical evaluation inadequate to determine which neonates at risk of SBI.

An acutely unwell or toxic-looking child may have signs of poor perfusion such as mottling, cool peripheries and delayed capillary refill time. They often dislike being disturbed and may lie still with alternating drowsiness and irritability. They refuse to feed. They may look pale or have a 'muddy' grey appearance or show signs of respiratory distress with rapid, laboured breathing with or without grunting.

In children presenting with a fever, the following should be recorded at the initial assessment:
- temperature
- heart rate
- respiratory rate
- blood pressure
- capillary refill time
- oxygen saturation
- assessment of conscious level

- pupil size and reaction
- the presence of a rash.

During the assessment of a child with fever, attention should be paid to:
- vital signs and changes in vitals
- overall appearance
- potential sites of infection.

A detailed history and examination, paying particular attention to the vital signs, overall appearance of the child and searching for potential sources of infection, can help guide further management and determine whether further investigations and treatment are required.

Normal vital signs in childhood			
Age (years)	Heart rate (beats/min)	Respiratory rate (breaths/min)	Systolic blood pressure (mmHg)
<1	110–160	30–40	70–90
1–2	100–150	25–35	80–95
2–5	95–140	25–30	80–100
5–12	80–120	20–25	90–110
Over 12	60–100	15–20	100–120

PHARYNGITIS

Children with pharyngitis are non-toxic and may present with a fever, sore throat and refusal to feed. Examination reveals an erythematous pharynx with cervical lymphadenopathy. The commonest causative agent is a common virus. Viral infections have a gradual onset. There may be associated coryzal symptoms, diarrhoea or non-specific generalised rash. Group A beta-haemolytic streptococcus accounts for approximately 15%–30% of cases. It has a rapid onset. With bacterial pharyngitis, coryzal signs are generally absent. There may be associated headache, abdominal pain, palatal petechiae, swollen and erythematous uvula and tonsillar exudates with tender cervical lymphadenopathy. Splenomegaly, palatal petechiae and generalised lymphadenopathy suggest Epstein–Barr virus infection.

Suppurative complications of group A beta-haemolytic streptococcal pharyngitis:
- otitis media
- sinusitis
- peritonsillar and retropharyngeal abscesses
- suppurative cervical lymphadenitis.

Non-suppurative complications of group A beta-haemolytic streptococcal pharyngitis:

- acute rheumatic fever
- acute glomerulonephritis.

ACUTE OTITIS MEDIA

Acute otitis media (AOM) is inflammation of the middle ear associated with fluid collection in the middle ear space (effusion) or a discharge (otorrhoea). Children may present with fever, ear pain (non-verbal infant may pull at his or her ears), anorexia and irritability. There may be associated coryzal symptoms or vomiting or diarrhoea. The normal tympanic membrane is pearly grey and translucent. With AOM, examination reveals a bulging, diffusely erythematous eardrum with loss of the light reflex and anatomical landmark. AOM is often over diagnosed. A red tympanic membrane is a common finding in children with viral upper respiratory tract infections (URTIs) and in the crying child.

Risk factors for otitis media include:

- younger age, because of an immature, short and more horizontal Eustachian tube
- immunodeficiency
- recurrent URTIs
- trisomy 21
- craniofacial abnormalities including cleft palate
- attendance at day care or crèche
- smoking in the home.

It can be difficult to distinguish bacterial from viral causes based on history and examination findings alone. Viral agents are implicated in up to 50% of cases. Common bacterial causes include *Streptococcus pneumoniae, Haemophilus influenzae* and *Moraxella catarrhalis*. If associated with pharyngotonsillitis it is likely to be secondary to *S. pneumoniae* and if associated with purulent conjunctivitis it is likely to be secondary to *H. influenzae*.

Following an episode of AOM, 70% of patients will still have an effusion at 2 weeks, 40% at 1 month, 20% at 2 months and 5%–10% at 3 months.

Complications of otitis media include:

- perforation resulting in ear discharge, which often relieves the pain
- conductive hearing loss
- acute suppurative labyrinthitis
- facial nerve palsies
- acute mastoiditis
- intracranial spread of infection: venous sinus thrombosis, meningitis, subdural or extradural abscess.

PNEUMONIA

Viruses are the most common causes of pneumonia in children less than 2 years of age. In school-age children *S. pneumoniae* and *Mycoplasma pneumoniae* are most common, but in 50% of children no clear aetiology can be discerned. Typically, the child presents with fever (sometimes rigors) that is associated with a new-onset cough, which may not be productive in the early stages. Chest pain reflects the pleural involvement and abdominal pain may reflect lower lobe disease. The typical child has difficulty in breathing and systemic symptoms of anorexia, lethargy and headache.

Physical examination reveals fever, tachypnoea and signs of accessory muscle use (intercostal retractions, and tracheal tug). The presence of consolidation is suggested on palpation by diminished chest expansion and increased tactile fremitus (if the child is old enough to co-operate), auscultation reveals diminished air entry, localised crackles, bronchial breathing and occasionally a pleural rub. The physician has to be patient in examining the child to elicit these physical signs. The finding of wheeze is suggestive of mycoplasma infections.

Routine chest X-ray is not necessary on all children with pneumonia. Pulse oximetry is recommended for those children with an elevated respiratory rate, to assess the need for supplemental oxygen.

Pneumonia is assessed as mild to moderate in infants if:

- temperature is <38.5°C
- respiratory rate is <50 breaths/min
- recession is mild
- the infant is taking full feeds.

Pneumonia is assessed as severe in infants if the following are present:

- temperature is >38.5°C
- respiratory rate >70 breaths/min
- moderate to severe recession
- nasal flaring
- cyanosis
- intermittent apnoea
- grunting respiration
- not feeding
- tachycardia – elevated for age and temperature
- capillary refill time ≥2 seconds.

In older children, pneumonia is assessed as mild to moderate if:

- temperature is >38.5°C
- respiratory rate is <50 breaths/min
- breathlessness is mild
- no vomiting is present.

Pneumonia is assessed as severe if the following are present:

- temperature is >38.5°C
- respiratory rate is >50 breaths/min
- severe difficulty in breathing
- nasal flaring
- cyanosis
- grunting respiration
- signs of dehydration
- tachycardia
- capillary refill time ≥2 seconds.

These clinical features represent a transitioning from mild to moderate to severe disease and referral to hospital for assessment is warranted at the moderate stage.

URINARY TRACT INFECTIONS

It is estimated that 8% of girls and 2% of boys will have a symptomatic UTI in childhood. The commonest causative organism is *Escherichia coli*. Infants present with non-specific symptoms and signs including fever, irritability, lethargy, poor feeding or febrile convulsions. However, the diagnosis of UTI in toxic infants does not out rule SBI elsewhere, including septicaemia. Children present with more classical symptoms of cystitis with dysuria, and urgency and frequency or a reluctance to void. There may be a return of enuresis. Fever is often absent or low grade. Children with pyelonephritis present with systemic symptoms including fever, vomiting and abdominal or flank pain.

Predisposing factors include:

- congenital structural abnormalities
- history of broad-spectrum antibiotics
- incomplete bladder emptying or infrequent voiding
- constipation.

In 30% of children with UTI, vesicoureteric reflux (VUR) is present. VUR is a developmental anomaly of the vesicoureteric junction. There is often a positive family history. There are five described grades of VUR.

> Grade I: reflux without dilatation into distal ureter
> Grade II: reflux with dilatation into proximal ureter
> Grade III: reflux into renal pelvis with dilatation
> Grade IV: further dilatation and distortion of calyces
> Grade V: hydronephrosis

MENINGOCOCCAL DISEASE

Meningococcal disease has two main clinical presentations: meningitis and septicae-mia, which often occur together. Septicaemia is more common and more dangerous. It is more likely to be fatal when it occurs without meningitis. Not all children with meningococcal disease present with a fever. The presentation of early meningococcal disease can be difficult to differentiate from common viral illnesses. Fifty per cent of children presenting to their primary care physician with meningococcal disease are sent home on their first visit. These children are more likely to die.

Meningitis can present with severe headache, neck stiffness, photophobia, decreased level of consciousness or seizures.

Septicaemia can present with a rash, tachycardia, tachypnoea, cool peripheries, prolonged capillary refill time, hypovolaemia, limb or joint pain, abdominal pain or decreased level of consciousness.

The presentation in infants is very non-specific and clinical expertise is required to recognise the infant with potentially life-threatening disease. There may be a history of poor feeding, irritability, a high-pitched cry, abnormal tone, lethargy, a tense and bulging fontanelle and/or cyanosis. Some children may complain of painful feet and be reluctant to walk.

The onset of the rash in meningococcal disease occurs at a median of 8 hours after the start of the illness in infants. The presence of purpura is highly predictive of meningococcal disease and should be considered an emergency requiring prompt evaluation and treatment. Purpura fulminans is a severe complication of meningo-coccal disease occurring in approximately 15%–25% of those with meningococcemia. It is characterised by the acute onset of cutaneous haemorrhage and necrosis due to vascular thrombosis and disseminated intravascular coagulopathy.

Long-term complications of meningococcal disease include:

- hearing loss and other sensory impairments
- neurological impairment including learning, motor and neurodevelopment deficits and epilepsy
- orthopaedic damage including amputation, growth plate damage and arthritis
- post-necrotic tissue/skin loss
- renal impairment
- psychiatric and behavioural problems.

The Glasgow Meningococcal Septicaemia Prognostic Score is used to assign a prognostic score to patients with meningococcal disease. It aims to identify patients, at the point of admission to hospital, most likely to suffer morbidity or mortality.

Glasgow Meningococcal Septicaemia Prognostic Score	
Observation	*Score*
Blood pressure <75 mmHg, age <4 years; or <85 mmHg, age >4 years	3
Skin/rectal temperature difference >3°C	3
Modified Glasgow Coma Scale score <8 or deterioration of >3 points in 1 hour	3
Deterioration in 1 hour before scoring	2
Absence of meningism	2
Extending purpuric rash or widespread purpura	1
Base deficit >8	1
Maximum total score	15

HISTORY

KEY POINTS				
Fever	Onset Pattern Response to antipyretics Method of temperature measurement Duration	**Dermatology and rheumatology symptoms**	Rash Limp Joint swelling Refusal to weight-bear Bone pain	**🡒 Red flags** Chronic or recurrent fever Marked change in temperament Meningeal symptoms Under 2 months of age Maternal infection before or during delivery Non-immunised child
Feeding	24 hour intake Interest in feeds Ability to feed	**Medical history**	Previous infections Previous hospitalisations Chronic diseases	
Behaviour	Lethargy Reaction to parents Cry: high-pitched, weak?	**Birth history (in neonates)**	Gestation Prolonged rupture of membranes Maternal pyrexia Maternal group B streptococcus Antibiotics required after birth	
Neurological symptoms	Headache Seizure Neck stiffness Photophobia	**Drugs**	Regular medications Recent antibiotic use	

(continued)

KEY POINTS				
Gastrointestinal symptoms	Vomiting Diarrhoea Abdominal pain	**Vaccinations**	Up to date	
Respiratory and ear, nose and throat symptoms	Cough Runny nose Wheeze Red or sticky eyes Shortness of breath Sore throat Ear pain or discharge	**Family history**	VUR or renal disease	
Renal symptoms	Dysuria Haematuria Frequency Urgency Loin pain Voiding pattern	**Social history**	Sick contacts Attendance at crèche or day care Foreign travel	

EXAMINATION

- Assess the overall appearance of child by observation: toxic or well looking?
- Expose the child fully and perform a head-to-toe examination
- Vital signs including temperature should be recorded
- Assess hydration status
- Assess for signs of meningism
- Ear, nose and throat: otitis media, pharyngitis, stomatitis, cervical lymphadenopathy
- Joint exam: swelling, erythema, paresis
- Skin exam: rash, erythema, tenderness
- Respiratory exam: signs of respiratory distress, wheeze, crepitations
- Gastrointestinal exam: abdominal tenderness, masses

Red flags

- Altered level of consciousness
- Respiratory distress
- Signs of impending shock
- Seizures
- Petechiae rash
- Meningism

DIFFERENTIAL DIAGNOSIS

Common causes	
Viral exanthems	Coryzal symptoms, rash, lymphadenopathy
Viral pneumonia	Temperature usually <38°C, gradual onset, bilateral crepitations, wheezing
Viral URTIs	Cough, runny nose
Pharyngitis	Sore throat, refusal to feed, erythematous pharynx, cervical lymphadenopathy
Otitis media	Irritable, vomiting or diarrhoea, pulling at ear, may present without fever, otorrhoea, associated coryzal symptoms
Viral gastroenteritis	Vomiting, watery diarrhoea, dehydration, absence of blood per rectum

Serious bacterial infections	
UTIs	Very non-specific presentations, may present without fever, failure to thrive, malodorous urine, poor feeding, vomiting, jaundice, family history of VUR
Bacterial pneumonia	Tachypnoea, signs of respiratory distress, localised crepitations
Meningococcal disease	Toxic, poor perfusion, lethargy, apnoea, bulging fontanelle, high-pitched cry, hypotonia, listlessness, poor feeding, seizures, fever or hypothermia, vomiting, cool peripheries
Encephalitis	Altered level of consciousness, seizures, headaches, irritability
Septic arthritis and osteomyelitis	Paresis, abnormal position of limb, pain elicited on passive movement, swelling
Cellulitis	Localised erythema, increased temperature
Bacterial gastroenteritis	Vomiting, bloody diarrhoea
Septicaemia	Toxic, poor perfusion, hypotension, altered level of consciousness
Orbital cellulitis	Erythema of eyelids, pain on eye movement, reduction in visual acuity, proptosis

Prolonged fever	
Infections	Epstein–Barr virus, malaria, Lyme disease, Rocky Mountain spotted fever, bacterial endocarditis, tuberculosis, rheumatic fever, cat scratch disease, HIV, abscesses, systemic fungal infection
Inflammation	Systemic juvenile idiopathic arthritis, systemic lupus erythematosus, Kawasaki's disease
Neoplasia	Leukaemias, lymphomas, metastases, solid organ tumours

Recurrent fever (occurring at regular intervals)	
PFAPA syndrome (periodic fever, aphthous ulcers, pharyngitis, cervical lymphadenopathy)	Fevers occur every 21–28 days
Cyclic neutropenia	Fevers occur every 21–28 days
Relapsing fever	Fevers occur every 14–21 days
Familial Mediterranean fever	Fevers occur every 7–21 days
Hyperimmunoglobulinaemia D syndrome	Fevers occur every 14–28 days
Epstein–Barr virus	Fevers occur every 6–8 weeks

INVESTIGATIONS

If meningococcal disease is suspected, what blood tests should be performed?

- Glucose
- Urea and electrolytes
- Full blood count (FBC)
- Coagulation screen
- Liver function tests
- Lactate
- Calcium, phosphate and magnesium
- Pneumococcal and meningococcal polymerase chain reaction testing
- Venous blood gas
- Blood cultures
- Group and hold

In a child with suspected meningococcal disease, what are the contraindications to lumbar puncture?

The contraindications to lumbar puncture are:
- prolonged or focal seizure
- focal neurological signs
- widespread purpuric rash
- Glasgow Coma Scale score <3
- impaired oculocephalic reflexes
- abnormal posture
- pupillary dilation
- signs of raised intracranial pressure
- coagulopathy

Cerebrospinal fluid (CSF) should be sent for:
- Gram stain and culture
- cell count and differential
- protein
- glucose
- bacterial and viral polymerase chain reaction testing

With bacterial meningitis, the CSF is cloudy and turbid. White cell count (WCC) is raised, with predominant neutrophils. The red cell count (RCC) is normal (unless traumatic tap), protein is raised and glucose is low or very low.

With viral meningitis, the CSF is clear and colourless; the WCC is raised with predominant lymphocytes. The RCC is normal (unless traumatic tap), protein is normal or high and glucose is normal or low.

In an unwell infant under 2 months of age with a fever, what investigations should be performed?

A full septic workup should be performed. However, decisions to treat for presumed sepsis should not be based on laboratory investigations alone. Decisions should be based on the clinical picture, i.e. a child who is clinically unwell and toxic should be commenced on antibiotics for presumed SBI, irrespective of whether the white cells or inflammatory markers are raised.

(continued)

INVESTIGATIONS (*cont.*)

- FBC: a child with a WCC of less than 15×10^9 is considered to have a lower risk of SBI
- A neutrophil count of $>10 \times 10^9$ is considered high-risk for SBI
- Urea and electrolytes: may show signs of dehydration
- C-reactive protein: may be raised
- Blood cultures may show growth of bacteria
- Lumbar puncture (*see* earlier)
- Clean-catch urinalysis and culture (*see* later)
- Chest X-ray: may show signs of consolidation or collapse

In children with a suspected UTI, what initial investigations should be performed?

A urine dipstick should be performed.
- Nitrates: are produced by bacterial reduction of urinary nitrates and are highly specific if strongly positive (but high false negative rate).
- Leucocyte esterase is an enzyme present in white blood cells and is frequently positive but has a low sensitivity and may be present because of contamination or other febrile illnesses.
- The presence of blood and protein are unreliable markers of infection.

Urine culture is required to confirm the diagnosis of infection.
- Confirmed UTI: pure growth of organism $>10^5$ CFU/mL

MANAGEMENT PLAN: THREE-STEP APPROACH

1. Clarifying and pitfall avoidance strategies
2. Treatment of fever
3. Treatment of specific conditions:
   a) recognising and treating the sick infant less than 3 months of age
   b) pharyngitis
   c) acute otitis media
   d) pneumonia
   e) urinary tract infections
   f) meningococcal disease and meningitis
   g) osteomyelitis and septic arthritis

Clarifying and pitfall avoidance strategies

- Explain to parents that fever is a symptom and not a disease. **Rationale**: fever is only one aspect of an illness and while parents can readily identify that their child is febrile this does not correlate with illness severity. Children with high fevers and a viral syndrome may appear quite well; however some children with mildly elevated temperatures may be miserable and become seriously ill. Parents should focus on the overall state of the child and not just the fever. Explain the role of fever in illness. **Rationale**: the presence of fever enhances enzyme systems, thus enhancing the body's response to illness.
- Define the parental response to fever. **Rationale**: evaluate for fever phobia (parental anxiety related to fever is amplified). Reinforce the value of fever and ensure that

parents do not exceed therapeutic recommendations of antipyretics. The effectiveness of antipyretic strategies must be explained (*see* Evidence 1)

- Parents and tepid sponging. **Rationale**: tepid sponging should be discouraged. Parents often use cool water and cause peripheral vasoconstriction of the skin, thus preventing heat loss through the skin. If the child is unable to defervesce, temperatures may rise.
- Fever of short duration. **Pitfall**: anxious parents may present early to their family doctors with their febrile child. If no cause is apparent, explain that symptoms may evolve over the following hours. Be explicit to the parent about when the child should be reviewed, especially in children under 1 year of age.

For the doctor, the febrile child represents a significant clinical challenge.

- Sick child and presence of fever. **Pitfall**: not all infants and children who are septic will be febrile. Fever must be considered in the context of other features inclusive of age, temperament and other specific features.
- Fever and the lack of specific symptoms and signs. **Rationale**: the occurrence of fever may reflect an illness in evolution; therefore, the absence of findings on initial examination does not preclude their evolution over the subsequent hours. Certain children with fever should be regarded as being at high risk and these include the following groups: those 1) <3 months of age, 2) with underlying immunodeficiency state, 3) with a chronic condition, for example, sickle cell disease or cystic fibrosis and, 4) who are on immunosuppressive treatment. Fever and the concept of disease evolution. **Pitfall**: Some children, especially infants, can deteriorate clinically after a few hours, therefore if a febrile infant clinically deteriorates advise the parents to bring the child to an emergency department for further assessment and laboratory tests.
- A febrile child with sepsis. **Pitfall**: Some children with sepsis will present with a normal or even low temperature therefore do not assume that all septic children will be febrile.
- All fever is reflective of infection. **Pitfall**: not all fever is reflective of infection. Clinical conditions such as Kawasaki's disease and collagen vascular disease present with fever and symptoms evolve over time.
- Recognising the sick child (Toxicity). **Rationale**: With the improvement in immunisation, the frequency of acute illness is lessening, and as a consequence recognising the evolution of the child from a well state to an illness state is becoming more of a diagnostic challenge. The Yale observation scale focuses on the appearance of the child and is a useful adjunct to the history, clinical examination and laboratory test for the febrile child younger than 24 months. The features assessed include 1) quality of the child's cry, 2) reaction to parents, 3) state variation, 4) colour, 5) hydration status and 6) response to overtures. Each item is ranked normal scoring 1, moderate scoring 3 and severe scoring 5. The maximum score is 30. If <10 the risk of serious illness is 2.7% and if 11–15 it is 26%, and if ≥16 it is 92%.[1]

These results may be modified by the immunisation status of the child. The ABCD mnemonic can also be used to assess toxicity where 'A' is for arousal, alertness or decreased activity, 'B' is for breathing difficulties (tachypnoea, increased work of breathing), 'C' is for poor colour (pale or mottled), poor circulation (cold peripheries, increased capillary refill time) or cry (weak or high pitched), and 'D' is for decreased fluid intake (less than half normal) and/or decreased urine output (fewer than four wet nappies per day). The presence of any of these signs places the child at high risk for serious illness.

- Fever in the child with incidental neutropenia. **Pitfall**: the finding of neutropenia in the child with fever may reflect severe sepsis; however, if the child is not clinically septic, careful follow-up is advised, as a percentage of these children will present with leukaemia within a few months.
- Fever in the child diagnosed with a malignancy who is neutropenic. **Pitfall**: treat this child with intravenous antibiotics promptly while awaiting culture reports (follow clinical protocol for antibiotic regimens). This is a clinical emergency.
- Fever and rash. **Pitfall**: Do not assume that all rashes are part of a viral syndrome. Doctors need to be familiar with specific rashes inclusive of erythema multiforme, erythema nodosum and those that reflect bacterial infections

Treatment of fever

Parents often focus on fever reduction as the sole goal of addressing the needs of the febrile child; however, for the doctor, fever most often reflects the presence of an illness, so discerning the aetiology is the primary focus, and subsequently the focus is on fever treatment. If the febrile child feels well then automatic reduction of the fever is not required. The two most common medications used to reduce fever are paracetamol and ibuprofen. Both are effective in fever reduction, and combined treatment or alternating treatment is more effective than single treatment (*see* Evidence 1); however, whether this translates into a clinically relevant practice is uncertain.

Treatment of specific conditions

Recognising and treating the sick infant less than 3 months of age

With the advances in immunisation the frequency of SBI has lessened over the past 2 decades, but the risk of SBI in infants younger than 3 months with fever is 8%. For the inexperienced doctor, febrile infants at this age represent a major diagnostic challenge. The Philadelphia protocol (*see* Evidence 2) and Rochester criteria (*see* Evidence 3) provide a clinical strategy for the evaluation and treatment of these infants. Given the risks associated with this group of infants, the high adherence rates are not surprising.

Pharyngitis

Viral pharyngitis requires nothing other than supportive treatment, which includes the maintenance of adequate hydration and temperature control. Group A beta-haemolytic streptococcal infection should be treated to minimise the risk of complication, reduce the duration of symptoms and shorten the infectious period.

Acute otitis media

Despite being a very common paediatric condition, there is no uniformity on the appropriate treatment strategy, with over 95% of affected children in the United States and Australia receiving antibiotic therapy compared with 30% in the Netherlands. Most cases of otitis media are viral in origin and will resolve spontaneously in 10–14 days provided adequate analgesia is provided. The case for routine antibiotic use is not proven (*see* Evidence 4) and watchful waiting is a more prudent approach (offer antibiotic treatment if no improvement after 3 days). Utilising the clinical otitis score allows the clinician to quantify the disease severity and modify the treatment strategy accordingly. Decongestants and antihistamines have no role in AOM treatment.

A percentage of children will develop persistent otitis media with effusion, which may impair their speech development because of associated hearing deficit, and these children require referral to an ear, nose and throat specialist. Ventilation tubes (VTs) offer a temporary solution for these children (*see* Evidence 5). Parents should be advised of the association between smoking and otitis media with effusion. Patients who have VTs inserted should not be restricted from swimming.

Parents of children with recurrent otitis media often seek a final solution to prevent the occurrence of infection and may inquire about a surgical solution in addition to VT placement. The performance of an adenoidectomy does not result in clinically relevant gain for the child (*see* Evidence 6).

Pneumonia

The diagnosis of pneumonia in children may trigger several reactions in the parent. Often they will wish for a chest X-ray to be performed, but this is not necessary if the history and examination are consistent with the diagnosis of pneumonia. Admission to hospital is determined by the clinical state of the child. Cough suppressant and decongestants are not warranted, but analgesia should be provided for fever and pain. Oral amoxicillin is effective for most children admitted to hospital and is not inferior to intravenous antibiotics (*see* Evidence 7). For those with suspected mycoplasma infection, erythromycin should be administered. For those children with community-acquired pneumonia, physiotherapy offers no advantage (*see* Evidence 8) and does not shorten the duration of the illness.

Urinary tract infections

In a child with a UTI, ensure that there is a positive urine culture to guide antibiotic treatment.
Ensure:
- high fluid intake
- avoidance of constipation

- regular voiding: at least five times a day
- complete bladder emptying
- recommend good perineal hygiene: girls should wipe from front to back, avoid soap, bubble bath, and shampoo in the perineal area and wear cotton panties.

If the child is toxic the physician may have a preference for intravenous antibiotics (penicillin and an aminoglycoside) rather than oral antibiotics such as cefixime or trimethoprim-sulfamethoxazole. However, there is growing evidence that oral therapy of serious infections, e.g. pyelonephritis is effective (*see* Evidence 9) and it is likely that this will become a more widely accepted strategy as more evidence accumulates.

In children who have recurrent UTIs parents will seek preventive strategies that do not employ antibiotic therapy. Cranberry juice has been shown to have a modest effect in the reduction of UTI frequency (*see* Evidence 10) but there were adherence issues in younger children.

In children with VUR the aim is to reduce UTI occurrence through the use of prophylactic antibiotics, to prevent further damage of renal function. The presence of significant adherence issues suggests that this is not an effective therapeutic manoeuvre (*see* Evidence 11).

Meningococcal disease and meningitis
(*See* Chapter 3: First Response)

Osteomyelitis and septic arthritis
(*See* Chapter 24: The Child with a Limp)

FOLLOW-UP
In children who are being discharged home, it is important to provide parents with a 'safety net'. Safety net arrangements should take into account the parents' anxiety and capacity to manage the situation, the proximity to medical care and any individual problems with access or transport.

- Encourage parents to trust their instincts and seek medical help again if the illness gets worse, even if this is shortly after the patient was seen.
- Provide information about symptoms and signs of serious illness, including how to identify a non-blanching rash and the tumbler test.
- It may be necessary to suggest follow-up within a specified period (usually within 4–6 hours).
- Ensure that the parents understand how to get medical help after normal working hours.

WHEN TO REFER?

- Under 2 months of age with a fever, there should be a very low threshold for referral to hospital
- Children with a clear history of fevers, in the absence of upper respiratory symptoms
- Fever with constitutional symptoms, e.g. anorexia, irritability
- Fever with petechiae

CLARIFICATION STATEMENTS FOR PARENTAL MISCONCEPTIONS

'I read fever can cause brain damage.'

Fever does not cause brain damage in children. Fever serves several physiological functions: (a) fever enhances the immune response, elevating the WBC, (b) fever prevents microbes from replicating and (c) fever results in children becoming less active. The brain internally regulates temperature so that temperatures beyond 40.5^0C are very rare.

'Getting the temperature reduction is my goal.'

Making the febrile child comfortable should be the goal. Aggressively treating fevers may result in the child suffering iatrogenic side effects.

'Febrile children require antibiotic treatment.'

The vast majority of fevers encountered in childhood are related to viral illness and antibiotics are not indicated. The indiscriminate use of antibiotics is leading to antibiotic resistance and producing further clinical challenges. Watchful waiting is the prudent strategy unless there is a clear bacterial focus for the disease.

SUMMARY PRACTICE POINTS

- Fever must be assessed in terms of the well-being of the child.
- Children with strep throat typically have no URTI symptoms and have tender cervical lymph glands.
- AOM is overdiagnosed.
- Antibiotic treatment for AOM is not routinely warranted provided adequate analgesia is offered.
- Oral antibiotic treatment is adequate for community-acquired pneumonias.
- Physiotherapy is of no proven benefit in previously well children with pneumonia.
- Obtain a urine culture prior to commencing children on antibiotics for UTIs.

● Meningococcal disease is often non-specific in its presentation – most children are irritable.

EVALUATING THE EVIDENCE

Evidence 1	
Theme E1	*Medication and the treatment of febrile children*
Question	Which is more effective in the treatment of fever: ibuprofen alone or in combination with or alternating with paracetamol?
Design	Randomised controlled trial
Level of evidence	Jadad 1
Setting	Department of paediatrics, academic medical centre, the United States
Participants	Children, previously healthy, without recent ingestion of antipyretic medications, with a fever >38°C, aged 6 months to 8 years were eligible for inclusion.
Intervention	Participants were allocated to one of three groups: (1) one dose of ibuprofen (10 mg/kg), (2) ibuprofen (dose 10 mg/kg) plus paracetamol (dose 15 mg/kg) at the same time or (3) ibuprofen (dose 10 mg/kg) followed by paracetamol 3 hours later. Temperatures were measured over a 6-hour period using a temporal artery thermometer.
Outcomes	The primary outcome was the absence of fever at 6 hours.
Main results	Sixty febrile episodes in 46 children were assessed. The most common diagnoses were upper respiratory tract infection (n = 27), fever without source (n = 12) and otitis media (n = 8). No subjects in the 'ibuprofen followed by paracetamol' group were febrile at hours 4, 5 or 6; in the ibuprofen group, febrile states were 30% at 4 hours (absolute risk reduction (ARR) = 30%; number needed to treat (NNT) = 4), 40% at 5 hours (ARR = 40%; NNT = 3) and 50% at 6 hours (ARR = 50%; NNT = 2). There was one febrile state present in the 'ibuprofen plus paracetamol' group.
Conclusion	Combined or alternating doses of ibuprofen and paracetamol are more effective than ibuprofen alone in producing antipyresis.
Commentary	Despite a lack of evidence to support their fears, many parents believe that fever can be dangerous and so wish to treat it aggressively. The focus on fever reduction is important, but equally valid outcomes that need to be assessed include reduction in discomfort and pain that the ill child experiences. The data indicating effectiveness of combined treatments is likely to encourage parents to use this strategy for their children prior to sleep and attendance at school or crèche. Recognising the real risk of parents being unable to accurately measure medication and the attendant risk of side effects, clear guidance should be offered on antipyretic therapy. The focus should not be exclusively on fever reduction but on improving the temperament of the child.
Reference	Paul IM, Sturgis SA, Yang C, *et al.* Efficacy of standard doses of ibuprofen alone, alternating, and combined with acetaminophen for the treatment of febrile children. *Clin Ther.* 2010; **32**(14): 2433–40.

Evidence 2	
Theme E2	*Recognition and treatment of febrile infants (FIs)*
Question	Can the Philadelphia protocol identify FIs at low risk of serious bacterial infection (SBI)?
Design	Consecutive cohort study
Level of evidence	
Setting	Emergency department, children's hospital, the United States
Participants	Four hundred and twenty infants aged 29–60 days with rectal temperature ≥38°C seen in an emergency department were enrolled.
Intervention	The Philadelphia protocol was used to stratify care rendered to FIs. This study evaluated adherence to the protocols of care.
Outcomes	The primary outcome was adherence rate to the treatment protocol for FIs 29–60 days of age and to its effectiveness in accurately predicting those infants at low risk for SBI.
Main results	During the 36-month study period, 422 FIs were managed in the emergency department. One hundred and one (23.9%) were low-risk FIs and 94 were managed in accordance with the protocol, seven were not (infants were admitted and treated with intravenous antibiotics for non-bacterial diseases). Three hundred and twenty-one (76.1%) were high-risk FIs and 300 (93.5%) were admitted as per protocol. Of the 21 remaining, managed outside the protocol, 11 were admitted but did not receive antibiotic treatment and 10 were managed without antibiotics as outpatients. Twenty-eight (6.6%) infants in total breached the protocol. The diagnoses in order of frequency were viral syndrome, 54%; non-bacterial gastroenteritis, 16.4%; aseptic meningitis, 11.8%; serious bacterial illness, 10.2%; bronchiolitis, 4.7%; pneumonia, 1.9%; otitis media, 0.5%; varicella, 0.2%; and conjunctivitis, 0.2%. Of the 47 (10.2%) FIs with SBI the aetiologies were urinary tract infection, 17; bacteraemia, 9; meningitis, 5; salmonella gastroenteritis, 5; cellulitis, 5; *Chlamydophila pneumoniae*, 2; necrotising enterocolitis, 1; osteomyelitis, 1; and septic arthritis, 1. The rate of SBI in the high-risk FI group was 14.6%.
Conclusion	The adherence rate to protocol management was 93.3%. The sensitivity was 100% in identifying FIs at low risk of SBI. One in six infants in the high-risk group had a SBI.
Commentary	The components of the Philadelphia protocol include infants >28 days, acute infantile observation score ≤10 (range, 5–30), no recognisable bacterial infection, laboratory values WBC <15 000, band to neutrophil ratio <0.2, WBC <10/mm^3 and a few bacteria per high-power field on microscopic exam of spun urine, no infiltrate on chest X-ray and stool smear negative for blood and few or no white blood cells (for infants with diarrhoea). The acute infantile observational scale consists of a scoring system of 1–5 on each of six items: tone, colour, activity, cry, irritability and state variation. In this study the emergency room physicians were unaware that they were taking part and thus the study accurately reflects their practice. Recognising the different aetiologies of SBI is important, as symptoms or signs maybe subtle or limited; therefore, a high index of suspicion is required for those deemed at high risk.

(continued)

Evidence 2

Theme E2	*Recognition and treatment of febrile infants (FIs)*
Commentary (*cont.*)	The results may have limited generalisability if the laboratory tests are not available to practitioners. The 'band to neutrophil ratio' represents the ratio of immature neutrophils to mature neutrophils, which is utilised in the United States.
Reference	Baker MD, Bell LM, Avner JR. The efficacy of routine outpatient management without antibiotics of fever in selected infants. *Pediatrics*. 1999; **103**(3): 627–31.

Evidence 3

Theme E3	*Externally evaluating criteria to define infants at low risk of serious bacterial infection (SBI)*
Question	Are the Philadelphia protocol and the Rochester criteria valid in determining infants at low risk of SBI?
Design	Prospective cohort study
Level of evidence	
Setting	Emergency department, children's hospital, the United States
Participants	Term infants less than 56 days of age who were febrile (temperature 100.6°F) were eligible for enrolment.
Intervention	An emergency room physician, prior to laboratory tests and physical examination, recorded the Infantile Observation Score and the Overall Impression of Sepsis scale (a three-item scale rating likelihood of sepsis as strong, ambivalent or negative). After the physical examination each infant had a full blood count, with manual differential, blood culture, serum glucose, lumbar puncture, urine culture and urinalysis from a specimen obtained by urethral catheterisation. Additional tests were optional and these were chest X-ray, respiratory syncytial virus assay and stool culture. A blinded investigator assigned a risk category based on the clinical and laboratory tests. Infants from birth to 56 days were evaluated on the Rochester criteria and those 29–56 days on the Philadelphia protocol. Infants who received a negative score on the Overall Impression of Sepsis scale were recorded as well on the Rochester criteria. Infants with bacteraemia, urinary tract infections (UTIs), bacterial meningitis or bacterial positive enteritis were considered to have a SBI.
Outcomes	The primary outcome was the sensitivity of the Rochester criteria and Philadelphia protocol in assessing febrile infants at low risk of SBI.
Main results	A total of 302 were enrolled, but full data were available in 259 (85.7%). There were 78 infants aged 28 days or younger and 181 aged 29–56 days. Of the 181 assigned to the Philadelphia protocol, 34 (18.7%) were assigned to low risk of SBI but one infant had a SBI. Of the 73 (28.1%) rated at low risk of SBI by the Rochester criteria, two had a SBI. Sixty-five (25%) infants were identified as having a SBI, including 51 with UTI, 5 with UTI and bacteraemia, 8 with bacteraemia and 1 with bacteraemia and meningitis. The sensitivity of the Philadelphia protocol was 0.98 (0.92, 1.00) and the negative predictive value was 0.99 (0.99, 1.0). For the Rochester criteria the sensitivity was 0.92 (0.84, 0.097) and the negative predictive value was 0.98 (0.97, 1.00).

(*continued*)

Evidence 3	
Theme E3	*Externally evaluating criteria to define infants at low risk of serious bacterial infection (SBI)*
Conclusion	Both the Rochester criteria and the Philadelphia protocol functions were to identify febrile infants at low risk of SBI. The occurrence of SBI rates of 25% is higher than previously reported.
Commentary	This study replicates the original work done and enhances the generalisability of the results. The doctor is offered a framework to assess febrile infants but familiarity with the criteria utilised is required. In the Rochester criteria the infant must appear well, and have been previously well as indicated by delivery ≥37 weeks, no exposure to perinatal antibiotic therapy, have an absence of unexplained hyperbilirubinaemia, have no previous hospitalisation, no chronic disease, no current antibiotic treatment and not to have been hospitalised longer than the mother. On examination there must be no evidence of skin, soft tissue, bone, joint or ear infection. The laboratory criteria include white blood cells (WBCs) of 5000–15 000, absolute band count of ≤1500/mm^3, ≤10 WBCs per high-power field on microscopic exam of spun urine and ≤5 WBCs per high-power field on microscopic exam of stool smear (for infants with diarrhoea). The Infantile Observation Score further aids recognising illness.
Reference	Garra G, Cunningham SJ, Crain EF. Reappraisal of criteria used to predict serious bacterial illness in febrile infants less than 8 weeks of age. *Acad Emerg Med.* 2005; **12**(10): 921–5.

Evidence 4	
Theme E4	*Treatment of acute otitis media (AOM)*
Question	In AOM, with adequate control of pain and fever, is antibiotic use superior to placebo?
Design	Randomised controlled trial
Level of evidence	Jadad 5
Setting	Emergency department, children's hospital and community clinics, Canada
Participants	Children aged over 6 months and <6 years who were previously well with middle ear effusion, defined as two or more of the following: opacity, impaired mobility on the basis of pneumatic otoscopy, and redness or bulging (or both) of the tympanic membrane. In addition, children had to have symptoms referable to the upper respiratory tract (for less than 4 days) and either ear pain or fever. Exclusion criteria included children with allergy to penicillin or amoxicillin and sensitivity to ibuprofen or aspirin.
Intervention	Each child received either amoxicillin (60 mg/kg/day) or placebo in three divided doses for 10 days. Parents were given a 5-day supply of antipyretics and analgesic medications in the form of ibuprofen (5 mg/kg per dose if <10 kg, 10 mg/kg per dose if >10 kg) to be taken every 8 hours as required for pain and fever, and a 48-hour supply of codeine (1 mg/kg) to be given as required for pain or fever. Each parent was contacted at days 1, 2, 3, 10 and 14. If in the first 3 days the child was not improving, a physician assessment was undertaken.

(continued)

Evidence 4

Theme E4	*Treatment of acute otitis media (AOM)*
Outcomes	The primary outcome measure was the clinical resolution of symptoms, defined as the absence of receipt of an antimicrobial (other than the amoxicillin in the treatment group) at 14 days. Antibiotic treatment was initiated on the basis of persistence or worsening of symptoms of fever, irritability with otoscopic signs of non-resolving otitis media, or complications, e.g. mastoiditis.
Main results	Of the 963 eligible patients, 432 were not randomised, as in 109 the doctor wanted to treat the infection or the doctor or parent did not want to treat, 237 parents refused consent and 50 for logistical reasons. Of the 531 randomised, 19 were withdrawn – 13 because of alternate diagnoses and 6 for incorrect randomisation. Two hundred and fifty-eight received amoxicillin and 254 received placebo. The mean age in the amoxicillin group was 3 years and in the placebo group, 2.9 years. Clinical resolution occurred in 92.8% of the amoxicillin group and in 84.2% of the placebo group (absolute risk reduction (ARR) = 8.4%; number needed to treat (NNT) = 12). In the intention-to-treat analysis, 89.9% of the amoxicillin group and 79.5% of the placebo group responded (ARR = 10.4%; NNT = 10). Abnormal tympanograms occurred in 65.5% of the amoxicillin group and in 57.9% of the placebo group. The mean otitis score was 5.2 for amoxicillin and 5.3 for placebo (*see* Commentary section). Pain rates were 27.5%, 22% and 17%, for days 1, 2 and 3 of amoxicillin treatment and 41.7%, 33.2% and 21.5 for days 1, 2 and 3 of placebo.
Conclusion	This study indicated that children in the placebo group were not significantly worse off than the amoxicillin group.
Commentary	This study utilised a clinical otitis score that is based on temperature (scoring 0 for <38°C, 1 for 38°C–38.5°C, 2 for 38.6°C–39.0°C, 3 for >39°C) and irritability, ear tugging and redness and bulging of the tympanic membrane (scoring for other signs and symptoms: 0 if absent, 1 if mild, 2 if moderate, 3 if severe). The episode is mild if the score is less than 3, moderate if the score is 3–7 and severe if the score is 8–15. Obtaining an aetiological diagnosis by tympanocentesis is not possible. AOM was probably overdiagnosed in this study, given the rates of abnormal tympanograms in both groups studied, but this has been previously reported. The non-resolution of symptoms at 14 days most likely represents a true clinical or bacteriological failure. This study offers an alternate strategy of reassessment rather than immediate antibiotic therapy in children with AOM, provided pain and fever are addressed appropriately. At day 2 pain was absent in 78% of the amoxicillin group compared with 66.8% of the placebo group (ARR = 11.2%; NNT = 12). The presence of pain may well influence the choice to commence treatment if a 'watch and wait' option is pursued. There is also added value if handheld tympanometers are used to aid diagnosis, as the presence of middle ear fluid predicts a greater response to antimicrobial treatment (odds ratio, 6.7).
Reference	Le Saux N, Gaboury I, Baird M, *et al.* A randomized, double-blind, placebo-controlled noninferiority trial of amoxicillin for clinically diagnosed acute otitis media in children 6 months to 5 years of age. *CMAJ.* 2005; **172**(3): 335–41.

Evidence 5	
Theme E5	*Persistent otitis media treatment options*
Question	In children with persistent otitis media with effusion, which is better: ventilation tubes (VTs) or watchful waiting (WW)?
Design	Randomised controlled trial
Level of evidence	Jadad 3
Setting	Ear, nose and throat clinics, the Netherlands
Participants	Three hundred and eighty-six infants diagnosed with persistent (4–6 months) bilateral otitis media by typanometry and otoscopy were eligible, with 187 being randomised, 93 to the VT group and 94 to the WW group. Both groups were followed for 1 year with 3-monthly typanometry and otoscopy measurements and audiometry every 6 months.
Intervention	There were two interventions: VTs at randomisation or WW.
Outcomes	The primary outcome was difference in hearing at 6 and 12 months between the two groups.
Main results	The mean age of the VT group was 19.5 months, compared with 19.4 in the WW group. In the VT group, 3 patients dropped out and eight required a second surgery for reinsertion of the VT. In the WW group, eight were lost to follow-up but ten received VTs. Bilateral otitis media with effusion was present in 27% and 27% of the VT group at 6 and 12 months, respectively, compared with 57% and 53%, respectively, of the WW group (absolute risk reduction (ARR) = 30%, number needed to treat (NNT) = 4; ARR = 26%, NNT = 4). The improvement in hearing at 6 months for the VT group was 10.2 dB, compared with 4.6 dB in the WW group. At 12 months the improvement in the VT group was 13.1 dB, compared with 8.5 dB in the WW group.
Conclusion	VTs had a beneficial effect on hearing in the short run at 6 months but this lessened at 12 months.
Commentary	The development of language in children is a marker of academic performance and its impairment will concern parents. In the patient with recurrent otitis media, hearing loss may contribute to a degree of language delay. The placement of a VT may offer a short-term solution but the tube must be functioning. In this study the percentage of VTs that remained functioning and in place were 92%, 76%, 56%, and 30% at 3, 6, 9 and 12 months, respectively.
Reference	Rovers MM, Straatman H, Ingels K, *et al.* The effect of short-term ventilation tubes versus watchful waiting on hearing in young children with persistent otitis media with effusion: a randomized trial. *Ear Hear.* 2001; **22**(3): 191–9.

Evidence 6	
Theme E6	*The role of adenoidectomy in conjunction with tympanostomy tubes in otitis media (OM)*
Question	How effective is adenoidectomy with tympanostomy tube insertion as compared with tympanostomy tube insertion alone in children with recurrent OM?
Design	Randomised controlled trial
Level of evidence	Jadad 3
Setting	Tertiary care centre, Finland
Participants	Children 1–4 years of age with recurrent acute otitis media (defined as three or more episodes of acute otitis media (AOM) during the preceding 6 months or five or more episodes of AOM during the preceding 12 months) or a suspicion of chronic otitis media with effusion, as judged by examination with a pneumatic otoscope, and no previous adenoidal surgery or tympanostomy tube placement, were eligible.
Intervention	Children were assigned to receive tympanostomy tube insertion alone or to have it combined with adenoidectomy.
Outcomes	The primary outcome was the number of episodes of OM in the 12-month follow-up period.
Main results	Of the 296 eligible patients, 79 parents refused consent and 217 were randomised. Of these patients, 109 were randomised to the 'adenoidectomy and tympanostomy' group, of whom 104 received the intervention and 102 completed the study; of the 108 in the 'tympanostomy alone' group, 103 received the intervention and 96 completed the study. The mean age in both groups was 1.9 years. The mean number of OM episodes in the 'adenoidectomy plus tympanostomy' group was 1.7 and 1.4 in the 'tympanostomy alone' group. The odds ratio of the difference in the mean number of episodes of OM was 1.11.
Conclusion	Adenoidectomy did not significantly reduce the incidence of OM in AOM-prone children aged 1–4 years.
Commentary	The lack of value of adenoidectomy in conjunction with tympanostomy tube placement is evident in this paper. Parents wish to be informed of the health gain that accrues from surgery. This intervention offers a small gain that most will be reluctant to undertake. The natural history of OM needs to be explained to parents as well.
Reference	Hammarén-Malmi S, Saxen S, Tarkkanen, *et al.* Adenoidectomy does not significantly reduce the incidence of otitis media in conjunction with the insertion of tympanostomy tubes in children who are younger than 4 years: a randomized trial. *Pediatrics.* 2005; **116**(1): 185–9.

Evidence 7	
Theme E7	**Antibiotic treatment of community-acquired pneumonia**
Question	Which are more effective in the treatment of community-acquired pneumonia: intravenous or oral antibiotics?
Design	Randomised controlled trial (non-inferiority)
Level of evidence	Jadad 3
Setting	Eight paediatric centres, general hospitals and tertiary hospitals, England
Participants	All children, previously well, admitted to hospital with pneumonia were eligible. The following criteria were used to define pneumonia: respiratory symptoms and signs, temperature ≥37.5°C or a history of fever at home, and a radiological diagnosis of pneumonia (defined as a confluent area of consolidation agreed subsequently by two independent radiologists). Children with oxygen saturations ≤85% in air, shock requiring >20 mL/kg fluid resuscitation, immunodeficiency, or pleural effusion at presentation requiring drainage were excluded.
Intervention	Participants were assigned to oral amoxicillin: 6 months to 12 years, 8 mg/kg three times per day; 12–16 years, 500 mg three times per day or intravenous (IV) benzylpenicillin, 25 mg/kg four times per day. If clinical improvement was not observed at 48 hours either oral erythromycin or IV clarithromycin was commenced.
Outcomes	The primary outcome measure was the time from randomisation until the temperature was <38°C for 24 hours continuously and oxygen treatment had ceased.
Main results	One hundred patients were randomised to the oral treatment group and 103 to the IV treatment group. The mean age of the oral treatment group was 2.4 years and the symptoms and signs included cough (89%), recession (42%), grunting (14%) and difficulty breathing (34%). In the IV group the mean age was 2.5 years and the symptoms and signs were cough (92%), recession (49.5%), grunting (24%) and difficulty breathing (32%). The median time for temperature to settle in both groups was 1.3 days. Three children in the oral treatment group were switched to IV antibiotics and seven children in the IV group were switched to other antibiotics (three because of empyema and four because of ongoing fever and worsening consolidation on chest X-ray). Six children in the oral treatment group and eight in the IV group received macrolide therapy.
Conclusion	Oral amoxicillin is effective for most children admitted to hospital with pneumonia.
Commentary	This study addressed the treatment of community-acquired pneumonia in an era of *Haemophilus influenzae* immunisation and a low incidence of tuberculosis. By its nature it would not be ethical to undertake a double-blind study requiring IV placement to administer placebo IV medications. The use of a radiological evidence of consolidation minimised the number of pneumonia cases with a viral aetiology. This study gives confidence to paediatricians that oral antibiotics are as effective as IV antibiotics in the treat of community-acquired pneumonia. The use of an initial temperature of ≥37.5°C to define temperature reflects the significant use of antipyretic medication by parents when their children are febrile.
Reference	Atkinson M, Lakhanpaul M, Smyth A, *et al.* Comparison of oral amoxicillin and intravenous benzyl penicillin for community acquired pneumonia in children (PIVOT trial): a multicentre pragmatic randomised controlled equivalence trial. *Thorax.* 2007; **62**(12): 1102–6.

Evidence 8	
Theme E8	***Physiotherapy in children with pneumonia***
Question	How effective is chest physiotherapy in children with community-acquired pneumonia?
Design	Randomised controlled trial
Level of evidence	Jadad 3
Setting	Tertiary care centre, Brazil
Participants	Children aged 1–12 years hospitalised with a clinically and radiologically confirmed diagnosis were eligible for enrolment. Clinical diagnosis criteria for pneumonia were cough, tachypnoea (respiratory rate ≥40 breaths/min in children aged 12–59 months and ≥30 breaths/min for children over >5 years of age) and fever. Radiological diagnosis of pneumonia required lobar, segmental or bronchopneumonia or pleural effusion on the chest X-ray within 48 hours.
Intervention	The physiotherapy intervention for children <5 years of age included being sat up and receiving manual thoracic vibration, thoracic compression, positive expiratory pressure and artificially stimulated cough with suction. In addition, children over 5 years of age undertook breathing exercises and a forced expiratory technique consisting of one or two 'huffing' breaths followed by relaxed, controlled diaphragmatic breathing. These were carried out three times a day. The control group were recommended to lie on their lateral side, to cough to clear secretions and to breathe deeply for 5 minutes a day.
Outcomes	The primary outcome was reduction in respiratory rate and score of severity. The severity score was based on the presence or absence (0 or 1) of tachypnoea (respiratory rate ≥40 breaths/min for children aged 12–59 months and ≥30 breaths/min for children aged 5–12 years), suprasternal, intercostal and subcostal recession, desaturation (transcutaneous oxygen ≥95%), fever (temperature ≥37.5°C) and pleural effusion on chest X-ray.
Main results	There were 362 potentially eligible patients. Of these, 262 did not fulfil the criteria and were excluded (97 with pneumonia, 48 with cerebral palsy, 34 with atelectasis on chest X-ray, 16 with intensive care unit hospitalisation, 10 with a chest drain in place, 16 with underlying pulmonary disease, 10 with heart disease, 9 with Down's syndrome and 22 for other reasons), 19 were lost before randomisation and two refused to participate. Seventy-two patients were randomised, 35 to the intervention group and 37 to the control group. Baseline characteristics were similar, with 71.4% in the intervention group and 75.7% in the control group aged 12–59 months. For the intervention group the baseline severity score and respiratory rate at baseline were 2.1 ± 1.6 and 39.1 ± 9.9, respectively, and at discharge were 0.57 ± 0.8 and 31.6 ± 6.9, respectively. For the control group, severity score and respiratory rate at baseline were 1.78 ± 1.1 and 38.4 ± 9.8, respectively, and at discharge were 0.41 ± 0.6 and 32.5 ± 8.3, respectively. There was no difference between the groups. Children in the control group were discharged on day 6 as opposed to day 8 for the treatment group.
Conclusion	Physiotherapy in children with community-acquired pneumonia did not show a clinical benefit when compared with controls.

(continued)

Evidence 8	
Theme E8	*Physiotherapy in children with pneumonia*
Commentary	The use of physiotherapy in the acute stages of pneumonia offered no advantage in terms of primary outcomes and lengths of stay. Those on the treatment did receive intensive treatment three times a day, with a compliance rate of 98%, a process that would be difficult to replicate in a general paediatric unit. Physiotherapy is utilised to improve the clearance of airway secretions from the lung and in the initial pneumonic state, with the absence of secretions in the airway, there is little biological plausibility to recommend its use. The determinants of the length of hospitalisations were not explained, and the lengths of stay at 6–8 days would appear excessive in European terms.
Reference	Lukrafka JL, Fuchs SC, Fischer GB, *et al.* Chest physiotherapy in paediatric patients hospitalised with community-acquired pneumonia: a randomised clinical trial. *Arch Dis Child.* 2012; **97**(11): 967–71.

Evidence 9	
Theme E9	*Intravenous versus oral antibiotic treatment for pyelonephritis*
Question	In the treatment of pyelonephritis, which is more effective: intravenous or oral antibiotic treatment?
Design	Randomised controlled trial (non-inferiority study)
Level of evidence	Jadad 3
Setting	Department of paediatrics in five academic medical centres, Switzerland
Participants	Children aged 6 months to 16 years with a community-acquired pyelonephritis, who had a positive urine culture that was obtained by urinary catheterisation, and who had acute lesions on DMSA scans were eligible to participate.
Intervention	Patients were randomised to receive oral ceftibuten (9 mg/kg/day) for 14 days or intravenous ceftriaxone (50 mg/kg once daily) for 3 days followed by ceftibuten for 11 days.
Outcomes	The primary outcome was rate of renal scaring determined by DMSA scan at 6 months' follow-up. In this non-inferiority study a maximal difference of 20% between the percentages of renal scarring of the two groups was considered acceptable.
Main results	Initially 365 patients were randomised (175 to oral treatment (PO), and 190 to intravenous and oral treatment (IV+PO)), 19 had no acute-phase scintigraphy, 127 had normal acute-phase scintigraphy, leaving 219 (63%) with lesion on acute-phase DMSA scans. However, 67 had no follow-up DMSA scans. Ultimately 152 had a second DMSA scan, 80 in the PO group and 72 in the IV+PO group. Renal scarring occurred in 20 (26.3%) of the PO group and 33 (45.8%) of the IV+PO group (absolute risk reduction = 19.5%; number needed to treat = 5, favouring PO treatment). Forty-four (55%) of the PO group and 47 (65.2%) of the IV+PO group were treated as outpatients.
Conclusion	Oral antibiotic treatment with ceftibuten is as effective as IV ceftriaxone plus PO ceftibuten in the treatment of pyelonephritis.

(continued)

Evidence 9

Theme E9	*Intravenous versus oral antibiotic treatment for pyelonephritis*
Commentary	In this study the diagnosis of pyelonephritis was considered probable in children with fever, an abnormal urinary dipstick test (leukocyte esterase ≥1, or nitrite positive) or microscopic urinalysis (pyuria with ≥10 white blood cells/µL) and serum C-reactive protein concentration >10 mg/L. Additional signs were not mandatory (e.g. abdominal or flank tenderness or flank pain in children old enough to report pain accurately, irritability, vomiting, diarrhoea, or feeding problems in infants). Urine cultures were obtained by catheterisation. In children with pyelonephritis, bacteraemia is rare beyond 6 months of age, but the prevalence in children under 2 months is up to 22%, and 9.3% in those children under 6 months.
Reference	Neuhaus TJ, Berger C, Buechner K, *et al.* Randomised trial of oral versus sequential intravenous/oral cephalosporins in children with pyelonephritis. *Eur J Pediatr.* 2008; **167**(9): 1037–47.

Evidence 10

Theme E10	*Prevention of urinary tract infections (UTIs) in children*
Question	Is cranberry juice effective in the prevention of UTIs in children?
Design	Randomised controlled trial
Level of evidence	Jadad 5
Setting	Paediatric departments, academic medical centres, Finland
Participants	Children aged 1–16 years with a verified UTI were eligible for inclusion.
Intervention	Participants were randomised to 5 mL/kg/day of cranberry juice to a maximum of 300 mL or an identical placebo for 6 months. Children who developed UTIs in the follow-up year were treated with antibiotics and if they developed three UTIs they were placed on prophylactic antibiotics.
Outcomes	The primary outcome was the occurrences of the first UTI episode during a 12-month follow-up period.
Main results	Two hundred and sixty-three children aged 1–16 years were eligible for randomisation. One hundred and twenty-nine were randomised to the cranberry juice, with data available in 126, and 134 received placebo therapy, with data available in 129. In the cranberry juice group 16% developed UTIs, compared with 22% in the placebo group (absolute risk reduction = 6%, number needed to treat = 17). Two children (1.4%) in the cranberry juice group were placed on prophylactic antibiotics, as opposed to seven (5.4%) in the placebo group. Thirty-seven per cent of the treatment group took <50% of the treatment doses, as opposed to 17% of the placebo group.
Conclusion	The use of cranberry juice to reduce the occurrence has a modest effect but issues of adherence in children lessen its impact.
Commentary	In this study the use of cranberry juice reduced the incidence of UTI and there were reduced numbers who had recurrent episodes of UTI as well. The preventive effect was more pronounced in the second 6-month period.

(continued)

Evidence 10	
Theme E10	*Prevention of urinary tract infections (UTIs) in children*
Commentary (*cont.*)	While it is known that cranberry juice can inhibit uropathogenic bacteria growth and adherence, the authors of the study suggest that cranberry juice may exert its effect through modification of gut bacteria. Adherence to the cranberry juice was an issue and may detract from its therapeutic usefulness, which must be raised with parents if recommending it as a treatment option, recognising that children with one proven UTI have a 30% risk of recurrence.
Reference	Salo j, Uhari M, Helminen M, *et al.* Cranberry juice for the prevention of recurrences of urinary tract infections in children: a randomized placebo-controlled trial. *Clin Infect Dis.* 2012; **54**(3): 340–6.

Evidence 11	
Theme E11	*Prevention of recurrent urinary tract infections (UTIs)*
Question	In children with vesicoureteric reflux and normal urinary tracts, do long-term, low-dose antibiotics prevent UTIs?
Design	Randomised controlled trial
Level of evidence	Jadad 5
Setting	Four children's hospitals, Australia
Participants	Children from birth to 18 years of age with one or more microbiologically proven UTI were eligible for inclusion.
Intervention	Children were randomised to receive trimethoprim (2 mg/kg) with sulfamethoxazole (10 mg/kg) or an identical placebo for 12 months after a 2-week run-in period.
Outcomes	The primary outcome was the development of a symptomatic UTI with a positive urine culture, defined as a pathogenic organism from a suprapubic bladder tap, or a colony-forming unit of 10^7 or more of a single organism per litre from a catheter sample, or of 10^8 or more of a single organism from a mid-stream voided urine sample.
Main results	A total of 576 underwent randomisation; the median age of entry was 14 months, and 64% of the patients were female. Of the 288 in the treatment group, 116 had ceased taking medications, 36 had UTIs, 4 experienced adverse drug reactions, 72 had other reasons, and 4 were lost to follow-up. In the placebo group of 288, 136 had ceased taking medications, 55 had UTIs, 10 experienced adverse drug reactions, 63 withdrew for other reasons and 8 were lost to follow-up. In the treatment group, 41% had no reflux, 20% had grade I–II reflux, 23% had grade III–V reflux and it was unknown in 16%. In the placebo group, 40% had no reflux, 20 had grade I–II reflux, 22% had grade III–V reflux and it was unknown in 18%. The rate of UTI in the placebo group was 19% and in the treatment group it was 12.5% (absolute risk reduction = 6.5%; number needed to treat (NNT) = 15).
Conclusion	Long-term low-dose trimethoprim-sulfamethoxazole was associated with a decreased number of UTIs in predisposed children.

(*continued*)

Evidence 11	
Theme E11	**Prevention of recurrent urinary tract infections (UTIs)**
Commentary	The use of low-dose antibiotics is offered to parents as a treatment strategy to reduce the occurrence of UTIs in children. However, this study suggests that adherence to the preventive treatment is a major challenge for parents. Parents stopped the treatment in 24% of cases in the first 6 months of treatment for reasons other than the occurrence of a UTI. Prior to commencing prophylactic treatment, parents must be counselled on the importance of treatment adherence. The gain that accrues from prophylactic treatment is modest (NNT = 15).
Reference	Craig JC, Simpson JM, Williams GJ, *et al.*; PRIVENT investigators. Antibiotic prophylaxis and recurrent urinary tract infection in children. *N Eng J Med.* 2009; **361**(18): 1748–59.

Reference

1. McCarthy PL, Lembo RM, Fink HD, *et al.* Observation, history, and physical examination in diagnosis of serious illnesses in febrile children less than 24 months. *J Pediatr.* 1987; **110**: 26–30.

THE CHILD WITH A FEVER: MULTIPLE-CHOICE QUESTIONS

Q1 Which of the following should be assessed in children presenting with fever?
   a) Heart rate
   b) Respiratory rate
   c) Rectal temperature
   d) Evaluate for a rash
   e) Blood cultures

Q2 Which of the following is/are associated with strep throat in children?
   a) Epigastric pain
   b) URTI
   c) Tender cervical lymphadenopathy
   d) Palatal petechiae
   e) A red rash with the texture of sandpaper

Q3 Risk factors for otitis media include which of the following?
   a) Recurrent URTI
   b) Trisomy 21
   c) Smoking at home
   d) Attendance at crèche
   e) Craniofacial abnormalities

Q4 Which of the following statements with regard to pneumonia is/are correct?
  a) Chest X-rays should be undertaken routinely to confirm the diagnosis.
  b) Intravenous antibiotics shorten the length of hospitalisation.
  c) Physiotherapy is beneficial.
  d) Consolidation is suggested by diminished chest expansion.
  e) Vomiting is a recognised presentation.

Q5 Which of the following statements with regard to pneumonia is/are correct?
  a) Chest pain reflects pleural involvement.
  b) Anorexia and headache are systemic manifestations of pneumonia.
  c) Wheeze is found in mycoplasma pneumonias.
  d) Inability to feed is an indicator of severe pneumonia in infants.
  e) No aetiology is discerned in 50% of children with pneumonia.

Q6 Which of the following statements is/are true of UTIs?
  a) Eight per cent of girls will have a symptomatic UTI.
  b) One per cent of boys will have a symptomatic UTI.
  c) Febrile seizure is a recognised presentation of UTIs.
  d) VUR is present in 3% of children with UTIs.
  e) Intravenous antibiotics are necessary in the treatment of pyelonephritis.

Q7 Which of the following is/are true of meningococcal disease?
  a) Meningococcal meningitis has a worse outcome than meningococcal septicaemia.
  b) The meningococcal rash is present within 4 hours of the illness commencing.
  c) Limb pain is a feature of meningococcal disease.
  d) Irritability is a common finding.
  e) Purpura fulminans occurs in 7.5% of children.

Q8 Illnesses that present with prolonged fever include which of the following?
  a) Tuberculosis
  b) Kawasaki's disease
  c) Bacterial endocarditis
  d) Epstein–Barr infections
  e) Systemic lupus erythematosus
  f) Systemic rheumatoid arthritis

Q9 Contraindications to lumbar puncture include which of the following?
  a) Focal seizure
  b) Purpuric rash in the distribution of the superior vena cava
  c) Glasgow Coma Scale score of 3
  d) Rigors
  e) Coagulopathy

Q10 Which of the following tests should be undertaken in a clinically unwell infant less than 2 months old?
a) Full blood count
b) C-reactive protein
c) Procalcitonin level
d) Lumbar puncture
e) Blood culture

Answers

A1	a, b, d	**A2**	a, c, d, e
A3	a, b, c, d, e	**A4**	d, e
A5	a, b, c, d, e	**A6**	a, c
A7	c, d	**A8**	a, b, c, d, e
A9	a, c, e	**A10**	a, b, d, e

SLIDES

1. Acute follicular tonsillitis
2. Atypical mycobacterium infection of cervical gland
3. Erythema multiforme
4. Erythema multiforme (target lesion)
5. Erythema nodosum
6. Orbital cellulitis
7. Periorbital cellulitis
8. Geographic tongue

Chapter Five

THE CHILD WITH RECURRENT INFECTIONS

COMMON SCENARIO

'My 5-year-old child has had four episodes of pneumonia in 10 months and I want further tests done to ensure he does not have a problem with his immune system.'

LEARNING OBJECTIVES

- Understand the frequency of infections in normal children
- Know the potential clinical indicators of immune deficiency states
- Understand the clinical presentations of the primary immunodeficiency disorders (PID)
- Understand the mechanisms of the clinical presentations
- Develop a rationale approach to investigation
- Understand treatment strategies

BACKGROUND

All children experience infections and for the majority the illnesses are short and the child returns to a normal state of health. The parents, however, may experience significant worry and distress when their child is ill and will visit their family doctor to allay their anxiety and seek clarification that their child is well and has no underlying medical condition. In general, children experience four to six infections each year for the first 3 years of life. Infection will occur more frequently in the winter months, if the child is in a day care environment and if the parents smoke (*see* Evidence 1).

Children who experience multiple infections present a challenge to the consulting doctor. Parents will be anxious and require assurance and will wish for investigations to be done to 'check their child's immune system'. After investigation it is reassuring to know that for 50% of cases no abnormality will be discerned and the child will be classified as normal but unlucky to acquire the infection; 30% will have atopy; 10%

will a chronic condition such as cystic fibrosis, gastro-oesophageal reflux, complex congenital heart disease or cerebral palsy with recurrent aspiration; and 10% will have an identifiable immune deficiency state either secondary, e.g. HIV, immunosuppression from malignancy or have a PID. There are in excess of 100 identified PIDs. The majority are rare. Children with secondary immune deficiency states are relatively easily recognised given their clinical presentations; however, this is not the case with the PIDs. This chapter will deal with children who have these conditions.

To aid recognition of PID the Jeffrey Modell Foundation (JMF) published 10 criteria as an aide-memoire to clinicians. The features include:

- four or more new ear infections in 1 year
- two or more sinus infections in 1 year
- two or more months on antibiotic treatment with little clinical effect
- two or more pneumonias in 1 year
- failure to thrive or gain weight normally
- recurrent deep skin or organ abscesses
- persistent thrush in the mouth or fungal infections on the skin
- the need for intravenous antibiotics to clear infections
- two or more deep-seated infections or septicaemia
- and a family history of primary immunodeficiency.

These features represent expert opinion and are not based on clinical trials (*see* Evidence 2). The JMF criteria are helpful, as physicians have very limited exposure to PIDs and delayed diagnosis is characterised by poorer outcome. With advances in knowledge, more and more individual immune deficiency states are recognised.

Various classifications of PIDS exist but it is useful to consider them in the following manner.

a) Predominant antibody deficiencies (65% of all PIDs):
   - X-linked agammaglobulinaemia (frequency 1:70 000)
   - autosomal recessive agammaglobulinaemia (rare)
   - common variable immunodeficiency (1:25 000)
   - selective IgA deficiency (1:500 but many asymptomatic)
   - IgG subclass deficiency (uncertain incidence, as most are asymptomatic)
b) Combined T- and B-cell deficiency (15% of all PIDs):
   - severe combined immunodeficiency (SCID) frequency (1:65 000)
   - Omenn's syndrome (rare)
c) Phagocytic defects (10% of all PIDs):
   - chronic granulomatous disease (1:200 000)
   - severe congenital neutropenia (1:300 000)
   - cyclical neutropenia (1:100 000)
d) Complement deficiency

e) Other well-defined cellular immunodeficiency:
  ○ Wiskott–Aldrich's syndrome (1:100 000)
  ○ DiGeorge's syndrome (chromosomal deletion 22q11) (1:4000)
  ○ ataxia telangiectasia (1:250 000)
  ○ hyper-IgE syndrome (1:100 000)

The frequency of the various conditions are estimates, with the exception of SCID, as screening programmes are not available and some children may die before their condition is recognised.

CLINICAL FEATURES OF SELECTED PRIMARY IMMUNODEFICIENCY STATES
Predominantly antibody deficiencies
X-linked agammaglobulinaemia
In this condition there is a profound defect in B-lymphocyte production and consequently severe hypogammaglobulinaemia occurs. Due to the presence of maternal antibodies clinical presentation is delayed until after 6 months and the child develops sinopulmonary infections and less commonly sepsis or meningitis. Mycoplasma infections are problematic but viral illnesses are handled normally with the exception of enteroviruses and hepatitis. Clinical examination reveals small or absence tonsillar tissue and non palpable lymph glands.

Common variable immunodeficiency
In this condition the B-cells are phenotypically normal but hypogammaglobulinaemia is present. The exact aetiology is as yet unknown. These children and adolescents present with sinopulmonary infections and may develop bronchiectasis. On clinical examination tonsils are present and may be enlarged and lymph nodes are enlarged. Twenty-five per cent of patients have splenomegaly.

IgA deficiency
This condition is extremely common but at least 80% of affected children are asymptomatic. When symptoms occur they include diarrhoea, which may be associated with *Giardia lamblia* infection.

Combined T- and B-cell deficiency (severe combined immunodeficiency)
In this condition there is a defect in T-lymphocyte development and function; however the T-cell may be unable to provide immunological support to the B-cell lines and thus there is impaired antibody production. Typical features include illness in the early months of life, with interstitial pneumonia, chronic diarrhoea, failure to thrive and chronic candidiasis. Life-threatening infection with common viruses such as respiratory syncytial virus, adenovirus, cytomegalovirus and opportunistic infections such as *Pneumocystis jirovecii* may occur. If the infant receives the bacillus

Calmette–Guérin immunisation, uncontrolled replication may occur and the infant will present clinically as a consequence. The presence of a low lymphocyte count (<2000 cells/μL) should serve as a clinical prompt for SCID to be considered as a clinical diagnosis. This condition can be diagnosed by screening and is treatable. In the absence of a screening programme a high index of suspicion is required, as infants can die of overwhelming sepsis.

Phagocytic defects

Chronic granulomatous disease

Children with this condition have neutrophils which are unable to generate superoxide ions and hydrogen peroxide, thus they are unable to kill intracellular microorganisms. The diagnostic test is the measurement of phagocyte oxidase. This condition should be considered in any child with recurrent deep-seated abscesses caused by *Staphylococcus aureus*, *Serratia marcescens*, *Burkholderia cepacia* and *Nocardia*.

Neutropenia

The occurrence of neutropenia as a primary event is rare compared with secondary causes. In PIDs the neutrophil function is impaired and patients may present with infections of the skin, mucous membranes and gums. The presence of fever and neutropenia is an emergency and treatment with antibiotics, after the appropriate cultures have been taken, is warranted.

Other cellular immunodeficiencies

Wiskott–Aldrich's syndrome

This syndrome is characterised by recurrent respiratory tract infections, eczema and thrombocytopenia. This is an X-linked condition and petechiae from the thrombocytopenia may be the first sign. The platelets may be small in size.

DiGeorge's syndrome

The classic features are recurrent infections related to thymic hypoplasia (T-cell deficiency), congenital heart disease and parathyroid hypoplasia, which may present as tetany or hypocalcaemic seizures in the newborn period.

Ataxia telangiectasia

These children present with progressive ataxia from infancy and develop both bulbar and cutaneous telangiectasia from 5 years onward. Many children have associated respiratory chest infections. In 95% of children the alpha-fetoprotein level is elevated.

Hyper-IgE

In this condition children have eczema, candidiasis, recurrent staphylococcal infections in the skin and lungs where pneumatocoeles develop. Non-immunological features include retained primary teeth, lax ligaments, bone fractures and craniosynostosis.

On the full blood count the eosinophils count is elevated and the serum IgE is markedly elevated.

INTERPRETING HALLMARK FEATURES OF PRIMARY IMMUNODEFICIENCY STATES

Recurrent sinopulmonary infections

Suspected immunodeficiencies that can present with sinopulmonary infections include antibody deficiencies, common variable immunodeficiency (CVID), neutropenia, Wiskott–Aldrich's syndrome and HIV. The types of organisms that cause these infections include non-typable *Haemophilus influenzae*, pneumococcus and less frequently *S. aureus*, meningococcus, *Mycoplasma pneumoniae*, enterovirus and *G. lamblia*. Infection with giardia can cause severe diarrhoea and lead to associated failure to thrive. Some adolescents with CVID may develop bronchiectasis. In children with agammaglobulinaemia, enteroviral meningoencephalitis may occur.

Failure to thrive

The development from early in infancy of failure to thrive suggests T-lymphocyte deficiency (HIV must also be excluded). The infecting organisms are mainly viruses (cytomegalovirus, Epstein–Barr virus, varicella zoster, and herpes simplex), fungi (superficial candidiasis, *P. jirovecii*), protozoal infections (toxoplasma, cryptosporidium). These infants can have severe diarrhoea, and the infections are either unexpected or unusually severe.

Recurrent pyogenic infections

The recurrence of pyogenic infections suggests a phagocyte deficiency, most commonly neutropenia and infrequently defects in phagocyte function. The most common organism is *S. aureus* and occasionally klebsiella, *Escherichia coli*. These children present with skin infections and may have abscesses in the lymph nodes or liver. Poor wound healing also occurs.

Unusual infections or unusual severe course of infection

These types of infections suggest T-lymphocyte deficiency (HIV must be excluded), WAS and hyper-IgE syndrome. The infecting organisms include mycobacterium, salmonella, viruses (cytomegalovirus, Epstein–Barr virus, varicella zoster, herpes simplex) and fungal infections (superficial candidiasis, aspergillus, *P. jiroveci*).

Recurrent infections with the same organism

The recurrence of intracellular bacteria infection (salmonella, mycobacterium) suggests T-lymphocyte deficiency, candidiasis suggests T-lymphocyte deficiency, *Neisseria meningitidis* infection suggests complement deficiency and pneumococcus suggests antibody deficiency.

Autoimmune or chronic inflammatory diseases

These presentations suggest antibody deficiency states (CVID, IgA deficiency) and complement deficiency T-cell-mediated deficiencies (WAS).

Clinical features of eponymous syndromes

The features of Wiskott–Aldrich's syndrome, DiGeorge's syndrome, ataxia telangiectasia and hyper-IgE syndrome have been described earlier.

Angioedema

The development of recurrent angioedema lasting more than 24 hours and which can mimic an acute abdomen can be related to a deficiency of C1 esterase.

HISTORY

KEY POINTS				
Infections increased frequency	Frequency, more than six a year	**Past medical history**	Occurrence of otitis media (more than four episodes a year in a child >4 years)	**🔍 Red flags** Recurrent sinopulmonary infections
			Pneumonia (more than two episodes a year)	Failure to thrive with diarrhoea
			Sinus infections (more than three episodes a year)	Recurrent pyogenic infections with same pathogen
			Use of preventive antibiotics	
			Hospital admissions	
Infection severity	Pneumonia with empyema, osteomyelitis, septicaemia	**Family history**	Family member with immunodeficiency, Consanguinity, Neonatal death unexplained Smoking	
Site of infection	Multiple sites should raise concern, especially if recurrent	**Social**	Attendance at crèche	
Age of the child	PIDs more common at specific ages	**Neonatal history**	Delayed separation of the umbilical cord	

(continued)

KEY POINTS				
Types of infecting organisms	Opportunistic infection *P. jirovecii*, deep fungal infection, mucocutaneous Candidiasis Bacillus Calmette–Guérin disease post vaccination Toxoplasma, cryptosporidium Virus that produces more severe disease than expected	**Systemic review**	Angioedema Occurrence of prolonged diarrhoea	
Antibiotic use	Clinical response to antibiotics, dose and timeliness of response, recurrence post cessation of antibiotics	**Immunisation**	Response to immunisation, complications	

EXAMINATION

- Height and weight centiles
- Dysmorphic features
- Skin: eczema, petechiae
- Molluscum contagiosum, candidiasis, telangiectasia
- Skin abscesses
- Albinism
- Cardiovascular: cardiac murmur (patent truncus arteriosus)
- Abdomen: hepatosplenomegaly
- Splenomegaly
- Central nervous system: ataxia, ocular telangiectasia

Red flags

- Failure to thrive
- Angioedema
- Absent lymphoid tissue
- Dysmorphic features
- Illness level disproportionate to infection type
- Eczema that is non-responsive to standard treatment

DIFFERENTIAL DIAGNOSIS

Differential diagnosis of recurrent infections	Features
The child with a normal immune system develops more frequent infections than expected, so is called normal but UNLUCKY Child The Child with a normal immune system but with an underlying chronic condition	Child has normal growth parameters, illness duration with normal limits, frequency of occurrence often explained by attendant risk factors Cystic fibrosis Gastro-oesophageal reflux Complex congenital heart disease Cerebral palsy with recurrent aspiration
Child with immunodeficiency state secondary to a primary condition	HIV Immunosuppression related to treatment for malignancy or autoimmune disease Nephrotic syndrome Asplenia or post splenectomy syndromes Sickle-cell disease
PID	Predominant antibody deficiencies (65% of all PID) Combined T- and B-cell deficiency (15% of all PID) Phagocytic defects (10% of all PIDs) Complement deficiency Well-defined cellular immunodeficiency: • Wiskott–Aldrich's syndrome • DiGeorge's syndrome • ataxia telangiectasia • Hyper IgE syndrome (*see* text for details of individual conditions)

INVESTIGATIONS

What is the value of a full blood count?

The total and absolute white blood cell count and absolute lymphocyte count should be assessed in terms of normative values for age. Lymphopenia is suggestive of SCID, especially in infancy; neutropenia may suggest cyclical neutropenia. Giant cytoplasmic granules in the white blood cell count suggest Chédiak–Higashi's syndrome. Thrombocytopenia and small platelets suggest WAS.

What is value of a chest X-ray?

Chest X-ray should be done on all children. Absence of thymus suggests DiGeorge's syndrome. It may also indicate the presence of pneumonia and may suggest the presence of bronchiectasis.

Should immunoglobulin levels be measured?

Assay of serum immunoglobulin types G, A, M and E should be done on children suspected of PID (screening test for B-cell defects)

(*continued*)

INVESTIGATIONS (*cont.*)

When is HIV testing warranted?

HIV testing is warranted in all infants with a suspected T-cell defect.

Should chromosome analysis be undertaken?

This should be undertaken if DiGeorge's syndrome is suspected or there is evidence of lymphopenia.

When should specific antibodies to vaccines be done (tetanus, H. influenzae type B and pneumococcus)?

In infants and children with low immunoglobulin levels, this assay should be performed 4 weeks after vaccination (test for B-cell defects).

What is the delayed-type hypersensitivity skin test?

This is an intradermal skin test with 0.1 mL heat-killed *Candida* (dilution 1:1000). It is an assessment of T-cell function.

Are there other tests of T-cell function that should be undertaken?

Yes, and these include T-cell subset analysis inclusive of CD3/total T-cell, CD4/helper, CD8/T-suppressor/cytotoxic counts. The interpretation of these tests should be done in conjunction with an immunologist or infectious disease consultant.

Respiratory burst assay

This is a screening test for phagocytic cell function and is required when the absolute neutrophil count is low. This test is not routinely done and the laboratory staff must be informed prior to the blood being drawn from the child.

CH_{50}

This is a screening test for complement deficiency.

MANAGEMENT PLAN: THREE-STEP APPROACH

1. Clarifying and pitfall avoidance strategies
2. Screening for primary immunodeficiency states
3. Therapeutic interventions:
   a) immunisation strategy
   b) prophylactic antibiotics
   c) immunoglobulin therapy.

Clarifying and pitfall avoidance strategies

- Outline the role of infection in the development of immunity. **Rationale**: the occurrence of illness in children is normal and allows for the development of immunity against bacterial and viral illnesses. Such immunity is protective for the child.
- Assess the impact of the infections in terms of the child's growth parameters. **Rationale**: the unlucky child will have normal growth parameters and the illness duration will be within normal limits, although the frequency will be increased.

The failure to maintain normal growth parameters should prompt evaluation for alternate explanations.

- Form an opinion as to the reason for the recurrence of infections. **Rationale**: parents will need an explanation as to whether the frequency is normal and if not, the potential reasons for the recurrence, e.g. crèche attendance, parental smoking, overcrowding or a chronic condition (e.g. cystic fibrosis) being present.
- Weigh and consider the pattern and type of infections in terms of PID presentations. **Rationale**: PID are individually rare, but with over a hundred conditions now being recognised, they are increasingly being diagnosed. Therefore, review the hallmark features of PID to determine if the child has one of them. The aim is to think about the possibility of a PID being present.
- If a PID is diagnosed, determine the impact on siblings. **Rationale**: many PID are inherited and consequently siblings need to be assessed as well.
- If PID is present, educate on and explain the importance of hand hygiene, infection avoidance and risk of infections recurring.
- Outline the impact of treatment of PIDs on the child or adolescent's life. **Rationale**: parents are likely to be devastated when their child is diagnosed with a PID; however, being able to inform them of the impact of this condition will reassure them (*see* Evidence 3).

Screening for primary immunodeficiency states

PIDS are individually rare but it is now possible to screen for SCID in the newborn period. Early diagnosis can change prognosis (*see* Evidence 4).

Therapeutic interventions

Immunisation strategy

Live vaccinations are contraindicated in children with immunodeficiency states. Inactivated vaccines are permissible.

Exposure to varicella must be avoided in those with immunodeficiency states, as they are at of increased risk of severe disease. Significant exposure includes (a) continuous household contact, (b) being indoors for more than 1 hour with a person with varicella, (c) having more that 15 minutes face-to-face contact with an infected person with varicella and (d) touching a varicella lesion. Varicella zoster immunoglobulin is effective if administered within 96 hours of exposure and provides protection for 3 weeks (varicella zoster immunoglobulin dosing is 125 IU/10 kg; to a maximum dose of 625 IU and with a minimum dose of 125 IU). Varicella vaccine within 3–5 days of exposure can prevent or reduce infection severity.

Prophylactic antibiotics

Prophylactic antimicrobials are used in children and adolescents with PID; however, these strategies are derived from expert opinion and not from studies. Due to the rarity of some of the PIDs it is not possible to perform clinical trials. Individual centres that deal with child PID may have practices specific to their unit.

In children with antibody defects, if they experience three or more infections per year then trimethoprim-sulfamethoxazole is used. For those with CVID and associated bronchiectasis, a macrolide three times a week is used as prophylactic treatment.

Immunoglobulin therapy

Immunoglobulin therapy, either intravenous or subcutaneous (*see* Evidence 5), is the cornerstone of treatment. The goal is the reduction of infections that would normally necessitate hospitalisation.

FOLLOW-UP

Children with diagnosed PID need to be followed up at a specialty clinic.

WHEN TO REFER?

- Eight or more infections within 1 year
- Two or more sinus infections or two pneumonias in 1 year
- Two or more months on antibiotics without improvement
- Failure to thrive despite adequate calorie intake
- Recurrent deep skin infections or organ abscesses
- Superficial candidiasis after 1 year of age that persists
- Complications associated with live vaccines

CLARIFICATION STATEMENTS FOR PARENTAL MISCONCEPTIONS

> *'My child's immune system must be weak, as he's always getting infections.'*

Frequent infections do not necessarily imply a deficiency in immune functioning. The occurrence of infection allows the immune system to become more competent and as long as the child is growing well there is little need to be concerned.

> *'What about vitamins to boost his immune system?'*

Vitamins per se will not correct immune deficiencies and are not a substitute for appropriate treatment.

> *'Can antibiotics damage his immune system?'*

Antibiotics kill bacteria, and allow the immune system to process the dead bacteria in an efficient manner, which results in the duration of the illness being reduced. They do not affect the immune system; however, inappropriate antibiotic use can lead to the development of bacterial resistance, which has clinical implications for the child.

SUMMARY PRACTICE POINTS

- Normal children experience up to 7 viral illnesses per year.
- Allergy and PID often coexist.
- Complication with vaccination should prompt consideration of PID.
- Failure to thrive with frequent infections should prompt consideration of PID.
- Lymphopenia should prompt consideration of SCID.
- Patients with PID need to be aware of the risks of varicella exposure.
- Persistent superficial candidiasis should prompt consideration of PID.

EVALUATING THE EVIDENCE

Evidence 1	
Theme E1	*The frequency of infections in children*
Question	What is the frequency of infections in the first 3 years of life?
Design	Prospective cohort study
Level of evidence	
Setting	Community setting, the United States
Participants	Parents of term infants born in Allegheny County, Pennsylvania, who were willing to be followed for 3 years and would maintain health records were recruited.
Intervention	This was an observational cohort study where the impact of home care, group care and day care on the frequency of infections in the first 3 years of life was recorded. Home care was defined as care provided for children of a single family in a residential setting. Group care was defined as care for a child and at least one non-family member in a group of two to six children for at least 20 hours per week in a residential setting. Day care was defined as care of a child in a group of at least seven children for at least 20 hours per week in a non-residential setting. Parents were contacted every 2 weeks and completed a standardised questionnaire that evaluated the type and severity (inclusive of hospitalisation) of infections.
Outcomes	The primary outcome was the frequency and severity of infections in the first 3 years of life.
Main results	Of the 244 enrolled subjects, 159 were in home care, 40 were in group care and 45 were in day care. Infection rates were 4.2/year for those in home care, 6.5/year for those in group care and 7.0/year for those in day care. Infections occurred most frequently in year 2. The percentage of children in year 2 having at least six infections was 50% for home care, 82% for group care and 75% for day care.

(*continued*)

Evidence 1	
Theme E1	*The frequency of infections in children*
Main results (*cont.*)	The reduction in infection for group care compared with home care was 32% (absolute risk reduction (ARR) = 32%; number needed to treat (NNT) = 4), and for day care compared with home care it was 25% (ARR = 25%; NNT = 4).
Conclusion	The frequency of infections in the first 3 years of life ranges from 4.2 per year for those looked after at home to 7.0 per year for those in day care.
Commentary	The data in this study indicate the frequency of infection in a predominantly middle-class population. When extrapolating these data to other populations the similarities need to be considered. Children in families that have poor housing, lower socio-economic status, presence of smoking in the home are likely to have increased numbers of infections. These normative data are useful in discussing with parents whether the numbers of infections their child is experiencing is actually increased or not and it can also prove useful when explaining the impact of location in addressing the child's care needs.
Reference	Wald ER, Guerra N, Byers C. Frequency and severity of infections in day care: three-year follow-up. *J Pediatr.* 1991; **118**(4 Pt. 1): 509–14.

Evidence 2	
Theme E2	*Evaluating patients for primary immunodeficiency*
Question	What symptoms and signs should prompt evaluation for primary immunodeficiency?
Design	Retrospective case series
Level of evidence	
Setting	Department of paediatric allergy and immunology, academic medical centre, the United States
Participants	Children and adolescents (birth to age 21), evaluated for a diagnosis of primary immunodeficiency disorder (PID) were included. Participants were only classified as having PID if they met the criteria specified in the Primary Immunodeficiency Practice Parameter.
Intervention	The 10 warning features of PID from the Jeffrey Modell Foundation (JMF) were evaluated against the clinical notes. The presence of allergy in children with PID was evaluated.
Outcomes	The primary outcome was the sensitivity, specificity, positive and negative predictive value of the JMF warning signs in children with a PID.
Main results	Of the 141 referred for evaluation, 104 (74%) met one or more of the 10 JMF warning criteria. A total of 32 (23%) were diagnosed with a PID. Of the 104 with positive JMF criteria, 20 were diagnosed with a PID, and of the 37 with negative JMF criteria, 12 were diagnosed with a PID sensitivity of 19%, specificity of 23%, positive predictive value of 66% and negative predictive value of 23%. Nine (31%) atopic patients were diagnosed with PID compared with 6 (9%) atopic patients who were PID negative.
Conclusion	The JMF criteria did not distinguish between non-PID and PID patients. Allergy and immunodeficiency may co-exist.

(*continued*)

Evidence 2	
Theme E2	*Evaluating patients for primary immunodeficiency*
Commentary	PIDs are a relatively rare and heterogeneous group of conditions. The JMF criteria were developed by an expert group to identify potential PID in individuals; however, they have not been prospectively validated. The features are four or more new ear infections in 1 year, two or more sinus infections in 1 year, 2 or more months on antibiotic treatment with little clinical effect, two or more pneumonias in 1 year, failure to thrive or gain weight normally, recurrent deep skin or organ abscesses, persistent thrush in the mouth or fungal infections on the skin, the need for intravenous antibiotics to clear infections, two or more deep-seated infections or septicaemia, and a family history of primary immunodeficiency. These 'warning signs' serve as clinical prompts to consider whether a child might have a PID or not. Positive predictive and negative predictive values of 66% and 23%, respectively, are low. The notion that allergy, as demonstrated by the presence of specific IgE, precludes PID is incorrect. This study indicates an overlap is present and that allergy presence makes PID more likely.
Reference	MacGinnitie A, Aloi F, Mishra S. Clinical characteristics of pediatric patients evaluated for primary immunodeficiency. *Pediatr Allergy Immunol.* 2011; **22**(7): 671–5.

Evidence 3	
Theme E3	*Quality of life in children and adolescents with chronic infections*
Question	What is the quality of life in children and adolescents with X-linked agammaglobulinaemia (XLA)
Design	Two groups were studied, one with XLA patients and the other with healthy controls.
Level of evidence	
Setting	Departments of paediatrics participating in the Italian Network for Primary Immunodeficiencies
Participants	Two groups were assessed that included children and adolescents aged 5–18 years with a definitive diagnosis of XLA in fair health (no hospital admissions in the month prior to the study) and a second group of healthy children and adolescents serving as the healthy control (HC) group. All patients with XLA were receiving intravenous immunoglobulin treatment in hospital every 21–28 days.
Intervention	The Pediatric Quality of Life Inventory (which evaluates physical, emotional, social and school domains on a five-point Likert scale plus three summary scores) was used to assess well-being for the 4 weeks prior to interview. Potential scores range from 0 to 100.
Outcomes	The primary outcome was the difference in quality-of-life measures between the two groups.
Main results	Twenty-five children and adolescents were assessed, with a mean age of 7.2 years (six were aged 5–7 years, eleven aged 8–12 years and eight aged 13–18 years). There were 80 control subjects, all aged between 8 and 14 years.

(*continued*)

Evidence 3	
Theme E3	***Quality of life in children and adolescents with chronic infections***
Main results (*cont.*)	Significant statistical differences were observed between XLA patients and the HC group in total scores (XLA, 75.8 ± 13.0; HC, 86.8 ± 9.5; $P < 0.001$), psychosocial health (XLA, 73.8 ± 14.2; HC, 86.5 ± 10.3; $P < 0.001$), emotional functioning (XLA, 68.6 ± 18.4; HC, 82.9 ± 16.2) and school functioning (XLA, 69.2 ± 21.0; HC, 84.6 ± 13). No differences were noted in physical health (XLA, 81.6 ± 15.3; HC, 87.7 ± 10.2; $P < 0.072$) and social functioning (XLA, 83.6 ± 16.7; HC, 92.0 ± 11.8; $P < 0.026$). There was a weak correlation between quality-of-life assessment compliance to treatment.
Conclusion	The global quality-of-life total score observed in XLA children and adolescents was lower than that observed for healthy controls.
Commentary	This study addressed quality-of-life measures in subjects with XLA and healthy controls. The subjects were not age matched and the influence that this may have had on the results is speculative but important. The findings of impairment in psychosocial health and school functioning rather than physical health require attention in the early school years by appropriate learning support structures and input from a psychologist. This study included previously published data on children and adolescents with rheumatic diseases and noted that those with XLA had a better quality of life (XLA, 77.3 ± 14.8; rheumatic diseases, 71.0 ± 18.49; $P = 0.025$). This is a reflection on the effectiveness of immunoglobulin treatment in those with XLA.
Reference	Soresina A, Nacinovich R, Bomba M, *et al*. The quality of life of children and adolescents with X-linked agammaglobulinemia. *J Clin Immunol*. 2009; **29**(4): 501–7.

Evidence 4	
Theme E4	***Screening for immunodeficiency***
Question	What is the effectiveness in screening for severe combined immunodeficiency?
Design	State-wide screening programme
Level of evidence	
Setting	State of Wisconsin, the United States
Participants	All infants born in the state of Wisconsin from January 2008 to December 2010 were included for screening.
Intervention	The newborn screening test used was the T-cell receptor excision circle (TREC). TRECs are small circular pieces of DNA that are formed during the differentiation of T-cell in the thymus and do not replicate with cellular division.
Outcomes	The primary outcome was to identify infants with severe combined immunodeficiency (SCID) and other forms of T-cell lymphopenia (TCL) by the TREC assay.
Main results	During the first 3 years of screening, 207 696 infants were screened. Seventy-two infants had an abnormal TREC assay on newborn screening. Thirty-three infants were found to have TCL of varying degrees (positive predictive value of TREC assay was 45.8%). The false positive rate was 0.018% and the specificity was 99.8%.

(continued)

Evidence 4	
Theme E4	*Screening for immunodeficiency*
Main results (*cont.*)	Of the 33 infants with TLC, five had SCIDs, 14 had chromosomal or metabolic anomalies, two had gastroschisis with necrotising enterocolitis, three had a lymphatic malformation, five had TCL that resolved and four had DiGeorge's syndrome.
Conclusion	The TREC assay is a sensitive and specific test to identify SCID and other forms of lymphopenia.
Commentary	Infants with SCID are typically normal at birth but are at high risk of developing life-threatening infections, a risk that is markedly increased once maternal transferred antibody levels have declined. While there are several forms of SCID, the severe deficiency of naïve T-cells is a universal finding. Detecting this abnormality prior to 14 weeks of life and before the occurrence of infections allows the child to undergo haematopoietic stem cell transplantation to correct the underlying immunodeficiency. If a child should have an abnormal TREC assay result, the chances of having SCID are 7% and those with abnormal assays will require further investigation to determine the significance of the finding.
Reference	Verbsky JW, Baker MW, Grossman WJ, *et al.* Newborn screening for severe combined immunodeficiency: the Wisconsin experience (2008–2011). *J Clin Immunol.* 2012; **32**(1): 82–8.

Evidence 5	
Theme E5	*Treatment of immunodeficiency states*
Question	Is subcutaneous immunoglobulin (SCIG) administration equivalent to intravenous immunoglobulin (IVIG) administered treatment?
Design	Prospective, open-label, single-arm study
Level of evidence	
Setting	Fifteen immunology clinics (paediatric and adult) across Europe
Participants	Persons with a primary immunodeficiency state (common variable immunodeficiency (CVID), X-linked agammaglobulinaemia and autosomal recessive agammaglobulinaemia) were eligible for inclusion.
Intervention	Patients previously on IVIG or SCIG were switched to Hizentra, which is a 20% IgG concentration product administered subcutaneously on a weekly basis. Due to its increased concentration and low viscosity, the product can be infused faster and quicker than the current 16% solutions.
Outcomes	The primary outcome was to compare IgG trough levels during 6 consecutive weeks of the study to three IgG trough levels from the patients' previous treatments.
Main results	Of the 53 patients screened, 51 were enrolled, of whom 31 had previously been on IVIG and 20 on SCIG (different product from Hizentra). Forty-six completed the wash-in/washout period (27 IVIG; 19 SCIG), 43 patients completed the study (24 IVIG; 19 SCIG). Seventeen (37%) were aged 2–11 years, five (10.9%) were aged 12–15 years and 24 (52.2%) were aged 16–64 years. The primary outcome was achieved as the pre-study mean IgG level in grams per litre was 7.49 ± 1.57 and the steady state study level was 8.10 ± 1.34.

(*continued*)

Evidence 5	
Theme E5	*Treatment of immunodeficiency states*
Main results (*cont.*)	No serious bacterial infections were reported during the study period. Local reactions were common with SCIG and 25 (49%) patients experienced 110 reactions during the study (rate: 0.06 per infusion).
Conclusion	The use of SCIG was effective in maintaining IgG levels and protected against infection.
Commentary	For patients with primary immunodeficiency the mainstay of treatment is replacement therapy with human polyvalent IgG. Heretofore IVIG has been the gold standard of therapy but with improved technology, subcutaneous IgG is being increasingly used. From the patients' experience the preference is limited school/work loss, convenience and therapeutic effectiveness. SCIG would appear to aid in achieving these goals.
Reference	Jolles S, Bernatowska E, deGracia J, *et al.* Efficacy and safety of Hizentra® in patients with primary immunodeficiency after a dose-equivalent switch from intravenous or subcutaneous replacement therapy. *Clin Immunol.* 2011; **141**(1): 90–102.

THE CHILD WITH RECURRENT INFECTIONS: MULTIPLE-CHOICE QUESTIONS

Q1 The JMF criteria for immunodeficiency screening include which of the following?
a) Eight or more ear infections per year
b) Four sinus infections per year
c) Two or more months on antibiotics treatment with little improvement clinically
d) Failure to thrive
e) Recurrent deep-seated infections

Q2 In children with primary immunodeficiency, which of the following is/are correct?
a) Antibody deficiency accounts for 30% of cases.
b) Selective IgA immunodeficiency occurs in 1:1500 children.
c) IgG subclass deficiency presents with recurrent pneumonias.
d) Children with X-linked immunodeficiency have large tonsils from recurrent infections.
e) Common variable immunodeficiency affects 1:25000 children.

Q3 Cellular immunodeficiency states include which of the following?
a) Williams's syndrome
b) Wiskott–Aldrich's syndrome
c) Ataxia telangiectasia
d) DiGeorge's syndrome
e) Hyper-IgE syndrome

Q4   In X-linked agammaglobulinaemia, which of the following is/are correct?
   a) The primary defect is related to the B-cell function.
   b) Symptoms usually begin at 18–24 months of age.
   c) Sinopulmonary infections are frequent.
   d) Enteroviral illnesses are unusually severe.
   e) Lymph glands are small.

Q5   SCID is associated with which of the following?
   a) An enhanced reaction to Bacillus Calmette–Guerin BCG
   b) Chronic candidiasis
   c) Failure to thrive
   d) Chronic diarrhoea
   e) Recurrent lobar pneumonias

Q6   Recognised features of hyper-IgE syndrome include which of the following?
   a) Lax ligaments
   b) Retained primary teeth
   c) Recurrent staphylococcal infections
   d) Eczema
   e) Chronic candidiasis

Q7   Which of the following statements is/are correct?
   a) Salmonella infections occur more frequently in T-cell deficiency states.
   b) Recurrent pneumococcal infections occur more frequently in complement deficiency states.
   c) Meningococcal infections occur more frequently in complement deficiency states.
   d) Candidiasis occurs more frequently in T-cell deficiency states.
   e) Rotaviral infections occur repeatedly in IgA deficiency states.

Q8   Clinical 'red flags' in children with recurrent infections include which of the following?
   a) Ataxia
   b) Eczema that responds well to treatment but recurs
   c) Absence of tonsillar tissue
   d) Cardiac murmurs
   e) Tetany

Q9   Which of the following statements is/are correct?
   a) In screening for SCID states, the T-cell receptor excision circle test is utilised.
   b) The positive predictive value of the T-cell receptor excision circle test to identify T-cell lymphopenia is 90%.
   c) SCID usually presents after 4 months of age.

d) In SCID the key abnormality is a deficiency of naïve T cells.

e) Bone marrow transplantation if successful is curative.

Q10 Which of the following statements is/are correct?

a) Immunoglobulin therapy for X-linked agammaglobulinaemia can be discontinued in adolescence if the patient is free of bacterial infection for 2 years.

b) Subcutaneous immunoglobulin infusion is equivalent to intravenous immunoglobulin treatment.

c) Quality-of-life studies suggest a better outcome for patients with X-linked agammaglobulinaemia than those with rheumatic conditions.

d) In children on treatment for X-linked agammaglobulinaemia, the risk of bacterial infection is more than 2 episodes per year.

e) Subcutaneous infusion of immunoglobulin is effective because of the reduced viscosity of the product compared with the intravenous preparation.

Answers

A1	c, d, e	A2	e
A3	b, c, d, e	A4	a, c, d, e
A5	a, b, c, d	A6	a, b, c, d, e
A7	a, c, d	A8	a, c, d, e
A9	a, c, d, e	A10	b, d, e

Chapter Six

THE AFEBRILE INFANT WITH EXCESSIVE CRYING

COMMON SCENARIO

'I don't know what's wrong with him, he's been crying for hours and he's normally such a quiet, well-tempered baby. I've tried everything, I've checked his temperature, I don't know what's wrong. It's like he's in pain and he just won't stop crying.'

LEARNING OBJECTIVES

- Understand the normal patterns of crying and variations of normal in infancy
- Recognise the importance of repeated observation of infants' behaviour in helping to detect warning signs of serious underlying pathology
- Recognise 'red flags' in the history or examination that require further investigation or treatment
- List the differential causes of excessive crying in an afebrile infant
- Determine what investigations should be performed
- Recognise non-accidental injury (NAI) patterns
- Develop a strategy to deal with colic in infancy

BACKGROUND

The crying afebrile infant represents one of the most challenging diagnostic dilemmas for practitioners. Crying is a normal part of infancy, representing an infant's means of communication. Crying can be due to hunger, excessive tiredness, discomfort from a wet or soiled nappy, need for attention or pain. Parents develop an intuitive sense as to what their infant's cry means and can distinguish different types of crying indicating the various needs of their child. They can distinguish between what they perceive as their child's 'normal' cry and an 'abnormal' cry.

However, when does crying become excessive? A normal healthy 2-week-old neonate cries for approximately 2 hours a day and this increases to 3 hours a day by

6–8 weeks of age, after which, there is a gradual steady decline in crying until about 4 months, when it tends to plateau. During the first 6 months of life, crying tends to be concentrated in the late afternoon and evening and in the second 6 months of life it occurs mainly at night. However, there is a huge amount of variability and no uniform consensus on when normal crying patterns become excessive, for both parents and health professionals. A crying infant is extremely stressful for parents, who, often by the time they present to their family practitioner or local emergency department are extremely anxious and distressed, sleep deprived and frustrated, having exhausted all their usual tried and tested consoling techniques.

The commonest cause of excessive crying in infancy is colic. The most widely used definition of colic is that proposed by Wessel *et al.* (1954)[1] which is referred to as the 'Rule of threes'. An infant can be considered to have colic if he or she cries for more than 3 hours a day for more than 3 days a week for 3 weeks. Infants with colic are well and thriving. Crying episodes start in the first few weeks of life and usually peak by 6–8 weeks of age. Episodes usually occur in the late afternoon or early evening and can last for hours. The child is typically inconsolable during episodes. The child may draw up his or her legs, clench fists, arch his or her back and grimace as if in pain. By 3–4 months of age, excessive crying usually resolves.

However, colic is a diagnosis of exclusion and infants presenting with an acute episode of crying require careful evaluation in order to ensure that serious or potentially life-threatening illness are not missed. Organic disease accounts for approximately 5% of cases of excessive crying. However, crying can be the presenting symptom of almost any pathological condition presenting in infancy. Clinically distinguishing a well child from a potentially unwell or toxic-looking child requires experience and an appreciation of early warning signs that may indicate serious pathology. Observation of the infant can provide valuable information and is the most important skill to master.

An acutely unwell child may have signs of poor perfusion such as mottling, cool peripheries and delayed capillary refill time. They often dislike being disturbed and may lie still with alternating drowsiness and irritability. They refuse to feed. They may look pale or have a 'muddy' grey appearance or show signs of respiratory distress with rapid, laboured breathing with or without grunting. In cases where there is no clear diagnosis or concerns regarding an underlying pathology, infants should not be discharged home; they should continue to be observed and reassessed. With continued observation, the infant will proclaim his- or herself as either well or unwell, and requiring further investigation or treatment.

The crying infant with bony or soft tissue injuries

NAI needs to be considered in infants presenting with excessive crying and with bone or soft tissue injuries on examination. Fractures occur in up to 25% of physically abused children, 80% of these fractures occur in children under 18 months of age. Although there are patterns of injury that are highly suggestive of abuse, there are no pathognomonic findings. Fractures that occur in children who are abused can also occur in children accidentally. Therefore a fracture, like any other injury, should never be interpreted in isolation. It must always be assessed in the context of a child's medical and social history, developmental stage and the explanation given. Fractures that are suggestive of NAI but not are pathognomonic include:

- posterior rib fractures
- fractures of the sternum, scapula or spinous processes
- multiple fractures in various stages of healing
- bilateral acute long bone fractures
- depressed skull fractures in children less than 18 months of age
- metaphyseal corner fractures.

In children less than 1 year of age, 60%–80% of femoral fractures are due to physical abuse.

Skull fractures that are suggestive of abuse:

- non-parietal fractures
- multiple or complex fractures
- depressed fracture
- involvement of more than single cranial bone
- associated intracranial injury.

Cutaneous manifestations of inflicted injuries are the most recognisable forms of NAI. Many cutaneous signs can, however, be the result of benign childhood injuries or medical conditions. It is therefore important to be able to distinguish between common cutaneous manifestations of NAI and benign injuries or medical conditions. Bruising is the commonest injury in children who have been physically abused. A bruise must never be interpreted in isolation and must always be assessed in the context of medical and social history, developmental stage, explanation given, full clinical examination and relevant investigations. Most accidental bruises occur over bony prominences. For example, a child who is pulling to stand may bump his or her head and sustain bruising to the head, usually the forehead.

Bruises that are suggestive of physical abuse include:

- bruising in children who are not independently mobile
- bruising in children under 6 months of age
- bruises that are seen away from bony prominences
- bruises to the buttocks, ears, abdomen and back
- multiple bruises in clusters
- multiple bruises of uniform shape
- bruises that carry the imprint of the implement used or a ligature.

HISTORY

KEY POINTS				
Crying	Onset Duration Frequency Ability to be consoled Previous episodes Diurnal variation	**Medical history**	Gastro-oesophageal reflux Constipation Urinary tract infection	**🔍 Red flags** Fever Poor feeding Per rectum bleeding Concern regarding social circumstances or mother's coping abilities
Associated symptoms	Fever Sleeping pattern Vomiting Diarrhoea Blood PR Coryzal symptoms Rash Breathing difficulties Apnoeic episodes	**Surgical history**	Previous abdominal surgeries Ventriculoperitoneal shunt	
Mother's perspective	What does she think is wrong? How is she coping? Has she adequate support at home? Postnatal depression	**Medications**	Medications tried Over-the-counter preparations Herbal remedies	
Birth and maternal history	Gestation Maternal drug use	**Social history**	Who lives at home? Who cares for child? Difficulties	
Feeding history	Difficult to wind Regurgitation Excessive flatulence Poor feeding Breathlessness with feeds Failure to gain weight or weight loss	**Growth and development**	Reaching milestones	
Family history	Food intolerance Vesicoureteric reflux	**Vaccinations**	Recent vaccinations	

It can be very difficult to distinguish between accidental and non-accidental burns in ambulatory children. However, burns that have a clear outline or which are on areas normally covered by clothing may arouse suspicion. Deliberate cigarette burns have a characteristic appearance, being clearly demarcated, round and deep. Non-accidental scalds are usually caused by dumping the child's limb or buttocks in hot water and leave a demarcated 'tide mark'.

EXAMINATION

- All babies should have their weight, length and head circumference plotted on an appropriate centile chart
- Assess the overall appearance of child by observation: toxic or well looking
- Expose the child fully and perform a head-to-toe examination
- Vital signs including temperature should be recorded
- Ear, nose and throat: otitis media, stomatitis, teething
- Eyes: corneal abrasions, retinal haemorrhages, corneal clouding
- Fingers, toes: swollen with constriction ring
- Cardiovascular: murmurs, tachycardia
- Respiratory: distress
- Gastrointestinal: masses, tenderness
- Neurological: tone, posture, abnormal movements
- Genitourinary exam: hernia orifices, genitalia
- Perianal exam: fissures
- Joint exam: swelling, erythema, paresis
- Skin exam: rash, bruising, scalds
- Head: size, fontanelle

🔱 Red flags

- Full fontanelle
- Fever
- Toxic-looking child
- Suspicious bruises or signs of trauma or neglect
- Failure to thrive
- Abnormal posturing or hypotonia
- Joint swelling

DIFFERENTIAL DIAGNOSIS

Gastrointestinal	
Gastro-oesophageal reflux disease	Increasing distress over several weeks, forceful vomits, back arching, refusal to feed, poor weight gain
Anal fissures	History of constipation, straining with defecation, blood streaks in nappy
Cows' milk allergy	Diarrhoea, vomiting, blood per rectum
Lactose intolerance	Watery diarrhoea, recent gastroenteritis, excess flatulence

Surgical	
Intussusception	Extreme irritability, flexing of legs, pallor, especially around mouth, increasing lethargy in between episodes of abdominal pain, vomiting, red current jelly stool (late sign), abdominal distension, sausage-shaped mass in right upper quadrant
Malrotation and volvulus	Bilious vomiting, signs of peritonitis
Incarcerated inguinal hernia	Males, usually right side, tender inguinal mass

Infection	
Meningitis	Toxic, poor perfusion, lethargy, apnoea, bulging fontanelle, high-pitched cry, hypotonia, listlessness, poor feeding, seizures, fever or hypothermia, vomiting, cool peripheries
Viral exanthems	Coryzal symptoms, rash, lymphadenopathy, fever
Otitis media	Irritable, vomiting or diarrhoea, pulling at ear, may present without fever, otorrhoea, associated coryzal symptoms
Septic arthritis and osteomyelitis	Paresis, abnormal position of limb, pain elicited on passive movement, swelling
Cellulitis	Localised erythema, increased temperature

Renal	
Renal calculi	Colicky abdominal pain, family history of stones, haematuria, associated urinary tract infection, history of prematurity
Urinary tract infection	Very non-specific presentations, may present without fever, failure to thrive, malodorous urine, poor feeding, vomiting, jaundice, family history of vesicoureteric reflux

Neurological	
Hydrocephalus and raised intracranial pressure	Macrocephaly, widely separated sutures, bulging anterior fontanelle, dilated scalp veins, sun setting eyes

Trauma	
Fractures	Paresis, refusal to move limb, pain on passive movement, swelling or deformity
Abusive head trauma	Limp, lifeless infant, seizure, extreme irritability, respiratory distress, retinal haemorrhages, full fontanelle
Bruising	Concerning in non-ambulatory child (*see* earlier section on bruising and NAI)
Burns and scalds	Concerning in non-ambulatory child (*see* earlier section on burns, scalds and NAI)

Dermatological	
Eczema	Eczematous plaques on cheeks, forehead, scalp and extensor surfaces, scratch marks, secondary infection
Nappy rash	Erythematous rash in nappy area, with irritant contact dermatitis may be associated fissures and erosions localised to areas covered by nappy and sparing skin folds, with candida infection satellite lesions may be seen, relatively sharp border, involvement of skin folds, may have history of recent antibiotic use
Epidermolysis bullosa	Blisters in lower limbs, extremely painful

Cardiac	
Supraventricular tachycardia	Heart rate >220 beats per minute, narrow QRS complex, absent p-waves on ECG
Total anomalous left coronary artery	Episodes of Irritability, poor feeding, crying after feeds, resting tachypnoea, diaphoresis with feeding, tachycardia Signs of decreased peripheral perfusion, pulmonary oedema Cardiomegaly on chest X-ray

Head, eyes, ears, nose and throat	
Corneal abrasion	Inability to open eye, watery eye, sensitivity to light, fingernail scratches on face
Stomatitis	Ulcers in mouth, drooling, refusal to feed
Teething	Eruption of teeth, gum swelling, drooling, may bite on fingers or toys
Oral thrush	Refusal to feed, white patches on buccal mucosa, tongue or palate that do not scrape off
Glaucoma	Corneal enlargement, haziness, tearing, blinking, sensitivity to light

Other	
First presentation of colic	Well child, normal exam, growing and thriving
Post immunisation	Normal examination, growing and thriving infant, recent immunisation, localised erythema or swelling at site of injection
Hair tourniquet syndrome	Affecting fingers, toes or genitalia, erythematous, swollen, tender with constriction ring, visible hair entangled
Neonatal abstinence syndrome	History of maternal drug ingestion, poor feeding, diarrhoea, vomiting, jitteriness, seizures, high-pitched cry, sneezing, increased muscle tone, apnoea, excessive sucking

INVESTIGATIONS

In a well-looking child, with no concerning features, what investigation if any should be performed?

A urinalysis should be performed to rule out a urinary tract infection.

Ideally a clean catch urine sample should be obtained. The infant's perineum should be wiped with water and wipes. They should be laid down on the bed, with the nappy open and offered a feed. The parents should be instructed to wait with an open sample jar and catch a mid-stream sample of urine when passed.

If a corneal abrasion is suspected, what further investigations are required?

- Topical application of fluorescein to the eye
- Visualising the cornea under cobalt-blue filtered light
- Abrasion appears green

In infants under 6 months of age, with a proven urinary tract infection, what radiological investigations should be performed?

- A renal ultrasound scan within 72 hours of admission
- A repeat renal ultrasound scan at 4–6 months post infection to look for evolving scars or a DMSA
- If vesicoureteric reflux is suspected, a micturating cystourethrogram between 3 and 6 months of age

If a fracture is suspected clinically, what radiological investigations should be performed?

- An anteroposterior and lateral X-ray of the injured area, above and below the joint, should be taken
- In children less than 2 years of age a skeletal survey should also be done
- A repeat skeletal survey or radionucleotide bone scan can be helpful if there is a high suspicion of abuse but the first skeletal survey is normal; there is no role for a babygram, i.e. one to two views of the entire body

In infants with bruising, what test should be done?

Every child should have a complete blood count, international normalised ratio/partial thromboplastin time done for bruising. Extended coagulation evaluation should be determined by the clinical situation. In children with retinal haemorrhages or intracranial haemorrhage glutaric aciduria should be considered and screening the urine for organic acids undertaken.

MANAGEMENT PLAN: TWO-STEP APPROACH

1. Clarifying and pitfall avoidance strategies
2. Treatment options and specific therapy

Clarifying and pitfall avoidance strategies

Infants and young children who present with acute afebrile crying are a diagnostically challenging group of patients; therefore, remember the following points.

- Parents are intuitively able to decide whether a cry is more intense than usual or is distinctly abnormal from before. Sometimes they will record the crying to document the distress their child is experiencing.
- Acknowledge what parents have done to console or soothe their baby. They are

attending the emergency or the outpatient department because they are worried or have been unsuccessful in their efforts.

- The causes of acute crying are varied (*see* Evidence 1), and consequently do *not* rush to a diagnosis of colic before completing your assessment. Remember not all crying is colic related.
- **Colic** is a diagnosis of exclusion and should not be the first diagnosis, unless the infant has met the diagnostic criteria. Where a diagnosis of colic is likely, the following are suggested:
  - ○ acknowledge how difficult it is to deal with a crying infant
  - ○ assess the fatigue and sleep deprivation level of the parents – in particular, the mother
  - ○ determine if the parents have had respite from the crying
  - ○ be prudent in ordering investigations
  - ○ give a specific treatment plan and outline specific strategies
  - ○ recognise that not all treatment strategies are equally effective
  - ○ when undertaking a treatment strategy, ensure that the parents log the crying, sleep and feeding pattern, to ensure that any improvement obtained can be objectively assessed
  - ○ explain the natural history of colic to the parents.
- The following approach will help in dealing with a potential **NAI** evaluation.
  - ○ State who you are and why you have been asked to assess the infant or child.
  - ○ Be non-judgemental in your assessment. **Rationale**: jumping to conclusions without supportive evidence does not serve any person's interest.
  - ○ Obtain the history from the parent or guardian and assess if it is compatible with NAI or not.
  - ○ Know your hospital protocol for suspected NAI, and inform the relevant team members early.
  - ○ Follow your radiology protocol for X-rays.
  - ○ Provide an explanation to the parents for the investigations being undertaken.
  - ○ A clear understanding of the risk associated with bruising (*see* Evidence 2) and potential abusive head trauma (*see* Evidence 3) is required.

Treatment options and specific therapy

There are many approaches to colic and parents may have tried several modalities, prior to their initial visit for a medical assessment, which may include:

- swaddling
- white noise – vacuum cleaner, washing machine or dishwasher
- going for a drive in the car with the infant in his or her car seat
- pushing the infant in his or her stroller or pram
- keeping the noise level and stimulation down
- bathing in a warm bath
- playing gentle music.

Specific evidenced-based approaches are as follows.

- Formula modification (*see* Evidence 4).
- Behavioural approaches which incorporated both parent and infant strategies together are successful (*see* Evidence 5). Essential to these strategies is effective care of the mother to reduce stress and enhance coping by having 'away time' from the baby.
- Probiotics taken by breastfeeding mother have been shown to be effective but the mechanism of action is unclear (*see* Evidence 6).
- Specific advice to breastfeeding mothers to modify their diet must be undertaken with caution (*see* Evidence 7).
- The management of organic causes of failure to thrive depends on the underlying pathology. Please refer to the relevant chapters for further information on the management of medical or surgical conditions that may present as excessive crying.

FOLLOW-UP

The infant with colic should be seen by the public health nurse and family doctor to ensure that (a) the parents are coping well, (b) the infant is thriving and (c) that no 'red flags' are evident.

WHEN TO REFER?

- An organic cause is suggested by the history or examination findings
- An unwell or toxic-looking child
- Abnormal examination findings
- Concern that the parents are not coping
- Concerns about possible NAI

CLARIFICATION STATEMENTS FOR PARENTAL MISCONCEPTIONS

'Should my baby receive analgesia for his crying? He looks to be in pain.'

There is no evidence that analgesia is effective for colic and consequently it is not recommended for routine administration.

'What test should be done for the child with colic?'

Colic is a diagnosis of exclusion and routine test are not warranted. If the child is thriving and there is an absence of 'red flags', devising an effective management strategy should be the goal. If this fails then the situation should be re-evaluated.

'So my 3-month-old baby has been crying for about 4 hours. It's the first time this has happened. I suppose this is the beginning of colic.'

Colic is a diagnosis of exclusion and specific criteria must be met. It is prudent to recall that only 11% of infants with excessive crying will have colic (*see* Evidence 1).

SUMMARY PRACTICE POINTS

- Parents can distinguish normal from abnormal crying.
- Colic is the most commonly applied diagnosis but the criteria need to be fulfilled.
- Colic is a diagnosis of exclusion.
- Crying with bruises suggests NAI.
- Infants with excessive crying require an urinalysis.
- Classify the crying child as well or unwell.
- Perform a full examination (*see* Evidence 1).
- Acknowledge the distress that crying causes parents.

EVALUATING THE EVIDENCE

Evidence 1	
Theme E1	**Acute crying in infancy**
Question	What is the aetiology of acute crying in infancy?
Design	Case series
Level of evidence	
Setting	Department of paediatrics, academic medical centre, the United States
Participants	Children from birth to 24 months were eligible for inclusion if they presented to the emergency department with acute, excessive, unexplained crying or fussiness. Patients were excluded if (a) they had a history of fever or were febrile at presentation, (b) if they had an acute illness in the previous 72 hours and (c) if they were previously diagnosed with a chronic condition that predisposed them to pain, e.g. colic, sickle-cell disease or hydrocephalus with shunt placement.
Intervention	All patients had a history and clinical examination performed. Further investigation was at the discretion of the medical staff assessing the infant.
Outcomes	The primary outcome was the aetiology of the acute crying.
Main results	During the 1-year study period, 56 infants were assessed. The age ranged from 4 days to 24 months, with a median age of 3.5 months and 75% were less than 8 months of age. The duration of crying was 1 hour to 5 days. Forty per cent of parents described the crying as constant and 60% as intermittent. Seventy-five per cent of parents described the crying as partially consolable, 20% said their child was inconsolable and 5% said their child was easily consoled.

(continued)

Evidence 1	
Theme E1	*Acute crying in infancy*
Main results (*cont.*)	The aetiologies of the acute excessive crying were idiopathic, ten (17.8%); colic, six (10.7%); infectious aetiologies, 16 (28.5%) (otitis media, ten; herpangina, one; herpetic stomatitis, one; urinary tract infection, one; viral syndrome, one); trauma related, 9 (16.1%) (corneal abrasion, three; foreign body eye, one; foreign body mouth, one; tibial fracture, one; clavicular fracture, one; spider bite, one; hair tourniquet syndrome of toe, one), gastrointestinal tract pathology, 5 (8.9%) (constipation, three; intussusceptions, one; oesophagitis, one), central nervous system pathology, three (5.3%) (subdural haematoma, one; encephalitis, one; pseudo-tumour cerebri, one); drug reactions, two (3.5%) (DTP reaction, one; inadvertent pseudoephedrine overdose, one); behavioural problems, two (3.5%) (night terrors, one; overstimulation, one); and cardiovascular aetiology, two (supraventricular tachycardia, two) and metabolic disease, one (1.7%).
Conclusion	Infants who present with acute crying can have a myriad of potential aetiologies therefore a careful history and a reflective clinical examination are necessary. The physical examination revealed the final diagnosis in 23 (41%) of infants and the history and clinical examination provided the diagnosis in 17 (30%).
Commentary	In this study the frequency of infants with acute excessive crying who presented to the emergency department was 1:400 attendances. The potential causes are extensive so that the importance of history and physical examination must be stressed. Colic accounted for <11% of aetiologies and doctors should be careful in ascribing this aetiology to crying especially on the first clinical presentation. For the practising doctor the question arises, what is excessive crying? This study suggests that crying be considered excessive if it lasts longer than 2 hours. In assessing the crying the concept of infant consolability must be assessed (the non-soothable infant needs careful assessment – review potential aetiologies from the results list). In this study the presence of (a) evidence of serious illness during the physical examination or (b) persistent crying in the emergency department beyond the initial assessment was predictive of serious illness (sensitivity, 100%; specificity, 77%; and positive predictive value, 87%).
Reference	Poole SR. The infant with acute, unexplained, excessive crying. *Pediatrics.* 1991; **88**(3): 450–5.

Evidence 2	
Theme E2	*Bruising and child abuse*
Question	Are there patterns of bruising that are diagnostic or suggestive of child abuse?
Design	Systematic review
Level of evidence	
Setting	
Participants	
Intervention	Systematic review to define abusive and non-abusive bruising

(*continued*)

Evidence 2	
Theme E2	*Bruising and child abuse*
Outcomes	Studies that defined patterns of bruising in abused and non-abused children and adolescents were eligible for inclusion.
Main results	*Bruising in non-abused children.* There were nine studies evaluated (two case controlled, four cross-sectional and three case series). Bruising is more common in boys than girls and more common in the summer months. Bruises are characteristically small (10–15 mm) and parents can give explanations [23 (72%) of parents in one study offered explanations]. Bruising is directly related to motor development (bruising in the non-mobile infant is very uncommon, <1%). With increasing mobility, lower limb bruises increase, especially over the knees and shins (bony prominences). Bruising on the head usually occurs on the forehead area. Areas where bruising was uncommon included back, buttocks, forearm, face, abdomen or hip, upper arm posterior leg, or foot. Bruising on the hands (<4 years) was not noted, nor was ear bruising. *Bruising in abused children.* There were 16 studies evaluated (two case control, 13 case series, and one cross-sectional study). In abuse situations bruising is common (depending on the study, it ranged from 28% to 98%). The mean number of bruises was variable. In the distribution of bruises the head was the most common site. Bruising to ear face, head and neck, trunk and buttocks and arms are common. Bruises often cluster and reflect defensive injuries. Sometimes the bruises may reflect an imprint of the implement used. The location of the bruises is away from bony prominences.
Conclusion	When abuse is suspected the medical, social and developmental history, the explanation offered and the patterns of non-abusive bruising must all be assessed when evaluating the child.
Commentary	Bruising is common in children. Seventeen per cent of infants who are starting to mobilise, 53% of walkers and the majority of school children have bruises. The majority of these will be small and located on the front of the body. For the doctor assessing bruising, there is a clear need to evaluate the child in the context of the history (inclusive of medical, social and developmental), physical examination and explanations offered. Ensuring the absence of underlying bleeding diatheses is essential and consequently such tests should be performed.
Reference	Maguire S, Mann MK, Sibert J, *et al.* Are there patterns of bruising in childhood which are diagnostic or suggestive of abuse? A systematic review. *Arch Dis Child.* 2005; **90**(2): 182–6.

Evidence 3	
Theme E3	*Head trauma related to abuse*
Question	Can the probability of abusive head trauma (AHT) be estimated from specific clinical features?
Design	Pooled analysis from six comparative studies
Level of evidence	
Setting	
Participants	Children under 3 years of age with intracranial injury were included for analysis. Criteria to define abuse were as follows: (a) abuse confirmed at case conference or civil, family, or criminal court or admitted by the perpetrator or independently witnessed or (b) abuse confirmed by stated criteria including multidisciplinary assessment.
Intervention	The relationship between AHT and the following clinical features was assessed: (a) apnoea; (b) retinal haemorrhage (RH); (c) rib, skull and long bone fractures; (d) seizures; and (e) head and/or neck bruises.
Outcomes	The probability of AHT based on the combination of six factors: (1) apnoea, (2) RH, (3) rib fractures, (4) long bone fractures, (5) seizures and (6) head and/or neck bruises.
Main results	A total of 1053 children (348 with AHT) were analysed. When a child had intracranial injury alone, the risk of AHT was 4%. When present with intracranial injury, the odds ratio (OR) for rib fractures was 44.7 (95% confidence interval (CI): 7.7–261), for long bone fractures was 13.7 (95% CI: 3.4–55), for RH was 33.7 (95% CI: 17.9–63.9), for head and/or neck bruising 4.3 (95% CI: 1.1–17), for apnoea 6.9 (95% CI: 2–22.9), for seizures 5.1 (95% CI: 2–12.9). When rib fractures or RH was present with any one other features the OR for AHT was >10 (positive predictive value: 0.85%). Any combination of three or more of the six features yielded an OR of >100 (positive predictive value >85%).
Conclusion	The probability of AHT can be estimated on the basis of different combinations of the clinical features.
Commentary	Central to determining the presence of AHT is the history provided by the carer. Some features that are noteworthy include (a) absence of trauma to account for the physical findings is frequent, (b) suggesting that the resuscitation process made a significant contribution to the physical findings and (c) the occurrence of persisting neurological finding in the presence of low or no impact trauma. Failure to seek medical attention may not be as strong a predictor as previously thought. The major benefit of this study lies in presenting evidence in court, where it is the 'balance of probabilities' that is being assessed. The physician in the context of the history can quantify the probability of AHT using the ORs. In the case of rib fracture the CIs are very wide and this reflects the small number of children who had this finding.
Reference	Maguire SA, Kemp AM, Lumb RC, *et al.* Estimating the probability of abusive head trauma: a pooled analysis. *Pediatrics.* 2011; **128**(3): e550–64.

Evidence 4	
Theme E4	**Colic and the use of hydrolysed infant formula**
Question	What is the impact of a hydrolysed formula in infants with colic?
Design	Randomised controlled trial
Level of evidence	Jadad 1
Setting	General paediatric practices and the department of paediatrics in an academic medical centre in Italy
Participants	Formula-fed infants less than 4 months of age with a diagnosis of colic, which was defined as three episodes of unexplained full-force crying lasting more than 3 hours a day on at least 3 days a week. Crying episodes were considered significant and recorded by parents when they endured more than 40 minutes.
Intervention	Infants were randomised to receive the study formula (hydrolysed whey proteins, prebiotic oligosaccharides, with a high beta-palmitic acid content) or standard formula and simethicone at a dose of 6 mg/kg/day (control treatment). The paediatrician assessed infants at days 7 and 14.
Outcomes	The primary outcome, record by the parents, was the reduction in the number of full-force inconsolable episodes lasting more than 40 minutes, so that the overall crying time endured less than 3 hours per day. These outcomes were evaluated at days 7 and 14.
Main results	Two hundred and sixty-seven infants were eligible for enrolment, 222 commenced the study and 199 completed it, with 103 in the control group and 96 in the study group. In the treatment group, crying episodes reduced from 5.99 ± 1.84 to 2.47 ± 1.94 at 7 days and to 1.76 ± 1.60 at 14 days – a reduction of 70%. In the control group, crying episodes reduced from 5.41 ± 1.88 to 3.72 ± 1.98 at 7 days and to 3.32 ± 2.06 at 14 days – a reduction of 38.6%. The reduction in crying episodes was 31.4% (number needed to treat = 4).
Conclusion	This new formula reduced the episodes of colic in infants when compared with the standard formula and simethicone.
Commentary	In this study of a partially hydrolysed formula supplemented with fructo and galacto oligosaccharides, there was an improvement in colic symptoms. However, the magnitude of the contribution related to each component cannot be defined. The potential impact from the visits to the paediatrician on days 7 and 14 was not explored.
Reference	Savino F, Palumeri E, Castagno E, *et al.* Reduction of crying episodes owing to infantile colic: a randomized controlled study on the efficacy of a new infant formula. *Eur J Clin Nutr.* 2006; **60**(11): 1304–10.

Evidence 5	
Theme E5	*Behavioural interventions for colic*
Question	What is the effectiveness of the REST Routine behavioural intervention for colic?
Design	Randomised controlled trial
Level of evidence	Jadad 2
Setting	Primary care setting
Participants	Participants were full-term healthy low-risk infants between the ages of 2 and 6 weeks, with an average of 3 hours unexplained crying over a 1- to 2-week period as a minimum. All infants were screened for illness and organic causes for their unexplained excess irritability.
Intervention	Participants were allocated to the REST Routine or standard well child care visit for a 4-week period. A third group was added, to explore change in the control group related to attention or developmental changes alone – this group received only one visit at week 8. The intervention consisted of the REST Routine, which included educational material, a video entitled *Fussy Babies and Frantic Families* and four visits by a masters-prepared paediatric nurse specialist over a 1-month time frame. The control group received routine or standard well child care for a 4-week period.
Outcomes	Outcomes were (a) reduction in crying hours and (b) resolution of irritability at 8 weeks (defined as an average of 1 hour or less per day of unexplained crying or fussiness).
Main results	The treatment group had 64 subjects: the control group 57 and the post-test-only group had 43. Initial unexplained infant crying in both treatment and control group was 5.9 ± 3.5 hours. At the 8-week follow-up for the treatment group it was 1.29 ± 1.21 and for the control group it was 2.94 ± 3.17 hours. For the post-test-only group it was 5.9 hours ± 4.3 hours. The resolution rate for irritability was 61.8% in the treatment group and 28.8% in the control group (absolute risk reduction = 33%; number needed to treat = 3).
Conclusion	The REST Routine and routine well child care were both effective in infants with colic that no intervention. However, the REST Routine was more effective than standard care.
Commentary	In this model the irritable or colicky infant has a disorganised or underdeveloped sleep–wake cycle that underlies the excessive crying and difficulty in initiating sleep. The REST programme is designed to regulate and reduce the infant's level of arousal by environmental and behavioural restructuring. The programme has two components: one for the infant and the other for the parent. For the infant it consists of Regulation (protecting from overstimulation), Entrainment (synchronising the sleep wave cycles with the environment), Structure and Touch. For the parents it consists of Reassurance, Empathy, Support and Time out (at least 1 hour per day). Daily routines that reinforce regularity and predictability in sleeping and feeding are central components to the management strategy.
Reference	Keefe MR, Lobo ML, Froese-Fretz A, *et al*. Effectiveness of an intervention for colic. *Clin Pediatr (Phila)*. 2006; **45**(2): 123–33.

Evidence 6	
Theme E6	*Treatment of breastfed infants with colic*
Question	What is the effect of *Lactobacillus reuteri* DSM 17938 in infantile colic?
Design	Randomised, double-blind, placebo-controlled trial
Level of evidence	Jadad 5
Setting	Paediatric practices and paediatric outpatient departments in an academic medical centre, Italy
Participants	Exclusively breastfed infants, diagnosed with colic defined as episodes of fussy crying that lasted more than 3 hours per day and episodes that lasted for 3 or more days in the week prior to enrolment. Mothers were requested to avoid cow's milk in their diet at enrolment.
Intervention	The study product consisted of a suspension of freeze-dried *L. reuteri* DSM17 938 in a mixture of sunflower oil and medium-chain triglycerides oil supplied in a 5 mL dark bottle fitted with a dropper cap. The placebo was identical but without the live bacteria. Five drops once a day were administered in the morning.
Outcomes	Primary outcome was defined as a reduction of average crying time to less than 3 hours per day on day 21. Secondary outcomes were the number of responders at days 7, 14 and 21. Response was defined as a reduction in crying time of 50% from baseline.
Main results	One hundred and twenty-six infants were eligible, 30 did not give consent and 46 did not meet the inclusion criteria. Fifty infants were randomised, 25 in each group. Forty-six completed the study, 25 in the intervention group and 21 in the control group. Twenty-one (84%) of the intervention group and nine (43%) of the control group had less than 3 hours of crying (absolute risk reduction (ARR) = 41%; number needed to treat (NNT) = 3). For secondary outcomes the response rate in the treatment group at day 21 was 96% versus 71% in the placebo group (ARR = 25%; NNT = 4). There were no adverse affects recorded.
Conclusion	The use of *L. reuteri* DSM 17 938 resulted in improved symptoms in infantile colic and was well tolerated.
Commentary	There is no accepted mechanism of action to explain the positive findings noted in this study. Gut motility and function may be improved and there may be an effect on visceral pain leading to a calming effect and reduction in crying. The clinical impact of the modification of gut microbial groups is uncertain.
Reference	Savino F, Cordisco L, Tarasco V, *et al. Lactobacillus reuteri* DSM 17938 in infantile colic: a randomized, double-blind, placebo-controlled trial. *Pediatrics.* 2010; **126**(3): e526–33.

Evidence 7	
Theme E7	*Maternal diet and colic*
Question	What is the impact of a maternal hypoallergenic diet in breastfed infants with colic?
Design	Randomised controlled trial
Level of evidence	Jadad 3
Setting	Australia
Participants	Exclusively breastfed healthy infants with colic <6 weeks of age participated. Colic was defined as crying for >180 minutes/24 hours on 3 days in the week prior to enrolment.
Intervention	Two maternal diets were used. The low allergenic diet removed dairy products, soy, wheat, eggs, peanuts, tree nuts and fish for 1 week. Calcium supplements were supplied. The control diet consisted of milk and soya powder supplements, with a requirement to eat wheat, peanuts (one serving per day), and one chocolate muesli bar per day. Adherence to diets was monitored through diaries.
Outcomes	The primary outcome was a reduction in cry of greater than 25% on days 8 and 9 compared with baseline at days 1 and 2.
Main results	Two hundred and eleven infants were eligible for enrolment, with 107 being randomised, 53 to the intervention group and 54 to the control group. Forty-seven (89%) of the intervention group and 43 (80%) of the control group completed the study. The primary outcome was achieved in 72% of the test group and 37% of the control group (absolute risk reduction = 37%; number needed to treat = 3). The adherence to the hypoallergenic diet was 98%.
Conclusion	The use of a hypoallergenic diet was effective in the treatment of infants with colic.
Commentary	There is as yet an incomplete understanding of the role of hypersensitivity to food proteins and its contribution to colic. The findings of a mean difference of 3 hours per 48 hours reduction in crying is clinically relevant but the negative impacts of such diets have not been explored.
Reference	Hill DJ, Roy N, Heine RG, *et al.* Effect of a low-allergen maternal diet on colic among breastfed infants: a randomized, controlled trial. *Pediatrics.* 2005: **116**(5); e709–15.

Reference

1. Wessel MA, Cobb JC, Jackson EB, *et al.* Paroxysmal fussing in infancy, sometimes called colic. *Pediatrics.* 1954; **14**: 421–35.

THE CRYING CHILD: MULTIPLE-CHOICE QUESTIONS

Q1   Which of the following conditions is a recognised cause or are recognised causes of acute crying in 4- to 24-month-old infants and children?
a) Colic
b) Supraventricular tachycardia
c) Otitis media
d) Corneal abrasion
e) Subdural haematoma

Q2   Signs of NAI include which of the following?
a) Anterior rib fracture
b) Fractures at various stage of healing
c) Bilateral acute long bone fractures
d) Metaphyseal corner fractures
e) Xiphoid sterna fractures

Q3   Bruising characteristics that suggest NAI include which of the following?
a) Bruise in non-mobile infants
b) Bruises away from bony prominences
c) Bruises over the ears
d) Multiple bruises of the same shape
e) Bruises over the tibial tuberosity

Q4   Recognised causes of irritability in children include which of the following?
a) Gastroenteritis
b) Lactose intolerance
c) Intussusception
d) Dislocation of the hip
e) Tongue tie

Q5   In an infant with an incarcerated hernia, which of the following is/are correct?
a) Vomiting is an early sign.
b) Hydrocoeles are frequently present.
c) Recurrent apnoea is a recognised presentation.
d) Testicular loss occurs in 20% of boys.
e) Bilateral hernias occur in 10%.

Q6   Infections that cause acute crying include which of the following?
a) Herpangina
b) Impetigo
c) Otitis media
d) Urinary tract infection
e) Osteomyelitis

Q7 Features of infantile colic include which of the following?
   a) It presents in the first 2 weeks of life.
   b) Crying typically occurs at night.
   c) Twenty-five per cent of infants have poor growth.
   d) Terminal vomiting with crying is common in 20%.
   e) Colic resolves often by 6 months of age.

Q8 Treatments of colic include which of the following?
   a) Maternal hypoallergenic diets
   b) Probiotics
   c) Gaviscon
   d) Behavioural interventions
   e) Lactulose

Answers

A1	a, b, c, d, e	**A2**	b, c, d
A3	a, b, c, d	**A4**	a, b, c
A5	a, c	**A6**	a, c, d, e
A7	e	**A8**	a, b, d

SLIDES

1. Bruising (Von Willebrand's disease)
2. Bruising of arm (haemophilia)
3. Non-accidental injury (NAI) bruise (pinna)
4. NAI (buttock bruising)
5. Normal bruising leg
6. Raccoon eyes (basal skull fracture)
7. Spider naevus
8. Hydrocephalus (dilated veins)
9. Hydrocephalus
10. Hydrocephalus (setting sun)

Chapter Seven

COMMON PROBLEMS WITH INFANT FEEDING

COMMON SCENARIO

'He's just not putting on weight, the public health nurse has been checking on him every week and his weight just isn't coming up. He just doesn't seem as hungry as my last child, he never wakes for feeds.'

LEARNING OBJECTIVES

- Know the benefits of breastfeeding
- Understand the types of infant formulas available
- Understand the weaning process
- Know the common problems associated with infant feeding
- Understand the impact of formula supplementation in breastfeeding mothers

BACKGROUND

Healthy eating for infants and toddlers means eating a combination of age-appropriate foods that provide sufficient energy and nutrients to allow for growth and development and which also help to optimise health and reduce the risk of disease. Exclusive breastfeeding for 6 months is the feeding option of choice for early infancy as it ensures protection against bacterial and viral infection in addition to its nutritional superiority. However, breastfeeding rates in many countries are low, with mothers opting to feed their children formula feeds. Infant formulae are based on modified cow's milk. Breast milk or infant-based formula should be the main milk drink for the first year of life and unmodified cow's milk should not be used as the main source of milk before 1 year of age. Feeding problems are a common reason for referral to general paediatricians. Frequent formula changes in the first few months of life are not uncommon and frequently unnecessary. Recognising when specialised formula is required is important and should only be used under medical supervision. Weaning the infant onto solids is not necessary before 6 months.

BREASTFEEDING

Breastfeeding has a diverse range of benefits for mothers, babies, families and society and is the optimal method of infant feeding. However breastfeeding has to be learnt and some women may encounter difficulties at the beginning. Ideally, breastfeeding education should start in the antenatal period. Practical assistance is essential after birth in order to ensure the baby is feeding well prior to discharge home. Correct attachment and positioning are fundamental to breastfeeding success. What a mother learns in hospital about breastfeeding and the quality of that experience will affect her breastfeeding skills for a long time and will strongly influence how she feeds her future children. Unfortunately, it is increasingly common for mothers to be discharged before breastfeeding difficulties have been diagnosed, leaving public health nurses, general practitioners and paediatricians with the task of identifying and rectifying feeding problems. Establishing breastfeeding can be a challenging time for mothers particularly if they have had difficulties in the past with breastfeeding, or are not receiving enough support or advice.

Breastfeeding is matched to the specific nutritional requirements of the growing infant and provides protection against infection. The optimal time to initiate breastfeeding is in the period immediately following delivery. The infant's sucking reflex is at its most intense within the first 2 hours after birth. The colostrum is the milk produced in the first 5 days and it contains large amounts of protein, IgA, immunoglobulins and lysozyme and provides immunity within minutes of birth. Milk yield increases gradually over the first 36 hours and this is followed by a dramatic increase during the next 48–96 hours. Breast milk consists of whey proteins in a 60:40 ratio, fat and essential fatty acids and carbohydrate, mainly in the form of lactose. Milk production will be initiated whether or not breastfeeding takes place. However, breastfeeding and milk removal are essential components for the continuation of lactation. Milk removal depends on effective maternal and infant breastfeeding techniques, combined with an intact milk-ejection reflex. (Breast milk is ejected in response to oxytocin secreted in response to suckling.)

Breastfed infants have reduced incidence of:

- acute otitis media and severe lower respiratory tract infections
- non-specific gastroenteritis
- atopic dermatitis and asthma (young children)
- obesity
- type 1 and type 2 diabetes
- necrotising enterocolitis.

Breastfed infants:

- perform better in intelligence tests
- have lower mean blood pressure and total cholesterol.

In addition, there are maternal benefits of breastfeeding including:

- lactational amenorrhoea
- return to pre-pregnant weight sooner
- improved bone remineralisation post-partum
- reduced incidence of:
  - type 2 diabetes
  - breast and ovarian carcinoma
  - early cessation of breastfeeding is associated with an increase incidence of post-natal depression.

Most infants will feed 8–12 times a day. Some infants, however, may develop a pattern of 'cluster feeding': feeding every hour for 2–3 hours, usually in the evening, and then sleeping for 4–5 hours at a time. A normal newborn infant, after the first few days of life, should have at least six wet nappies a day, which is a good indication of their hydration status. On days 3–5 of life, their stools usually change colour from green-black meconium to yellow, seedy mustard-like stools. It is important to remember that in the first couple of weeks of life, breastfed infants tend to have more frequent and higher volume stools than formula-fed infants. Normal babies sleep for 14–16 hours a day, wake for feeds every 2–4 hours and take approximately 20–30 minutes to feed.

Monitoring the infant's weight is extremely important. Babies of first-time breast-feeding mothers should be weighed weekly until breastfeeding is well established. If discharged early, i.e. in the first 24–48 hours of life, babies should be weighed within 2–3 days. Infants lose weight in the initial period after birth; however, most infants should start to regain weight by the end of the first week. By days 10–14 infants should have returned to their birthweight; they subsequently gain 20 g/kg/day.

An infant who is latching on correctly should have his or her mouth wide open before latching on. The infant's mouth should cover the entire nipple and almost all of the areola. The infant's chin should be touching the breast. Brief pauses in the sucking swallowing motion can be observed and heard. Finally the infant's breathing should be co-ordinated with the suck–swallow cycle.

FORMULA FEEDING

Infants who are not breastfed should be fed infant formula for the first year of life. Formula brands are generally divided into two types, depending on whether they are whey or casein protein dominant. Whey-dominant formula has a whey to casein ratio of 60:40. These formulae are made from cow's milk that has been modified to reflect the composition of breast milk. Therefore, they are recommended as 'first milks' for babies who are not being breastfed. Whey-based formula can be used up to 1 year of age.

The second type of infant formula available is casein dominant. This formula, also known as 'second milk', has a whey to casein ratio of 20:80. These formulae are made from cow's milk that has been modified to reflect the protein composition in full-cream cow's milk. These milks are marketed for hungrier babies. Casein-based formula has a similar calorie content to whey-based formula, but the larger casein protein fraction takes longer to digest and so the baby may feel fuller or more satisfied for longer.

The third milk group available is follow-on milks; these again are made from modified cow's milk and contain extra iron, minerals and vitamins. They have been marketed for the older baby – for an infant over 6 months of age. These milks are designed to discourage mothers from feeding unmodified cow's milk to infants less than 1 year of age. However, if the baby is content and gaining weight well, there is no reason to change from a first milk to a follow-on milk. When bottle-feeding, it is better to avoid constantly switching formula feeds every few months. Frequent changes form one brand of formula milk to another is strongly discouraged, as it carries a real possibility of error in preparation and is of questionable usefulness.

After the first few days of life, formula-fed infants take up to 100 mL per kilo per day (1 fluid ounce = 30 mL) and may later settle on 100–120 mL per kilo per day. Fruit drinks should not be given in lieu of milk feeds or at bedtime. Tea, mineral water or fizzy drinks are not suitable drinks for infants. Breast or formula milk should remain the main milk of choice for the first 12 months of life, as cow's milk is too low in iron. Cup drinking should be introduced from after 6–7 months of age and the limiting of bottle feeds should be commenced at this stage.

Average number and volume of formula feeds in infancy		
Age	Feed volume	Number of feeds in 24 hours
1–2 weeks	60 mL	7–8
2–6 weeks	90–120 mL (3–4 oz)	6
2 months	120–180 mL (4–6 oz)	5–6
3 months	180–210 mL (6–7 oz)	5
6 months	210–240 mL (7–8 oz)	4

WEANING TO SOLIDS

Weaning to solid foods should commence from 6 months of age. Infants usually begin with small spoonfuls of a cooked cereal or potato mixed with their usual milk to the consistency of runny yogurt. Expressed breast milk (EBM), infant formula or cooled, boiled water should be used to mix the foods. First feeds should be pureed and be of a soft, runny consistency, without lumps. Once the infant has mastered the art of spoon-feeding, pureed fruit or vegetables can be added. Foods should be introduced one at a time, leaving a few days between addition of each new food. Recommended first foods include gluten-free cereals such as baby rice, mashed potato, pureed fruit with little or no added sugar and pureed vegetables. Pureed meat can be added later on, once weaning is established. Honey carries a small risk of botulism and is not recommended until after 1 year of age. Peanut butter may be included after 6 months of age unless there is a family history of nut allergy or severe atopic disease. By 7–8 months, most infants should be established on a routine of three meals a day. At this stage, infants can begin chewing soft lumps and then progress to mashed and chopped food. By 11–12 months of age, the infant should have progressed to eating the family meals.

COMMON PROBLEMS WITH FEEDING

Jaundice

There are two types of jaundice that can occur in breastfed infants. The first breast-feeding jaundice or exaggerated physiological jaundice may develop in infants due to inadequate milk intake usually on the second or third day of life, before the mother's milk supply comes in. The decrease in caloric intake causes increased entero-hepatic circulation of bilirubin, which leads to jaundice. Jaundice usually resolves by improving milk supply. Jaundice becomes clinically apparent when the serum level of bilirubin rises above 85 µmol/L. There is a normal progression of the depth of jaundice from head to toe as the level of bilirubin rises (the Kramer Rule); however, clinical estimation of jaundice is difficult, particularly in dark-skinned infants. Physiological jaundice does not occur before 24 hours of age.

Prolonged jaundice refers to jaundice persisting beyond the first 2 weeks of life in the term neonate. Breast milk jaundice occurs in 20%–30% of breastfeeding infants and is a diagnosis of exclusion. Breast milk jaundice causes prolonged jaundice in a healthy, thriving newborn, with normal stools and urine. The jaundice resolves gradually over a period of weeks; however, it may persist for up to 3 months. Although there are many causes of prolonged jaundice such as hypothyroidism and infection, the most important cause to rule out is biliary atresia, which presents with pale stools and dark urine.

Dehydration

One of the most serious consequences of inadequate breast milk intake is hypernatraemic dehydration. It is a potentially devastating condition, which can lead to seizures, permanent neurological and vascular damage if not recognised and treated early. It is defined as a serum sodium of greater than 145 mmol/L. It is caused by a deficit of total body water relative to total body sodium levels due to loss of free water. A weight loss of 10% should be considered a warning sign that an infant is not receiving enough milk.

Failure to thrive

Insufficient milk supply can result in both hypernatraemic dehydration and failure to thrive. If failure to thrive alone is present, then milk is adequate to maintain the infant's hydration but insufficient to allow adequate growth and development. Failure to thrive in an infant should not be attributed to breastfeeding without an exploration of other differential diagnoses unrelated to feeding, such as urinary tract infection, cardiac disease, oral thrush or severe gastro-oesophageal reflux.

Gastro-oesophageal reflux

Most normal babies have some degree of gastro-oesophageal reflux. In the vast majority of cases it is benign and resolves by 6–12 months of age. Reflux presents with 'spitting up' or regurgitation, which is the passive return of gastric contents up into the oesophagus. Infants with simple reflux gain weight normally and do not have signs or symptoms of oesophagitis or any systemic signs.

Lactose intolerance

Lactose is a disaccharide present in milk. Lactase, a duodenal brush border enzyme, is needed in order to digest lactose and break it down into glucose and galactose, which can be absorbed into the blood stream. Symptoms of lactose intolerance generally occur within a couple of hours of ingestion of milk. Symptoms include frequent watery stools, irritability or colic, abdominal distension and weight loss. The occurrence of primary lactose intolerance is extremely rare; however infants can develop secondary lactose intolerance after gastroenteritis. Symptoms generally last only a few weeks. Although investigations can be performed, they are generally not recommended in young infants as they are rarely diagnostic and can often be misleading.

Cow's milk protein allergy

Cow's milk allergy can be difficult to diagnose, it is often confused with lactose intolerance and colic. It is estimated that the prevalence of cow's milk protein allergy is only 2%–7%. Cow's milk protein allergy is caused by an immunological reaction to one or more proteins present in milk. It includes both IgE-mediated reactions, which are immediate, and non-IgE-mediated reactions, which are delayed. Cow's milk protein allergy can range from mild to severe. Symptoms and signs are varied, but include frequent regurgitation, vomiting, diarrhoea with blood in the stool, colic or persistent distress, atopic dermatitis and in severe cases failure to thrive and anaphylactoid reactions.

Mastitis

Correct positioning skills will minimise problems such as sore and cracked nipples, breast engorgement and mastitis. Mastitis is localised inflammation of the breast accompanied by flu-like signs and symptoms. The incidence of mastitis in lactating women varies from 10% to 33%. It is more likely to occur within the first 12 weeks of breastfeeding. It occurs as a result of incomplete removal of milk from the breasts, which may or may not be accompanied by or progress to infection. It is more likely to occur if nipples are cracked, as this provides a portal of entry for bacteria. The commonest causative organism is *Staphylococcus aureus*.

BREASTFEEDING HISTORY

KEY POINTS				
Birth history	Gestation Birth weight Discharge weight Complications at birth Admission to special care baby unit or neonatal intensive care unit Ventilation Nasogastric feeds	**Maternal education and support**	Ever breastfed before? Received breastfeeding education Aware of support groups	**🔍 Red flags** Lack of antenatal education Poor peer or family support especially if breastfeeding Reduced volume of milk intake Excessive time spent feeding the infant Maternal fatigue
Breastfeeding	Frequency of feeds Duration of feeds Night-time feeds 'Clustering of feed' Ability to latch on	**Maternal concerns**	Nipple pain Cracked nipples	
Stooling and voiding	Number of wet and dirty nappies Colour and consistency of stool	**General health**	Content after feeds Restless or crying Waking for feed Good suck Level of alertness	
Weight	Weight loss in first 10 days of life Average weekly weight gain Vomiting Regurgitation			

EXAMINATION

- Weight, length and head circumference should be plotted on appropriate centile chart
- If possible, observe a feed
- Assess level of alertness, tone and posture
- Signs of jaundice
- Signs of dehydration

- Examine the oral cavity
- Examine for hepatosplenomegaly

 Red flags
- Dehydration
- Failure to thrive
- Lethargy
- Jaundice

INVESTIGATIONS

If jaundice is clinically suspected, what investigations should be performed?

Transcutaneous bilirubin measurements can be used in the initial assessment of jaundice. This is a fast, non-invasive means of determining the need for further evaluation. It correlates well with serum bilirubin levels but is inaccurate at high levels.

Total serum bilirubin, direct Coombs' test, blood group, full blood count and urea and electrolytes should be taken.

What investigations should be performed in infants with gastro-oesophageal reflux?

In general, if the child is thriving, no investigations are required. The gold standard investigation for infants with suspected gastro-oesophageal disease is a 24-hour pH oesophageal monitor. It measures the frequency and duration of acid reflux episodes into the oesophagus.

MANAGEMENT PLAN: TWO-STEP APPROACH

1. Clarifying and pitfall avoidance strategies:
   a) mother
   b) doctors
2. Common feeding problems:
   a) management of insufficient breast milk supply
   b) maternal breastfeeding problems
   c) jaundice
   d) secondary lactose intolerance
   e) gastro-oesophageal reflux
   f) cow's milk allergy

Clarifying and pitfall avoidance strategies

Mother

- Prenatal education. **Rationale:** to enhance success rates at breastfeeding, the attendance at prenatal educational classes is beneficial. While the focus of these classes traditionally has been on labour and delivery, postnatal issues are now incorporated into the curriculum. Providing anticipatory information to mothers better prepares them for breastfeeding and addresses the challenges that it may present. Unfortunately the lack of standardised education leads to postpartum difficulties (*see* Evidence 1).

- Breastfeeding and formula supplementation. **Rationale and Pitfall**: healthcare providers are divided on the best strategy to address this issue. This can be frustrating for parents. One option, to aid mothers who are experiencing difficulties, is early limited formula use (*see* Evidence 2).
- Weaning. **Rationale**: the best method of weaning is not known. In infant-led weaning (gradual weaning), mothers take their cues from the baby and start the process as the amounts and types of complementary foods increase. This weaning process is complete by 2–4 years. In mother-led weaning (planned weaning), the process is initiated by the mother without receiving cues from the infant.
- Allergy prevention and breastfeeding. **Rationale**: breastfeeding reduces the risk but does not prevent the occurrence of allergic disorders. If breastfeeding mothers wish to reduce the risk of allergic disease when they stop breastfeeding, the use of extensively hydrolysed formulas is helpful (*see* Evidence 3).
- Soother use by parents. **Rationale**: while soother use is not encouraged, they are used and mothers are not influenced by the views of healthcare providers (*see* Evidence 4). The use of soothers may reflect maternal concerns with regard to the baby's temperament or feeding difficulties.

Doctors

- Breastfeeding and supplementation. **Pitfall**: the lack of a uniform response to supplementation by the breastfeeding mother is a cause of confusion for parents. The difference between protocols and practice adds to the confusion (*see* Evidence 1).

Common feeding problems

Management of insufficient breast milk supply

Ensuring a correct feeding pattern and feeding technique can resolve most cases of perceived insufficient milk supply. Breastfeeding mothers should be encouraged and supported. A feed should be observed to assess technique and identify problems such as latching on difficulties; this enables practitioners to give advice on positioning and attachment. Mothers should be given advice about the frequency and duration of feeds and the need to wake sleepy or 'undemanding' babies at regular intervals for feeding.

If increasing the frequency of breastfeeding does not lead to an increased milk supply, mothers should be advised to start expressing milk after feeding and offer EBM as top-ups after breastfeeds. Mothers may express milk by hand or by using an electric pump. Mothers should be directed to use the pump to express milk from the breast after the baby has breastfed. They should pump for approximately 10–15 minutes, ideally using a dual collection system that allows drainage of both breasts simultaneously. This allows the mother to maintain an adequate milk supply and provides breast milk supplements as top-ups.

Despite establishing a correct feeding pattern and feeding technique, approximately 5% of breastfeeding mothers will not produce enough milk to provide adequate nutrition for their infant. Mothers should continue breastfeeding; however they will need additional supplementation with formula.

If failure to thrive is secondary to insufficient milk supply then mothers should be encouraged to continue breastfeeding every 3 hours, EBM top-ups should be given. If EBM top-ups do not result in adequate weight gain then supplementation with formula is needed. Infants need close monitoring and regular weight checks to ensure that supplementation results in improved weight gain.

Maternal breastfeeding problems

Mild degrees of breast engorgement in the mother can be managed by ensuring that the infant feeds both effectively and frequently to aid breast emptying. Ensuring correct breastfeeding technique can prevent cracked nipples.

The four principles of treatment for mastitis are:
1. supportive counselling
2. effective milk removal
3. antibiotic therapy
4. symptomatic treatment.

Mothers should be provided with ongoing support and reassured about the value of continued breastfeeding. As stasis increases the risk of abscess formation, mothers should be advised to increase the frequency of feeds in order to empty the breasts; if necessary, milk may need to be expressed. The condition can be extremely painful and distressing for mothers; therefore, regular analgesia is needed. Flucloxacillin is the first-line antibiotic for the treatment of mastitis. As short courses of antibiotics are associated with a higher incidence of relapse, the recommended duration of treatment is 10–14 days.

Jaundice

Breastfeeding jaundice is managed by increasing the frequency and duration of breastfeeding to increase milk ingestion and improve caloric consumption. Neonates may require intensive phototherapy if bilirubin levels are above the treatment line on standard normographs used to monitor bilirubin levels.

Secondary lactose intolerance

If symptoms are severe, a trial of lactose-free formula can be given for a few weeks until the brush border enzymes recover.

Gastro-oesophageal reflux

Most infants with uncomplicated gastro-oesophageal reflux do not require treatment and respond to conservative measures alone. Feeds can be thickened with formula thickeners such as carobel or commercially available formulas can be utilised (*see*

Evidence 5). These formulas are of normal consistency, but thicken on contact with stomach acid.

Cow's milk allergy

Infants with severe symptoms require specialist referral; however, those with mild to moderate symptoms can be managed by an elimination diet, which should be given for at least 2–4 weeks to assess response. If symptoms improve or disappear on an elimination diet, an open challenge should be performed. Milk challenges should be performed according to local protocols and under medical supervision with resuscitation facilities. If symptoms reappear, then the diagnosis of cow's milk protein allergy is confirmed and the infant should be maintained on an elimination diet for at least 6 months or until the child is 9–12 months of age, at which time the challenge should be repeated. Children who do not develop either immediate or delayed symptoms after the milk challenge can resume a normal diet. Extensively hydrolysed formulas are the first choice for an elimination diet. An amino acid formula is indicated if the child refuses to drink the hydrolysed formula or if symptoms do not improve on the hydrolysed formula.

FOLLOW-UP

- All infants discharged from the maternity hospital should have a follow-up weight check with their public health nurse within 2–3 days.
- If there is concern about poor weight gain, infants should continue to be followed up until weight gain improves.
- Infants who are discharged home with mild jaundice should be followed up to ensure it does not progress.

WHEN TO REFER?

- An infant who has lost more than 10%–12% of his or her birthweight
- Jaundiced infant with pale stools and dark urine needs urgent referral
- If there is concern that the level of jaundice may be high or increasing
- An unwell infant with signs or symptoms of sepsis or dehydration

CLARIFICATION STATEMENTS FOR PARENTAL MISCONCEPTIONS

'If breastfeeding is so natural, why am I experiencing difficulties?'

Breastfeeding is described as natural, but this does not imply easy. First-time mothers require support if they are experiencing difficulties. The importance of prenatal education to effect successful breastfeeding cannot be underestimated. Institutions need to ensure that support is offered to mothers, especially out of hours.

'Why am I getting such confusing advice about supplementation with formula? What's the problem?'

Breastfeeding supplementation is controversial. The 'Baby Friendly Hospital Initiative' campaign has been developed to increase breastfeeding rates and it recommends the reduction or avoidance of formula supplementation. There is no agreed national policy on supplementation but evidence is evolving that some supplementation is required for specific infants if mothers are to continue to breastfeed.

'So if I breastfeed, my baby won't get eczema.'

Not quite – breastfeeding reduces the risk of allergic disorders but it does not guarantee their prevention.

'It can't be normal for babies to spit up; maybe he is allergic to the formula!'

Spitting up is normal and occurs in the majority of infants. Cow's milk allergy should be considered in the differential diagnosis of those infants who have symptoms of gastro-oesophageal reflux disease.

SUMMARY PRACTICE POINTS
- Breastfeeding education should start antenatally.
- Breast milk volume increases gradually over the first 36 hours and dramatically from day 3–4 onwards.
- Jaundice on day 1 is never physiological.
- The degree of jaundice cannot be reliably assessed from examination of the skin.
- There is a marked difference between the symptoms of gastro-oesophageal reflux and gastro-oesophageal reflux disease.
- Inadequate breast milk intake can lead to hypernatraemic dehydration.
- Mothers do not rely on healthcare professionals when deciding on soother use.
- Soother use may indicate feeding difficulties; therefore, ask why mother has instigated its use.
- Early limited formula use should be considered for a breastfeeding mother whose infant is experiencing weight loss.

EVALUATING THE EVIDENCE

Evidence 1	
Theme E1	***Supplementation of breastfeeding infants***
Question	What are the beliefs and practices of doctors and nurses relating to supplementation of breastfeeding infants?
Design	Design cross-sectional cohort study
Level of evidence	
Setting	Maternity and paediatric departments, academic medical centre, Canada
Participants	All nurses and attending (consultant) paediatricians working in postpartum wards and level 2 nurseries in five hospitals were invited to participate.
Intervention	Questionnaire completion was the intervention in this study.
Outcomes	The primary outcomes were (a) methods of supplementation used, (b) decision-making on the use of supplementation and (c) safety and convenience of breastfeeding supplementation.
Main results	A convenience sample of 87 nurses and 16 paediatricians responded to the survey. With regard to institutional practices, postpartum and neonatal nurses reported as follows: (a) cup feeding 96% and 73% (b) bottle feeding 96% and 90% (c) nasogastric feeding 17% and 100% (d) finger feeding 96% and 44% (e) other type of feeding 37% and 32%. The supplementation actually performed by the postpartum and neonatal nurses were: (a) cup feeding 68% and 46% (b) bottle feeding 59% and 87% (c) nasogastric feeding 6.5% and 97.3% (d) finger feeding 58% and 11%. Persons involved in the decision on the type of supplementation method (multiple input possible): nurse leadership 14%, nurses 77%, paediatrician 42%, resident (Non-Consultant Hospital Doctor) 14% and others 58%. Cup feeding and finger feeding were deemed unsafe by nurses (43% and 18%, respectively). Finger feeding and cup feeding were deemed unsafe by 41% and 61% of doctors. With regard to supplementation with bottle feeding and occurrence of nipple confusion, 15% of neonatal nurses agreed, compared with 44.4% of postpartum nurses and 56.2% of paediatricians. Parental involvement in the decision to offer supplements was 81.2% for most of the time (sometimes, 16.5%; rarely, 2%).
Conclusion	There is considerable variation in the beliefs and practices surrounding the supplementation methods in breastfeeding mothers.
Commentary	The issue of nipple confusion is not resolved and this study outlines diverse methods of supplementation. The difference between institutional practice and healthcare provider preference is obvious, and can lead to difficulty for the breastfeeding mother, as advice may not be consistent. The situation is further confounded due to a lack of evidence that can support a specific practice.

(*continued*)

Evidence 1	
Theme E1	***Supplementation of breastfeeding infants***
Reference	Al-Sahab B, Feldman M, Macpherson A, *et al*. Which method of breastfeeding supplementation is best? The beliefs and practices of paediatricians and nurses. *Paediatr Child Health*. 2010; **15**(7): 427–31.

Evidence 2	
Theme E2	***Formula supplementation and breastfeeding***
Question	What is the effect of early limited formula supplementation in breastfed infants?
Design	Randomised controlled trial
Level of evidence	Jadad 5
Setting	Department of paediatrics, academic medical centre, the United States
Participants	Infants of exclusively breastfeeding infants were eligible for enrolment if they (a) were 37 weeks or older, (b) had lost ≥5% but ≤10% body weight before 36 hours and (c) were 24–48 hours old at enrolment. Exclusion criteria included formula or water usage.
Intervention	After enrolment the early limited formula intervention group received 10 mL of extensively hydrolysed formula (Nutramigen), by syringe and performed by the mother, after each breastfeed until mature milk production began, and the control group was taught infant soothing techniques for 15 minutes (and continued exclusive breastfeeding until mature milk production began).
Outcomes	The primary outcomes were formula supplementation at 1 week and exclusive breastfeeding at 3 months
Main results	Twenty infants were enrolled in each group, and the mean weight loss was 6.0% ± 0.9%. Lactogenesis stage II occurred at a mean of 3.1 ± 1.2 days in both groups. In the treatment group 90% of mothers were exclusively breastfeeding at 1 week compared with 53% in the control group (absolute risk reduction (ARR) = 37%; number needed to treat (NNT) = 3), at 3 months 79% of the intervention group were exclusively breastfeeding compared with 42% of controls (ARR = 37%; NNT = 3).
Conclusion	Early limited formula supplementation lessens formula feeding rates at 1 week and increases breastfeeding rates at 3 months. Early limited formula may be a useful temporary coping strategy for the breastfeeding mother until mature milk production begins.
Commentary	At birth, mothers do not produce copious volumes of mature milk but instead begin with the secretion of 1–5 mL of colostrum per feed. While healthcare providers may attempt to reassure mothers, this may be unsuccessful and they may believe that their milk supply is insufficient. Usually formula supplementation is not recommended in breastfeeding mothers and is associated with early reduction of breastfeeding rates.

(continued)

Evidence 2	
Theme E2	*Formula supplementation and breastfeeding*
Commentary (*cont.*)	However, this intervention was carefully crafted: (a) volumes were small (10 mL/post breastfeed), (b) a syringe was used to deliver the formula (to avoid confusion associated with bottle's nipple) and (c) it was time limited. The results are important, given the current public health emphasis on formula reduction in hospitals. The use of early limited formula in targeted cases could well increase breastfeeding success rates. The sample size of this study is small and a large study is warranted to confirm the clinical gain achieved.
Reference	Flaherman VJ, Aby J, Burgos AE, *et al.* Effect of early limited formula on duration and exclusivity of breastfeeding in at-risk infants: an RCT. *Pediatrics.* 2013; **131**(6): 1059–65.

Evidence 3	
Theme E3	*Allergy and formula ingestion: can allergy be prevented in infants with formula?*
Question	Can allergy be prevented in infants with formula?
Design	Randomised controlled trial
Level of evidence	Jadad 5
Setting	Community-based setting, two regions in Germany
Participants	Parents with a healthy newborn and at least one family member (mother, father or biological sibling) with an allergic disease were eligible for inclusion.
Intervention	Patients received one of the following: (a) cow's milk formula (CMF), (b) partially hydrolysed whey formula (pHF-W), (c) an extensively hydrolysed whey formula (eHF-W) and (d) a lactose-free, extensively hydrolysed casein formula (eHF-C).
Outcomes	The primary outcome was the presence of an allergic manifestation in the first 12 months of life. Allergic manifestations were categorised as allergic dermatitis, allergic urticaria or food allergy with gastrointestinal manifestation.
Main results	Study formula was given to 1249 infants but 166 (13%) dropped before the 12 months' follow-up and 138 of 1083 (13%) were non-compliant. The following are the number and completion rate for each formula: (a) CMF commenced 328, full data available 256 (78%) (b) pHF-W commenced 315, completed 241 (76.5%) (c) eHF-W commenced 302 completed 236 (78.4%) (d) eHF-C commenced 304 completed 210 (69%). The allergic manifestations in the CMF were 16%, and 9% in the EHF-C (absolute risk reduction (ARR) = 7%; number needed to treat (NNT) = 13) and reduced by 5% in the pHF-W group (ARR = 5%; NNT = 20).
Conclusion	In families with allergic diseases, modifying the occurrence of allergic disease is feasible by dietary interventions.
Commentary	Parents are keen to eliminate, if possible, disease states in their children and some will wish to resort to modified formula use to reduce their risk. Parents will view the odds of 6:1 as high and modifying them to 10:1 will be seen as acceptable.

(*continued*)

Evidence 3	
Theme E3	*Allergy and formula ingestion: can allergy be prevented in infants with formula?*
Commentary (*cont.*)	The most effective formula had the highest dropout rate and this is related to its lack of palatability. In those fed CMF the occurrence of allergic manifestations, in 40 patients, was as follows: allergic dermatitis, 38; urticarial, one; and food allergy with gastrointestinal manifestation, one.
Reference	Von Berg A, Koletzko S, Grübl A, *et al*. German Infant Nutritional Intervention Study Group. The effect of hydrolyzed cow's milk formula for allergy prevention in the first year of life: the German Infant Nutritional Intervention Study, a randomized double-blind trial. *J Allergy Clin Immunol*. 2003; **111**(3): 533–40.

Evidence 4	
Theme E4	*Pacifier use by parents*
Question	What are the predictors of and reasons for pacifier use in first-time mothers?
Design	Cohort study
Level of evidence	
Setting	Department of dietetics, academic medical centre, Australia
Participants	In total, 670 first-time mothers were recruited to complete a questionnaire regarding infant feeding and pacifier use.
Intervention	The intervention was an evidence-based and expert opinion survey related to pacifiers.
Outcomes	The primary outcomes were (a) age of commencement of pacifier use, (b) frequency of use, (c) those persons, if any, who advise its use and (d) reason for use.
Main results	Of the 698 enrolled, full data were available on 670 (97.2%). The mean age of infants at baseline was 18.6 weeks and 97% were still breastfeeding to some extent. Five hundred and thirty-two (79%) had used a pacifier and 464 (69%) were currently using one. The median age of pacifier introduction was 2 weeks of age, with two-thirds commencing prior to 4 weeks. Three hundred and ninety-five (85.1%) were using pacifiers daily. Those who advised use were (a) no one (30.6%); (b) mother or mother-in-law (28.7%); (c) midwife (22.7%); (d) friends (20.25%); (e) other family member (16.6%); (f) husband (16.6%); (g) child health nurse (9.8%); and (h) doctor/general practitioner (3.2%). Multiple responses were allowed. The main reasons for use included: (a) soothe infant (78.3%); (b) aid sleeping (57.4%); (c) comfort or keep baby quiet (40.4%); (d) natural for babies to suck (21.9%); and (e) stretch time between feeds (12.6%). Pacifier use before 4 weeks and used on most days were associated with reduced breastfeeding (adjusted hazard ratio = 3.67 and 3.28, respectively).
Conclusion	This study identified the reasons for pacifier use and the potential negative impact on breastfeeding rates.
Commentary	The 'Baby Friendly Hospital Initiative' campaign actively discourages pacifier use. For breastfeeding parents the use of pacifiers may reflect difficulties in or reduced motivation to breastfeed. This may in turn lead to early weaning.

(*continued*)

Evidence 4

Theme E4	Pacifier use by parents
Commentary (cont.)	Parents need counselling on appropriate soothing techniques when their baby exhibits signs of fussiness. The relationship between pacifier use and otitis media is unclear. Pacifier sucking may impair Eustachian tube functioning, but the mechanism triggering otitis media is uncertain. Pacifiers should not be covered with sugar or honey. Dental caries, malocclusion and gingival recession only occur with pronged use (>5 years) and with the use of sweetened pacifiers.
Reference	Mauch CE, Scott JA, Magarey AM, et al. Predictors of and reasons for pacifier use in first-time mothers: an observational study. BMC Pediatr. 2012; 12: 7.

Evidence 5

Theme E5	Infant regurgitation and formula thickeners
Question	What is the effect of cornstarch thickening to feeds of infants who have vomiting related to gastro-oesophageal reflux?
Design	Randomised controlled trial
Level of evidence	Jadad 5
Setting	Department of paediatrics, academic medical centres, Belgium, Greece, France, Morocco
Participants	Healthy infants with vomiting and excessive regurgitation were eligible for inclusion. If infants were very irritable, had haematemesis, passed black stool, had chronic cough or episodes of cyanosis, they were excluded.
Intervention	Infants were randomised to receive regular infant formula or cornstarch thickened casein predominant formula. The caloric content of both formulas was identical. Monitoring of pH was undertaken both at baseline and at 1 month.
Outcomes	The primary outcome was the change in baseline symptoms of vomiting and regurgitation from baseline to assessment at 1 month post intervention.
Main results	Ninety-six infants, 45 in the regular formula group (mean age 95 ± 32 days) and 51 in the thickened formula group (mean age 92 ± 35 days), were enrolled. For the thickened formula group, baseline symptoms of regurgitation/day reduced from 5.6 ± 4.15 to 2.56 ± 2.71 (54%) at 1 month; in the regular formula group, baseline symptoms reduced from 4.77 ± 2.35 to 4.31 ± 2.01 (9.6%) at 1 month (absolute risk reduction (ARR) = 44.4%; number needed to treat (NNT) = 3). With regard to vomiting episodes, the thickened formula group reduced from 4.34 ± 2.42 to 1.45 ± 1.65 (31%) and the regular formula group reduced from 3.09 ± 1.24 to 2.74 ± 1.37 (11%) (ARR = 20%; NNT = 5). The reflux index for thickened formula changed from 14.9 ± 10.9 to 6.8 ± 6.2 at 1 month (54% reduction) compared with the standard formula, where the reflux index was 13.3 ± 6.4 at baseline to 11.4 ± 7.0 at 1 month (14% reduction) (ARR = 40%; NNT = 3).
Conclusion	A casein-dominant formula thickened with specifically treated cornstarch reduces the frequency of clinical symptoms of gastro-oesophageal reflux and reduces oesophageal acid exposure.

(continued)

Evidence 5	
Theme E5	Infant regurgitation and formula thickeners
Commentary	This study confirms the benefit of thickened feeds (in this study with cornstarch) in the reduction of symptoms of gastro-oesophageal reflux. Infants with gastro-oesophageal reflux DISEASE were not included. Gastro-oesophageal reflux is defined as the involuntary passage of gastric contents into the oesophagus. The frequency of regurgitation peaks at 3 months and usually resolves by 12 months (when the child is walking). Thickening formulas with cornstarch, potato starch, rice and bean gum have been developed commercially. The cornstarch used in the thickened formula was re-gelatinised cornstarch, which had previously been shown to decrease regurgitation and vomiting as well as episodes of acid reflux. When commencing thickened feeds, for gastro-oesophageal reflux, it is best to advise that symptom reduction is the most likely outcome rather that no symptoms.
Reference	Xinias I, Mouane N, Le Luyer B, et al. Cornstarch thickened formula reduces oesophageal acid exposure time in infants. Dig Liv Dis. 2005; **37**(1): 23–7.

INFANT FEEDING: MULTIPLE-CHOICE QUESTIONS

Q1 The benefits of breastfeeding include which of the following?
a) Reduction in incidence of otitis media
b) Reduction in allergic dermatitis
c) Reduced obesity levels
d) Reduction in occurrence of croup
e) Reduced incidence of asthma

Q2 Which of the following statements with regard to exaggerated physiological jaundice is/are true?
a) It is associated with reduced milk intake.
b) It is manifest at 24 hours of age.
c) The direct serum bilirubin is usually >85 mmol/L.
d) Its severity can be estimated clinically as mild, moderate or severe.
e) There is enhanced enterohepatic circulation of bilirubin.

Q3 Which of the following statements is/are true of prolonged jaundice?
a) It occurs after 6 weeks of age.
b) It occurs in 2% of breastfed babies.
c) The stools are normal.
d) The urine is dark.
e) Biliary atresia is a cause of 1% of cases.

Q4 Which of the following is/are features of cow's milk protein allergy?
a) Colic
b) Blood in the infant's stools
c) Gastro-oesophageal reflux disease
d) Urticaria
e) Atopic dermatitis

Q5 Features of gastro-oesophageal reflux include which of the following?
a) Weight loss
b) Arching of the back
c) Regurgitation
d) Vomiting
e) Excessive weight gain

Q6 Which of the following is/are correct, regarding soother use in infants and children?
a) Soothers are usually recommended by healthcare professionals
b) Complication include malocclusion
c) Complications include caries
d) Soother use may reflect a feeding difficulty
e) Adding sugar to a soother is useful to promote sucking

Answers

A1	a, b, c		**A2**	a, e
A3	c		**A4**	a, b, c, d, e
A5	c, d		**A6**	d

Chapter Eight

FOOD ALLERGY IN CHILDREN

COMMON SCENARIO

'After he ate the peanut he began to feel unwell, he developed hives on his skin and he became wheezy. It was really scary.'

LEARNING OBJECTIVES

- Understand the causes of food allergy
- Understand the mechanisms of food allergy
- Know the clinical presentations of food allergy
- Understand the value of the test for food allergy
- Be able to counsel and advise parents to deal with allergic reactions

BACKGROUND

The prevalence of food allergies is increasing in industrialised countries, most likely as a consequence of changes in dietary habits and a reduction in exposure to early childhood infections. The mechanism of food allergies is IgE mediated, non-IgE mediated or a combination of both. Surprisingly, only eight foods (cow's milk, soy, hen's eggs, peanuts, tree nuts and seeds, wheat, fish and shellfish) account for 90% of all food allergies in the population. In children, allergies to milk, peanuts and eggs are the most frequent and, as a consequence, parents will require specific information on them. Fortunately, good-quality data can be provided to parents on these topics.

Cow's milk allergy

Cow's milk allergy has a prevalence of 2.2%–2.8% at 1 year of age and about 60% of reactions are IgE mediated. Casein and whey proteins account for 80% and 20%, respectively, of the milk protein. The most important whey allergens are alpha lactoglobulin and beta lactoglobulin, the allergenicity of which is reduced by cooking. Skin prick testing (SPT) is useful in assessing cow's milk allergy; in children younger than 2 years of age, a weal >6 mm or a cow's milk-specific IgE level >5 kUA/L is predictive; for children older than 2 years, a wheal of >8 mm is predictive. From a prognosis perspective, 64% of children will develop tolerance by 12 years of age, which has significant dietary and lifestyle implications.

Peanut allergy

Peanut allergy has a prevalence of 1.6%. The proteins that trigger peanut allergy in North America are Ara h1, Ara h2 and Ara h3, but in southern Europe they are Ara h8 and Ara h9. Peanut allergy typically occurs before 2 years of age, often with significant respiratory symptoms; however the source of the peanut is often obvious, in that the child may have had it as a snack. Peanut allergy often occurs with other atopic conditions including atopic dermatitis, allergic rhinitis and asthma. Children with peanut allergy have a skin prick test of >6 to 8 mm to peanut or a peanut-specific IgE level >14 to 25 kUA/L. Children can outgrow peanut allergy and should be followed up with yearly IgE levels for subsiding reactions. In children with peanut allergy, asthma control must be optimal. Despite a significant amount of research, the mechanism that determines the severity of the peanut reaction is still poorly understood.

Egg allergy

In children with egg allergy the responsible proteins are Gal d1 to Gal d5, which are found in the egg white. Ovomucoid is the dominant egg allergen, probably related to its heat stability. Typically, the first clinical symptoms occur at 6 months of age. Sensitisation may have occurred with atopic dermatitis, or through breast milk protein. Symptoms occur within 2 hours of ingestion and typically include urticarial, respiratory and gastrointestinal (GI) symptoms (acute vomiting). In known asthmatics anaphylaxis often occurs. SPT aids the diagnosis (in conjunction with the history of ingestion) if the wheal is >5 mm for a child younger than 2 years and >7 mm for a child older than 2 years. Egg-specific IgE level is usually >7 kUA/L if older than 2 years and >2 kUA/L if younger than 2 years. Test results unfortunately do not correlate with the clinical reaction severity. Over time most children can tolerate extensively heated or baked eggs. The natural history of egg allergy is variable, with 4% having resolution at 4 years, 12% at 6 years, 37% at 10 years and 68% at 16 years.

Definition of terms
- **Food allergy**: this is defined as an adverse reaction health effect arising from a specific immune response that occurs reproducibly on exposure to a given food.
- **Food intolerance**: this relates to the production of symptoms through non-immunological mechanisms (e.g. lactose intolerance due to the absence of the enzyme lactase).
- **Tolerance**: this term denotes that an individual is symptom free after consumption of a food to which there were symptoms in the past (i.e. has outgrown food allergy).

Presentations of food allergy

- Food-induced anaphylaxis
- GI food allergies:
  - immediate GI hypersensitivity
  - eosinophilic oesophagitis
  - eosinophilic gastroenteritis
  - food protein-induced allergic proctocolitis
  - food protein-induced enterocolitis syndrome
  - oral allergy syndrome
- Cutaneous:
  - acute urticaria
  - angioedema
  - atopic dermatitis (atopic eczema)
  - allergic contact dermatitis
  - contact urticaria
- Respiratory symptoms:
  - Heiner's syndrome

HISTORY

KEY POINTS				
Food ingested	8 foods account for 90% of food allergies Specific questions related to the food ingested: Has it caused similar symptoms in the past? What quantity was ingested? Have the symptoms been present in the absence of the food ingested?	**Past medical history**	History of urticarial (recurrent or contact urticaria) Atopic dermatitis Gastro-oesophageal reflux not responding to standard antireflux therapy Colic Asthma	**❶ Red flags** Anaphylaxis recurrent Especially urticaria with respiratory or cardiovascular symptoms Collapse History of acute vomiting on exposure to a specific food Contact urticaria Atopic dermatitis aggravated by food ingestion
Onset of symptoms	Symptoms less 2 hours after ingestion of potential allergen What treatment was given and what was the response?	**Dietary history**	Ingestion of potentially allergenic foods and impact Do family avoid specific foods and why (may have had reaction in past)?	

(continued)

KEY POINTS				
Skin	Urticaria acute onset Urticaria on direct contact with the skin Tingling of lips Swelling of lips	**Parental beliefs about allergy**	Check if parents or other siblings have allergy, check timelines to occurrence of symptoms	
Respiratory	Stridor Wheeze Feeling of dyspnoea Feeling of impending doom	**Drug history**	What medication did child take to address the symptoms? Has the child been given antihistamines?	
GI tract	Acute vomiting Itchy throat Abdominal pain	**Central nervous system**	Unresponsive state	
Ear, nose and throat	Clear rhinorrhoea sometimes profuse	**Cardiovascular**	Increase in heart rate, feeling light-headed	

EXAMINATION

- Ask the patient how he or she is feeling – if they say scared, presume they are hypoxic
- Height and weight (estimate if emergency state)
- Skin: check for urticaria, location (around the mouth or generalised), angioedema
- Cardiovascular: heart rate, blood pressure, perfusion status (capillary refill)
- Respiratory rate, stridor (inspiratory, expiratory or both),
- Wheeze pitch (inspiratory, expiratory or both), air entry
- Assess abdomen
- Level of consciousness

Red flags

- Feeling anxious
- Unable to speak or sounding hoarse
- Stridor, hypotension, collapsed state

DIFFERENTIAL DIAGNOSIS

Clinical condition	Feature of allergy	Differentiating features
Food intolerances (lactose intolerance)	Diarrhoea, abdominal discomfort	Absence of cutaneous and respiratory manifestations
Urticaria	Skin has flares and wheals	Only cutaneous features, no history of ingestion
Vasovagal syncope	May have hypotension, nausea, vomiting and sweating	No rash, no tachycardia (often bradycardia)
Vocal cord dysfunction	May simulate asthma	Have distinctive cough
Panic attack	Tachypnoea, tachycardia,	Perioral tingling, tingling of fingers, difficulty breathing in No cutaneous signs, no wheeze or stridor
Gastroenteritis	Vomiting with history of allergic food ingestion within 2 hours	History of contact with infected person more than 8 hours before symptoms
Drug side effect – vancomycin	Cutaneous erythema	History of drug administration

Food allergy conditions with mechanism and symptoms		
Condition	**Mechanism**	**Symptoms**
Food-induced anaphylaxis	IgE	Anaphylaxis symptoms
GI food allergies		
immediate GI hypersensitivity	IgE	Anaphylaxis, acute vomiting
eosinophilic oesophagitis	IgE, non-IgE	Dysphagia, food impaction in adolescents
eosinophilic gastroenteritis	IgE, non-IgE	Depends on location in gut, may have abdominal pain and nausea; if diarrhoea occurs, may have weight loss In infants, often present with projectile vomiting Adolescents' symptoms and signs akin to irritable bowel disease
food protein-induced allergic proctocolitis		Flecks of blood, or blood mixed with mucus in the stool (occurs in breastfed infants)
food protein-induced enterocolitis syndrome	Non-IgE	Chronic vomiting, diarrhoea, failure to thrive A small number present with acute dehydration secondary to vomiting
oral allergy syndrome	IgE	Itching of lips, tongue, roof of mouth and throat; swelling may be evident

(continued)

Food allergy conditions with mechanism and symptoms		
Condition	**Mechanism**	**Symptoms**
Cutaneous		
acute urticaria	IgE usually	Irregular pruritic wheals, post ingestion of food trigger
angioedema	IgE	Skin and subcutaneous tissues have non-pruritic, non-pitting well-defined areas
atopic dermatitis (atopic eczema)	IgE, non-IgE	Food-sensitised patients may get urticaria, itching and eczematous flares that aggravate the atopic dermatitis (which may not respond to eczema therapy)
contact urticaria	IgE, non-IgE	Contact with skin by food trigger causes urticaria (direct histamine release)
Respiratory manifestations		
respiratory symptoms	IgE	Many symptoms occur with anaphylaxis. Occasionally asthma and rhinitis symptoms may be related to a food allergy
Heiner's syndrome	Non-IgE	Constellation of symptoms, with respiratory symptoms, GI symptoms, failure to thrive and iron-deficiency anaemia being present

INVESTIGATIONS

Skin prick test

SPT determines whether a child has been sensitised to an allergen, by re-exposing him or her to a minute amount of allergen. The trace amount of allergen is introduced into the skin by a lancet, which has a guard, thereby limiting the depth of skin penetration. SPT assesses IgE-mediated responses.

Prior to undertaking SPT, the following precautions should be observed:
- the person undertaking the test is trained appropriately
- emergency equipment is available
- commercially available standardised extracts are used or else fresh food extracts
- a positive control (histamine) and negative control are used
- ideally the testing is done on normal skin
- the patient is checked for dermatographism
- antihistamines are discontinued before testing.

Common errors in SPT include:
- antigen solution should be tested 2 cm apart
- if bleeding should occur, this may lead to false positive results.

What is the value of SPT? If the skin prick test is positive and this coincides with the clinical history of exposure, the need for a food challenge is lessened. SPT is positive in 59% of food challenges with commercial extracts and positive in 92% when fresh foods are used.

A clinically positive response to SPT is a weal >3 mm and a flare of >10 mm. However, relating the result to the clinical history is paramount. If the skin prick test is negative but the history is suggestive of allergy, a food challenge is required to establish causality.

(continued)

INVESTIGATIONS (*cont.*)

Patch testing

Patch testing is not generally recommended and when positive, it reflects non-IgE-mediated food allergy (delayed-type sensitivity). Like SPT, there must be a clinical history that supports the diagnosis of food allergy.

Food-specific IgE

Increased levels of serum IgE specific antibodies indicate sensitisation to a food, and the results must be used in the context of the clinical history. Periodically repeating these tests is required to assess clinical progress.

Food challenges

Indications for food challenges include (a) a history suggestive of food allergy but SPT and IgE are unhelpful (patients with recurrent flares with atopic dermatitis, children with oral symptoms, e.g. itching of the throat), (b) excessive dietary restrictions based on vague symptoms and (c) to determine if tolerance has occurred.

Open food challenge: in open food challenges the food being tested is given in a small amount (less than that which provokes a reaction) and the amount is incremented after a waiting time usually 15–30 minutes. The dose is increased in increments to a full serving, over five to seven increments. A positive test is the occurrence of an objective reaction. If no reaction occurs, the patient is observed for a further period and then allowed home.

Double-blind placebo-controlled food challenge (DBPCFC): DBPCFCs are undertaken when the symptoms are ambiguous or the family is extremely anxious. A DBPCFC is conducted in two parts. The test food is mixed in a food that the patient tolerates well, to ensure that it is masked in terms of taste and colour. The tolerated food serves as the control. Neither the patient nor the doctor is aware of the order in which the foods are given (double-blind). The interval between preparation of the foods varies with the food being tested and the responses that are being evaluated. When a DBPCFC is being undertaken, medical staff need to be on hand with the appropriate rescue medications (antihistamines, adrenaline) and the patient should have intravenous access established.

Serum tryptase

Serum tryptase peaks at 90–120 minutes post anaphylaxis, but clinical relevance is uncertain and it is unlikely to modify subsequent investigation or treatment.

MANAGEMENT PLAN: FIVE-STEP APPROACH

1. Clarifying and pitfall avoidance strategies:
   a) for the parents
   b) for the doctor
2. Allergen avoidance by families
3. Recognition of anaphylaxis by parents and child
4. Oral immunotherapy
5. Acute anaphylaxis in the emergency department

Clarifying and pitfall avoidance strategies

For the parents

- Define what the parents mean by allergy. **Rationale**: parents overestimate the presence of food allergies in their children (*see* Evidence 1). When present, they must be carefully assessed, but when absent, inappropriate food restriction must be avoided.
- Obtain temporal relationship between ingestion and symptom expression. **Rationale**: history taking is central to risk assessing children and adolescents with allergy. Failure to undertake this step results in incorrect conclusions being inferred.
- Assess parental view of allergy. **Rationale**: parents worry that their child may develop allergic diseases (atopic eczema and asthma) and restrict the child's diet unnecessarily (*see* Evidence 2).
- Tell the parents a second allergic reaction is more likely to result from eating a snack or accidental ingestion of a trace amount of allergen. **Rationale**: parents need to be aware that despite their best efforts it is not possible to prevent food reactions, and when they occur, often it is an accidental occurrence (nobody is at fault).
- Discuss openly with parents their anxiety related to food allergies, but actively educate them to lessen the risk and to treat anaphylaxis, should it occur.

For the doctor

- Consider allergy as aetiology of symptoms. **Rationale**: in children with (a) uncontrolled asthma despite optimal adherence to the treatment programme or (b) with eczema that does not respond to treatment, and (c) the infant who presents with acute collapse; these clinical scenarios may reflect allergic reactions amplifying their symptoms.
- Be specific in your discussions with parents with regard to allergic reactions and prognosis. **Rationale**: the cornerstone of allergy treatment is trigger avoidance. Therefore, if possible give, in percentage terms, allergy resolution rates (*see* Background section and Evidence 3).
- Ensure that allergies are documented in the hospital chart. **Rationale**: allergy avoidance is required to prevent unnecessary harm accruing to the child.
- Separate allergic reaction from drug side effect. **Rationale**: many antibiotics have side effects; ascribing the reaction as a 'drug allergy' should only be done having taken a comprehensive history.
- Training the parents and child to deal with allergy. **Rationale**: both parents and child (if old enough) must demonstrate competence in the emergency treatment of anaphylaxis by being able to inject adrenaline (*see* Evidence 3).

Allergen avoidance by families

To achieve this, parents must become adept at label reading. In the United States food labels list the eight major allergens (milk, eggs, peanut, tree nuts, fish, crustaceans, wheat and soy). In the European Union the list also includes all gluten-containing products (wheat, rye, barley, oats, spelt and their hybridised strains), celery, mustard, sesame seeds and sulphites. The allergen presence must be stated, regardless of amount. Label reading, by itself, does not identify the risk level that is present to the child. Words such as 'may contain' does not necessarily mean there is less risk than when a comment states that 'shared manufacturing equipment was used'.

Preparation of meals at home also raises challenges in avoiding potential allergen exposure. Cross-contamination of utensils can occur; therefore, diligence is required in food preparation and in washing up afterwards. Often it is best to prepare the allergic child's meal first. Food storage in the refrigerator must ensure that contamination does not occur. The use of specific containers or colour coding can be useful.

Dining out in restaurants can be challenging and potential allergic exposure must be ascertained before ordering food. At the child's school both teachers and carers must be aware of potential triggers, and attempts to minimise potential exposure must be undertaken. Teachers and carers must be aware of anaphylaxis symptoms and the necessary treatment. Having the appropriate medications (antihistamines and adrenaline) on hand is essential.

Recognition of anaphylaxis by parents and child

Explaining to the parent both verbally and by providing definite information on the recognition and treatment of anaphylaxis is essential to ensure the safety of the child. Parents are likely to recognise the symptoms once their child has experienced one reaction, but parents must have a specific action plan. The Food and Allergy Plan (available at www.foodallergy.org/faap provides a systematic approach to the symptoms and signs. The way to use the adrenaline pen must be demonstrated to the parents and they should be comfortable in its administration. However, this is not usually the case and adrenaline rescue treatment is not used appropriately by those experiencing an anaphylactic reaction (*see* Evidence 4). People who have experienced an anaphylactic reaction or food allergic reactions should also carry antihistamine, so that immediate treatment can be given.

Food allergies should be reviewed on a yearly basis and periodically assessed to determine whether the severity of the reactions is decreasing or not.

Oral immunotherapy

Oral immunotherapy may well represent an important advance in treatment of children with allergy (*see* Evidence 5), but the mechanism of action is not currently known.

Acute anaphylaxis in the emergency department

(*See* Chapter 3: First Response)

FOLLOW-UP

- Explain prognosis (*see* Background section text)

The natural history of food allergy is variable but most children will eventually tolerate cow's milk, hen's egg, soy and wheat; however, far fewer will eventually tolerate peanuts and tree nuts.

WHEN TO REFER?

- Children with anaphylaxis should be referred for assessment
- Children with an unclear history but who have been placed on an elimination diet
- Children with atopic dermatitis that does not improve with treatment
- Children with asthma in whom allergies seem to be present
- Non-responding gastro-oesophageal reflux (to standard treatment)
- Colic (non-resolving)

CLARIFICATION STATEMENTS FOR PARENTAL MISCONCEPTIONS

> *'I am sure that he is allergic to this food, because he has dark circles under his eyes and also he gets a rash.'*

Temporal relationships do not prove causation. A detailed history needs to be taken especially as it relates to the rash to decide if it is urticarial or not. The dark circles occur in upper airways cough syndrome and are related to venous congestion.

> *'How can my child have allergies? I exclusively breastfed him.'*

In breast milk, intact food proteins may be present and contribute to the development of allergic symptoms. Infants may respond to maternal elimination diets. In general, breastfeeding reduces the risk of allergic diseases.

> *'But hives must mean he has an allergy.'*

Only 20% of children presenting with urticaria will have food aetiology. Checking the history for one of the eight common foods helps to unlock the history. Extensive testing with skin prick test or IgE specific antibodies is of no value in the absence of a credible history.

> *'If my child has egg allergy, is it safe to give the measles, mumps, rubella and varicella vaccine?'*

Even in the presence of egg allergy it is safe to give the MMR and the MMRV to children. The benefits of such vaccinations far outweigh the risks.

SUMMARY PRACTICE POINTS

- Up to 20% of allergic reactions do not involve a skin reaction.
- SPT is only useful in assessing IgE-mediated responses.
- The temporal relationship between food exposure and the resulting symptom complex that occurs is pivotal in making the diagnosis of food allergy.
- Parents and the child with food allergy should be aware of the symptoms of allergic reaction and the necessary treatment.
- Parents, the child if old enough and carers must be able to administer an adrenaline pen when necessary.
- Checking skin prick test responses and food-related IgE every 2 years is prudent to determine if the food allergy is waning.
- The offending allergen is often hidden in the ingested food, so look for it.
- Blood tests in the acute phase, e.g. serum tryptase, are unlikely to aid diagnosis.

EVALUATING THE EVIDENCE

Evidence 1	
Theme E1	*The frequency of food hypersensitivity (FHS) in children*
Question	What is the frequency of FHS in children?
Design	Cohort study
Level of evidence	
Setting	Community setting, Isle of Wight, England
Participants	The parents of 6-year-old children in a geographically defined region (Isle of Wight) were invited to complete a questionnaire to assess the prevalence of food sensitisation, reported adverse reactions to food and food avoidance.
Intervention	All those consenting to participate were offered skin prick testing (SPT) to a predefined panel of food allergens (milk, wheat, cod fish, peanut and sesame) and aeroallergens (house dust mite, cat, grass pollen). SPT was also offered to other reported allergens. Children with a history suggestive of adverse reactions to food regardless of SPT, or those with a positive skin prick test but no definite prior exposure to the relevant food, were invited for food challenges. Prior to food challenges, children avoided the offending food for 4 weeks and in the case of food additives, they avoided them for 2 days.
Outcomes	The primary outcomes were reported sensitisation rates, sensitisation rates based on a predefined panel of foods and rates based on food challenges.

(continued)

Evidence 1

Theme E1	*The frequency of food hypersensitivity (FHS) in children*
Main results	The target eligible population was 1440 children; however, only 798 (55.4%) consented to be included in the study. Ninety-four (11.4%) children had a reported problem with a food or food ingredient, and for 30 (32%) it was to more than one food (milk and dairy), 38 (40%); peanut, 15 (16%); egg, 15 (15%); additives and colouring, 13 (14%); tree nuts, 11 (12%); wheat, 10 (11%); strawberry, 6 (6%); sesame, 5 (5%); fish, 2 (2%); others, 59 (63%).
	A total of 700 (87.8%) agreed to SPT, with 25 (3.6%) sensitised to the predefined panel and 29 (4.1%) sensitised to other foods (total, 54 (7.7%)). Of the 94 who reported specific food problems, SPT was undertaken in 83, with 12 having a positive skin prick test to the food to which they reported a problem.
	Of the 94 children with reported food problems, only 28 were regarded as eligible for food challenges. Nineteen children underwent open food challenges, with ten having positive results; however, only six underwent a double-blind placebo-controlled food challenge, with three having positive results (milk = 2; wheat = 1). Based on open food challenges and/or suggestive history and skin tests, the prevalence of FHS was 2.5%, but when based on a double-blind placebo-controlled food challenge, a clinical diagnosis or suggestive history and positive skin tests, the prevalence was 1.6%.
Conclusion	Parental perception rates of FHS are higher than SPT prevalence rates and FHS rates based on food challenges. Milk, peanut and wheat are the key allergens triggering a positive food challenge.
Commentary	Food allergy accounts for a significant proportion of anaphylaxis in children; therefore, the correct identification of these children is essential. In this study, parents overestimated the presence of FHS in their children. When children present with potential food allergy the temporal relationship between cause and effect must be established and a specific treatment plan must be put in place, which includes medication strategies and trigger avoidance. A limitation of this study is the response rate of 55.4%; however, the authors did contact 103 non-responders to determine reasons for non-engagement and the majority indicated that they were not interested.
Reference	Venter C, Pereira B, Grundy J, *et al.* Prevalence of sensitization reported and objectively assessed food hypersensitivity amongst six-year-old children: a population-based study. *Pediatr Allergy Immunol.* 2006; **17**(5): 356–63.

Evidence 2

Theme E2	*Allergenic food and allergy symptoms development*
Question	Is the early introduction of allergenic food associated with the development of eczema or wheeze?
Design	Cohort study
Level of evidence	
Setting	Urban centre, the Netherlands

(*continued*)

Evidence 2

Theme E2	*Allergenic food and allergy symptoms development*
Participants	This was a population-based study that incorporated 6905 preschool children and their parents.
Intervention	When children were 6 and 12 months of age, their parents were questioned regarding the age of first introduction of cow's milk, hen's eggs, peanuts, tree nuts, soy and gluten into their child's diet. Short food diaries were also obtained. Data from the parent reports (on first introduction of allergenic foods) were cross-checked against the food diaries.
Outcomes	The primary outcome was the occurrence of eczema and wheeze at 2, 3 and 4 years of age, which was assessed though an adapted version of the International Study of Asthma and Allergies in Childhood questionnaire.
Main results	Wheezing was reported in 31%, 14% and 14% of all children aged 2, 3 and 4 years, respectively. The percentages for eczema were 38%, 20% and 18%. There was not a significant relationship between the introduction of allergenic food before 6 months and the development of wheezing or eczema.
Conclusion	There is no evidence to suggest that delaying the introduction of potentially allergenic food beyond 6 months of age will protect against the development of atopic diseases.
Commentary	This is a large observational study based on questionnaire data that were obtained retrospectively. The absence of strict criteria for eczema and wheezing may have led to an over-reporting of these conditions (e.g. eczema, 38% at age 2 years). Ideally a physician should confirm the diagnosis of both wheeze and eczema, but this is not practicable in population-based studies. The data provided by this study can offer reassurance to parents who may have concerns related to the introduction of allergic food into their child's diet lest they develop eczema or asthma. The development of wheeze in early infancy is not a strong predictor of asthma in later childhood.
Reference	Tromp II, Kiefte-de Jong JC, Lebon A, *et al.* The introduction of allergenic foods and the development of reported wheezing and eczema in childhood: the Generation R study. *Arch Pediatr Adolesc Med.* 2011; **165**(10): 933–8.

Evidence 3

Theme E3	*Long-term allergy management*
Question	In children with peanut allergy, what are the components of effective care?
Design	Longitudinal prospective study and case-controlled study
Level of evidence	
Setting	Department of allergy, academic medical centre, England
Participants	Children referred to the allergy clinic were eligible if they had typical features of an acute allergic reaction occurring within 1 hour of ingestion of a food known to contain a nut, and evidence of nut-specific IgE by positive skin prick testing (≥3 mm). Reactions were graded 1–5.

(continued)

Evidence 3	
Theme E3	*Long-term allergy management*
Intervention	A specific management plan consisting of (a) advice on nut avoidance, (b) provision of rescue medication based on defined criteria to allow for the early initiation of treatment of reactions by parents or school staff and (c) providing reinforcement and retraining at follow-up annually. Nut avoidance education consisted of verbal and written information inclusive of the principles of understanding labelling, eating in restaurants or on school trips. For medication, antihistamines were offered to all and injectable adrenaline was offered to three specific groups: (1) those with grade 4 and 5 reactions, (2) those with reactions to trace nut ingestion (as risk of severe reaction present in future) and (3) those with asthma. At annual follow-up reactions were graded, skin prick testing repeated and re-education undertaken. The case control component of the study matched those with follow-up reactions to those who did not.
Outcomes	The primary outcome was the frequency in reduction of allergic reaction to peanuts.
Main results	From the initial 747 children, 615 (82.3%) were followed-up prospectively. The age range was 10 months to 15 years (41% were <5 years, 39% were 5–9 years and 20% were ≥10 years). Co-existing asthma was present in 338 (55%). The mean skin prick test weal diameter was 8.4 mm (95% confidence interval (CI): 7.8–8.9) for peanut and 7.9 mm (95% CI: 7.4–8.5) for tree nut. Before enrolment, reaction severity was as follows: 64%, mild; 28%, involving airway narrowing; 8%, severe. At follow-up (mean of 3.3 years) only 131 (21%) had a further reaction (74% had one reaction, 15% had two reactions and 11% had three or more reactions). There was a 60-fold reduction in severe reactions (grade 5) and only two children received adrenaline. Of the 115 mild and moderate reactions, 96 (83%) received oral chlorpheniramine and 19 (16.8%) received no treatment. In the case control component, cases had 1.5 times more reactions pre-enrolment than controls.
Conclusion	Formal management plans that are followed reduce the frequency and severity of further reactions.
Commentary	This study gives a clear guide to inform practice. Reactions were classified as mild (grade 1) if there was local erythema, urticaria or angioedema; mild (grade 2) if there was generalised erythema, urticaria or angioedema; mild (grade 3) if there were at least one or two plus gastrointestinal or rhinoconjunctivitis symptoms; moderate (grade 4) if there was mild laryngeal oedemas or mild asthma; and severe (grade 5) if there was pronounced dyspnoea or hypotension. Clear management plans both verbal and written and with school involvement are essential. No child with an initial mild reaction proceeded to a severe reaction. The majority of severe reactions were triggered by snacks and accidental contact. In this study injectable adrenaline was not provided to those with mild reactions unless there was concurrent asthma or if the sensitivity was unknown (trace ingestion triggering a reaction). All patients were required to carry antihistamines at all times to ensure their ability to respond to an allergic reaction. Providing both parent and child with the data from this study may well modify their adherence to the treatment plan.
Reference	Ewan PW, Clark AT. Efficacy of a management plan based on severity assessment in longitudinal and case-controlled studies of 747 children with nut allergy: proposal for good practice. *Clin Exp Allergy*. 2005; **35**(6): 751–6.

Evidence 4	
Theme E4	*Adrenaline auto-injector use in anaphylaxis*
Question	When and why do children and adolescents with anaphylaxis use adrenaline auto-injectors?
Design	Prospective cohort study
Level of evidence	
Setting	Fourteen paediatric allergy clinics, England
Participants	Children and adolescents attending allergy clinics who were prescribed adrenaline auto injectors for anaphylaxis were eligible for inclusion.
Intervention	Participants completed a pretested questionnaire that requested data on demographic information, atopic status, and details of allergic reactions (inclusive of cause and symptoms) in the previous year and the treatment received (specifically adrenaline use).
Outcomes	The primary outcome was adrenaline usage for episodes of anaphylaxis (clinical features included difficulty in breathing, itchy throat or throat tightness, changing voice, vomiting, diarrhoea, difficulty in swallowing, wheezing, dizziness and loss of consciousness).
Main results	Of a total of 1304 screened, 969 (74.3%) were eligible, all of whom participated. About half had co-existing asthma and most had co-existing eczema. The most prevalent allergens were peanuts and tree nuts and all but two had been prescribed EpiPens. A total of 466 participants experienced allergic reactions, of whom 245 (52.5%) met the criteria for anaphylaxis, but only 41 (16.7%; 95% confidence interval: 11.7–21.3) received adrenaline, and 83.3% received antihistamine therapy. Six (2.7%) who did not meet the criteria for anaphylaxis were given adrenaline. For 204 (83%) the reasons cited for non-use of adrenaline were as follows: unnecessary (54.4%), unsure if necessary (19.1%), ambulance called (7.8%), device not available (5.4%), too scared (2.5%), not trained (2.5%), attended emergency department (1.5%) and device out of date (1%). Thirteen participants (31.7%) required a second dose of adrenaline. Adrenaline was administered by parents in 26 (55%) cases, health professionals in 18 (38%) cases and the patients themselves in two (4%) cases.
Conclusion	Adrenaline auto-injectors are underused by patients experiencing anaphylaxis in the community, despite appropriate instruction in the method and indications for their use. If not rectified, this situation may have adverse effects on patient outcome.
Commentary	Adrenaline auto-injectors were prescribed for previous anaphylaxis, reaction to trace amount, food allergy with asthma and nut allergy. Of the 245 with symptoms of anaphylaxis, 150 (61.2%) had wheezing, 130 (53.1%) had urticaria, 125 (58.7%) had difficulty breathing, 99 (40.4%) had throat tightness, 20 (8.2%) had feelings of impending doom and 12 (4.9%) had loss of consciousness, yet only 41 (16.7%) used an appropriate treatment strategy that was recommended. This mismatch needs to be corrected. One possible option is education in real-time simulation technology, where the patient's original experience of anaphylaxis could be incorporated into the educational event to enhance the relevance of the educational experience.

(*continued*)

Evidence 4	
Theme E4	*Adrenaline auto-injector use in anaphylaxis*
Commentary (*cont.*)	It is prudent to prescribe a second adrenaline auto-injection, as one-third will require a second dose to effectively treat anaphylaxis.
Reference	Noimark L, Wales J, Du Toit G, *et al*. The use of adrenaline autoinjectors by children and teenagers. *Clin Exp Allergy*. 2012; **42**(2): 284–92.

Evidence 5	
Theme E5	*Oral immunotherapy and allergy*
Question	Is oral immunotherapy effective in the treatment of egg allergy in children?
Design	Randomised controlled trial
Level of evidence	Jadad 5
Setting	Department of paediatrics, multiple academic medical centres, the United States
Participants	Children with known egg allergy (allergic symptoms within minutes to 2 hours of egg ingestion and serum egg-specific IgE >5 kU/L for those older than 6 years and >12 kU/L for those 5 years of age) were eligible for participation if between 5 and 18 years of age.
Intervention	Children were randomised to receive, on a daily basis, egg white powder or cornstarch. Food challenge occurred at 10 months (after which the placebo group discontinued their cornstarch) and at 22 months. Those who were successful avoided eggs for 4–6 weeks and then had another food challenge (which included the ingestion of 10 g of egg white powder and a cooked egg) at 24 months. Those who passed this test were allowed to eat eggs in an unrestricted fashion and were reassessed at 36 months.
Outcomes	The primary outcome was the ability of patients who were previously designated as having an egg allergy to eat eggs at 36 months (the final end point of the study).
Main results	Of the 420 screened, 365 were excluded (136 declined, 136 had insufficient history, 39 had asthma, 18 had incorrect age and 36 were excluded for other reasons) and 55 were randomised: 40 to the intervention group and 15 to placebo. Of the 15 in the placebo group, 13 had a food challenge at 10 months with a 0 (0%) pass rate. Two patients dropped out (one allergic reaction, one because of no transportation). Of the 40 in the intervention group there were five withdrawals (four allergic reactions and one anxiety state), therefore 35 had the 10-month food challenge with 22 (55%) pass rate (absolute risk reduction = 55%; number needed to treat (NNT) = 2), with 30 (75%) desensitised at 22 months. At the 24-month food challenge 11 (28%) had sustained unresponsiveness to eggs (NNT = 4).
Conclusion	Oral immunotherapy resulted in sustained unresponsiveness in 28% of those treated with egg white powder, which is clinically relevant, as egg avoidance is the only treatment option for these children and adolescents.

(*continued*)

Evidence 5	
Theme E5	*Oral immunotherapy and allergy*
Commentary	Egg allergy is common, with a cumulative prevalence of 4%, and a relatively small dose (80 mg) can precipitate anaphylaxis. This study avoided several pitfalls, one of which was to exclude children whose symptoms could have improved over the period of the study. The results are promising but the mechanism of action of the treatment is not understood yet. The occurrence of allergic reactions (significant to cause withdrawal from the study) is significant at 15%. It is likely that with further study, oral immunotherapy will become an established treatment for allergy.
Reference	Burks AW, Jones SM, Wood RA, *et al*. Consortium of Food Allergy Research (CoFAR). Oral immunotherapy for treatment of egg allergy in children. *N Engl J Med.* 2012; **367**(3): 233–43.

FOOD ALLERGY: MULTIPLE-CHOICE QUESTIONS

Q1 Which of the following is/are correct with regard to cow's milk allergy?
   a) The prevalence is 2.5% at 1 year of age.
   b) Sixty per cent of reactions are IgE mediated.
   c) The major allergen is whey alpha and beta lactoglobulin.
   d) A wheal of >6 mm in a child younger than 2 years is predictive.
   e) Sixty-five per cent develop tolerance at 12 years of age.

Q2 Which of the following statements is/are correct with regard to peanut allergy?
   a) The prevalence is 1.5%.
   b) The major antigens in North America are Ara H8 and Ara H9.
   c) The onset is usually at under 2 years of age.
   d) The symptoms are mostly respiratory on presentation.
   e) In peanut allergy, asthma control must be optimal.

Q3 Which of the following statements is/are correct as they relate to egg allergy?
   a) Egg allergy occurs at 6 months of age.
   b) Sensitisation occurs through breast milk protein.
   c) Recognised presentation includes acute vomiting.
   d) Symptoms usually occur with 2 hours of ingestion.
   e) The major allergenic proteins are Gal d1 to d5.

Q4 In egg allergy, which of the following is/are correct?
   a) A skin prick test >5 mm at younger than 2 years is diagnostic.
   b) Skin prick tests correlate with allergic reaction severity.
   c) Resolution rates of egg allergy are 4% at 4 years of age.
   d) Resolution rates of egg allergy are 40% at 10 years of age.
   e) Egg allergy in asthmatic children presents with urticaria.

Q5   Respiratory symptoms of food allergy include which of the following?
   a) Wheeze
   b) Acute cough
   c) Feeling of impending doom
   d) Choking
   e) Transient stridor

Q6   Which of the following statements regarding SPT is/are correct?
   a) Histamine control is required.
   b) Placebo control is required.
   c) SPT is IgE mediated only.
   d) Antihistamines must be discontinued 72 hours before testing is undertaken.
   e) Inhaled steroids should be discontinued 24 hours prior to testing.

Q7   In SPT, which of the following statements is/are correct?
   a) Skin prick tests should be administered 2 cm apart.
   b) A positive response is a wheal >3 mm and a flare >6 mm.
   c) SPT should not be done in a child with eczema.
   d) In SPT, fresh food extracts are superior to commercial extracts.
   e) SPT is contraindicated in children with psoriasis.

Q8   Indications for food challenge include which of the following?
   a) Positive history of allergy but negative skin prick test
   b) Recurrent flares of atopic dermatitis
   c) Atopic dermatitis not responsive to topical steroids
   d) Children with excessive dietary restrictions based on vague symptoms
   e) Children with colic

Q9   Which of the following statements is/are true in regard to food protein-induced enterocolitis?
   a) Chronic vomiting occurs.
   b) Hypocalcaemia is a feature.
   c) Failure to thrive occurs.
   d) Ten per cent of infants experience urticaria.
   e) Acute dehydration occurs from acute vomiting.

Q10 Which of the following statements is/are true as they relate to the oral allergy syndrome?
   a) It is IgE mediated.
   b) Urticaria occurs in 25% of patients.
   c) Itching of the lips occurs.
   d) The roof of the mouth is itchy.
   e) Stridor is pronounced.

Answers

A1	a, b, c, d, e	**A2**	a, c, d, e
A3	a, b, c, d, e	**A4**	a, c, d
A5	a, c	**A6**	a, b, c
A7	a, d	**A8**	a, b, d
A9	a, c, e	**A10**	a, c, d

Chapter Nine

THE CHILD WITH VOMITING

COMMON SCENARIO

'There was a vomiting bug going around the crèche earlier in the week and last night he just woke up and started vomiting continuously. I've been trying to give him fluids all day but he's just not keeping them down.'

LEARNING OBJECTIVES

- Understand the pathophysiology of vomiting
- Recognise the signs and symptoms of dehydration
- List the differential causes of acute and recurrent or chronic vomiting
- Determine what investigations should be considered based on likely differential diagnosis

BACKGROUND

Vomiting is the forceful propulsion of gastric contents out of the mouth. It is co-ordinated by the vomiting centre in the medulla oblongata of the brainstem. Vomiting may be triggered by both central and peripheral stimuli.

Central stimuli:

- cortical – due to pain, emotions, taste and smell
- drugs – chemotherapy, opiates, antibiotics
- metabolic – acidosis, uraemia, hyperthyroidism, hypercalcaemia
- vestibular – motion sickness, vertigo
- infections – septicaemia, gastroenteritis or non-gastrointestinal (GI) infections.

Peripheral triggers:

- pharyngeal stimulation
- gastric mucosal irritation
- abdominal distension.

The vomiting response cause the abdominal, thoracic and diaphragm somatic muscles to contract against a closed glottis. This increases intra-abdominal pressure, reversing the normal negative oesophageal pressure and forcing gastric contents upwards. Vomiting is one of the commonest presenting complaints in childhood. However, vomiting does not mean that pathology is limited to the GI tract. The differential diagnosis of a child with vomiting is vast. It can be secondary to GI pathology or disease in distant organs, secondary to drugs or toxins or psychiatric illness. A detailed history and examination will often narrow the differential and guide further management. There are two key questions to ask, regarding the nature of the vomitus: Does it contain blood or bile? Is this an acute or recurring episode?

Some clinical clues are as follows.

- Episodes triggered by acute illnesses, fasting or high protein meal may indicate an underlying metabolic condition.
- Children with vomiting secondary to raised intracranial pressure may have papilloedema or focal neurological signs.
- In girls of childbearing age, it is important to consider pregnancy in the differential diagnosis.
- Bilious vomiting implies obstruction distal to the ampulla of Vater.
- Constipation alone is a rare and unlikely cause of vomiting.

The most serious immediate complications of vomiting are dehydration and electrolyte disturbances. Compared to adults, children younger than 4 years and especially infants are at increased risk of dehydration. This is due to several factors, including higher body water contents in children and infant. Most of the volume loss in dehydration is from the extracellular space (plasma, lymph and interstitial fluid).

Signs and symptoms	Mild (<5%)	Moderate (6%–10%)	Severe (11%–15%)
Level of consciousness	Alert	Lethargic	Obtunded
Capillary refill time	<2 seconds	2–4 seconds	>4 seconds
Mucous membranes	Normal	Dry	Parched
Tears	Present	Decreased	Absent
Skin turgor	Normal	Slow	Tenting
Fontanelle in infants	Normal	Depressed	Sunken
Eye appearance	Normal	Sunken	Very sunken
Urine output	Decreased	Oliguric	Anuric
Heart rate	Mild increase	Moderate increase	Severe increase
Pulse volume	Normal	Thready	Faint
Blood pressure	Normal	Normal or low	Low

SOME IMPORTANT CAUSES OF VOMITING IN CHILDHOOD

Many of the causes of vomiting have already been discussed in previous chapters. This section will therefore focus on important common and rare conditions not previously addressed.

Gastroenteritis

Viral gastroenteritis is the commonest cause of acute vomiting in children; however, it is important not to conclude that the diagnosis is gastroenteritis without reflecting on alternate possibilities. In temperate climates, it is caused by a virus in over 80% of cases and is self-limiting. Rotavirus is the most common causative agent. Vomiting usually precedes the onset of diarrhoea. There may be associated low-grade fever and abdominal pain. In most cases, vomiting lasts for 1–2 days, with diarrhoea persisting for 5–7 days.

Pyloric stenosis

Pyloric stenosis is due to hypertrophy of the pylorus muscle, which obstructs the pyloric lumen and leads to almost complete gastric outlet obstruction. It classically presents with increasingly projectile vomiting in newborns 3–5 weeks of age. It is more common in males and firstborn infants. In 15% of cases there is a positive family history. Despite vomiting with every feed that infant remains hungry. Infants may present with signs of dehydration, weight loss, failure to thrive and jaundice. Examination may reveal visible gastric peristalsis passing from left to right. Palpation of an olive-shaped pyloric mass in the midline or right upper quadrant during a test feed is diagnostic.

Gastro-oesophageal reflux and gastro-oesophageal reflux disease

Gastro-oesophageal reflux (GER) is associated with transient relaxation of the lower oesophageal sphincter. Typical symptoms include regurgitation or spitting up, which occurs in 50% of infants. Reflux can be associated with vomiting, which is defined as a forceful expulsion of gastric contents. Regurgitation and vomiting need to differentiated from rumination (which is where recently ingested food is effortlessly regurgitated into the mouth, masticated and re-swallowed). Features of gastro-oesophageal reflux disease (GERD) in infancy include feeding refusal, recurrent vomiting, poor weight gain, irritability, sleep disturbance and respiratory symptoms; in children and adolescents, features include abdominal pain/heartburn, recurrent vomiting, dysphagia, asthma, recurrent pneumonia and upper airway symptoms (chronic cough, hoarse voice). Certain paediatric populations are at high risk for GERD, including those with neurological impairment, obesity, achalasia, hiatus hernia, and those with chronic respiratory disorders such as bronchopulmonary dysplasia and cystic fibrosis.

There is no ideal test to diagnose GERD and tests available include oesophageal pH monitoring, endoscopy, and gastro-oesophageal scinitigraphy. Upper GI tract radiography is not appropriate to diagnose GER and GERD. The natural history of GER is to resolve once the child is walking.

Cyclical vomiting syndrome

Cyclical vomiting syndrome is characterised by recurrent, self-limiting, stereotypic episodes of nausea and vomiting. Stereotypical episodes simply mean that the episodes are similar each time in terms of their onset, intensity, duration, frequency and associated signs and symptoms. The child is well and asymptomatic in between episodes. Vomiting typically begins in the morning, with episodes lasting from hours to days. There may be prodromal symptoms or triggers, which are often similar to the prodromal symptoms and triggers of migraine attacks. There may be associated headache, photophobia, pallor and low-grade pyrexia. A family history of migraine or irritable bowel syndrome is common. Dehydration is common. Most cases resolve by early puberty.

According to the diagnostic criteria for children with Cyclic Vomiting Syndrome, suggested by the North American Society for Pediatric Gastroenterology, Hepatology and Nutrition Consensus Statement, all of the following criteria must be met to meet the definition of cyclical vomiting syndrome:

- at least five attacks in any interval, or a minimum of three attacks during a 6-month period
- episodic attacks of intense nausea and vomiting lasting 1 hour to 10 days and occurring at least 1 week apart
- stereotypical pattern and symptoms in the individual patient
- vomiting during attacks occurs at least 4 times an hour for at least an hour
- return to baseline health between episodes
- not attributable to another disorder.

Pelvi-ureteric junction obstruction

Pelvi-ureteric junction (PUJ) obstruction is impediment to urinary flow from the renal pelvis to the ureter. It should be considered in a child with intermittent abdominal pain and vomiting. It may present with a palpable flank mass, intermittent abdominal pain and vomiting, and haematuria; however, in the majority of cases it is diagnosed antenatally. It occurs more commonly in boys than girls and is more likely to affect the left kidney. In 10%–40% of cases it is bilateral.

Nephrolithiasis

Renal stones or nephrolithiasis can present acutely with vomiting and abdominal pain or renal colic. There may be associated haematuria and/or dysuria. However, the commonest presentation of nephrolithiasis in children is with a urinary tract infection. Stones can be made up of:

- magnesium-ammonium phosphate
- calcium phosphate
- urate
- xanthine

- cysteine
- oxate.

Calcium stones are the most common. Approximately 50% of children with renal stones have an identifiable metabolic abnormality, the likelihood of which is increased with bilateral stones.

Pancreatitis

Pancreatitis is inflammation of the parenchyma of the pancreas and is extremely rare in paediatrics. It can be acute (reversible) or chronic (irreversible). The majority of cases are idiopathic; however, it can be secondary to drugs or alcohol, cholelithiasis, injury, multisystem disease, metabolic diseases or infections. The presenting signs are non-specific; children commonly present with epigastric abdominal pain, nausea and vomiting. Pain is typically sharp in nature, aggravated by eating and may be relieved by drawing up the knees to the chest. Examination may reveal generalised abdominal tenderness that is worse in the epigastric region, with quiet bowel sounds and fever.

Idiopathic intracranial hypertension

Idiopathic intracranial hypertension is characterised by signs and symptoms of raised intracranial pressure, headache, tinnitus, a sixth nerve palsy, papilloedema and visual loss. The computed tomography and magnetic resonance imaging scan is normal and there is an elevated opening pressure on lumbar puncture. The cause of idiopathic intracranial hypertension is usually unknown. Conditions associated with idiopathic intracranial hypertension include hypervitaminosis A, obesity, steroid therapy or withdrawal, chronic otitis media with lateral sinus thrombosis and Guillain–Barré syndrome. Visual loss is the major complication, as chronic papilloedema may lead to permanent damage to the optic nerve.

Bilious vomiting in neonates

Bilious vomiting in a neonate suggests bowel obstruction and requires urgent surgical consultation. If there is associated abdominal distension it implies that the level of obstruction is distal and may be secondary to low jejunoileal atresia, meconium ileus or malrotation with volvulus. The absence of associated distension suggests proximal obstruction that may be found in duodenal atresia or stenosis and high jejunal atresia.

HISTORY

KEY POINTS				
Vomiting	Onset Duration Time of day when starts Projectile Blood Bile Frequency of vomits Relationship to feeds Previous episodes	**Medical and surgical history**	Recent head trauma Previous abdominal surgery Diabetes Psychiatric history	**❓ Red flags** Haematemesis Bilious vomiting Lethargy Recurrent early-morning vomiting Temperament change Refusal to drink
Associated symptoms	Diarrhoea: blood or mucus Fever Abdominal pain Vertigo Sore throat Headache Rash Breathing difficulties	**Family history**	Migraine Diabetes Kidney stones or disease Metabolic disease Parental consanguinity	
Hydration status	Lethargy Urine output Fluid intake Anorexia Weight loss	**Social history**	Recent travel Sick or infectious contacts Concerns about weight gain	
Birth history	Polyhydramnios Gestation Passage of meconium	**Medications**	Over-the-counter drugs Prescribed drugs Herbal remedies	
Gynaecological history (in girls of childbearing age)	Last menstrual period Sexually active			

EXAMINATION

- All children should have their height, weight and head circumference plotted on an appropriate centile chart
- Vital signs including temperature should be recorded
- Assess level of dehydration or signs of hypovolaemia
- Assess for meningism
- Assess level of consciousness
- Head and neck: neck stiffness, otitis media, bulging fontanelle in infants, tonsillitis

- Abdominal exam: masses, organomegaly, tenderness, guarding, rigidity, presence of bowel sounds
- Respiratory exam: decreased air entry, wheeze or crepitations
- Neurological exam: papilloedema, positive Kernig's sign or Brudzinski's sign, focal neurological signs
- Skin exam: rash

ℚ   Red flags›

- Weight loss
- Bilious vomiting
- Persistent tachycardia or hypotension
- Meningeal signs
- Severe dehydration
- Signs of raised intracranial pressure
- Abdominal tenderness or peritionitis

DIFFERENTIAL DIAGNOSIS

Bilious vomiting in neonates
Duodenal atresia
Malrotation with volvulus
Meconium ileus
Necrotising enterocolitis
Jejunoileal atresia
Hirshsprung's disease

Children and adolescents acute vomiting
Injury: head injury
Non-GI infections: meningitis, encephalitis, otitis media, tonsillitis, urinary tract infection, pneumonia, non-specific, viral infections, sepsis
Endocrine: diabetic ketoacidosis
Respiratory: post-tussive vomiting, pneumonia
Cardiovascular: supraventricular tachycardia
Neurological: hydrocephalus with shunt obstruction, subdural haematoma, labyrinthitis
Surgical: adhesions, intussusception, strangulated hernia, appendicitis, pancreatitis, pyloric stenosis
Drugs and toxins: antibiotics, anti-epileptics, opiates, chemotherapy, illicit drugs, organophosphates, arsenic
Renal: nephrolithiasis
Metabolic: first presentation of metabolic disease

Recurrent vomiting
Metabolic disease: fatty acid oxidation disorders, acute intermittent porphyria, urea cycle defects, mitochondrial disease
GI: gastro-oesophageal reflux disease, gastritis, peptic ulcer disease, cyclical vomiting syndrome, recurrent pancreatitis
Psychiatric: anorexia nervosa, bulimia nervosa
Neurological: idiopathic intracranial hypertension, migraine, space occupying lesion
Endocrine: Addison's disease
Renal: hydronephrosis secondary to PUJ obstruction
Other: pregnancy, drugs

INVESTIGATIONS

In severely dehydrated children requiring intravenous fluids, what investigations should be performed?
- A full blood count, urea and electrolytes, blood glucose and venous blood gas

The clinical picture and the differential diagnosis will guide further investigations.
- Blood glucose may be low
- A full blood count may show high white cells indicating infection or a raised haematocrit secondary to volume depletion
- A urea and electrolytes may show (a) hypokalaemia secondary to GI and renal losses and decreased oral intake of potassium, (b) hypochloraemia secondary to GI losses
- The venous blood gas may show metabolic alkalosis due to retention of bicarbonate and volume contraction

Patients with uraemia or Addison's disease may have normal or even high serum potassium, despite vomiting.

In suspected pyloric stenosis, what investigations should be performed?
- Urea and electrolytes, blood glucose, and venous blood gas: the classic finding in pyloric stenosis is hypochloraemic, hypokalaemia metabolic alkalosis
- Urine should be analysed to rule out an infection
- With pyloric stenosis the urine may show a paradoxical aciduria
- Abdominal ultrasound scan: indicates muscle hypertrophy of pylorus muscle

If PUJ obstruction is suspected, what radiological investigations should be performed?
- A renal ultrasounds scan to assess the degree of pelvic dilatation
- A MAG 3 (functional test of renal tract) gives differential duction of the kidneys by generating a tracer curve – a flat or rising curve indicates obstruction

In children with suspected renal calculi, what investigations should be performed?
- Renal USS: may show dilatation or presence of stone or nephrocalcinosis
- Abdominal X-ray: may show radiopaque stone

MANAGEMENT PLAN: THREE-STEP APPROACH

1. Clarifying and pitfall avoidance strategies
2. Management of dehydration
3. Management of specific conditions:
   a) pyloric stenosis
   b) gastro-oesophageal reflux
   c) cyclical vomiting
   d) pelvi-ureteric junction obstruction
   e) bilious vomiting in the neonate

Clarifying and pitfall avoidance strategies

- The presence of vomiting does not always mean gastroenteritis. **Pitfall**: vomiting has an extensive differential diagnosis; therefore, exclude other conditions through an appropriate history, physical examination and tests as indicated.
- In the vomiting infant and young child, always enquire as to recently ingested formula or food. **Rationale**: Overfeeding is a frequent cause of vomiting in newborn infants (normal volume is 150 mL/kg/day of formula).
- For parents: vomiting and seeking medical advice. **Pitfall**: children with an inability to keep fluids down for 8 hours due to vomiting should be medically assessed for dehydration. Those with vomiting for 24 hours but able to hold fluids down should also be assessed.
- The parental response to vomiting. **Rationale**: ideally the infant and child with acute vomiting should be fed as normal. Breastfeeding or formula feeding should be continued. Oral rehydration fluid is also appropriate.
- **Pitfall**: offering a vomiting infant or child a non-physiological fluid, e.g. tea, is not appropriate. The fluid offered to any vomiting child must be documented. Such practices lead to electrolyte disturbances.
- Medication usage by parents. **Pitfall**: check if the parents have administered paracetamol or ibuprofen to treat their child (these medications are often used by parents when their child is unwell).
- Doctors and the vomiting child. **Pitfall**: Gastroenteritis is very common; however, to assume that all vomiting is gastroenteritis is a major error.
- Conceptualising vomiting as a symptom. **Rationale**: decide (a) if this is an acute illness and whether the child is febrile or not; (b) if chronic, decide if intermittent – child has periods of well-being between the vomiting episodes; and (c) if chronic persistent or progressive, child is not normal between episodes.
- Chronic vomiting. Define the impact of the vomiting in terms of weight loss and the child's sense of well-being. **Rationale**: The doctor must determine an aetiology in this group.
- Metabolic impact of vomiting. **Rationale**: clinically significant vomiting will lead to a hypochloraemic metabolic alkalosis.
- Ensure a full examination is performed, inclusive of 'red flag' assessments.

- Antibiotic use and gastroenteritis. **Pitfall**: antibiotic treatment is not usually indicated in gastroenteritis.
- Use of anti-nausea medications in the vomiting child. **Rationale**: Dimenhydrinate is not useful in children with vomiting (*see* Evidence 1) but oral Ondansetron is (*see* Evidence 2).

Management of dehydration

Children who are hypovolaemic require fluid resuscitation with 20 mL/kg boluses of normal saline, repeated until hypovolaemia is corrected and urine output is established. Dehydration and electrolyte disturbance should be corrected. Most children with mild to moderate dehydration can be managed at home with oral rehydration solution (*see* Chapter 11: The Child With Diarrhoea). If they are unable to tolerate oral fluids after a suitable trial period of oral rehydration solution, hospital admission is required. In breastfed infants, feeding should continue with oral rehydration solution supplementation. Parents should be educated about the importance of hydration, the signs and symptoms of dehydration, the likely duration of the illness and when to seek medical advice. The use of anti-emetics is generally not recommended. They may mask a more serious underlying cause of vomiting, distract from the appropriate fluid management and are associated with extrapyramidal side effects and dystonic reactions.

Management of specific conditions

The management of vomiting will depend on the underlying cause. The management of many conditions that can cause acute and recurrent or chronic vomiting in children have been dealt with in previous chapters. Therefore, this section will focus only on important conditions that have not been considered elsewhere.

Pyloric stenosis

Pyloric stenosis is not a surgical emergency; the first priority is to correct any fluid and electrolyte abnormalities with intravenous fluids and added potassium. Once the infant has been resuscitated adequately, a surgical pyloromyotomy is performed. The traditional approach is a right upper quadrant midline incision. However, surgical approaches have advanced over the years and many surgeons now access the pylorus laparoscopically or via a periumbilical incision. The pylorus is incised along its long axis and the hypertrophied muscle fibres are split while carefully avoiding breaching the mucosa. Feeding is usually recommended 24 hours after surgery and the majority of infants are discharged home well within 2–3 days.

Gastro-oesophageal reflux

Infants with GER, or 'happy spitters', need no specific therapy; however, if parents want an intervention then thickening of feed is reasonable and effective (useful in those with mild GERD symptoms). In infants with GERD who are breastfed, a maternal milk and egg exclusion diet is recommended for 2–4 weeks, as the symptoms of GERD may reflect milk protein allergy. If bottlefed then a trial of extensively hydrolysed protein or amino acid formula is warranted.

In young children antacids are used to directly buffer the acid (*see* Evidence 7) as are histamine$_2$ receptor antagonists (H2RA). The use of H2RA medication has improved the treatment of GERD; however, there are limitations due to the development of tachyphylaxis (increasing doses are required to produce the same effect). Proton pump inhibitors (PPIs) are effective (*see* Evidence 8). PPIs must be administered at the correct time, i.e. 30 minutes before a meal. The side effect profile needs to be considered when prescribing PPIs with headaches, nausea, diarrhoea and constipation occurring in 14% of children.

Cyclical vomiting syndrome

Management focuses on prevention and treatment of episodes. The first step is learning to recognise any triggers associated with episodes and the avoidance of identified trigger factors. If stress is an identified trigger, counselling and stress reduction techniques may be helpful. Prophylactic treatment is indicated if the child is having more than one episode per month, episodes last more than 24 hours, are severe enough to require hospitalisation or fail to respond to abortive treatments. Treatment options include anti-migraine agents, prokinetic medications and anticonvulsants. Children with a history of migraine or a family history of migraine often respond well to anti-migraine prophylaxis and so should be started on this as first line. Sumatriptan, taken at the onset of symptoms, has been shown to decrease the frequency, duration and intensity of episodes. Ondansetron can be given to reduce the severity of vomiting. The main complication is the risk of dehydration. Families should be educated about the signs of dehydration and when to seek medical attention.

Pelvi-ureteric junction obstruction

PUJ obstruction may resolve or increase over time. Long-term ultrasound follow-up is therefore required. Indications for surgery (pyeloplasty) include:

- progressive dilatation
- severe dilatation >30 mm
- calyceal dilatation
- decrease in renal function
- recurrent symptoms: pain, haematuria, urinary tract infections.

Bilious vomiting in the neonate

The neonate should be placed nil by mouth and a nasogastric tube should be inserted to decompress the bowel and prevent further vomiting. Intravenous access should be obtained and fluid resuscitation followed by maintenance fluids commenced. Further management is guided by the underlying cause.

FOLLOW-UP

Most cases of vomiting in childhood are secondary to acute, self-limiting infections, affecting either the GI tract or non GI organs. These children do not require long-term follow-up. However, parents should be advised to seek medical attention if the vomiting persists or there are signs of dehydration.

Children with cyclical vomiting require long-term follow-up to enable continued management of the disease, ensure response to treatment and ensure that no new symptoms or signs that suggest an alternative diagnosis develop.

WHEN TO REFER?

- Children with severe dehydration or signs of hypovolaemia require admission to hospital for fluid management and correction of associated electrolyte imbalances
- Severe abdominal pain or tenderness
- Parent unable to manage the child at home
- Children or infants with bilious vomiting
- Chronic vomiting that does not have a clear diagnosis

CLARIFICATION STATEMENTS FOR PARENTAL MISCONCEPTIONS

'If my child is vomiting, surely he has a tummy bug.'

No, vomiting does not always indicate gastroenteritis. This is a frequent error made by doctors and parents alike. Often the cause of the vomiting is remote from the stomach, and failure to undertake a detailed history can lead to a poorer outcome for the child.

'Flat carbonated drinks are best for 'gastro' – that's what my mother used when I was sick and it worked then.'

While carbonated drinks were used in the past, this reflects custom and practice of a former era, but evidence now suggest that this is a suboptimal treatment strategy. If the child is dehydrated then oral rehydration therapy should be used, but if the infant is breastfed this should be continued. Inappropriate solutions such as carbonated drinks may prolong the illness state, as they are not physiological solutions.

'I have had to use this ORT solution for 3 days because of this gastro bug.'

ORT is oral rehydration therapy, it is not oral maintenance therapy, and once the child is dehydrated he or she should commence a regular diet as recommended by guideline or refeeding post gastroenteritis. Small numbers may require lactose-free milk for a short period because of lactose intolerance.

'What about antibiotic treatment for gastroenteritis?'

Since most causes of gastroenteritis are related to viruses, antibiotic treatment is not indicated and if used can prolong symptoms due to medication side effects.

SUMMARY PRACTICE POINTS

- Vomiting often precedes diarrhoea in gastroenteritis.
- Pyloric stenosis presents with non-bilious vomiting in the first 3–4 weeks of life.
- GER occurs in 50% of children and resolves when they walk.
- GERD is associated with poor feeding, food refusal, recurrent vomiting, poor weight gain and poor sleep.
- PUJ is diagnosed antenatally in 40%.
- Idiopathic intracranial hypertension is diagnosed by an increased pressure of the cerebrospinal fluid at lumbar puncture; visual loss also occurs with it.
- Bilious vomiting in a neonate is an emergency.
- Recurrent episodes of vomiting, with mild illnesses, may indicate the presence of a metabolic disease.
- Ondansetron is useful to reduce the vomiting associated with gastroenteritis.

EVALUATING THE EVIDENCE

Evidence 1	
Theme E1	*The use of oral dimenhydrinate in children with gastroenteritis*
Question	How effective is oral dimenhydrinate in children with gastroenteritis?
Design	Randomised controlled trial
Level of evidence	Jadad 5
Setting	Paediatric emergency department, academic medical centre, Canada
Participants	Children, previously well, aged 1–12 years with some physician-assessed dehydration related to gastroenteritis were eligible if they presented with more than five episodes of vomiting in the preceding 12 hours.
Intervention	The intervention consisted of the administration of placebo or oral dimenhydrinate at a dose of 1 mg/kg/dose every 6 hours for four doses. Fifteen minutes post administration oral rehydration fluid was offered at a rate of 0.2 mL/kg/minute. During the emergency department stay, the degree of dehydration, number of vomits and diarrhoeal episodes, quantity of fluid consumed and the need for intravenous fluids were recorded.
Outcomes	The primary outcome was treatment failure defined as two or more episodes of vomiting in the 24 hours after administration of the first dose of medication.

(continued)

Evidence 1

Theme E1	*The use of oral dimenhydrinate in children with gastroenteritis*
Main results	Of the 209 patients who were eligible, 152 were randomised (50 refused and seven were missed): 76 to oral dimenhydrinate, with two lost to follow-up, and 76 to placebo, with six lost to follow-up. Baseline characteristics were similar. The proportion with two or more vomits in the treatment group was 31% and in the placebo group, 29% (95% confidence interval: −0.12 to 0.17) (absolute reduced risk (ARR) = 2; number needed to treat (NNT) = 50).
Conclusion	The use of oral dimenhydrinate did not significantly reduce the frequency of vomiting in gastroenteritis compared with placebo.
Commentary	This study reiterates the lack of effectiveness of oral dimenhydrinate in the treatment of vomiting related to gastroenteritis. The main adverse affect attributed to dimenhydrinate was drowsiness in 42%. Only 4% of the treatment group and 8% of the control group had an intravenous cannula inserted, and none of the treatment group and only 2% of the placebo group were admitted. The article reinforces the effectiveness of oral rehydration therapy.
Reference	Gouin S, Vo TT, Roy M, *et al.* Oral dimenhydrinate versus placebo in children with gastroenteritis: a randomized controlled trial. *Pediatrics.* 2012; **129**(6): 1050–5.

Evidence 2

Theme E2	*Pharmacological reduction of vomiting in gastroenteritis*
Question	What is the effectiveness of oral ondansetron for gastroenteritis in children?
Design	Randomised controlled trial
Level of evidence	Jadad 5
Setting	Emergency department in a children's hospital, the United States
Participants	Previously well children aged 6 months to 10 years with at least one non-bloody, non-bilious vomit within 4 hours of triage and one or more episodes of loose stools. Dehydration was assessed using a 7-point scale which was based on expert opinion and clinical studies).
Intervention	Subject received a 4 mg orally dissolvable tablet of ondansetron or placebo 15 minutes prior to the commencement of oral rehydration therapy (ORT). ORT was administered at a rate of 30 mL every 5 minutes for 1 hour, at which time a physician reassessed dehydration status.
Outcomes	The primary outcome was vomiting while receiving ORT. A vomit was defined as a forceful expulsion of stomach contents. Episodes of vomiting within a 2-minute period were considered as one episode. Secondary outcomes were the frequency of vomiting and the rate of intravenous fluid administration. The drug safety profile was evaluated.
Main results	Two hundred and forty-three were asked to enrol, and 214 were correctly randomised: 107 in the ondansetron group and 107 in the placebo group. The vomit rates for ondansetron and placebo were 14% and 35%, respectively (absolute risk reduction (ARR) = 22%; number needed to treat (NNT) = 5).

(continued)

Evidence 2	
Theme E2	***Pharmacological reduction of vomiting in gastroenteritis***
Main results *(cont.)*	For ondansetron and placebo, the intravenous fluid rate was 5% and 17%, respectively (ARR = 12%; NNT = 8). The most common side effect reported was diarrhoea.
Conclusion	Ondansetron facilitated oral rehydration due to a reduction in vomiting episodes.
Commentary	The use of ondansetron facilitated increased rates of ORT but did not decrease admission rates to hospital (the study was not powered to answer this question). Children were only allowed 1 hour for ORT in the emergency department (to simulate actual clinical practice). The use of ondansetron would appear to make economic sense, given its cost, and consideration should be given to its use to enhance ORT success in the emergency department. The authors did not use the World Health Organization dehydration scale, as most of the children had mild to moderate dehydration.
Reference	Freedman SB, Adler M, Seshadri R, *et al.* Oral ondansetron for gastroenteritis in a pediatric emergency department. *N Eng J Med.* 2006; **354**(16): 1698–705.

Evidence 3	
Theme E3	***Dehydration assessment in children***
Question	Is the clinical dehydration scale (CDS) valid in the assessment of children with acute gastroenteritis?
Design	Prospective cohort study
Level of evidence	
Setting	Emergency department, academic medical centre, Canada
Participants	Children aged 1 month to 5 years with a discharge diagnosis of acute gastroenteritis, gastritis or enteritis in whom the CDS had been completed were eligible for inclusion. These inclusion criteria reflect the population in whom the CDS had been derived.
Intervention	Trained triage nurses undertook a dehydration assessment on any child presenting with vomiting, diarrhoea or both who were between the ages of 1 month and 5 years. From these data, those participants who had a diagnosis of gastroenteritis, gastritis or enteritis were extracted.
Outcomes	The primary outcome was the association between length of stay in the emergency department and the CDS for children.
Main results	The CDS was measured in 279 patients but only 150 were included in the analysis as 46 patients did not have a final diagnosis of gastroenteritis, 32 were >5 years of age, 31 left the department prior to physician assessment and 20 had a previous visit to the ED within the study period. Fifty six patients had no dehydration, 74 had some dehydration and 20 had moderate to severe dehydration. Severity of dehydration, based on the CDS, was correlated to increased length of stay in the ED. The median length of stay for no dehydration was 54 minutes, for some dehydration was 128 minutes and for severe dehydration was 425 minutes.

(continued)

Evidence 3

Theme E3	Dehydration assessment in children
Conclusion	The CDS is a good predictor of length of stay in the emergency department post physician assessment. This study validated the CDS in a different paediatric centre from where it was developed.
Commentary	The CDS consists of four characteristics that are scored 0, 1, 2 (a score of 0 represents no dehydration; 1–4, some dehydration; 5–8, severe dehydration). The characteristics are GENERAL APPEARANCE (score 0, normal; 1, thirsty, restless or lethargic but irritable when touched; 2, drowsy, limp, cold or sweaty with or without comatose state), EYES (score 0, normal; 1, slightly sunken; 2, very sunken), MUCOUS MEMBRANES (tongue), (score 0, moist; 1, sticky; and 2, dry) and TEARS (score 0, tears; 1, decreased; 2, absent tears).
Reference	Bailey B, Gravel J, Goldman RD, *et al.* External validation of the clinical dehydration scale for children with acute gastroenteritis. *Acad Emerg Med.* 2010; **17**(6): 583–8.

Evidence 4

Theme E4	Oral rehydration in the treatment of gastroenteritis
Question	Which is more effective in moderately dehydrated children: oral or intravenous (IV) rehydration?
Design	Randomised controlled trial
Level of evidence	Jadad 3
Setting	Emergency department of a children's hospital, the United States
Participants	Children, previously well, aged 8 weeks to 3 years, moderately dehydrated (dehydration scores ≥3 and <7) with a diagnosis of probable gastroenteritis (more than three watery stools in the previous 24 hours).
Intervention	Oral rehydration treatment (ORT) was evaluated against IV fluid. The ORT group received Pedialyte at 50 mL/kg orally over 4 hours if their baseline dehydration scores were 3, 4, or 5, and at 75 mL/kg if their baseline dehydration score was 6. The fluid was administered in equal aliquots every 5 minutes. For the IV fluid group an IV line was placed and two 20 mL/kg fluids boluses were administered over the first hour and patients were the encouraged (but not required) to drink over the next 3 hours. All emesis were recorded. Infants were weighed and assessed for dehydration (by a blinded physician) at time 0, 2 and 4 hours. ORT failure was defined as >25% vomit of hourly fluid requirement or six consecutive refusals to drink.
Outcomes	The primary outcome was resolution of moderate dehydration (dehydration score ≤2, weight gain, urine production and absence of emesis). A secondary outcome was the time to initiation of therapy.
Main results	Three hundred and fifty-five patients were assessed for eligibility (246 did not meet criteria, and 36 refused to participate). Seventy-three were randomised, 36 to the ORT group and 37 to the IV group. Study completion rates were 33(92%) for ORT and 34(92%) for IV groups.

(*continued*)

Evidence 4	
Theme E4	*Oral rehydration in the treatment of gastroenteritis*
Main results (*cont.*)	Successful rehydration rate at 4 hours for ORT was 55.6% and for IV fluids was 56.8% (absolute risk reduction (ARR) = 0.2%; number needed to treat (NNT) = 500). Secondary outcome mean time to initiate treatment for ORT was 15 minutes and for IV fluids it was 36 minutes.
Conclusion	ORT is as effective as IV fluids in the correction of moderate dehydration related to gastroenteritis in the emergency department.
Commentary	This study provides practical insights into ORT versus IV fluid rehydration. Six (15.2%) subjects in the ORT group were unable to perform ORT; however, nasogastric tube placement was not allowed in the protocol (a measure that could have increased success rates of rehydration). In the IV fluid group, 19 (51.4%) had a cannula placed successfully on the first attempt, 7 (18.9%) on the second attempt and ten (27%) required three to eight attempts. Hospitalisation was rarest for the ORT group, at 22.7%, and for the IV fluid group it was 50% (ARR = 27.3%; NNT = 5).
Reference	Spandorfer PR, Alessandrini EA, Joffe MD, *et al.* Oral versus intravenous rehydration of moderately dehydrated children: a randomized, controlled trial. *Pediatrics.* 2005; **115**(2): 295–301.

Evidence 5	
Theme E 5	*Rehydration treatment in gastroenteritis*
Question	In a child with dehydration, which is superior: standard or rapid rehydration?
Design	Randomised controlled trial
Level of evidence	Jadad 5
Setting	Emergency department in children's hospital, Canada
Participants	Participants were children aged greater than 90 days with dehydration secondary to gastroenteritis who failed oral rehydration therapy. There were exclusion criteria underlying surgical condition. Participants had a clinical dehydration score of greater than 3 and were prescribed intravenous fluids by a physician.
Intervention	Rapid 60 mL/kg versus 20 mL/kg of 0.9% NaCl over 1 hour.
Outcomes	Primary outcome was the degree of clinical dehydration present, assessed by a validated tool at 2 hours.
Main results	At 2 hours, 41 (36%) of the rapidly hydrated and 33 (29%) of the standard hydrated were clinically dehydrated. The absolute risk reduction was 6.5%, and number needed to treat was 16. The secondary outcome of time to discharge was 6.3 versus 5 hours.
Conclusion	No clinically relevant benefit to child in the use of rapid dehydration correction
Commentary	The use of rapid dehydration confirms no increased benefit to children with dehydration who are haemodynamically stable. If it were to be used, serum electrolytes should be measured; however, this is only performed in 30% of children with gastroenteritis attending emergency departments.

(*continued*)

Evidence 5

Theme E 5	*Rehydration treatment in gastroenteritis*
Commentary (*cont.*)	In this study, to decrease the need for intravenous fluids, 5 mL every 5 minutes of flavoured oral rehydration solution was given to the child through a syringe and oral ondansetron was also administered. Caution is advocated in the use of rapid rehydration of febrile children in developing countries, as it is associated with an increased mortality.
Reference	Freedman SB, Parkin PC, Willan AR, *et al.* Rapid versus standard intravenous rehydration in paediatric gastroenteritis: a pragmatic blinded randomised trial. *BMJ.* 2011; **343**: d6976.

Evidence 6

Theme E 6	*Change in paediatric practice*
Question	Can treatment practices be modified? (Oral rehydration for gastroenteritis)
Design	Audit of practice (cross-sectional sample analysis)
Level of evidence	
Setting	Department of paediatrics, academic medical centre, Wales
Participants	Children admitted to hospital with a clinical diagnosis of acute gastroenteritis and who were younger than 5 years of age were eligible. Four cross-sectional samples were chosen in the years 1999, 2002, 2004 and 2009.
Intervention	The intervention undertaken after 2002 included an educational programme with a written guideline on the management of gastroenteritis, utilising oral rehydration treatment, carried out over a 1-month period with nursing staff. The guideline was reinforced with each child who was admitted with gastroenteritis and with nursing staff at handover rounds. The aim was to produce a culture change.
Outcomes	The primary outcome was the assessment of impact of an implementation strategy after the first audit in 1999, which focused on the use of oral rehydration therapy in the treatment of children admitted with gastroenteritis.
Main results	Four cross-sectional cohorts of children were reviewed. The dehydration status was documented in 86% in 1999, in 69% in 2002, in 86% in 2004 and in 74% in 2009. In 1999, of 106 subjects, 38% were dehydrated, with 20% (of total) receiving intravenous fluid therapy. In 2002, of 153 subjects, 19% were dehydrated, 15% (of total) received intravenous fluids and 48% of dehydrated subjects received intravenous fluid and 0% received nasogastric rehydration. In 2004, of 99 subjects, 28% were dehydrated, 4% (of total) received intravenous fluids, 14% of the dehydrated subjects received intravenous fluids, and 39% of dehydrated subjects received nasogastric rehydration. In 2009, of 89 subjects, 25% were dehydrated, 6% (of total) received intravenous fluids, 18% of those who were dehydrated received intravenous fluids and 23% received nasogastric fluids.
Conclusion	The implementation programme resulted in a change in practice that has been sustained.

(*continued*)

Evidence 6

Theme E 6	Change in paediatric practice
Commentary	Producing practice change is difficult, as is evident from the multiplicity of guidelines that are not followed. The success of this project lies in targeting those at the front line, i.e. nurses, and ensuring the active support of clinical decision-makers. The effectiveness in the culture change lies in the non-requirement for ongoing targeted education. The authors suggest that the succinctness of the guideline may have been a contributing factor to its success.
Reference	Fox J, Richards S, Jenkins HR, *et al.* Management of gastroenteritis over 10 years: changing culture and maintaining the change. *Arch Dis Child.* 2012; **97**(5): 415–17.

Evidence 7

Theme E 7	Gaviscon and gastro-oesophageal reflux
Question	What is the effectiveness of Gaviscon in the treatment of gastro-oesophageal reflux?
Design	Randomised controlled trial (crossover design)
Level of evidence	Jadad 5
Setting	Department of paediatric gastroenterology, academic medical centre, England
Participants	Infants less than 12 months of age were eligible if they had symptoms suggestive of gastro-oesophageal reflux (GOR) (e.g. regurgitation more than three times a day, any amount, or more than once a day, half the feed), were over 2 kg in weight, were exclusively bottle-fed formula or expressed breast milk, and had no signs of acute infection. Prior to enrolment, acid suppression medications or prokinetic agents were discontinued.
Intervention	During a 24-hour period, six random administrations (3 + 3) of Gaviscon Infant (625 mg in 225 mL of milk) or placebo (mannitol and Solvito N to ensure similar taste and appearance, 625 mg in 225 mL of milk) were given in a double-blind fashion and the impact on GOR assessed using a combined pH probe and intraluminal oesophageal impedance measurement. This technique allows detection of acid and non-acid reflux episodes.
Outcomes	The primary outcomes were the number of reflux events per hour, acid reflux events per hour and reflux height.
Main results	Twenty infants were included in this study, with a mean age of 163.5 days (range 34–319). There were 747 reflux events, of which 518 (69%) were non-acid and 229 (31%) were acidic (pH <4). The median number of reflux events per hour was 1.58 for Gaviscon and 1.68 for placebo (no difference). Acid reflux events per hour were 0.26 for Gaviscon versus 0.43 for placebo (no difference). Reflux height for Gaviscon was 66.6% versus 77.3% for placebo of oesophageal length (clinical relevance is uncertain).
Conclusion	The clinical relevance of the height difference of the reflux between Gaviscon Infant and placebo is uncertain. The clinical value of Gaviscon is unproven based on this study.

(continued)

Evidence 7	
Theme E 7	*Gaviscon and gastro-oesophageal reflux*
Commentary	GOR is a frequent occurrence with a propensity to improve once the child is ambulant. This study utilised combined pH and impedance procedure to detect the presence of both acid and non-acid reflux (the latter goes undetected with conventional pH-metry). Other authors have recognised that non-acid reflux is clinically relevant and accounts for 78% of apnoeas attributed to reflux. Liquid Gaviscon (sodium alginate and potassium bicarbonate) acts as a raft floating on the stomach contents, and then coats the oesophagus, where it acts as a movable neutral sealant that occupies the oesophageal space as a wave of reflux enters it from the stomach. Gaviscon Infant does not contain bicarbonate and consequently does not form a raft but acts as a thickening agent. The sodium content of adult Gaviscon is high and is unsuitable for infants.
Reference	Del Buono R, Wenzl TG, Ball G, *et al.* Effect of Gaviscon Infant on gastro-oesophageal reflux in infants assessed by combined intraluminal impedance/pH. *Arch Dis Child.* 2005; **90**(5): 460–3.

Evidence 8	
Theme E 8	*Proton pump inhibitors and gastro-oesophageal reflux (GERD)*
Question	How effective are proton pump inhibitors in the treatment of GERD?
Design	Randomised controlled trial
Level of evidence	Jadad 5
Setting	Thirty-three paediatric centres, the United States, France, Germany and Poland
Participants	Patients aged 1–11 months were eligible for inclusion if they had diagnosis of GERD based on symptoms, endoscopically proven GERD, or an investigator determined diagnosis of GERD based on patient's history, physical examination, laboratory tests, or findings from diagnostic tests. Patients were required to have at least one of the symptoms of GERD: vomiting or regurgitation, irritability, supra-oesophageal symptoms of GERD (cough, wheezing, stridor, laboured breathing), feeding difficulties (food refusal, gagging or choking, hiccoughs for more than 1 hour/day) at least twice per week in a 4-week period.
Intervention	After screening, patients entered the open-label phase of the study, where they all received Esomeprazole once a day based on weight (2.5 mg for 3–5 kg infant, 5 mg if >5–7.5 kg and 10 mg if >7.5–12 kg) for 14 days and those who responded as indicated by an improvement of the physician's global assessment scores for GERD in at least one category were eligible for the double blind phase of the study. Patients were randomised to Esomeprazole or placebo for up to 4 weeks. Symptoms were assessed utilising the modified Infant Gastroesophageal Reflux Questionnaire, which formed the basis of the physician's global assessment.
Outcomes	The primary outcome was time from randomisation to discontinuation owing to symptom worsening in the double-blind phase.
Main results	Of the 98 who entered the study, 95 (97%) were enrolled in the open-label phase and had data available on symptom severity at baseline and at the end of the open-label phase.

(*continued*)

Evidence 8	
Theme E 8	*Proton pump inhibitors and gastro-oesophageal reflux (GERD)*
Main results (*cont.*)	The proportion of patients with moderate to severe GERD decreased from 92.6% to 21.1%. A total of 81 (82.7%) patients had an improvement of at least 1 grade in the physician's global assessment score. The primary analysis revealed symptom worsening leading to discontinuation of placebo in 20 (48.8%) and of Esomeprazole in 15 (39%) (hazard ratio: 0.69; 95% confidence interval: 0.35%–1.35%; $P = 0.28$). A hazard ratio is an expression of the hazard or chance of an event occurring in the treatment group as a ratio of the chance of the event occurring in the control group. Infants on Esomeprazole had a 31% reduced risk of discontinuing from the study due to symptoms worsening compared with placebo.
Conclusion	The discontinuation rates owing to symptom worsening did not differ significantly between the two groups.
Commentary	The study has some intriguing results: in the open-label component there was symptom improvement noted in 71.5% of patients on Esomeprazole treatment but the time to symptom resolution was not evaluated. The overall results were equivocal; however, specific subgroups did respond well to Esomeprazole and these included those infants with symptoms of crying for more than 1 hour with medium to large vomited volumes. In the first 2 weeks after randomisation, five (12.8%) of the Esomeprazole group and nine (22.2%) of the placebo group discontinued treatment because of symptom worsening. Given that these were post hoc analyses (and not pre-planned) they should be viewed with caution. A central difficulty in assessing infants with GERD is the absence of a specific test that can be utilised to define the population; such a test would more accurately allow the impact of acid suppression therapy to be assessed.
Reference	Winter H, Gunasekaran T, Tolia V, *et al.* Esomeprazole for the treatment of GERD in infants ages 1–11 months. *J Pediatr Gastroenterol Nutr.* 2012; **55**(1): 14–20.

VOMITING: MULTIPLE-CHOICE QUESTIONS

Q1 Recognised causes of vomiting in childhood include which of the following?
  a) Acidosis
  b) Hypercalcaemia
  c) Pelvi-ureteric obstruction
  d) Chronic renal failure
  e) Hypothyroidism
  f) Supraventricular tachycardia

Q2 Which of the following statements regarding pyloric stenosis is/are correct?
  a) It presents in the first 2 weeks of life.
  b) The vomiting is projectile and bilious in nature.
  c) Weight loss is a common feature.
  d) An olive-shaped mass is palpable in 75% of patients.
  e) The infant refuses to feed.

Q3 Features of cyclical vomiting include the presence of which of the following?
a) Five attacks per 6 months
b) At least six vomits per hour for at least 1 hour
c) Intense nausea during an attack
d) Similar features for each occurrence
e) The finding of gallstones in 3% of patients

Q4 Which of the following statements regarding paediatric pancreatitis is/are correct?
a) Most cases are idiopathic.
b) Clinical features include epigastric pain, nausea and vomiting.
c) Alcohol ingestion is a recognised risk factor.
d) Cholelithiasis is a recognised cause.
e) It accounts for 3% of epigastric pain admitted to hospital.

Q5 Non-GI causes of vomiting include which of the following?
a) Diabetic ketoacidosis
b) Otitis media
c) Meningitis
d) Pneumonia
e) Tonsillitis

Q6 Which of the following are risk factors for GERD?
a) Obesity
b) Cystic fibrosis
c) Bronchopulmonary dysplasia
d) Pneumonia
e) Cerebral palsy

Q7 Diseases that cause acute recurrent vomiting include which of the following?
a) Urea cycle defects
b) Mitochondrial disease
c) Fatty acid oxidation defects
d) Acute intermittent porphyria
e) Hypoglycaemia

Q8 Which of the following statements are correct?
a) ORT is contraindicated in severe dehydration.
b) Giving 50 mL/kg over 4 hours for moderate dehydration is appropriate.
c) The failure rate of ORT (due to refusal to drink) is 6%.
d) The success rate of ORT is 90%.
e) ORT is contraindicated in febrile children.

Q9 Which of the following statements is/are correct?
  a) Ondansetron is effective in 90% of vomiting children.
  b) Oral dimenhydrinate is superior to placebo in vomiting children with dehydration.
  c) Ondansetron and dimenhydrinate are equally effective in the vomiting child.
  d) Nasogastric fluid administration is contraindicated in vomiting children.
  e) Dimenhydrinate causes drowsiness in 40% of children.

Q10 Appropriate tests for GERD include which of the following?
  a) Barium studies
  b) Chest X-ray
  c) Endoscopy
  d) pH monitoring studies
  e) Ultrasound

Answers

A1	a, b, c, e	A2	c
A3	c, d	A4	a, b, c, d
A5	a, b, c, d, e	A6	a, b, c, e
A7	a, b, c, d	A8	b
A9	e	A10	c, d

SLIDES

1. Addison's disease 1
2. Addison's disease 2
3. Intestinal obstruction (neonatal)

Chapter Ten

THE CHILD WITH ABDOMINAL PAIN

COMMON SCENARIO

'At first I thought he was just trying to get out of going to school, but he's been complaining of tummy pain all day now and hasn't eaten a thing. It just suddenly got worse in the last hour and has moved to the right side.'

LEARNING OBJECTIVES

- Understand the medical and surgical causes of abdominal pain in children
- Recognise 'red flags' in the history or examination that require investigation or urgent treatment
- Develop a strategy to counsel parents of children with functional abdominal pain (FAP)
- Develop a treatment strategy to treat medical and surgical causes of abdominal pain

BACKGROUND

Abdominal pain in childhood can be classified as acute or chronic. It is one of the commonest presenting complaints of childhood. There are several important surgical causes of acute abdominal pain that must be recognised and treated to minimise morbidity. The history and examination are the most important steps in the evaluation of a child with abdominal pain. In the clinical setting acute surgical conditions present with pain followed by vomiting, whereas a medical cause presents with vomiting as the presenting feature. In a child presenting with an acute onset of abdominal pain, simple observation of the child provides valuable information, e.g. the child with peritonitis may be unable or refuses to walk, lies motionless and has decreased or absent abdominal wall movements with respiration.

There are three recognised types of abdominal pain: visceral, somatic and referred. Visceral pain is a dull, aching, midline pain that is not necessarily located over the site of pathology. It is typically felt in the midline according to the level of dermatome innervations and can be epigastric, periumbilical or suprapubic. Visceral pain becomes somatic if the affected viscus involves a somatic organ, i.e. the peritoneum or abdominal wall. In contrast, somatic pain is localised, sharp and aggravated by movement or coughing. Referred pain is pain referred from the parietal pleura to the abdominal wall. Abdominal pain radiating to the back is suggestive of cholecystitis or pancreatitis.

Features that suggest a surgical cause:

- bilious vomiting
- bloody stool
- localised tenderness
- guarding or rebound tenderness
- palpable mass
- inguinoscrotal pain or swelling.

Important surgical causes of acute abdominal pain

Intussusception

Intussusception is invagination of the proximal bowel into distal bowel, usually the ileum into the caecum. There may be a history of a recent upper respiratory tract infection (URTI) or gastroenteritis, recent weaning onto solids or vaccination. It classically presents at 2 months to 2 years of age. A lead point for invagination is usually hypertrophy of Peyer's patches in the terminal ileum. It presents as sudden, severe, spasmodic colicky pain. The child is extremely irritable, pulls up his or her legs and goes pale, particularly around the mouth. Episodes typically last 20 minutes and the infant becomes increasingly lethargic and listless in between episodes. There may be associated vomiting or the passage of red currant jelly stool, which is considered a late sign indicating infarction. Examination may reveal abdominal distension, tenderness and a sausage-shaped mass in the right upper quadrant, with an impression of emptiness in the right lower quadrant. Coma is a rare presentation of intussusception.

Testicular torsion

Testicular torsion can be intra- or extravaginal. Intravaginal torsion occurs in older children and is due to torsion within the tunica vaginalis secondary to anomalous testicular suspension or the 'bell and clapper' deformity. Classically it presents with the sudden onset of severe scrotal pain with or without vomiting. Alternatively, it may present as referred pain to the flank or lower abdomen. Examination reveals a swollen, erythematous and extremely tender testis with absent cremasteric reflex. The contralateral testis may show a 'bell and clapper' deformity, i.e. lying horizontally rather than vertically. Extravaginal torsion occurs in the neonatal period because of twisting of the cord proximal to attachment of the tunica vaginalis. Neonates are asymptomatic and present immediately after birth with a non-tender bluish-black scrotal mass. Unfortunately, 75% of neonatal torsions occur antenatally and there is a poor salvage rate, even when the condition occurs in the neonatal period.

Malrotation and volvulus

Malrotation is a congenital abnormal position of the bowel within the peritoneal cavity, usually involving both the small and the large bowel. Fixation may be absent or abnormal and predisposes to volvulus. Volvulus is obstruction caused by twisting of the intestines around the axis of the mesentery. This obstructs the bowel and blood flow in the superior mesenteric artery and vein. Sixty per cent of cases present in the first month of life, 20% between 1 month and 1 year, and the remainder after the first year of life. In the neonatal period it presents with bilious vomiting. In the infant and child it may present with severe abdominal pain with or without vomiting. As the bowel becomes ischaemic, signs of peritonitis may be found.

Appendicitis

Appendicitis is the commonest cause of acute abdominal pain in children requiring surgical intervention. It is extremely rare in neonates and uncommon in children under 3 years of age. The rate of perforation is 80%–100% for children younger than 3 years and <10%–20% for children aged 10–16 years. Children present with a history of vague central abdominal pain preceded by anorexia and vomiting. The pain then shifts and localises to right lower quadrant as the parietal pleura becomes involved. The usual history is less than 48 hours. Examination may reveal a child who is reluctant to move and unable to stand up straight, with low-grade pyrexia, tachycardia and rebound tenderness over McBurney's point (two-thirds of the way between the umbilicus and the right anterior superior iliac spine).

Gallstones

Gallstones may develop at any age, with pigment stones predominating in the first decade of life and cholesterol stones accounting for 90% of gallstones in adolescence. Most children are asymptomatic. For those children with symptomatic gallstones, the dominant symptoms are acute or recurrent episodes of severe, sharp right upper quadrant or epigastric pain. Rarely children may present with a history of jaundice, back pain or generalised abdominal discomfort associated with pancreatitis and usually due to a stone in the common bile duct. Pain episodes may occur after ingestion of fatty foods. The risk groups for gallstones include children with haemolytic anaemia, adolescents with rapid weight loss, patients with Crohn's disease or cystic fibrosis and infants with prolonged parenteral nutrition.

Meckel's diverticulum

Meckel's diverticulum occurs in 2% of the population, making it the commonest congenital defect of the gut. It is a remnant of the vitellointestinal duct, which in the developing embryo connects the yolk sac to the gut, providing nutrition until the placenta is established. It usually involutes at 5–7 weeks' gestation. It is located in the distal ileum on the anti-mesenteric border, within 100 cm of the ileocaecal valve. Fifty per cent of diverticula contain ectopic gastric, pancreatic or colonic tissue. In the majority of cases it is asymptomatic if not lined by ectopic mucosa. Between 40% and 60% of symptomatic patients have painless rectal bleeding. Intestinal obstruction can occur as a result of ileocolic intussusception.

Important medical causes of recurrent abdominal pain

Functional abdominal pain

According to Apley's criteria, functional or recurrent abdominal pain (RAP) is defined as at least three discrete episodes of pain of sufficient severity to interrupt routine activities over a period of at least 3 months. RAP affects 5%–15% of children between the ages of 5 and 15 years and is more common in girls. It can lead to considerable morbidity and loss of school days. In less than 10% of cases an organic cause is found, with the majority of cases being classified as recurrent abdominal pain syndrome. The pain is periumbilical, self-resolving, unrelated to activities and has no impact on growth and no abnormal examination findings.

According to the Rome II criteria, RAP or FAP can be subcategorised into five distinct groups based on the symptoms:
1. functional dyspepsia
2. irritable bowel syndrome
3. abdominal migraine
4. FAP
5. functional abdominal pain syndrome.

These are explained as follows.
- **Functional dyspepsia**: diagnostic criteria include persistent or recurrent pain or discomfort centred in the upper abdomen (above the umbilicus), that is not relieved by defecation or associated with the onset of a change in stool frequency or stool form (i.e. not irritable bowel syndrome). There is no evidence of an inflammatory, anatomic, metabolic or neoplastic process that explains the symptoms.
- **Irritable bowel syndrome**: abdominal discomfort or pain associated with two or more of the following features at least 25% of the time: improved with defecation or associated with a change in stool frequency or appearance. There is no evidence of an inflammatory, anatomic, metabolic or neoplastic process that explains the symptoms.
- **Abdominal migraine**: paroxysmal episodes of intense, acute, periumbilical pain lasting for 1 or more hours. Pain associated with anorexia, nausea, vomiting, headache, photophobia or pallor. Criteria fulfilled two or more times in the preceding year. The child is healthy and asymptomatic in between episodes. There is no evidence of an inflammatory, anatomic, metabolic or neoplastic process that explains the symptoms.
- **FAP**: episodic or continuous abdominal pain with insufficient criteria for other functional gastrointestinal disorders. There is no evidence of an inflammatory, anatomic, metabolic or neoplastic process that explains the symptoms.

- **Functional abdominal pain syndrome**: FAP and at least 25% of the time have one or more of the following; daily functioning or additional somatic feature: headache, limb pain, difficulty sleeping.

When evaluating a child with abdominal pain, the clinical features that suggest an organic cause include:
- night-time pain that awakens the child
- pain with a consistent focal location, especially pain that is localised away from the umbilicus
- altered bowel habit, rectal bleeding or vomiting
- pain in children less than 5 years of age
- a positive family history of peptic ulcer disease or inflammatory bowel disease
- weight loss or anorexia
- associated fever, mouth ulcers, arthralgia, rash, uveitis
- pain radiating to back, shoulder or lower limbs.

Inflammatory bowel disease

Crohn's disease is a chronic inflammatory disease of the bowel involving anywhere from the mouth to the anus. The terminal ileum and colon are involved in 50% of cases, the small bowel in 35% and perirectal disease is found in 20% of cases. Clinical features include abdominal pain, diarrhoea, weight loss, growth failure and anaemia. Extraintestinal manifestations include joint disease and ankylosing spondylitis, skin manifestations (erythema nodosum, erythema multiforme and pyoderma gangrenosum), liver disease (sclerosing cholangitis, chronic active hepatitis and cirrhosis), uveitis and episcleritis and osteoporosis. Complications include severe perianal disease, enteroenteral fistulas, short bowel syndrome, growth retardation and delayed puberty, nephrolithiasis and abscess formation.

Ulcerative colitis is characterised by diffuse mucosal inflammation limited to the colon. Children classically present with bloody diarrhoea and abdominal pain. Eighty per cent of children have a pancolitis at presentation, compared with 30% in adults. Both ulcerative colitis and Crohn's disease can present insidiously with weight loss, anorexia and growth failure.

HISTORY

KEY POINTS				
Pain features	Location Radiation Duration Onset Quality Severity Timing Aggravating and relieving factors Constant or intermittent	**Medical history**	Sickle-cell anaemia Haemolytic anaemias Cystic fibrosis Malignancy Renal disease	**🔍 Red flags** Fever Severe diarrhoea and vomiting Gastrointestinal bleeding Chronic right iliac fossa or right upper quadrant pain Weight loss
Associated symptoms	History of trauma Vomiting (bile, blood) Increased flatulence Altered bowel habit Per rectum bleeding or mucus Fever Rash Anorexia Urinary symptoms Arthralgia Visual disturbance	**Surgical history**	Previous abdominal surgery	Family history of inflammatory bowel disease Back or flank pain Nocturnal abdominal pain
Impact on child	School days lost Participation in extracurricular activities	**Medications**	Use of analgesia and their impact Regular medications	
Family history	Inflammatory bowel disease Migraines Peptic ulcer disease Coeliac disease Irritable bowel syndrome Renal stones	**Social history**	Stressors at school or at home Bullying or teasing	
Gynaecological history in females	Last menstrual period Sexually active Vaginal discharge	**Growth and development**	Weight loss Energy levels	
Birth history	Delayed passage of meconium Prolonged total parenteral nutrition			

EXAMINATION

- Observe overall appearance of child for signs of peritonitis: ability to walk and hop, with comfort, posture
- Assess vital signs including temperature and hydration status
- Plot height and weight on appropriate centile charts

Examine:
- abdomen: signs of tenderness, rebound, guarding or rigidity, swellings, masses, discoloration or distension (Cullen's and Grey Turner's sign)
- hands: clubbing
- signs of anaemia: pallor of palmar creases and conjunctiva
- oral cavity: ulcers
- perianal area: skin tags, fissures, fistulae
- respiratory exam: crepitations, decreased air entry.

❗ Red flags

- Growth impairment (check previous growth pattern)
- McBurney's point tenderness
- Abdominal bruising
- Pallor
- Failure to thrive
- Guarding
- Abdominal masses
- Clubbing

DIFFERENTIAL DIAGNOSIS FOR ACUTE ABDOMINAL PAIN

Some conditions causing abdominal pain are universal affecting all age groups, whereas others are age specific. Therefore a useful approach to narrowing the differential causes of abdominal pain in childhood is to consider the age of the child and the pathologies that are more likely to occur in that age group.

Birth to 1 year	
Infantile colic	Diagnosis of exclusion, inconsolable crying, normal physical exam
Intussusception	Colicky abdominal pain, flexing of legs, lethargy, vomiting, red current jelly stool (late sign)
Hirschsprung's enterocolitis	Delayed passage of meconium, abdominal wall erythema, tenderness, distension, blood in stools
Volvulus	Bilious vomiting

2–5 years	
Pharyngitis	Sore throat, fever, cervical lymphadenopathy
Henoch–Schönlein purpura	Joint pain or swelling, palpable purpuric rash on extensor surface
Mesenteric lymphadenitis	Presents similar to appendicitis but prodromal URTI, fever, diffuse pain, no signs of peritonitis, lymphadenopathy, absence of rigidity
Trauma	Bruising, bleeding or laceration
	Cullen's sign (blue purple periumbilical discoloration) and Grey Turner's sign (blue purple flank discoloration) indicate retroperitoneal haemorrhage
Diabetic ketoacidosis	History of polyuria and polydipsia
Meckel's diverticulum	Intermittent painless rectal bleeding, may present with partial obstruction or may resemble acute appendicitis

6–11 years	
FAP	First presentation of FAP, otherwise well child, normal physical examination
Pneumonia	Cough, shortness of breath, focal findings on chest examination
Mesenteric lymphadenitis	Presents similar to appendicitis but prodromal URTI, fever, diffuse pain, no signs of peritonitis, lymphadenopathy, absence of rigidity
Diabetic ketoacidosis	History of polyuria and polydipsia
Trauma	Bruising, bleeding or laceration. Cullen (blue purple periumbilical discoloration) and Grey Turner's (blue purple flank discoloration) signs indicate retroperitoneal haemorrhage
Crohn's disease	First presentation of inflammatory bowel disease, poor growth, short stature, weight loss, anorexia
Henoch–Schönlein purpura	Joint pain or swelling, palpable purpuric rash on extensor surface
Pharyngitis	Sore throat, fever, cervical lymphadenopathy
Testicular torsion	Loss of cremasteric reflex, horizontal testis

12–16 years	
Appendicitis	Vague central abdominal pain, anorexia, pain shifts and localises to right lower quadrant, rebound tenderness over McBurney's point
Ectopic pregnancy	Sexually active, amenorrhea or vaginal bleeding
Ovarian cyst or torsion	Tender pelvic mass, nausea and vomiting
Testicular torsion	Loss of cremasteric reflex, horizontal testis
Mittelschmerz	Midcycle pain (2 weeks after first day of menstrual cycle), history of previous similar episodes
Dysmenorrhoea	Begins before onset of menstruation, crampy pain

All ages	
Gastroenteritis	Low-grade fever, vomiting and diarrhoea
Appendicitis	Vague central abdominal pain, anorexia, pain shifts and localises to right lower quadrant, rebound tenderness over McBurney's point
Urinary tract infection	Haematuria, frequency, urgency, pyrexia, loin pain
Incarcerated inguinal hernia	Males, usually right side, tender mass

Special considerations	At-risk groups
Nephrolithiasis	Crohn's disease, renal disease, positive family history, metabolic disease
Gallstones	Haemolytic anaemia, cystic fibrosis, Crohn's disease, prolonged parenteral nutrition,
Splenic infarction	Sickle-cell anaemia, bacterial endocarditis, malignancy

INVESTIGATIONS

What investigations should be performed in a child presenting with acute abdominal pain?

The decision to perform investigations is largely guided by the history and clinical examination findings.

- Children with gastroenteritis generally do not require investigations apart from a stool culture to confirm the diagnosis and a urea and electrolytes test if there are concerns about significant dehydration
- A urinalysis should be performed in all patients. White cells in the urine could indicate an infection. Blood present in urine may indicate stones or trauma. Blood glucose should be checked to rule out diabetic ketoacidosis.
- A raised C-reactive protein level may indicate an inflammatory process.
- A full blood count may show anaemia which may indicate an underlying illness or acute blood loss; a raised white cell count may be seen with infection.
- If pneumonia is suspected a chest X-ray may show consolidation.

If malrotation is suspected, what radiological investigation should be performed?

An upper gastrointestinal study should be performed if malrotation is suspected but there are no clinical signs of an acute abdomen (which requires urgent surgery). With malrotation, the position of the duodenojejunal flexure is abnormally low and to the right of the midline. If volvulus is present, the corkscrew sign may be seen and represents a surgical emergency. Ultrasound, evaluating the position of the superior mesenteric vein in relation to the superior mesenteric artery, can also aid the diagnosis of malrotation.

In children with chronic abdominal pain, what investigations should be performed?

If there are no 'red flags' in the history or examination and the practitioner is confident with the diagnosis, no investigations apart from routine urinalysis and stool for occult blood is required. Over-investigation contributes to more anxiety and may exacerbate the situation.

The only investigation worth considering is a coeliac screen (anti-transglutaminase type 2 IgA and IgA), which can present with similar non-specific abdominal symptoms.

(continued)

INVESTIGATIONS (*cont.*)

In a child with suspected intussusception, what tests should be utilised?

Ultrasound of the abdomen is the best test to diagnose intussusception in a child. This test may not always be available, especially at night. Plain film of the abdomen can be useful in excluding intussusception (*see* Evidence 1).

In children with suspected inflammatory bowel disease, what investigations should be performed?

- Full blood count, C-reactive protein, erythrocyte sedimentation rate, liver function tests may show anaemia, raised inflammatory markers and hypoalbuminemia
- Stool culture: to rule out infection with shigella, salmonella, campylobacter, yersinia, entamoeba
- Faecal calprotectin: assesses presence of intestinal mucosal inflammation; high sensitivity for Crohn's disease and ulcerative colitis
- Perinuclear antineutrophil cytoplasmic antibody may be positive in ulcerative colitis
- Anti-*Saccharomyces cerevisiae* antibody may be positive in Crohn's disease
- Upper and lower gastrointestinal endoscopy with multiple biopsies is the gold standard
- Barium meal and follow through should be performed in children with Crohn's disease, to assess involvement of the small bowel

Additional investigations:
- white cell scanning can help define disease extent
- ultrasound scan can identify bowel wall thickening, abscesses or free fluid in the abdomen
- computed tomography or magnetic resonance imaging to evaluate complications such as fistula.

MANAGEMENT PLAN: THREE-STEP APPROACH

1. Clarifying and pitfall avoidance strategies:
   a) acute abdominal pain
   b) chronic abdominal pain
2. Surgical management:
   a) acute appendicitis
   b) intussusception
   c) volvulus
   d) testicular torsion
   e) Meckel's diverticulum
3. Medical management:
   a) functional abdominal pain
   b) inflammatory bowel disease: Crohn's disease
   c) inflammatory bowel disease: ulcerative colitis

Clarifying and pitfall avoidance strategies

Acute abdominal pain

In the child who presents with abdominal pain, explain to parents that not all abdominal pain is appendicitis (*see* Differential Diagnosis). Indicate that potential aetiologies are varied and that the progression of symptoms is often required to establish a diagnosis, hence the need for repeated physical assessment.

FOR THE DOCTOR

- The aetiology of the abdominal pain is always in the abdomen. **Pitfall**: pneumonia that involves the diaphragm can present with abdominal pain.
- All presentations of appendicitis are the same. **Pitfall and Rationale**: retroiliac location of the appendix leads to poor pain localisation; appendix location in the paravertebral gutter leads to flank pain; pelvic appendix location leads to diarrhoea by directly irritating the sigmoid colon (*see* Evidence 2).
- Children with abdominal pain do not require analgesia. **Pitfall**: analgesia is required by children with abdominal pain and does not interfere with clinical assessment (*see* Evidence 3).
- Clinical deterioration always occurs immediately with perforation of the appendix. **Pitfall**: some children, immediately after the appendix perforates, will feel very well but their heart rate will remain unchanged (an important clinical finding). They will clinically deteriorate in the following hours and have clear signs of peritonitis.

Chronic abdominal pain

When dealing with FAP the following strategies are suggested.

WITH THE CHILD

- Validate the child's experience. **Rationale**: explain the brain gut axis and the role of visceral hyperalgesia and gut motility in the development of FAP.
- Encourage the child to explore potential triggers. **Rationale**: ask the child to explore potential triggers. Using the analogy of the child being a detective is helpful.
- Define the impact on the child's life of the pain, school loss, absence from sports and so forth.
- Determine the parental response. **Rationale**: how the parents respond is likely to serve as role modelling for the child.

WITH THE PARENTS

- Determine the parental beliefs, especially the mother's.
- Check for the presence of irritable bowel disease in the family.
- Determine the parental response to the pain. **Rationale**: the parental response to the FAP is a major determinant of outcome (*see* Evidence 4).
- Determine the interventions pursued by the family and include dietary restriction and the use of a modified coeliac diet. **Rationale**: this will aid in assessing the parents belief system and give insight if they will accept the concept of FAP.
- Clearly explain the concepts of FAP. Using specific screening questionnaires can be of value (*see* Evidence 5).
- Check for secondary gain being achieved by the FAP. **Rationale**: the occurrence of secondary gain will make symptom resolution more difficult.

FROM THE DOCTOR'S PERSPECTIVE

- Mention what limited tests should be undertaken. **Rationale**: explain the reason for performing test (tests are used to modify the degree of uncertainty that the clinician may have. If the diagnosis is clear-cut from the history and examination, then tests are of limited value).
- Avoid the urge to over-investigate. **Rationale**: it will not reassure the family and may engender more anxiety.
- Ensure that there are no 'red flags' (*see* examination section). **Rationale**: FAP is a diagnosis of exclusion but the criteria used are specific (*see* Evidence 5).
- At each visit check height, weight and plot percentiles.
- Respond if symptoms change.
- Outline the lack of benefit of analgesia. **Rationale**: excessive amounts of ineffective analgesic medication may lead to side effects.

Surgical management

Surgical approaches and the timing of surgery are dependent on the underlying pathology.

Acute appendicitis

Children should be commenced on intravenous fluids to correct fluid and electrolyte abnormalities, prophylactic intravenous antibiotics should be started and an open or laparoscopic appendectomy performed. Of children undergoing appendectomy for appendicitis, 10%–40% will have a normal appendix. In girls the threshold for appendectomy is lower because of the risk of infertility associated with peritonitis.

Intussusception

Infants should be first resuscitated with adequate fluid and the abdomen should be decompressed with the insertion of a nasogastric tube. First-line treatment is non-operative radiological air reduction, which is successful in 90% of cases. If this fails or is contraindicated because of sepsis or peritonitis, surgical laparotomy is indicated. Very occasionally Peutz-Jeghers syndrome presents with intussusception (check for lip pigmentation)

Volvulus

Emergency Ladd's procedure surgery to de-rotate the bowel, relieve the obstruction and divide adhesions and broaden the mesenteric base.

Testicular torsion

Detorsion needs to occur within 6 hours to salvage the testis. The tunica is opened and the testis exposed and untwisted. The contralateral testis should be fixed to the dartos muscle or scrotal septum.

Meckel's diverticulum

Diagnosis is made on the basis of a Meckel's scan (gastric mucosa) and surgery is required.

Medical management

Functional abdominal pain

The primary goal is to return the child to normal function rather than complete disappearance of pain. The first step is explanation and education regarding the benign nature of the problem to both the child and parents. Patient information leaflets should be provided. They should be reassured that the pain is real but that there is no underlying organic cause. Parents and child need to be encouraged not to let the condition interfere with daily activities. School attendance and participation in extra-curricular activities should be encouraged. Parental factors and reaction to pain are more important than psychological characteristics of the child in predicting persistence of abdominal pain; therefore, it is essential that parents accept the benign nature of the condition.

There is no evidence to support dietary measures to treat FAP; however, if it associated with irritable bowel syndrome, probiotic therapy is of benefit (*see* Evidence 6). The role of cognitive behavioural therapy in FAP is established (*see* Evidence 7); however, it may not be readily available. In 50% of cases, symptoms will resolve rapidly, in 25% of cases resolution is slower and in 25% of cases symptoms will persist or recur in adulthood.

Inflammatory bowel disease: Crohn's disease

The aims of treatment are:
- induce and maintain remission
- facilitate normal growth and development
- prevent complications
- improve quality of life.

ACUTE-PHASE TREATMENT
- Oral steroids (prednisolone or prednisone) are effective in inducing remission. Potential side effects are excessive weight gain, hypertension and steroid facies.
- Controlled ileal release of budesonide for terminal ileum or right colon disease is effective.
- Exclusive enteral feeding with a polymeric formula. Fifty per cent of patients can drink it orally but the other half require nasogastric placement.
- Anti-tumour necrosis factor alpha antibodies (infliximab) is effective in inducing remission.

MAINTENANCE TREATMENT

- Immunoregulatory drugs such as methotrexate and 6 mercaptopurine are used for maintenance treatment.
- Anti-tumour necrosis factor alpha antibody therapy is also being used with increased frequency. Parents must be counselled on the risk of infection, tuberculosis reactivation. Physicians need to be aware of unusual infections such as *Listeria monocytogenes* and histoplasmosis that can occur with this treatment. Assessing varicella status prior to commencement of treatment and ensuring that no live vaccine is administered while on treatment is prudent.

Inflammatory bowel disease: ulcerative colitis

As for Crohn's disease, the aims of treatment are:
- induce and maintain remission
- facilitate normal growth and development
- prevent complications
- improve quality of life.

ACUTE-PHASE TREATMENT

- Most patients require oral steroid therapy as the disease is more severe than in adults. Only 30% of children are effectively managed with oral 5-aminosalicylic acid plus or minus adjunctive per rectum treatment.
- Recently infliximab has been used with good effect in children and adolescents with moderate to severe ulcerative colitis and this is likely to modify future practice.

MAINTENANCE TREATMENT

- Unlike Crohn's disease, oral 5-aminosalicylic acid or sulfasalazine is effective in the maintenance of remission.

Surgery due to disease severity or failure to respond to medical therapy is necessary in some children.

FOLLOW-UP

- Infants with colic should be followed up to ensure that parents are coping with colic and the infant continues to thrive.
- FAP should be followed up to ensure that the child is returning to normal functioning and no new symptoms which would suggest an alternative diagnosis develop.

WHEN TO REFER?

- Children with an acute surgical abdomen or acute abdominal pain for more than 4 hours should be urgently referred to a paediatric surgeon for review.

- Children with signs or symptoms suggesting inflammatory bowel disease or gall-stones should be referred to a paediatric gastroenterologist.
- Children with nephrolithiasis should be referred to a paediatric nephrologist.
- FAP can be managed within the primary care setting.

CLARIFICATION STATEMENTS FOR PARENTAL MISCONCEPTIONS

'Surely, if she is having ongoing episodes of tummy pain she needs to have some tests done or a scan of her tummy.'

(Respond to the parent focusing on the condition, the clinical state of the child, and use I statements to indicate willingness to re-evaluate the diagnosis)

RAP is common in childhood and there is no underlying pathology or disease that is causing the pain. It is important to realise that the pain is real, but not the result of any disease within her abdomen. Fortunately she is growing and developing normally and importantly her clinical examination is entirely normal and there are no worrying signs or symptoms that would suggest an underlying cause. Her symptoms are typical of many children with RAP that we see on a daily basis. Over-investigating can lead to more distress and anxiety and in all cases of RAP the results are normal. If I were worried about any underlying cause, then yes certainly I would request investigations. However, what's important now is learning how to live with the pain, which will lessen as she gets back to school and her extracurricular activities, which she certainly seems to have enjoyed in the past. I'll continue to follow her up on a regular basis and if at any point her symptoms or signs change or there is any concern regarding an underlying cause then and only then would it be appropriate to put her through any investigations.

'Surely this pain must be related to a food allergy.'

When presented with a parent who believes the RAP is caused by allergy, check what food and what other symptoms are present. Make sure the diet is safe and that the child has not been restricted by his parent. Encourage food challenges if dietary restrictions have occurred inappropriately. Also explain coeliac disease as parents may have placed the child on a coeliac diet in an attempt to improve their child's symptoms.

'How could the perforated appendix have been missed? It was obvious.'

Perforation rates for appendicitis are high especially if under 3 years of age. The occurrence of perforation does not imply poor care per se.

SUMMARY PRACTICE POINTS

- Pain followed by vomiting is characteristic of surgical aetiologies of abdominal pain.
- Bilious vomiting is typical of surgical aetiologies.
- Inguinal orifices should be assessed in all patients with abdominal pain.
- Lethargy in a young child with abdominal pain is a worrying feature.
- Clinical prediction rules are useful in assessing a child for appendicitis.
- The aetiology of RAP is organic in <10% of cases.
- Pain at night suggests an organic aetiology.

EVALUATING THE EVIDENCE

Evidence 1

Theme E1	X-rays in intussusception
Question	Can plain film radiographs exclude the diagnosis of intussusception?
Design	Prospective cross-sectional study
Level of evidence	
Setting	Departments of paediatrics and radiology, academic medical centre, the United States
Participants	Children aged 3–36 months seen in the emergency department who were evaluated for suspected intussusception were eligible for inclusion.
Intervention	All children underwent a three-view abdominal radiograph (supine, prone, left lateral decubitus) as part of their assessment for the presence of intussusception.
Outcomes	The primary outcome, determined by a radiologist, was the presence of air in the ascending colon of all three X-rays. A secondary outcome was the presence of air in the transverse colon of the supine X-ray film. The diagnosis of intussusception was confirmed by ultrasound, air enema or operative procedure. Ultrasound is regarded as the definitive procedure with sensitivities of 95.5%–100% and specificities of 88%–100%.
Main results	Of 190 eligible patients, 146 were enrolled (but 18 were lost to follow-up) and full data were available on 128 (67.3%), of whom 19 (14.8%) had intussusception. The sensitivity of the three-view abdominal X-rays was 100% (95% confidence interval (CI): 79–100), the specificity was 17.4% (95% CI: 11.1–26.1), the negative predictive value was 100% (95% CI: 79.1–100) and the positive predictive value was 17.4%. The sensitivity of the air in the transverse colon on the supine abdominal X-ray was 84.2% (95% CI: 67.8–100), the specificity was 63.3% (95% CI: 54.2–72.4) and the negative predictive value was 95.5% (95% CI: 91.2–100).
Conclusion	The presence of air in the ascending colon on the three-view abdominal radiograph significantly reduces the likelihood of intussusception.
Commentary	Ileocolic intussusception is a common cause of intestinal obstruction in children 3 months to 3 years that occurs with a frequency of 1–4/1000 live births. When diagnosed within 24 hours the success rate with air enema is 80%–85%.

(continued)

Evidence 1	
Theme E1	*X-rays in intussusception*
Commentary (*cont.*)	The presentation of intussusception is variable and only 20% present with the classic triad of abdominal pain, palpable abdominal mass and red currant jelly stools. The use of three-view abdominal radiograph is very helpful in excluding the diagnosis of intussusception but many centres will only use the supine view. Consequently for the practising clinician, if the clinical suspicion is present, an ultrasound will be required to modify the diagnostic uncertainty. If the risk of the pretest probability of intussusception is low, X-ray finds may suffice. Expertise is required in assessing abdominal X-rays, as these authors have noted.
Reference	Roskind CG, Kamdar G, Ruzal-Shapiro CB, *et al.* Accuracy of plain radiographs to exclude the diagnosis of intussusception. *Pediatr Emerg Care.* 2012; **28**(9): 855–8.

Evidence 2	
Theme E2	*Diagnosing appendicitis in children*
Question	How effective is a clinical prediction rule (CPR) in indentifying children at low risk for acute appendicitis?
Design	Prospective cohort study
Level of evidence	
Setting	Departments of emergency medicine, surgery and radiology, academic medical centre, the United States
Participants	Children and adolescents aged 3–18 years who underwent surgical consultation for appendicitis were eligible for inclusion.
Intervention	This study was undertaken in two phases: first the clinical prediction rule was derived and then it was prospectively assessed.
Outcomes	The primary outcome measure was the presence or absence of appendicitis. Appendicitis was confirmed histologically and a perforated appendix was determined at surgery. The absence of appendicitis was confirmed by telephone follow-up at 2–4 weeks post hospital assessment.
Main results	Over a 15-month period, 4140 patients aged between 3 and 18 presented to the emergency department with abdominal pain, of whom 767 (19%) were referred for a surgical consultation to evaluate the patient for potential appendicitis. Six hundred and one patients were enrolled (425 in the derivation of the CPR and 176 in the validation process). Six items were incorporated into the CPR and given a weighting: nausea (2 points), history of focal right lower quadrant pain (2 points), migration of the pain (1 point), difficulty walking (1 point) and absolute neutrophil count $>6.75 \times 10^3\,\mu$L (6 points). A score of ≤5 had a sensitivity of 96.3% (95% confidence interval (CI): 87.5–99.0), negative predictive value of 95.6% (95% CI: 90.8–99), and a negative likelihood ratio of 0.102 (95% CI: 0.026–0.405). After assessment in the emergency department, 507 (84%) underwent diagnostic imaging, with 416 (69%) having a computed tomography (CT) scan, 219 (36.4%) having an ultrasound and 128 (21%) having both.

(*continued*)

Evidence 2	
Theme E2	*Diagnosing appendicitis in children*
Main results (*cont.*)	After evaluation, 303 (50%) were discharged home, of whom six returned and four underwent appendectomy, and 221 (37%) had surgery, of whom 17 (8%) had a normal appendix. Seventy-seven were admitted for observation. Through the use of recursive partitioning the authors were able to further refine the characteristics of the low-risk patient as follows: with the absolute neutrophil count <6.75 × 10^3/μL, absence of nausea (or emesis or anorexia) and the absence of maximal tenderness in the right lower quadrant essentially excluded appendicitis.
Conclusion	The derived rules predict children at low risk of appendicitis and many can be safely observed rather than have imaging.
Commentary	Clinical prediction rules are to be used in conjunction with good history taking and appropriate physical examination. They can modify the doctor's clinical uncertainty experienced when presented with a child who appears to be at low risk of acute appendicitis. A value of clinical prediction rules is the impact that they can have (if applied) in relation to the ordering of tests. Data from this study suggest that CT scan requisitioning would have been reduced by 20% if the rules were applied. Despite the increase in CT scanning for children with acute abdominal pain, negative appendectomy rates and perforation rates remain unchanged. Investigation is not a substitute for history taking and physical assessment.
Reference	Kharbanda AB, Taylor GA, Fishman SJ, *et al.* A clinical prediction rule to identify children at low risk for appendicitis. *Pediatrics.* 2005; **116**(3): 709–16.

Evidence 3	
Theme E3	*Treatment of abdominal pain*
Question	Is oxycodone safe and effective in children with acute abdominal pain?
Design	Randomised controlled trial
Level of evidence	Jadad 5
Setting	Emergency department, academic medical centre, Finland
Participants	Children aged 4–15 years with undifferentiated abdominal pain of <7 days duration and an intensity of 5 or higher on a visual analogue scale measuring 10 cm (scores were rated 1–10) were eligible for inclusion. Children with hypotension (BP <90 mmHg), abdominal trauma or who had received analgesia prior to the emergency department arrival were excluded.
Intervention	Participants were randomised to receive either 0.1 mg/kg^{-1} of oxycodone hydrochloride sublingually or placebo, which in this study was normal saline. They were examined before administration of medication by a surgeon and were reassessed 1 hour later. The follow-up data were recorded on each occasion of fever, migration of pain, vomiting, right lower quadrant pain, abnormal bowel sounds, rebound tenderness, guarding and pain score (rated 1–10.)

(*continued*)

Evidence 3	
Theme E3	*Treatment of abdominal pain*
Outcomes	The primary outcome measure was the summed pain intensity difference, measured over a 3.5-hour period through seven observations. The pain intensity was measured on a visual analogue scale, rating 1–10 (in centimetres). The presence of guarding before and after medication was assessed, as was the diagnostic accuracy between the oxycodone group and placebo.
Main results	One hundred and four patients were eligible, with 63 being randomised (41 excluded; 31 did not meet inclusion criteria and 10 refused to participate). Of the 32 in the oxycodone group, 15 were observed and had a nonspecific pain aetiology; 17 underwent laparotomy with 12 having appendicitis, one with an ileal perforation and four a normal appendix. There were 31 in the placebo group, with 17 being observed of whom 16 had a non-specific abdominal pain, and one had an unnecessary laparotomy at 3 weeks; 14 underwent a laparotomy, of whom nine had appendicitis, one had a bowel obstruction and four had unnecessary surgery. The mean summed pain intensity difference for oxycodone was $22 \pm 18\,cm$ compared with $9 \pm 12\,cm$ for placebo. The diagnostic accuracy in the oxycodone group changed from 72% to 88% after medication administration but remained unchanged at 84% in the placebo group.
Conclusion	Early administration of buccal oxycodone provides analgesia for children without modifying the clinical presentation of clinical signs or of obscuring surgical diagnosis.
Commentary	Classic teaching suggests that the provision of analgesia to children with abdominal pain can mask surgical conditions and potentially lead to adverse outcomes. This study indicates that buccal oxycodone does not mask important clues to surgical diagnosis (an important consideration if a surgical condition is present) and also provides good analgesia (reducing pain scores from 7 to 4.5 within 30 minutes. The use of buccal oxycodone is easier to administer that intravenous morphine and is less sedating and should be considered in children with significant abdominal pain.
Reference	Kokki H, Lintula H, Vanamo K, *et al.* Oxycodone vs placebo in children with undifferentiated abdominal pain: a randomized, double-blind clinical trial of the effect of analgesia on diagnostic accuracy. *Arch Pediatr Adolesc Med.* 2005; **159**(4): 320–5.

Evidence 4	
Theme E4	**Parents influencing perception of abdominal pain in children**
Question	Can a parent's response influence the perception of abdominal pain in children with functional abdominal pain (FAP)
Design	Randomised controlled trial
Level of evidence	Jadad 3
Setting	Department of psychology, academic medical centre, the United States
Participants	Children and adolescents aged 8–16 referred with abdominal pain were eligible, provided they:
	• had at least three episodes of periumbilical or lower abdominal pain during the previous 3 months
	• had no chronic illness or disability
	• were living with a parent
	• had no organic disease revealed in a medical examination by a paediatric gastroenterologist.
	Control participants were recruited from a nearby school and were eligible if they were 8–16 years of age, had no more than two episodes of abdominal pain in the last 23 weeks and scored below the mean on the Children's Somatization Inventory.
Intervention	All participants underwent the water load symptom provocation test (WLSPT). In this test participants drink from a tube connected to a reservoir that is hidden from view (preventing visual cues on the amount imbibed) until they experience symptoms of fullness. The WLSPT produces symptoms similar to, but less intense than, those experienced during episodes of abdominal pain. Parent of the participants were randomised and trained to interact in one of three ways: (1) focus the child's attention on the pain, (2) distract the child or (3) offer no intervention (no instruction) for a 5-minute period. All parents were coached to render appropriate responses to their child, depending on which group they were assigned and the interaction were videotaped. Children completed a self-report on gastrointestinal symptoms before and after the intervention. Children thought that parents were present while their physiological measures were being recorded.
Outcomes	The change in children's symptom complaints was the primary outcome.
Main results	One hundred and ninety-eight participants with abdominal pain were eligible, of whom 110 (56%) were recruited, with full data available on 104 (95%). One hundred and eighty-nine control participants were contacted of whom 120 (63%) participated and full data were available on 119. Compared with NO INSTRUCTION condition, symptom complaints by pain patients and well children nearly doubled in the ATTENTION condition and were reduced by half in the DISTRACTION group. However parents of pain patients rated distraction as having greater potential negative impact on their children than attention. Girls with FAP are particularly vulnerable to the symptom-reinforcing effects of parental attention.
Conclusion	Parents' responses to symptoms can significantly increase or decrease symptoms. Distraction techniques are effective in dealing with FAP but are not preferred by parents.

(continued)

Evidence 4	
Theme E4	*Parents influencing perception of abdominal pain in children*
Commentary	The WLSPT can simulate the symptoms of FAP in children and adolescents. This study offers several insights inclusive of (a) the parental response to FAP, which is important; parents may focus the child's attention on the somatic complaint and have inadvertently rewarded such expressions, and (b) drawing attention to the somatic complaint may cause the child to evaluate their discomfort and perceive it as more sinister. The impact on symptoms was reduced fourfold when distraction was used compared to attention; which should form part of the discussion with parents but the parental reluctance to accept such a strategy must be discussed.
Reference	Walker LS, Williams SE, Smith CA, *et al.* Parent attention versus distraction: impact on symptom complaints by children with and without chronic functional abdominal pain. *Pain.* 2006; **122**(1–2): 43–52.

Evidence 5	
Theme E5	*Evaluating children for functional gastrointestinal disorders (FGIDs)*
Question	What is the clinical utility of the Rome II criteria in managing FGIDs in paediatric primary care?
Design	Prospective cohort study
Level of evidence	
Setting	Primary care paediatric practices, Italy
Participants	Children and adolescents aged 0–14 years attending 21 primary care practices were eligible for inclusion.
Intervention	All participants were evaluated over a 3-month period to determine if they met the Rome II criteria for FGIDs and if so were seen at 1-, 3- and 12-month intervals. All family practitioners received formal training in addressing FGID symptoms.
Outcomes	The primary outcomes were (a) to assess FGID prevalence, (b) to assess diagnosis and management of FGID with the exception of cyclical vomiting, (c) to verify how family practitioners comply with a predefined diagnostic/treatment protocol for managing FGID and (d) to assess the success of reassurance using the biopsychosocial model.
Main results	A total of 9291 participants were evaluated from 21 family practices, with 261 (2.6%) meeting the Rome II criteria, of whom 58 (0.62%) had functional abdominal pain (FAP) and 20 (0.21%) had functional dyspepsia. In the FAP group 20 had ultrasounds performed, all normal (this is deemed acceptable by the Rome II criteria), three had a barium study of the gastrointestinal tract and one had an endoscopy. Four (7%) had alarm symptoms (*see* Commentary). In those with FAP, full data sets were available in 56, of whom 25 (44.5%) had no pain, 19 (34%) were much improved, six (10.5%) had mild improvement, six (10.5%) had no change and none had worsened. Of the 261 participants initially diagnosed with FGID, only four (1.6%) had their diagnoses modified at the end of the study period.

(continued)

Evidence 5

Theme E5	*Evaluating children for functional gastrointestinal disorders (FGIDs)*
Conclusion	FGIDs can be diagnosed and managed in primary care. Use of the Rome II criteria facilitate clear diagnosis, with restriction of testing to those appropriate while proving a list of 'red flags' when the protocols can be modified.
Commentary	In children who present with features of FGID, appropriate blood tests include full blood count, erythrocyte sedimentation rate, urinalysis, faecal search for ova cysts and parasites, and an evaluation for coeliac disease. Ultrasound if desired is deemed acceptable (however, in this study it did not modify the diagnosis in any case). Alarm symptoms in FGID include localised pain, nocturnal pain or diarrhoea, weight loss, rectal bleeding, haematemesis, arthritis, delayed puberty and a family history of inflammatory bowel disease. Family practitioners successfully managed these patients through the use of a structured process, which incorporated education from a clinical leader in the topic.
Reference	Primavera G, Amoroso B, Barresi A, *et al.* Clinical utility of Rome criteria managing functional gastrointestinal disorders in pediatric primary care. *Pediatrics.* 2010; 125: e155–61.

Evidence 6

Theme E6	*Treatment of recurrent abdominal pain with probiotics*
Question	In children with functional abdominal pain (FAP) what is the impact of probiotic treatment?
Design	Randomised controlled trial
Level of evidence	Jadad 4
Setting	Department of paediatrics, academic medical centre, Italy
Participants	Children aged 5–14 years with a diagnosis of irritable bowel syndrome (IBS) or FAP were eligible for inclusion (provided the Rome II criteria were met and baseline studies were negative) and they experienced pain at least once per week.
Intervention	After a baseline period of 4 weeks, patients received either oral Lactobacillus GG (LGG) or placebo three times a day for 8 weeks. Outcome was assessed 8 weeks later.
Outcomes	The primary outcome was the change in abdominal pain (frequency and severity) according to the visual analogue scale. The secondary outcomes included (a) a decrease of at least 50% in the numbers and intensity of pain (treatment success), (b) a decrease in the perception of the children's pain according to the parents and (c) modification of the intestinal permeability.
Main results	Of 353 potential participants, 141 met the diagnostic criteria and 71 were randomised to the LGG group and 70 to the placebo group. Eighty-three participants had IBS and 58 had FAP. In the IBS group the pain intensity at baseline was 4.4 ± 2.1 and at 20 weeks was 1.8 ± 0.3, but for placebo the baseline was 4.6 ± 2.8 and at week 20 it was 3.3 ± 1.5. Treatment success was 72% versus 46% (absolute risk reduction (ARR) = 28%; number needed to treat (NNT) = 4), respectively.

(*continued*)

Evidence 6	
Theme E6	**Treatment of recurrent abdominal pain with probiotics**
Main results (*cont.*)	The frequency of the pain in the IBS group was 3.4 ± 2.3 at baseline and 0.9 ± 0.2 at week 20 for LGG but was 4.0 ± 3.5 at baseline and 1.6 ± 0.9 at week 20 for placebo. Treatment success for LGG was 82% versus 50% for placebo (ARR = 32%; NNT = 4). There was no significant change in the FAP group with LGG. For secondary outcomes parents rated a 70% improvement in pain in the LGG group compared with 55% in the placebo group (ARR = 15%; NNT = 7). The LGG group had a significant reduction in intestinal permeability compared to the placebo group. Only five patients withdrew from the study and adherence rate to LGG was 89% and to placebo was 86%.
Conclusion	LGG reduces the frequency and intensity of IBS symptoms in children.
Commentary	While this study title relates to FAP it was children with IBS that had a clinical improvement with LGG (bearing in mind that the placebo response was significant). The safety profile of probiotics suggests that they are an attractive therapeutic option for those with IBS. There are a need to standardise preparation to ensure a reproducible therapeutic effect. The authors suggest that the Probiotic effect is related to enhancing the mucosal epithelial cell barrier but the specific mechanism of IBS is not currently defined.
Reference	Francavilla R, Miniello V, Magistà AM, *et al*. A randomized controlled trial of Lactobacillus GG in children with functional abdominal pain. *Pediatrics*. 2010; **126**(6): e1445–52.

Evidence 7	
Theme E7	**Treatment of recurrent abdominal pain (RAP)**
Question	Is cognitive behavioural therapy (CBT) effective in the treatment of RAP?
Design	Randomised controlled trial
Level of evidence	Jadad 3
Setting	Children's hospital, the United States
Participants	Children attending the outpatient clinics of four paediatric gastroenterologists or diagnosed by their primary care physicians were eligible for inclusion.
Intervention	In this study the impact of short-term CBT with standard medical treatment (SMT) was evaluated against SMT in terms of effectiveness and efficiency. The major goal of the CBT was to explain RAP to the parent and child, while instructing the children in active management of the pain episodes and practicing pain management relief techniques. Three to five sessions were offered bimonthly until the child–parent dyad was proficient. SMT included physician follow-up with education and instructions to maintain a high-fibre diet. Medical treatment not outlined was available to all participants.
Outcomes	The primary outcome was (a) reduction in the sensory aspects of pain, including intensity, frequency, and the duration of the abdominal pain, and (b) the lessening of perceived interference in the activities of daily living.

(*continued*)

Evidence 7	
Theme E7	**Treatment of recurrent abdominal pain (RAP)**
Outcomes (*cont.*)	This was assessed using the Abdominal Pain Index (Child and Parent versions), where scores could range from 2 to 50. Outcome was assessed at baseline and 6–12 months post treatment.
Main results	One hundred and eight families were eligible for inclusion, of whom 86 were randomised (coin toss method), 46 were allocated to the CBT plus SMT, with 40 completing the study, and 40 were allocated to the SMT group, with 29 completing the study. The adjusted mean score for the parent API in CBT plus SMT at baseline was 24.7 at 3 months, and 15.8 at 6–12 months and for the SMT was 27.9 at baseline and 22 at 6–12 months (difference of 3 points). In the API for children the CBT plus SMT was 24.1 at baseline and 15 at 6–12 months, whereas the API baseline for SMT was 24.1 at baseline and 22.2 at 6–12 months (difference of 7.2). These results were clinically important, with a number needed to treat = 3 (95% confidence interval: 1.1–4.4).
Conclusion	This study indicates the effectiveness of CBT in reducing the sensory effects of RAP.
Commentary	Children and adolescents with RAP are challenging patients as there is no proven effective management for their symptoms. Frequently their symptoms lead to excessive school loss and there is an association between their childhood symptoms and the development of functional symptoms in adulthood. In this study one child was withdrawn due to an organic cause being diagnosed, which supports the importance of a prudent history. Stating the importance of coping mechanisms for children with RAP needs to be discussed early with the parents in the clinical engagement and not after investigation, which yields no organic aetiology for the child's symptoms.
Reference	Robins PM, Smith SM, Glutting JJ, *et al.* A randomized controlled trial of a cognitive-behavioral family intervention for pediatric recurrent abdominal pain. *J Pediatr Psychol.* 2005; **30**(5): 397–408.

ABDOMINAL PAIN: MULTIPLE-CHOICE QUESTIONS

Q1 Features associated with abdominal pain that suggest a surgical cause include which of the following?

a) Bilious vomiting

b) Vomiting followed by abdominal pain

c) Localised tenderness

d) Palpable mass

e) Inguinoscrotal swelling

Q2 Which of the following statements is/are correct with regard to intussusception?

a) The ileum invaginates into the caecum most often.

b) The lead point most often is related to hypertrophy of Peyer's patches.

c) The passage of red currant jelly stools is a rare finding.

d) A sausage-shaped mass in the left upper quadrant is typical.

e) Coma is a rare presentation.

Q3 Which of the following statements is/are true of testicular torsion?

a) Extravaginal torsion occurs in the neonatal period.

b) Seventy-five per cent of neonatal torsions occur antenatally.

c) In the older child, testicular torsion occurs with severe abdominal pain and nausea.

d) The cremasteric reflex is present on the affect side.

e) The affected testicle is tender.

Q4 In malrotation of the bowel, which of the following is/are correct?

a) The bowel twists around the axis of the inferior mesenteric artery.

b) Sixty per cent of infants and children with volvulus present in the first month of life.

c) In the neonatal period bilious vomit is a key feature.

d) The duodenal jejunal flexure is to right of the midline.

e) An emergency Ladd's procedure is the treatment of choice.

Q5 Which of the following statements is/are correct with regard to acute appendicitis?

a) Acute appendicitis is common in children under 3 years of age.

b) Pain localises to the right iliac fossa with involvement of the parietal peritoneum.

c) The perforation rates are 10% for 10- to 15-year-old children and adolescents.

d) Immediately after perforation children can improve transiently but still have an elevated heart rate.

e) The threshold for appendectomy is lower in girls than boys.

Q6 Which of the following statements is/are correct with regard to gallstones?

a) Cholesterol gallstones account for 90% of adolescent gallstones.

b) Most children are asymptomatic with gallstones.

c) Gallstones are found in children with haemolytic anaemias.

d) Gallstones are found in patients with cystic fibrosis.

e) Gallstones are found in infants with prolonged parenteral nutrition.

Q7 Which of the following statements is/are true with regard to Meckel's diverticulum?

a) Meckel's diverticulum occurs in 0.2% of the population.

b) It is a remnant of the vitello-intestinal duct.

c) Fifty per cent of Meckel's diverticulum have ectopic gastric mucosa present.

d) Sixty per cent present with painless rectal bleeding.

e) If not lined with gastric mucosa, Meckel's diverticulum is asymptomatic.

Q8 Subcategories of Functional Abdominal Pain include which of the following?
   a) Functional dyspepsia
   b) Irritable bowel syndrome
   c) Abdominal migraine
   d) Functional Abdominal Pain
   e) Functional abdominal pain syndrome

Answers

A1	a, b, d, e		**A2**	a, b, e
A3	a, b, e		**A4**	b, c, d, e
A5	b, c, d, e		**A6**	a, b, c, d, e
A7	b, c, d, e		**A8**	a, b, c, d, e

SLIDE

1. Peutz-Jeghers

Chapter Eleven

THE CHILD WITH DIARRHOEA

COMMON SCENARIO

'He picked up a gastro bug from crèche last month. The vomiting settled down within a couple of days, but his nappies are still really loose and runny. I thought it would settle down, but it's been 4 weeks now.'

LEARNING OBJECTIVES

- Understand the causes of acute and chronic diarrhoea
- Describe the pathophysiology of chronic diarrhoea
- Assess the severity of dehydration
- Understand the use of oral rehydration therapy for the management of acute diarrhoeal illness
- Determine what investigations are required in the assessment of chronic diarrhoea

BACKGROUND

Diarrhoea is an increase in the frequency, volume or liquidity of the bowel movement relative to the usual habit of the individual. Worldwide, it is one of the commonest causes of morbidity and mortality in children, especially in developing countries. At some point in childhood, almost every child will experience an episode of diarrhoea. Diarrhoea results when the normal absorptive processes in the small and large bowel are disrupted or the secretory processes are abnormally upregulated. Disorders that interfere with absorption in the small bowel tend to produce high-volume stools, as the small bowel absorbs the majority of water that reaches the intestine. In contrast, disorders that interfere with absorption in the large bowel produce lower-volume stools, which may be bloody. Dehydration, which may be associated with electrolyte disturbances, is the most frequent complication of acute diarrhoeal illnesses. Malnutrition is the major complication of chronic diarrhoea. Signs of dehydration in children and infants include absence of tears, sunken eyes, sunken fontanelle, decreased skin turgor, decreased urine output, weight loss, lethargy and dry mucous membranes. Children under 1 year of age are more at risk of dehydration. Signs of hypovolaemia include weak pulses, tachycardia, tachypnoea, delayed capillary refill time, hypotension, mottling of the skin, cool peripheries and decreased level of consciousness.

Acute diarrhoea usually lasts less than 2 weeks, it is usually due to an infection and it usually self-resolves. Most infectious organisms are spread via the faecal–oral route or through contaminated food or water. Chronic diarrhoea is diarrhoea that has been present for 4 weeks or more. There may be associated signs and symptoms of weight loss, anorexia and lethargy. Chronic diarrhoea shortly after birth suggests a congenital disorder such as ion transporter defects and ultrastructural abnormalities of enterocytes. Steatorrhoea is suggestive of generalised or selective fat malabsorption. Stools are large, offensive, oily or greasy and pale.

The pathogenesis of diarrhoea can be osmotic, secretory, inflammatory or secondary to altered bowel motility.

Osmotic diarrhoea

Osmotic diarrhoea is caused by failure to digest or absorb normal nutrients or ingestion of non-absorbable solutes (e.g. lactulose). The unabsorbed solute creates an osmotic load and causes stools to be watery, highly acidic and loose. Stools are positive for reducing substances with absent leucocytes. Perianal excoriations are common because of the passage of frequent and acidic stools. With fasting the diarrhoea stops. Examples include lactose intolerance, glucose–galactose malabsorption, lactulose or laxative abuse and rotavirus infection.

Inflammatory diarrhoea

Inflammatory diarrhoea is characterised by the presence of blood, mucus and leukocytes in the stool. Infections with salmonella or *Campylobacter jejuni* cause inflammation with high fevers, pus and bloody stools. Inflammation can also be due to chronic diseases such as inflammatory bowel disease (IBD) (*see* Chapter 10: The Child with Abdominal Pain), coeliac disease or secondary to allergic colitis.

Secretory diarrhoea

Secretory diarrhoea results from a disturbance in the balance between absorption (villous epithelial cells) and secretion (crypt cells). Stools are watery, with no leucocytes. With fasting the diarrhoea persists. Causes include bacterial enterotoxins, cholera, enterotoxigenic *Escherichia coli*, shigella and salmonella, *Clostridium difficile*, neuroendocrine tumours, VIPomas and congenital chloride-losing diarrhoea.

Altered bowel motility

Diarrhoea is secondary to decreased transit time in the gut. It may be due to toddler's diarrhoea, hyperthyroidism or irritable bowel syndrome.

IMPORTANT CAUSES OF DIARRHOEA IN CHILDHOOD

Acute gastroenteritis

Acute gastroenteritis is characterised by the rapid onset of diarrhoea with or without vomiting, fever and abdominal pain. Viruses, bacteria or parasites can cause it. Rotavirus is the most common cause of acute diarrhoea. The incubation period is 1–3 days. It commonly occurs in children aged 6 months to 2 years. There is a seasonal variation, with peaks during the winter months in temperate climates. Children in day care are more likely to suffer from acute gastroenteritis. It usually resolves within 2 weeks; however, protracted diarrhoea can occur in malnourished children, those with an underlying immunodeficiency and in children who develop secondary infections.

Post-gastroenteritis syndrome

The post-gastroenteritis syndrome occurs when an acute episode of gastroenteritis is followed by a period of prolonged diarrhoea. It occurs in approximately 5% of cases and is largely due to carbohydrate malabsorption. There may be associated protein malabsorption.

Antibiotic-associated diarrhoea

Antibiotic-associated diarrhoea is defined as diarrhoea occurring during or after antibiotic administration for which no other cause of diarrhoea is identified. The exact pathophysiology is unknown; however, it is thought to be related to alterations in normal bowel flora. It is more common in children under 2 years of age and the risk is higher with different antibiotic classes, particularly broad-spectrum antibiotics. Symptoms can range from mild diarrhoea, to colitis to pseudomembranous enterocolitis.

Coeliac disease

Coeliac disease is a gluten-sensitive enteropathy that causes villous atrophy and reduces the intestinal absorptive surface area. There is an increased prevalence of other autoimmune conditions including diabetes, hypothyroidism, pernicious anaemia and Addison's disease. Traditionally, coeliac disease has been described as presenting after weaning onto solids, with failure to thrive and chronic diarrhoea with offensive stools. There may be associated lethargy, irritability and anorexia. Examination may reveal pallor, short stature, wasting of the buttocks and abdominal distension. Older children may present with short stature, delayed puberty and unexplained iron deficiency. More recently, a review of 50 patients suggested a change in clinical presentations of coeliac disease that included diarrhoea, 36%; targeted screening, 26%; non-specific abdominal pain, 16%; constipation, 8%; faltering weight, 6%; short stature, 4%; recurrent mouth ulcers, 2%; and persistent iron-deficiency anaemia, 2%.

Cow's milk protein allergy

Cow's milk protein allergy is due to an immunological reaction to one or more milk proteins. It may be IgE mediated (type I hypersensitivity reaction) or non-IgE mediated (type III or IV hypersensitivity reactions). IgE-mediated allergy presents acutely after ingestion of cow's milk with urticaria, angioedema, exacerbation of eczema, vomiting and/or wheezing. Non-IgE-mediated reactions present with diarrhoea, vomiting and colicky abdominal pain. It is the most common food allergy in infancy, affecting approximately 2%–7% of infants. It gradually resolves by 1–3 years of age.

Lactose intolerance

Lactose is a disaccharide sugar made of glucose and galactose. Absorption of lactose requires normal lactase activity in the small intestinal brush border, which hydrolyses the disaccharide. Symptoms usually begin 30 minutes to 2 hours after eating or drinking foods containing lactose. Common symptoms include abdominal cramps, bloating, flatulence, nausea and diarrhoea. Lactase deficiency can be primary or secondary.

Primary lactase deficiency is relative or absolute absence of lactase. The prevalence and age of onset varies according to ethnicity. It is rare in northern Europeans and uncommon in all populations before 3 years of age. It develops slowly over several years and is not usually apparent until late adolescence or adulthood. The threshold for lactose tolerance varies between individuals.

Secondary lactase deficiency is lactase deficiency secondary to small bowel injury such as acute gastroenteritis, which causes loss of lactase-containing epithelial cells from the villi. Post-gastroenteritis lactase deficiency is transient and resolves without treatment. Secondary deficiency can also occur with coeliac disease, IBD and enteropathy related to immunodeficiency.

Congenital lactase deficiency is rare and presents with life-threatening diarrhoea in the first few hours of life after ingestion of the first milk feed.

Toddler's diarrhoea

Toddler's diarrhoea is known by a variety of different terms including functional diarrhoea, chronic non-specific diarrhoea and rapid transit diarrhoea. It occurs in healthy children 1–3 years of age who pass 3 or more large, painless, unformed stools per day, for at least 4 weeks due to shortened colonic transit time. The mechanisms underlying the condition are largely unknown. It is the commonest cause of chronic diarrhoea in children without failure to thrive. The child is otherwise well, with no nocturnal symptoms and no abnormal examination findings. It is associated with excessive consumption of fruit juices and a diet low in fat and fibre. Stools may contain undigested food particles or the 'peas and carrots' syndrome.

HISTORY

KEY POINTS				
Stooling pattern	Normal stool pattern Onset Duration of diarrhoea Frequency of defecation Pain with defecation	**Family history**	Lactose intolerance IBD Coeliac disease Autoimmune disease Allergies	**🔖 Red flags** Nocturnal diarrhoea Bloody, mucousy or fatty stools
Stool characteristics	Consistency: formed, semi-formed, watery Blood Mucus Fatty	**Surgical history**	Previous bowel operations	
Associated symptoms	Bloating Excess flatulence Vomiting Abdominal pain Relationship to lactose ingestion	**Medications**	Recent antibiotic use Laxative use	
Dietary history	Age at weaning onto solids Fluid intake Fruit juices Fats Fibre	**Social history**	Foreign travel Day care or crèche	
Symptoms of dehydration	Number of wet nappies or times voided Lethargy	**Growth and development**	Reaching milestones Temperament	
Medical history	Constipation Immunodeficiency or recurrent infections Recent gastroenteritis Atopic disease: asthma, eczema, hay fever			

EXAMINATION

- All children should have their height and weight plotted on appropriate centile charts
- Vitals including temperature should be recorded
- Examination of stool

Assess for:

- Signs of dehydration or hypovolaemia
- Signs of weight loss: loose skin folds, wasting of buttocks
- Hands: clubbing
- Signs of anaemia: pallor of conjunctiva or palmar creases
- Perianal disease
- Abdominal exam: tenderness, masses
- Examine for lymphadenopathy.

❶ Red flags

- Failure to thrive
- Weight loss (falling from percentiles)
- Growth failure
- Steatorrhoea, mucousy or bloody stools
- Hypovolaemia
- Clubbing
- Perianal disease
- Abdominal mass
- Visceromegaly or generalised lymphadenopathy
- Abdominal distension
- Mouth ulceration

DIFFERENTIAL DIAGNOSIS

Common causes

- Gastroenteritis
- Antibiotic-associated diarrhoea
- Excessive intake of fruit juices or sugary fluids
- Toddler's diarrhoea
- Irritable bowel syndrome
- Post-gastroenteritis syndrome
- Constipation with overflow
- Lactose intolerance

Less common causes

- IBD
- Coeliac
- Cow's milk protein intolerance

Rarer causes

- Fat malabsorption: cystic fibrosis, Shwachman–Diamond's syndrome
- Carbohydrate malabsorption syndromes: lactose, fructose, glucose–galactose
- Liver disease: primary bile acid malabsorption, cholestatic jaundice
- Immunodeficiency syndromes: severe combined immunodeficiency, acquired immunodeficiency syndrome, hypogammaglobulinaemia
- Surgical conditions: Hirschsprung's enterocolitis, appendicitis, intussusception
- Malignancies: VIPomas
- Endocrine: hyperthryroidism, diabetes mellitus, congenital adrenal hyperplasia
- Short bowel syndrome: previous resection, congenital short bowel syndrome
- Metabolic disorders: acrodermatitis enteropathica
- Congenital alterations in electrolyte transport: congenital chloride diarrhoea

INVESTIGATIONS

What investigations should be performed in children with acute diarrhoea?

For many children with acute diarrhoea, the likeliest cause is viral gastroenteritis. Systemically well children who are normovolaemic and not clinically severely dehydrated do not require investigations.

In children with severe dehydration or signs of circulatory compromise the following investigations should be performed:
- urea and electrolytes
- venous blood gas
- full blood count
- C-reactive protein/erythrocyte sedimentation rate
- blood culture
- urine culture
- stool culture
- random blood glucose.

How is coeliac disease diagnosed?

Screening tests for coeliac disease: anti-transglutaminase type 2 IgA and IgA (false negatives can occur if IgA deficient) or alternatively anti-transglutaminase IgG. Diagnosis requires a small intestinal biopsy. Prior to the biopsy the child must remain on a gluten diet with a least one daily meal containing gluten for the 6 weeks prior to the biopsy.

Biopsy findings of coeliac disease:
- sub-total villous atrophy
- crypt hyperplasia
- increased intraepithelial lymphocytes
- inflammatory cells in lamina propria.

A definitive diagnosis is confirmed when symptoms resolve following treatment with a gluten-free diet in a previously symptomatic individual with characteristic changes on small intestinal biopsy.

HLA (human leukocyte antigen) typing is mainly associated with HLA-DQ8 and HLA-DQ2. The absence of the antigens virtually excludes the presence of coeliac disease.

(continued)

How is lactose intolerance diagnosed?

Lactose intolerance is usually diagnosed by a dietary challenge. If suspected clinically, based on the history, a 2-week trial of a strict lactose-free diet should be introduced. The diagnosis is confirmed with resolution of symptoms during the 2-week trial and recurrence of symptoms after reintroduction of lactose-containing foods.

If the dietary challenge is inconclusive, further investigations can be performed, including a hydrogen breath test or lactose tolerance test.

The faecal reducing substances test detects presence of lactose, glucose and fructose in a stool sample. A positive test suggests the absence of the corresponding enzyme. A trace of positive reducing substances is normal in healthy breastfed infants.

In stool pH testing, a pH <5 suggests lactose intolerance.

In children with suspected gastroenteritis, when should stool cultures be sent?
- Stool should be sent for culture if there is uncertainty about the diagnosis
- A history of foreign travel
- Unwell child with suspected septicaemia
- Presence of blood or mucus in the stool
- Immunocompromised children
- Persistent diarrhoea after 7 days

A stool for ova, cysts and parasites test should be done if diarrhoea is recurrent or persistent. Viral antigen tests can be done for adenovirus and rotavirus.

MANAGEMENT PLAN: THREE-STEP APPROACH
1. Clarifying and pitfall avoidance strategies
2. Rehydration
3. Treatment of specific conditions:
   a) functional diarrhoea
   b) cow's milk allergy
   c) lactose deficiency
   d) coeliac disease

Clarifying and pitfall avoidance strategies
- Think of diarrhoea as follows: (1) acute, (2) chronic with normal growth or (3) chronic with systemic symptoms, e.g. weight loss.
- Define what the parents or child mean by the symptom diarrhoea. **Rationale**: it is best to clinically characterise 'diarrhoea' as stool that takes the shape of the container in which it is placed. This allows the parents and child to relate to the concept.
- Ensure that the diarrhoea is not constipation with overflow. **Rationale**: parents usually are unaware of the frequency of their child's bowel movements and may not realise that their child is constipated. Ask specifically if the diarrhoea alternates with periods of no stool or large-calibre stool. Often the parents will have to

record the stool frequency to determine if constipation with overflow is present, or at least reflect before offering a response.

- Exclude spurious diarrhoea. **Rationale**: spurious diarrhoea results from excessive juice intake and does not require investigation if the juice is discontinued, as the diarrhoea then abates. In many paediatric gastroenterology clinics this is standard practice prior to children being reviewed.
- Evaluate parental response to diarrhoea. **Rationale**: specifically check for anti-diarrhoeal medications (*see* Evidence 1) and dietary modification.
- For children with acute diarrhoea check antibiotic usage. **Rationale**: unfortunately, children with diarrhoea are placed on antibiotics and the diarrhoea as a consequence becomes worse.
- Probiotics and acute diarrhoea (*see* Evidence 2).
- Ensure appropriate hand washing is in place. **Rationale**: hand washing reduces the risk of transmission of infectious disease and should be undertaken rigorously (*see* Evidence 3).
- If the child has had severe abdominal pain suggestive of appendicitis and presents afterwards with diarrhoea, consider pelvic abscess if the child is unwell.
- Ask about travel. **Rationale**: travel is undertaken frequently and as a consequence infectious diseases are a hazard of such travel and need to be considered in the differential diagnosis.
- If a child has bloody diarrhoea that is not infectious, think of IBD and perform a faecal calprotectin early (*see* Evidence 4).
- Immunisation against infectious diseases – in particular, rotavirus – reduces the hospitalisation rates for children (*see* Evidence 5).

Rehydration

In most cases of acute diarrhoea secondary to infectious agents, the only treatment that is required is supportive, replacing fluid and electrolytes to prevent dehydration. Children with acute gastroenteritis should be rehydrated (*see* Chapter 9: The Child with Vomiting) with oral rehydration solution over 3–4 hours. Children who are dehydrated are thirsty and normally do not refuse oral fluids. However, if the child is vomiting, small amounts, i.e. 5 mL every 3–5 minutes, should be given. Children with mild to moderate dehydration require 30–80 mL/kg over 3–4 hours. Children with severe dehydration require 100 mL/kg over 3–4 hours.

European oral rehydration solutions contain:
- 60 mmol/L sodium
- 90 mmol/L glucose
- 20 mmol/L potassium
- 10 mmol/L citrate
- low osmolarity of 240 mmol/L.

Feeds should be reintroduced early. Breastfeeding should continue through rehydration and in formula-fed infants full-strength feeds should be restarted after completion of rehydration. Fruit juices, sugary drinks and fatty foods should be avoided until the diarrhoea has stopped. There is no role for anti-diarrhoeal agents in the management of gastroenteritis. They may potentially worsen inflammatory bacterial gastroenteritis causing toxic megacolon and haemorrhage. Children should not go to school or day care until 48 hours after their last episode of diarrhoea or vomiting.

Children who are severely dehydrated with signs of circulatory compromise require intravenous fluid resuscitation with boluses of 20 mL/kg of normal saline to restore circulation. Ongoing fluid management will be dependent on their response to fluid replacement.

Treatment of specific conditions

Functional diarrhoea

Management is largely conservative, reassuring the parents that the child is growing and developing normally and that the diarrhoea will gradually improve with time. Juice and sugary drinks should be avoided. Restrictive diets should be avoided to ensure that the child continues to meet his or her calorific requirements.

Cow's milk allergy

Cow's milk allergy requires elimination of all milk and all foods containing cow's milk protein.

Lactose deficiency

Tolerance of lactose varies; some children may tolerate up to two glasses of milk a day and remain asymptomatic, while others may not be able to tolerate a bar of milk chocolate. Therefore, the degree of avoidance of lactose depends on individual thresholds. To induce remission, children should be started on a lactose-free diet and then gradually introduce small amounts of lactose as tolerated.

Coeliac disease

Coeliac disease is managed with a gluten-free diet, excluding wheat, rye, barley and oats from the diet. Strictly adhering to a gluten-free diet can be difficult for families. They should be given written advice regarding selecting gluten-free foods and making gluten-free meals. There are various gluten-free products, including breads and biscuits, now available in many supermarkets, and gluten-free options on many restaurant menus. Ensuring compliance is important, as continuing to eat gluten increases the risk of developing small intestinal lymphoma, nutritional deficiencies, other autoimmune diseases and osteoporosis.

FOLLOW-UP

- Children with chronic condition, e.g. coeliac disease, need to be followed up for their growth parameters and to ensure dietary adherence.
- Children with IBD require subspecialist follow-up.
- Children with acute condition, provided appropriate advice is offered, do not need follow-up.

WHEN TO REFER?

- Acute bloody diarrhoea
- Chronic diarrhoea (for more than 4 weeks)
- Diarrhoea with weight loss or systemic symptoms
- Diarrhoea with faltering growth
- Child with family history of coeliac disease and diarrhoea
- Night-time diarrhoea
- Child with a history of constipation and diarrhoea

CLARIFICATION STATEMENTS FOR PARENTAL MISCONCEPTIONS

'Why does he need to go through so many investigations to know whether or not he has coeliac disease?'

The first step is to take a blood test to measure the levels of a certain antibody – anti-tissue transglutaminase – in the blood. The antibody test measures your child's immune system response to gluten, which is found in common foods such as wheat, rye, barley and oats. The test results will help determine whether a biopsy is needed; however, the test is only a screening test and cannot diagnose coeliac disease. Coeliac disease is a life-long condition; therefore, it is important that we are certain about the diagnosis, and the only way to confirm it is to take a small tissue sample or biopsy of the small intestine. In the meantime, he should continue on his normal diet and should have gluten in at least one meal for a minimum of 6 weeks. The tissue will be examined to see if eating gluten has damaged the surface of the small intestine. To get the tissue sample a gastroscope will be passed into the mouth, down into the small intestines.

'Why are you blaming the juice for his diarrhoea? After all, it is natural.'

Excessive juice intake causes diarrhoea. Fruit juices are high in sorbitol and some have a high fructose to glucose ratio. The sorbitol and the limited ability of toddlers to absorb fructose contribute to the diarrhoea.

'I take medication when I get diarrhoea, so why can't my child take it? Diarrhoea is not a pleasant symptom and I want him to get better quickly.'

While medications for diarrhoea are acceptable in adults, children are not little adults. Many of the anti-diarrhoeal medications are ineffective and those that are effective have significant side effects (*see* Evidence 1).

SUMMARY PRACTICE POINTS

- Osmotic diarrhoea is improved by fasting.
- Bloody diarrhoea suggests salmonella, campylobacter or IBD.
- Excess juice intake post gastroenteritis aggravates symptoms.
- The pattern of coeliac disease is changing (1/4 now diagnosed by targeted screening and 1/6 have non-specific abdominal pain).
- Primary lactose is rare in Europeans.
- Children with toddler's diarrhoea have undigested food in their stools (peas and carrots) but normal growth.
- If IgA deficiency is present, a screening test for coeliac disease needs to be evaluated with caution.
- Children with constipation can present with symptoms of diarrhoea.
- Avoid antibiotic use in children if acute diarrhoea is present.
- Immunisation for rotavirus significantly reduces rates of admission to hospital.
- Appropriate hand washing is essential if in contact with a child with acute diarrhoea.

EVALUATING THE EVIDENCE

Evidence 1	
Theme E1	**Drug treatment for acute diarrhoea in children**
Question	In infants and young children, how effective is loperamide?
Design	Randomised controlled trial
Level of evidence	Jadad 5
Setting	Department of paediatrics, academic medical centre, South Africa
Participants	Infants and young children aged 3–18 months with acute diarrhoea and dehydration requiring hospital admission were eligible to participate.
Intervention	Patients were randomised to receive loperamide 0.8 mg/kg/day in three divided doses to a maximum of six doses or placebo in addition to continuous nasogastric tube infusion of an oral rehydration fluid (ORF). Treatment failure was defined as >72 hours of ORF or if they developed persisting vomiting or ileus. The degree of dehydration was determined from the difference between admission and discharge weight.

(continued)

Evidence 1	
Theme E1	*Drug treatment for acute diarrhoea in children*
Outcomes	The duration of hospitalisation until fit for discharge – defined as being clinically hydrated, taking oral feeds and being able to maintain body weight without additional ORF – was the primary outcome.
Main results	Ninety-one patients were assigned to the loperamide arm, with a mean age of 8.25 (3–18) months, a mean degree of dehydration of 5.7% (0%–13%), and a mean duration of hospitalisation of 34 (14–72) hours; there were 12 (13%) treatment failures. In the placebo group 94 patients were assigned, with a mean age of 7.38 (3–18) months, a mean degree of dehydration of 5.5% (4%–14%), and a mean duration of hospitalisation of 36 (16–72) hours; there were nine (10%) treatment failures. No patient had persistent vomiting or ileus noted. Fifty per cent of patients had no pathogen isolated and in both groups rotavirus was isolated in approximately 25%, campylobacter in 15% and salmonella in 10%.
Conclusion	There was no difference between groups in terms of outcomes. Loperamide did not reduce the number of treatment failures in this study and thus it is not recommended in the treatment of diarrhoea in infants and young children.
Commentary	This study addressed length of stay in hospital as a marker of loperamide effectiveness and did not address the impact on the duration of diarrhoea. A recent meta-analysis on loperamide therapy for acute diarrhoea in children demonstrated a shorter duration of diarrhoea of 0.8 days (95% confidence interval (CI): 0.7–0.9). However, serious adverse effects, defined as ileus, lethargy or death, occurred in 8 of 927 children (0.9%; 95% CI: 0.4–1.7), usually occurring in children <3 years of age. Consequently, even at low doses ≤ 0.25 mg/kg/day the adverse effects outweigh the benefits (Su-Ting *et al.*, 2007).
References	Bowie MD, Hill ID, Mann MD. Loperamide for treatment of acute diarrhoea in infants and young children: a double-blind placebo-controlled trial. *S Afr Med J.* 1995; **85**(9): 885–7.
	Su-Ting T, Grossman DC, Cummings P. Loperamide therapy for acute diarrhea in children: systematic review and meta-analysis. *PLoS Med.* 2007; **4**(3): e98.

Evidence 2	
Theme E2	*Probiotic therapy and acute diarrhoea*
Question	What is the impact of probiotic treatment in children with acute diarrhoeal illnesses?
Design	Randomised controlled trial
Level of evidence	Jadad 1
Setting	Department of paediatrics, academic medical centre, Italy
Participants	Children aged 6–36 months with diarrhoea (defined as three or more outputs of loose stool or liquid stools a day for less than 48 hours. Children with malnutrition, severe dehydration or acute co-existing systemic conditions were excluded from this study.

(*continued*)

Evidence 2	
Theme E2	**Probiotic therapy and acute diarrhoea**
Intervention	All children received oral rehydration therapy for 3–6 hours and were then re-fed on full-strength formula containing lactose or cow's milk, depending on age. Children were randomised to group 1, oral rehydration therapy alone; group 2, *Lactobacillus* GC; group 3, *Saccharomyces boulardii*; group 4, *Bacillus clausii*; group 5, mixture of *Lactobacillus delbrueckii*, *Streptococcus thermophilus*, *Lactobacillus acidophilus* and *Bifidobacterium* bifidum and group 6, *Enterococcus faecium* strain SF68. Probiotics were prescribed for 5 days and administered in 20 mL of water.
Outcomes	The primary outcome was the duration of diarrhoea.
Main results	Six hundred child were assessed for eligibility, with 571 being randomised: 92 to group 1, 100 to group 2, 91 to group 3, 100 to group 4, 97 to group 5 and 91 to group 6. The mean duration of diarrhoea in group 1 was 115.5 (95.2–127) hours. Shorter durations were noted in group 2, with −32 (−41 to −23) hours and in group 5 with −37 (−47 to −25) hours.
Conclusion	Not all commercially available probiotics are effective in reducing the duration of acute diarrhoea.
Commentary	Two preparations of probiotics reduced the duration of diarrhoea by more than a day and the frequency of stools also reduced after the first 24 hours of administration; these are clinically relevant outcomes for parents of children with diarrhoea. In this study, it was the investigators assigned to collecting the reporting forms who were blinded. The aetiology of diarrhoea was not investigated with stool culture and they were treated as outpatients. A presumption of viral aetiology was made. Prior to recommending probiotics for acute diarrhoea there is a need to be specific in the type recommended, as three of the five were equivalent to the control group. No adverse effects were reported.
Reference	Canani RB, Cirillo P, Terrin G, *et al*. Probiotics for treatment of acute diarrhoea in children: randomised clinical trial of five different preparations. *BMJ.* **335**(7615): 340.

Evidence 3	
Theme E3	**Hand hygiene and infectious diseases**
Question	What is the effect of hand washing on infectious disease risk in the community?
Design	Meta-analysis
Level of evidence	
Setting	Studies performed in a community setting
Participants	
Intervention	Electronic search of four databases (PubMed, 1960–2007; Embase, 1980–2007; the Cochrane Library, 1988–2007; and the United Kingdom National Health Service Database of Abstracts of Review of Effects to evaluate studies that evaluated hand hygiene interventions in the reduction of gastrointestinal and respiratory illnesses and to identify the interventions with greatest efficacy.

(continued)

Evidence 3	
Theme E3	**Hand hygiene and infectious diseases**
Outcomes	To quantify the effect of hand hygiene interventions on rates of gastrointestinal and respiratory illnesses.
Main results	Studies evaluated were restricted to those undertaken in the community and those that employed a randomised or quasi-experimental design. From an initial search of 5378 articles, 30 were evaluated for meta-analysis. The proportion of gastrointestinal illnesses prevented was 31% (95% confidence interval (CI): 19–42). The use of non-antibacterial soap with education prevented 39% (95% CI: 12–57) of gastrointestinal illnesses, compared with no intervention in the control group. Hand hygiene education resulted in the prevention of 31% (95% CI: 5–50) of gastrointestinal illness, compared with no intervention. The prevention of respiratory illness prevented by all hand hygiene interventions was 21% (95% CI: 5–34).
Conclusion	Hand hygiene is effective against gastrointestinal disease and, to a lesser extent, respiratory disease.
Commentary	The importance of hand hygiene cannot be overstated in the reduction of transmission of infectious diseases. Despite the evidence, the ongoing difficulty is ensuring adherence from healthcare personnel.
Reference	Aiello AE, Coulborn RM, Perez V, *et al*. Effect of hand hygiene on infectious disease risk in the community setting: a meta-analysis. *Am J Public Health*. 2008; **98**(8): 1372–81.

Evidence 4	
Theme E4	**Tests for inflammatory bowel disease (IBD)**
Question	What is the value of faecal calprotectin (FC) in children with suspected IBD?
Design	Retrospective case-control study
Level of evidence	
Setting	Department of paediatrics, gastroenterology, academic medical centre, Scotland
Participants	Children and adolescents with FC measured prior to full endoscopic evaluation for suspected IBD were eligible.
Intervention	FC levels were obtained prior to endoscopy, as were haemoglobin levels, total white cell count, platelets, erythrocyte sedimentation rate, albumin and C-reactive protein.
Outcomes	Diagnostic accuracy of FC in differentiating IBD from non IBD
Main results	One hundred and ninety patients met the inclusion criteria (91 IBD and 99 non-IBD). The median FC for those diagnosed was 1265 µg/g (interquartile range (IQR): 734–2024 µg/g), compared with 65 µg/g (IQR: 20–235 µg/g) for those diagnosed with non-IBD. Of the 99 non-IBD patients the diagnoses were irritable bowel syndrome (33%), non-specific (12%), no pathology identified (11%), post-infectious enteropathy (11%), cow's milk or wheat intolerance (8%), pinworms (7%), allergic enteropathy (5%), coeliac disease (3%), miscellaneous (11%).
Conclusion	FC is an invaluable tool in determining those children who require endoscopy for suspected IBD, given the lack of overlap in values for IBD and non-IBD.

(continued)

Evidence 4	
Theme E4	*Tests for inflammatory bowel disease (IBD)*
Commentary	FC is a calcium-binding protein found in neutrophilic granulocytes. Its stability and convenience of collection make it a suitable surrogate indicator for the assessment of IBD. In the control population, symptoms and signs that suggested IBD were altered bowel habit (76%), abdominal pain (55%), rectal bleeding (48%), growth distortion (10%), recurrent mouth ulcers (3%) and iron-deficiency anaemia (2%). As a consequence of FC levels, the paediatrician can be more selective in referral patterns for endoscopy and be assured that IBD is not missed. Fortunately, FC is not influenced by age, sex, type and location of IBD, further enhancing its utility. For the secondary care paediatrician or general practitioner, FC can be used to assess relapse if subtle symptoms of IBD recur, thus allowing for prompt reassessment by the paediatric gastroenterologist.
Reference	Henderson P, Casey A, Lawrence SJ, *et al.* The diagnostic accuracy of fecal calprotectin during the investigation of suspected pediatric inflammatory bowel disease. *Am J Gastroenterol.* 2012; **107**(6): 941–9.

Evidence 5	
Theme E5	*Rotavirus infection and the impact of immunisation*
Question	What has been the impact of rotavirus immunisation on diarrhoea-associated hospitalisation?
Design	Cohort study
Level of evidence	
Setting	Sixty-two paediatric hospitals in America
Participants	Children aged 5 years or younger, admitted to 62 paediatric hospitals with diarrhoea-associated hospitalisations in three prevaccine seasons, 2003–06, and in two post-vaccine seasons, 2007–08 and 2008–09.
Intervention	The primary intervention was the administration of rotavirus vaccine.
Outcomes	The primary outcome was the reduction in diarrhoea-associated hospital admissions in the three defined periods.
Main results	Sixty-two acute care paediatric hospitals provided continuous data from 2003 to 2009 and of these, six were located in the North East, 21 in the Mid West, 24 in the South and 11 in the West. The median number of hospitalisations for 2003–06 was 15 645; this was reduced to 7760 (50%) in the 2007–08 season and an 11 039 (29%) reduction in the 2008–09 season. The rotavirus-coded admissions for 2003–06 were 4393; they were reduced to 760 (83%) for the 2007–08 season and to 1476 (66%) for the 2008–09 season.
Conclusion	Compared with the prevaccine era for rotavirus, hospitalisation for diarrhoea-associated and rotavirus-associated illnesses were reduced. Continued surveillance is required to assess the full impact of rotavirus immunisation.

(continued)

Evidence 5	
Theme E5	*Rotavirus infection and the impact of immunisation*
Commentary	The introduction of the rotavirus in infancy has markedly reduced the number of hospitalisations for diarrhoea-associated illnesses. The data provided for rotavirus reduction may not be fully accurate, as not all stools would have been sent for analysis for rotavirus. The issue of vaccine-related intussusceptions has recently been evaluated. In a case control study of 615 cases and 2050 controls in Mexico and Brazil, an annual excess of 96 cases of intussusceptions were identified in days 1 to 7 after the second dose of RV1 (rotavirus vaccine), with six deaths. This translates into an incidence of 1 per 51 000 infants in Mexico and 1 per 68 000 infants in Brazil; however, the vaccine prevented 80 000 hospitalisations and 1300 deaths in these countries (Patel *et al.*, 2011).
References	Yen C, Tate JE, Wenck JD, *et al.* Diarrhea-associated hospitalizations among US children over 2 rotavirus seasons after vaccine introduction. *Pediatrics.* 2011; **127**(1): e9–15.
	Patel MM, López-Collada VR, Bulhões MM, *et al.* Intussusception risk and health benefits of rotavirus vaccination in Mexico and Brazil. *N Eng J Med.* 2011; **364**(24): 2283–92.

DIARRHOEA: MULTIPLE-CHOICE QUESTIONS

Q1 The causes of bloody diarrhoea in childhood include which of the following?
a) Ulcerative colitis
b) Rotaviral diarrhoea
c) Campylobacter
d) Giardiasis
e) Helicobacter infections

Q2 Features of Crohn's disease include which of the following?
a) Mouth ulcers
b) Nocturnal pain
c) Perianal abscesses
d) Anorexia
e) Weight loss

Q3 Which of the following are recognised presentations of coeliac disease?
a) Constipation
b) Iron-deficiency anaemia
c) Short stature
d) Bloody diarrhoea
e) Abdominal distension

Q4 Which of the following statements is/are correct as they relate to coeliac disease?
a) Gluten sensitivity is the primary trigger.
b) Autoimmune diseases are associated with coeliac disease.
c) Coeliac disease is associated with HLA-DQ8 and HLA-DQ2.
d) Histological features include crypt hyperplasia.
e) Delayed puberty is a recognised presentation.

Q5 Which of the following statements is/are true with regard to secretory diarrhoea?
a) The aetiology is an imbalance between absorption of the villous epithelial cells and secretions from the crypt cells.
b) The stools do not contain leukocytes.
c) Aetiologies include shigella and cholera.
d) The diarrhoea abates with fasting.
e) Blood is present in 20% of cases.

Q6 Which of the following statements is/are correct?
a) Lactose is a monosaccharide.
b) Lactase deficiency causes lactose malabsorption.
c) Symptoms of lactose intolerance include abdominal pain, and crampy abdominal pain.
d) Primary lactase deficiency is rare in European populations.
e) Primary lactase deficiency typically presents at 9 months of age.

Q7 Which of the following statements on toddler's diarrhoea is/are correct?
a) It typically occurs at less than 1 year of age.
b) It is associated with failure to thrive in 15% of children.
c) It is associated with nocturnal pain which occurs in 20% of those affected.
d) It is associated with the presence of undigested food in the stool.
e) It is associated with a reduced transit time in the colon.

Q8 Which of the following is/are correct with regard to the diagnosis of lactose intolerance?
a) It is usually diagnosed by dietary challenge.
b) The hydrogen breath test is useful in diagnosis.
c) Stool for reducing substances is helpful in making the diagnosis.
d) Stool pH of <5 suggest lactose intolerance.
e) Urine for reducing substances are positive in 80% of cases.

Answers

A1	a, c	**A2**	a, b, c, d, e
A3	a, b, c, e	**A4**	a, b, c, d, e
A5	a, b, c	**A6**	b, c
A7	d, e	**A8**	a, b, c, d

SLIDES

1. Crohn's disease (perianal)
2. Dermatitis herpetiformis
3. Subtotal villous atrophy

Chapter Twelve

CONSTIPATION IN CHILDREN

COMMON SCENARIO

'I've tried everything, he just won't eat any fruit or vegetables and he hates water. He's even started soiling his pants at school. It's gotten so bad that the other children have started teasing him and calling him a baby ... there must be some investigations you can do. I'm certain there must be something wrong with his bowel.'

LEARNING OBJECTIVES

- Understand the terminology used to describe constipation in children
- Identify key points in a history or examination which point to a diagnosis of functional constipation
- Recognise 'red flags' in the history or examination that require further investigation
- Distinguish between functional versus organic causes of constipation
- Explain what investigations are indicated in children with constipation
- Construct a treatment plan for the effective management of childhood functional constipation
- Evaluate the available evidence to support your treatment options

BACKGROUND

Chronic constipation and faecal incontinence commonly present to general practitioners. They account for 5% of paediatric outpatients referrals, and make up 35% of the workload of a paediatric gastroenterologist. Up to 10% of children have experienced constipation. Constipation with faecal incontinence soiling occurs in 4% of preschool children (male to female ratio of 1:1) and 2% of school children (male to female ratio of 3:1).

Normal stool pattern varies with age. A newborn may stool four or more times per day, depending on whether he or she is breast- or bottle-fed. By 4 months of age, stool frequency reduces to two stools and to one per day by 4 years.

Constipation refers to the passage of infrequent hard stools causing distress to a child. However, the terminology can be confusing. The Paris Consensus on Childhood Constipation Terminology (PACCT) has therefore simplified the terminology defining the criteria for diagnosis.

Suggested terminology	PACCT definition
Chronic constipation	The occurrence of two or more characteristics in the past 8 weeks: • fewer than three bowel movements per week • more than one episode of faecal incontinence per week • large stool in the rectum • passing of stool that obstructs the toilet • display of retentive posturing with withholding behaviours • pain on defecation
Faecal incontinence (replaces soiling and encopresis)	The passage of stool in an inappropriate place. This may be due to: • organic faecal incontinence, e.g. anal sphincter abnormalities • functional faecal incontinence – which can be constipation-associated faecal incontinence or non-retentive (non-constipation-associated) faecal incontinence
Constipation-associated faecal incontinence	Functional faecal incontinence associated with the presence of constipation
Non-retentive faecal incontinence	The passage of stools in an inappropriate place, occurring in children with a mental age of 4 years and older, with no evidence of constipation based on history and/or examination
Faecal impaction	Large faecal mass in either the rectum or the abdomen is present which is unlikely to be passed on demand; the faecal impaction can be demonstrable by abdominal or rectal examination or other methodology
Pelvic floor dyssynergia	Inability to relax the pelvic floor when attempting to defecate

Functional constipation (no organic cause) can be considered a 'learnt phenomenon'. If a child experiences a painful bowel movement, they may voluntarily withhold defecation. Stool passage is delayed by voluntary contraction of the levator ani and external anal sphincter muscles. Hardened stool, which is more difficult to pass, accumulates in the rectum; thus the cycle of painful defecation and withholding continues. The lower colon gradually distends with accumulated stool and the urge to defecate becomes irregular due to decreased rectal sensation. When the rectum is sufficiently distended, softer stool leaks around the bulk of hard stool. The passage of soft stool is not sensed by the child until soiling has actually occurred. Recognised triggers that allow the constipation cycle to continue include difficulties with toilet training, school or home stresses, inter-current illnesses, avoidance of public toilets and/or hectic lifestyles. Once initiated, the constipation cycle is difficult to break. However, with effective diagnosis and proper treatment, the condition can be successfully managed in the primary care setting.

Anal fissures are commonly associated with constipation. Often the passage of a hard stool can cause a linear tear in the distal anal canal. There may be a history of painful defecation associated with bright red blood on the stool, in the nappy or on toilet paper. On examination, a small skin tag or 'sentinel pile' may be observed at the 12 o'clock or 6 o'clock position. Provided the stool is kept soft, anal fissures usually heal spontaneously.

HISTORY

KEY POINTS				
Stool pattern	Frequency of defecation Consistency of stool (use Bristol Stool Chart) Soiling or incontinence	**Factors relating to current episode**	Time of onset Trigger factors Illnesses Change in school Concerns at home	🔍 **Red flags** Weight loss or poor weight gain Anorexia Vomiting Symptoms present from birth or from first few weeks of life Failure or delay in passage of meconium Excessive milk ingestion
Symptoms associated with defecation	Bleeding per rectum Pain or distress Straining	**Treatments tried**	Medications tried Response to medications Duration of treatment Reason discontinued	
Behaviour	Withholding behaviour Reluctance to defecate Retentive posturing (straight-legged, tiptoe and back arching)	**General health and development**	Energy levels Episodes of weakness Weight loss Appetite Developmental concerns	
Past history	Previous episodes Previous anal fissure Passage of meconium after birth	**Dietary history**	Meal patterns Fluid intake Fibre intake	

EXAMINATION

All children presenting with constipation should have a full systemic examination, including height and weight measurement.

- Height and weight should be plotted on appropriate centile charts.
- The back and spine should be examined for any anomalies.
- The ankle jerks should be elicited.
- The abdomen should be palpated for masses.
- The perianal area should be inspected for evidence of anal fissures.

Red flags

- Abdominal distension, tenderness
- Spinal abnormalities such as sacral dimple, tuft of hair, naevi or sacral lipoma
- Abnormal neurological examination
- Abnormal perianal area, e.g. abnormal position, bruising

DIFFERENTIAL DIAGNOSIS

Between 90% and 95% of constipation is functional. In approximately 5% of cases an organic cause can be found. The frequency is not well defined; however, in the neonatal period an organic cause is more likely.

Common organic causes	Warning signs or symptoms
Anorectal malformations	Abnormal appearance or position of the anus
Neurological conditions	Abnormal tone, e.g. cerebral palsy or Down's syndrome
Hirshsprung's disease	Delayed passage of meconium (>48 hours)
	Passage of ribbon-like stool
	Failure to thrive
	Abdominal distension
Hypothyroidism	Bradycardia
	Lethargy
	Cold intolerance
Spinal cord abnormalities	Sacral dimple, tuft of hair, lipoma
Drugs	Opiates, anticholinergics, phenobarbital, antihypertensives

Other less common causes of organic constipation	
Metabolic conditions	Hypercalcaemic, hypokalaemia, diabetes mellitus, diabetes insipidus
Connective tissue disorders	Ehlers–Danlos's syndrome
	Systemic lupus erythematosus
	Scleroderma
Abnormal abdominal musculature	Gastroschisis
	Prune belly syndrome
Other	Cystic fibrosis, coeliac disease, heavy metal poisoning, child sexual abuse

INVESTIGATIONS

In what circumstances should a digital rectal examination be performed?

In children with functional constipation, digital rectal examinations are often unnecessary. However, in cases where the diagnosis is unclear, a digital rectal examination can help distinguish functional from organic constipation and can alter the course of therapy. As the examination is often poorly tolerated by children, it should be performed only once. It should only be undertaken by physicians who are competent in their ability to interpret the clinical findings. Therefore, in most cases, the examination will be performed by the specialist to whom the child has been referred.

Do plain films of the abdomen aid in the diagnosis of constipation?

Plain film of the abdomen may show a rectal faecal mass but there is little correlation between the clinical picture and radiological diagnosis. Routine radiography is therefore not routinely recommended. However, for those patients with a history of infrequent bowel movements but no objective findings of constipation, an evaluation of colonic transit time with radiopaque markers may be useful in selected cases.

Is urinalysis required?

Urinalysis must be carried out to exclude urinary tract infection. Constipation with a dilated rectum causes the same pattern of voiding dysfunction as that encountered in children with persistence of an unstable bladder. Effective treatment of the constipation results in normalisation of bladder function and cessation of urinary tract infections.

Should stool routinely be tested for occult blood?

It is recommended that a test for occult blood in the stool be performed in all infants with constipation, as well as in any child who also has abdominal pain, failure to thrive, intermittent diarrhoea, or a family history of colon cancer or colonic polyps.

When is a rectal biopsy indicated?

Rectal biopsy is rarely required unless there are symptoms of intractable constipation from birth with associated abdominal distension and a delayed passage of meconium. Rectal biopsy is done to exclude Hirschsprung's disease (a rare condition occurring in 1 in 7000 births).

MANAGEMENT PLAN: FOUR-STEP APPROACH

1. Clarifying and pitfall avoidance strategies:
   a) parent
   b) doctor
2. Education
   a) dietary modification
   b) bowel fitness training
3. Disimpaction
4. Maintenance

Clarifying and pitfall avoidance strategies

Parent

- Symptom recall of constipation. **Pitfall**: if the parent asks the child during the consultation how often they pass a bowel movement, the information is likely to be unreliable. Children usually do not keep track of this type of information. Prospectively get the parents to log the bowel movement frequency – the Bristol stool chart is a useful aid to clarify the stool type.
- Diarrhoea in the child with constipation. **Rationale**: parent will assume that diarrhoea occurring in a child with constipation is related to an episode of gastro-enteritis. It often reflects overflow of the constipated stool.
- This child who soils his underwear. **Rationale**: this is an indicator of constipation with overflow.
- The parental response to soiling. **Rationale**: parents are often very surprised that their child passes some stool in their underwear and does not recognise that the event has occurred especially when the parent has recognised the smell of faeces (faecal incontinence). Often their first response is disbelief, then they may become annoyed or believe that the child is soiling to get attention, prior to seeking a medical opinion. There is little secondary gain to be achieved from soiling.
- Stool avoidance practices. **Rationale**: in all children with constipation parents should be questioned regarding withholding manoeuvres (parents sometimes see these as attempts at defecating but they rarely take place in the bathroom – rather, the child hides).
- Constipation and the presence of psychological problems. **Pitfall**: effective treatment of constipation should be the first recommendation to parents of a child with constipation. If effectively treated, it is uncommon to find underlying psychological problems.
- Dependency on laxatives. **Rationale**: parents are often concerned that their child will become dependent on laxatives. There is no evidence to support this view.

Doctor

- If parents have used suppositories define the treatment response. **Pitfall**: the passage of thin ribbon-like stools in response to a suppository should prompt consideration of short segment Hirschsprung's disease.
- The non-responding child. **Rationale**: if the child does not respond to therapy once adherence has been assured rethink the diagnosis of constipation and seek secondary causes (coeliac disease hypothyroidism or polyuric states).
- Medication usage by the parent. **Pitfall**: transit studies are useful in the child who is not responding to medication where there are concerns of medication non-administration.
- Weight gain and poorly controlled constipation. **Rationale**: check the diet for 'junk foods' and strongly encourage a reduction in consumption.

- Examination of the anal region. **Pitfall**: Every child presenting with constipation should have the anal region inspected. If soiling is present then constipation with overflow is likely. Inspect the anus and assess anal tone by gently stretching the buttocks apart. If the anus opens then the tone is reduced. Always elicit the corrugator cutis ani reflex. Check for the presence of haemorrhoids and an anal fissure.

Education

Dietary modification

In order to encourage the production of soft bulky stool, children need to have adequate amounts of fibre in their diet. It has been shown that the Irish paediatric population does not take adequate fibre. High fibre intake with regular meals should be encouraged along with 6–8 cups of water-based fluid per day. For children older than 2 years of age the amount of fibre (in grams) that they should be eating daily can be calculated as follows:

Age in years + 5 = grams of fibre per day.

Foods high in fibre that should be recommended	
Breakfast	All-Bran Bran Flakes, All-Bran, Sultana Bran, Weetabix, Shreddies, muesli and porridge oats
Lunch	Brown bread, wholemeal and granary bread
Dinner	Wholegrain pasta and rice
	Vegetables, e.g. baked beans, kidney beans, sweet corn and peas
	Legumes, e.g. lentils
Snacks	Dried apricots, prunes, raisins and figs
	Fruit such as blackberries, raspberries, strawberries, passion fruit and kiwi fruit

Bowel fitness training

Bowel fitness training is essential to re-establish normal bowel habits. However, regular sits on the toilet pose compliance issues. Star charts can provide a useful means of improving compliance. Bowel fitness training works by exploiting the gastro-colic reflex, therefore the best time for children to sit on the toilet is after meals, particularly breakfast. A regular programme of three 5- to 10-minute sits per day on the toilet after each home meal is recommended. It is equally important to ensure that children are in a comfortable position when sitting on the toilet. Therefore, children should have a footstool to ensure the hips can be fully flexed during sits.

The success or failure of the whole treatment programme rests with the child's adherence to this sitting regime. Bowel fitness training needs to continue for at least 6 months until the normal sensory feedback in the lower colon has returned.

Disimpaction

Disimpaction can be carried out through the oral or rectal routes, with oral being the preferred route. Polyethylene glycol 3350 plus electrolytes or Movicol should be used as first-line treatment for disimpaction. An escalating dose regimen should be used. If there is no response to treatment after 2 weeks, a stimulant or osmotic laxative (e.g. lactulose) can be added. In order to help ensure compliance, it is important that both children and parents are informed that disimpaction treatment can cause abdominal pain and discomfort. The regime should be reviewed once disimpaction has occurred. This is usually indicated by the passage of a large stool. Movicol dosage should then be reduced by two sachets per day till soft stool is being passed. This dose of Movicol can then be used as maintenance dose.

Number of sachets of Movicol Paediatric Plain per day for faecal impaction							
Age (years)	Day 1	Day 2	Day 3	Day 4	Day 5	Day 6	Day 7
2–4	2	4	4	6	6	8	8
5–12	4	6	8	10	12	12	12
Number of sachets of Movicol Adult preparation per day for faecal impaction							
>12	4	4	6	6	8	8	7

Maintenance

Once disimpacted, maintenance therapy aims to allow the muscles and nerves of the lower bowel to recover by promoting regular toileting and preventing further impaction. Movicol is a safe and effective maintenance treatment for constipation in children to achieve this goal. The dose should be adjusted according to stool consistency and frequency. For children 1–6 years of age, the usual dosage is one sachet daily; however, doses up to a maximum of four sachets daily can be used. For children 6–12 years of age, the usual dosage is two sachets daily; however, up to a maximum of four sachets daily can be used. For children >12 years of age, Movicol Adult preparation can be used. The usual dosage is one to three sachets daily.

In order to ensure compliance and prevent impaction, it is important to explain to parents that their child may be on this treatment for a prolonged period of time and that the medication should not be stopped abruptly.

For those children who cannot tolerate Movicol, there are a number of alternative treatment options available, including osmotic and stimulant laxatives. Long-term use of stimulant laxatives is not recommended. Lactulose is licensed for use in children from 4 weeks of age. Dosage should be adjusted according to stool consistency and frequency; however, the usual dose for children is as follows.

- 1 month to 1 year: 2.5 mL twice daily
- >1–5 years: 2.5–5 mL twice daily
- >5–18 years: 5–20 mL twice daily

FOLLOW-UP

- Children require regular GP or outpatient visits to monitor and adjust their medications.
- Medication should be continued until a regular bowel pattern is established.
- In order to ensure that a relapse of constipation does not occur, the child should continue to be monitored when stopping or reducing medication.
- In those children who continue to soil, non-compliance with the sitting regimen is the most important contributory factor.
- In extreme cases a short admission to hospital may be required.

WHEN TO REFER?

- All children with 'red flags' in the history or examination should be referred for further assessment.
- In order to out rule an organic cause, children under 1 year of age who do not respond to optimum treatment within 4 weeks should be referred to a specialist.

Clarification statements for parental misconceptions

> *'My baby is nearly 4 months old and is breastfeeding. The problem is that his bowel movements seem to be very erratic. He might not have a motion for 3 days at a time. Why is he constipated?'*

Your baby's bowel movements are normal. Breastfed babies tend to be very irregular for the first few months. Some babies can pass several bowel motions a day; others may only pass a bowel motion every 3–4 days. What is important is the fact that your baby is thriving.

> *'Surely some tests are needed to make sure it's only constipation?'*

Constipation is extremely common in childhood and diagnosing it is extremely straightforward. I have no concerns regarding an underlying problem. An X-ray will merely show me the stool, which I can already feel in his tummy, and a blood test or further scans are only indicated in children who have concerning signs or symptoms.

> *'She soils her underpants nearly every day. I've tried cutting out dairy from her diet but it has made no difference to the diarrhoea.'*

Although it may seem like diarrhoea, she is actually constipated. Soiling is what happens when softer stool leaks around the hard mass of stool that has built up in her rectum. Firstly we need to soften her stool to make it easier for her to pass that hard stool. The best way to do this is by ensuring that she takes her prescribed medication every day. Once she has passed that hard stool, we then need to ensure that it doesn't build up again; we need to break the constipation cycle. First, we need to keep her stool soft. The best way to do this is by ensuring that she takes her prescribed medication regularly. Second, you need to look at her diet. She needs to drink 6–8 cups of water during the day and you need to increase the amount of fibre that she is getting in her meals. By tackling her diet now, it will help ensure that she will maintain healthy bowel habits in the future. At the same time you have to start encouraging her to sit on the toilet for 5–10 minutes after every meal. Star charts or rewards systems can be very helpful, and provide a way for you to monitor her progress.

SUMMARY PRACTICE POINTS

- Constipation is common in children.
- The vast majority of children who soil have chronic constipation.
- Very few children require investigations.
- Stool softening with Movicol Paediatric or lactulose forms the basis of medical treatment
- Regular sits for 5–10 minutes after meals is essential for resolution.
- The vast majority of cases can be managed by the general practitioner.

EVALUATING THE EVIDENCE

Evidence 1	
Theme E1	**Formula and its impact on constipation**
Question	Among infants with constipation does Nutrilon Omneo formula result in improvement in constipation?
Design	Randomised controlled trial with crossover design
Level of evidence	Jadad 5
Setting	Paediatric gastroenterology department, the Netherlands
Participants	Participants were 35 babies aged 3–20 weeks receiving at least two bottles of infant formula per day without an organic cause for constipation. Constipation was defined as one of the following: • fewer than three bowel movements per week • painful defecation (crying) • abdominal or rectal palpable mass.
Intervention	Nutrilon Omnio formula or standard formula for 3 weeks with crossover. Potential differences in taste were eliminated. Stool passage and consistency were based on four validated photographs.
Outcomes	• Bowel movements frequency • Stool consistency as per the four validated photographs • Reduction in painful bowel movements or decreased abdominal or rectal mass

(*continued*)

Evidence 1	
Theme E1	**Formula and its impact on constipation**
Main results	After the first 3 week period here was no change in defecation frequency between the two groups. Improvement of hard stool consistency to soft stool consistency was noted more often in the intervention group but did not reach statistical significance. There was no change in painful defecation or in the presence of abdominal or rectal masses.
	At the study conclusion the only clinical finding of relevance was the presence in four (17%) infants of soft stools on the Nutrilon Omnio formula and hard stools on the standard formula, while no infant had soft stools on the standard formula and hard stools on the Nutrilon Omnio formula ($P = 0.045\%$).
Conclusion	The formula did not result in an improvement in constipation, but there was some improvement in stool softness.
Commentary	This study was originally designed as a randomised control trial with crossover but the high dropout rate in the crossover prevented the study being completed as planned and thus the trial is a simple two-group parallel study. The explanation for the high dropout rate may reflect parental lack of satisfaction with immediate results in therapy.
	The mechanism of action of this formula is interesting in that human milk is high in oligosaccharides, which resist digestion in the small intestine and reach the colon unaltered, where they serve as probiotics. As these oligosaccharides are non-digestible they may be considered to be a form of soluble fibres and contribute as softness stools produced in breastfed infants.
Reference	Bongers ME, de Lorijn F, Reitsma JB, *et al*. The clinical effect of a new infant formula in term infants with constipation: a double-blind, randomized cross-over trial. *Nutr J.* 2007; **6**: 8.

Evidence 2	
Theme E2	**Fibre and constipation**
Question	Does increased fibre in the diet improve intestinal transit time and constipation in children with idiopathic chronic constipation?
Design	Randomised, double-blind controlled trial
Level of evidence	Jadad 1
Setting	Academic centre, Spain
Participants	Fifty-six children aged 3–10 years with constipation defined by the Rome II criteria, that is at least 12 weeks (non-consecutive in the previous 12 months) with two of the following: • straining in greater than 25% of defecation • lumpy or hard stools in greater than 25% of defecation • a sensation of incomplete evacuation in greater than 25% of defecation • a sensation of anorectal obstruction/blockage in greater than 25% of defecations • a need for manual manoeuvres to facilitate greater than 25% of defecations (e.g. digital evacuation, support of the pelvic floor) • less than three defecations per week.

(continued)

Evidence 2	
Theme E2	*Fibre and constipation*
Participants (*cont.*)	Exclusion criteria were: • faecal impaction that required enema 7 days before the start of the study • treatment with a dietary fibre or bulk forming agents or laxatives 2 weeks prior to the study • history of organic aetiology for constipation.
Intervention	All children had a standard toileting procedure and the experimental group received coco husk fibre in sachets weighing 4 g or placebo with the same weight. Children aged 3–6 years received two sachets and those aged 7–10 years received four sachets, dissolved in 200 mL of water.
Outcome	Colonic transit time was the primary outcome measurement to verify the efficacy of therapy, which was measured after the intake of 10 radiopaque markers.
Main results	There was no change in colonic transit time between the coco husk fibre and placebo. There was no significant change in bowel movement frequency. There was a reduction in hard stool frequency from 90% to 41.7% in the intervention group and 90% to 75% in the placebo group ($P = 0.017$; absolute reduced risk = 33.3%; number needed to treat = 3).
Conclusion	There was no major impact on constipation or transit time. There was a change in stool consistency, which may be of benefit to some children where hard stool is a primary feature.
Commentary	This was a short study where the compliance with fibre intake was good at 80%. The success is probably related to the chocolate flavouring of the husks. The introduction of fibre was not associated with side effects such as abdominal pain, bloating or excessive gas production.
Reference	Castillejo G, Bulló M, Anguera A, *et al.* A controlled, randomized, double-blind trial to evaluate the effect of a supplement of cocoa husk that is rich in dietary fiber on colonic transit in constipated pediatric patients. *Pediatrics.* 2006; **118**(3): e641–8.

Evidence 3	
Theme E3	*Polyethylene glycol (PEG) 3350 in the treatment of constipation*
Question	Is PEG plus electrolytes (+ E) safe and effective in the treatment of children with chronic constipation?
Design	Randomised, double-blind, placebo-controlled crossover trial
Level of evidence	Jadad 5
Setting	Academic medical centre, the United Kingdom
Participants	Participants were 51 children aged 2–11 years with a history of constipation for 3 months, defined as fewer than three bowel movements per week, plus one of the following: 25% bowel movements with staining; 25% of bowel movements hard or lumpy stool. Children with history of faecal impaction or organic constipation were excluded.
Intervention	PEG + E or placebo for 2 weeks followed by 2 weeks' placebo washout period and then alternating treatments for 2 weeks.

(*continued*)

Evidence 3	
Theme E3	**Polyethylene glycol (PEG) 3350 in the treatment of constipation**
Outcomes	The primary outcome was the mean number of complete defecations per week. Secondary outcomes included: • total number of defecations per week • pain on defecation • straining on defecation • stool consistency and the percentage of hard stools.
Main results	The mean number of complete defecations per week increased by 1.67 in the treatment group versus placebo (based on an intention-to-treat analysis). When only those who completed the protocol were analysed, the difference increased to 1.96. The safety profile of this survey was excellent: 41% of PEG + E and 45% of placebo experience side effects – most noticeably abdominal pain, which was ranked mild to moderate.
Conclusions	PEG + E is both safe and effective.
Commentary	This study demonstrates the efficacy of PEG + E in the treatment of constipation in children. The crossover design study can lead to concerns about a carry-over effect but this was reduced by 2-week washout phases
	The study also offers a useful protocol for clinicians in using PEG + E: in children 2–6 years of age, on days 1 and 2, one sachet; days 3 and 4, two sachets taken together; days 5 and 6, three sachets – two in the morning and one in the evening; and days 7 and 8, four sachets – two in the morning and two in the evening. In children 7–9 years of age, on days 1 and 2, two sachets; days 3 and 4, two sachets; days 5 and 6, five sachets – two in the morning and three in the evening; days 7 and 8, six sachets – three in the morning and three in the evening. In either group with the occurrence of diarrhoea the sachet frequency should be decreased by two or a day's therapy should be missed. If stools are loose then the sachet frequency should be reduced by one.
Reference	Thomson MA, Jenkins HR, Bisset WM, *et al.* Polyethylene glycol 3350 plus electrolytes for chronic constipation in children: a double blind, placebo controlled, crossover study. *Arch Dis Child.* 2007; **92**(11): 996–1000.

Evidence 4	
Theme E4	**Oral polyethylene glycol (PEG) 3350 and enemas in the treatment of constipation**
Question	In children with constipation who have rectal faecal impaction, which is better: high-dose oral PEG or enemas?
Design	Randomised controlled trial
Level of evidence	Jadad 1
Setting	Academic centre, the Netherlands
Participants	Participants were 90 children aged 4–16 years with symptoms of constipation for greater than 8 weeks and who had defecation fewer than three times per week, more than one episode of faecal incontinence per week, a history of retentive posturing or excessive volitional stool retention, a history of painful or hard defecation and a history of large-diameter stools that may have obstructed the toilet.

(*continued*)

Evidence 4

Theme E4	*Oral polyethylene glycol (PEG) 3350 and enemas in the treatment of constipation*
Participants (*cont.*)	Children with organic causes of constipation or colorectal surgery were excluded.
Intervention	Rectal enema for 6 days verses PEG 3350 at a dose of 1.5 g/kg for 6 days. Maintenance therapy consisted of PEG plus electrolytes for more than 2 weeks.
Outcome measure	The primary outcome was successful disimpaction. Secondary outcome measures included defecation and faecal incontinence frequency, abdominal pain, watery stools and transit time values.
Main results	Thirty-seven of 46 (80%) children had successful disimpaction with enemas and 30 of 44 (68%) had successful disimpaction with PEG (absolute risk reduction (ARR) = 12%; number needed to treat (NNT) = 8). Pertaining to secondary outcome measures there was more incontinence and watery stools with PEG therapy. However, 95% of children experience fearful behaviour with enemas as opposed to 81% with PEG (NNT = 6; ARR = 14%; number needed to harm = 8).
Conclusion	Enemas and PEG were equally effective in the treatment of rectal faecal impaction.
Commentary	PEG is a soluble inert polymer that acts by hydrogen bonding water molecules to expand the volume in the large intestine resulting in softer and more watery stools.
	In this study, 90 of 622 children with constipation had rectal faecal impaction on presentation.
	When discussing enemas or PEG therapy it is important to inform parents and children that disimpaction with oral PEG treatment is likely to result in more episodes of faecal incontinence.
Reference	Bekkall NL, van den Berg M, Dijkgraaf MG, *et al.* Rectal fecal impaction treatment in childhood constipation: enemas versus high doses oral PEG. *Pediatrics.* 2009; **124**(6): 1108–15.

Evidence 5

Theme E5	*Oral polyethylene glycol (PEG) 3350 and lactulose in the treatment of constipation*
Question	In the treatment of children with functional constipation, which is more effective: PEG therapy or lactulose?
Design	Parallel double-blind, randomised prospective multicentre comparison trial
Level of evidence	Jadad 5
Setting	Academic centre in the Netherlands
Participants	Participants were 100 children aged 6 months to 15 years with constipation defined as having at least two of four of the following symptoms for the last 3 months: 1. fewer than three bowel movements per week 2. encopresis more than once a week 3. large amounts of stool every 7–30 days (large enough to clog the toilet) 4. palpable abdominal or rectal mass on physical examination. Children with organic causes for constipation were excluded.

(continued)

Evidence 5	
Theme E5	***Oral polyethylene glycol (PEG) 3350 and lactulose in the treatment of constipation***
Intervention	Patients randomised to receive either lactulose (6 g sachet) or PEG 3350 (2.95 g sachet). In the run-in phase of 1 week, no oral laxatives were allowed; however, at the end of this phase patients received one enema daily for 3 days to clear any rectal faecal impaction.
Outcome	The primary outcomes were: • frequency of stools • frequency of encopresis • overall treatment success at 8 weeks.
Main results	The success rate of PEG therapy was 56% versus 29% for lactulose (absolute reduced risk = 27%; number needed to treat = 4). Fewer side effects were noted in the PEG group except for the higher instance of poor palatability. Twenty-six patients were treated for greater than 1 year with constipation prior to entry to this study. Fourteen per cent and 33% were treated successfully with lactulose and PEG, respectively.
Conclusion	PEG therapy has a higher success rate and fewer side effects than lactulose and should be the laxative of first choice in the treatment of childhood constipation.
Commentary	Despite the effectiveness of PEG in this study, 20% of patients needed other laxatives during the intervention phase. This is in contrast to the adult experience.
Reference	Voskujil W, de Lorijn F, Verwijs W, et al. PEG 3350 (Transipeg) versus lactulose in the treatment of childhood functional constipation: a double blind, randomised, controlled, multicentre trial. *Gut.* 2004: **53**(11): 1590–4.

CONSTIPATION: MULTIPLE-CHOICE QUESTIONS

Q1 Constipation is a recognised presentation of which of the following conditions?
   a) Hypercalcaemia
   b) Hypokalaemia
   c) Diabetes mellitus
   d) Diabetes insipidus
   e) Hyperuricaemia

Q2 Which of the following statements relating to constipation is/are correct?
   a) Organic aetiologies account for 5% of children with constipation.
   b) Constipation occurs with increased frequency in Down's syndrome.
   c) Constipation is associated with posterior anal displacement.
   d) Organic causes occur more frequently in the neonatal period.
   e) Constipation is associated with daytime wetting.

Q3 Features of Hirschsprung's disease include which of the following?
a) Delayed passage of meconium
b) Enterocolitis
c) Scaphoid abdomen
d) Passage of ribbon-like stools
e) Failure to thrive

Q4 Features of chronic constipation include which of the following?
a) More than one episode of faecal soiling per week.
b) Passage of stool that blocks the toilet.
c) Displaying retentive postures.
d) Fewer than five bowel movements per week.
e) Presence of large amounts of stool in the rectum.

Q5 Effective treatment strategies for constipation include which of the following?
a) Increase fluid intake
b) Fibre intake of 1.5 g/kg/day if greater than 18 months
c) Movicol on a daily basis
d) Lactulose
e) Liquid paraffin

Q6 In the examination of a child with constipation, which of the following should specifically be evaluated?
a) Ankle reflexes
b) Palpation for a mass in the right iliac fossa
c) Assessment of anal tone
d) Assessment of the corrugator cutis ani reflex
e) Inspection of the spine

Q7 Constipation is a recognised feature of which of the following?
a) Coeliac disease
b) Vesicoureteric reflux
c) Systemic lupus erythematosus
d) Hereditary spherocytosis
e) Ehlers–Danlos's syndrome

Q8 Side effects of Movicol in the treatment of constipation include which of the following?
a) Nausea
b) Abdominal distension
c) Hiccoughs
d) Polyuria
e) Abdominal pain

Q9 In children with faecal incontinence (encopresis), which of the following statements is/are true?
a) Twenty per cent have psychological problems.
b) The child is aware that the soiling has occurred before the parent or guardian is aware.
c) Diarrhoea is a recognised presentation.
d) The anal tone is lax.
e) High-fibre diet is the preferred treatment with counselling.

Q10 Red flags, clinical symptoms and signs in children with constipation include which of the following?
a) Abdominal pain with fever
b) A history of tripping
c) A hairy tuft on the child's back
d) Epigastric tenderness
e) Growth failure

Answers

A1	a, b, c, d	A2	a, b, d, e
A3	a, b, d, e	A4	a, b, c, e
A5	c, d, e	A6	a, c, d, e
A7	a, b, c, e	A8	b, e
A9	b, c, d	A10	a, b, c, e

Chapter Thirteen

FAILURE TO THRIVE (INCLUSIVE OF EATING DISORDERS)

> **COMMON SCENARIO**
>
> 'She just doesn't seem to be able to put on weight. I've tried everything. She's not interested in her dinner, she just takes the bottle and that's it.'

LEARNING OBJECTIVES

- Understand normal growth in infancy and childhood
- Recognise the causes of failure to thrive (FTT)
- Understand the classification of eating disorders
- Recognise 'red flags' in the history or examination that require further investigation
- Construct a treatment plan for the management of non-organic FTT
- Construct a treatment plan for the adolescent with eating disorders

BACKGROUND

FTT is a state of undernutrition when a child's rate of growth fails to meet the potential expected for a child of that age. Many healthcare professionals solely identify FTT as a child's weight falling below the 0.4th centile on standardised growth charts; however, this can be misleading, as some children are constitutionally small and may be growing healthily along their centile line. In addition, larger children who are dropping centiles may not be identified. Therefore a more appropriate means of identifying FTT is weight that is showing a downward trend on centile charts. The key to diagnosing FTT is regular documentation of a child's height and weight at every opportunity – only then can worrying trends be recognised. It is important that FTT is recognised early to avoid subsequent growth delay, compromised immune function and impairment of cognitive development. The exact incidence of FTT is unknown, but it is estimated that FTT affects 5%–10% of children.

Standardised centile charts allow a child's growth to be compared with normal growth. Modified growth charts exist for specific populations, e.g. Down's syndrome. In the first 6 weeks of life, crossing of centiles is more common, as lower birthweight infants tend to grow faster and higher birthweight infants grow slower (regression towards the mean). Nutrition is the main driver of growth in the first 2 years of life. During the first year of life, an infant's weight increases by 300%. During the first 3 months of life, infants gain approximately 1 kg a month, from 3–6 months of age, they gain an average of 0.5 kg a month and from 6–9 months of life they gain an average of 0.33 kg a month. Children aged 1–5 years typically gain 1–3 kg per year.

Eating disorders do not fall into an easy classification system and a high index of suspicion is necessary to recognise the early symptoms and signs, to ensure a favourable outcome. In anorexia nervosa there is a refusal to maintain weight that is consistent with health for age, height and gender (<85% of expected). The child or adolescent has a fear of gaining weight or of becoming fat and has a distorted body image (this is evident if the patient draws an image of themselves). In adolescent girls menstrual periods cease (more than three consecutive periods missed is defined as amenorrhoea).

In children with bulimia nervosa there are recurrent episodes of binge eating (large amounts of food in a short period of time and a feeling of being out of control. To prevent weight gain, self-induced vomiting occurs; some may use laxatives while others resort to intense exercise. The child and adolescent are overly influenced by body shape and weight. In this group the weight is often within normal limits. Some children and adolescents do not fit neatly into either group.

Normal calorie requirements in childhood	
Age	Calorie requirement (kcal/kg/day)
Premature infants	120–140
0–6 months	108
6–12 months	98
1–3 years	102
4–6 years	90
7–10 years	70

Traditionally, the causes of FTT have been classified as organic or non-organic. However, this approach is not useful, as most cases have mixed aetiologies and it overemphasises organic causes, which account for only 5% of cases. Organic disease is unlikely in children who are asymptomatic and well on examination. A useful approach to determine the cause of FTT is to consider the pathophysiology. Is it secondary to:

- inadequate caloric intake?
- increased losses?
- excessive caloric expenditure?

A careful history and examination can help identify the cause of FTT. Ideally, a feed or meal should be observed and a home visit scheduled by the public health nurse or other appropriate health professionals. In many cases, no one cause is identified. Poor calorific intake can occur unintentionally with breastfeeding difficulties, errors with formula preparation, delayed weaning onto solids and poor parental understanding of calorie requirements in infancy and early childhood. A wide variety of psychosocial factors can contribute to FTT, including stresses in the home (e.g. recent death, divorce, financial difficulties) maternal depression or psychiatric problems and lack of support. Any number of factors can negatively impact on the child–parent relationship, which can in turn lead to maladaptive feeding behaviours including food refusal.

Child abuse and neglect are rare causes of FTT; however, they remain important to consider, particularly if there is concern regarding deliberate withholding of food or the family is resistant to interventions or there is failure to respond to appropriate interventions. Risk factors for possible neglect include:

- drug or alcohol misuse
- mental health problems
- parental history of abuse as a child
- domestic violence
- socio-economic disadvantage
- social isolation
- previous abuse in the family.

When interviewing adolescents the HEADS framework is useful. **H** refers to the **home** situations, with a focus on relationship with parents and family members, the degree of support available and an evaluation of stresses if present. **E** stands for **education** (school performance, career goal, part-time employment, if occurring) and **eating** (changes in weight, food preferences, views on dieting, weight control and exercise). **A** refers to **activities** (hobbies, sports, and activities with friends) and **adherence** (medication usage). **D** refers to **drugs** (smoking, alcohol, street drugs, best to ask first about friends or family usage prior to asking the adolescent). **S** refers to **sexuality** (sexual activity, birth control, best to explore what friends do first, then refer to adolescent but clarify what he or she means by sexual activity), **suicide** (evaluate 'mood', presence of disturbed sleep, examples of low energy, thoughts on self-harm) and **safety** (presence of bullying at school or at home, sexual abuse/date rape).

DIFFERENTIAL DIAGNOSIS

Organic causes of failure to thrive

Inadequate caloric intake	
Mechanical causes	Cleft lip or palate
Central nervous system or neuromuscular	Hypotonia
	Cerebral palsy
Chronic illness	Anorexia secondary to chronic illness
Drugs	Anorexia secondary to medications
Iatrogenic	Fluid restriction post cardiac surgery
Increased losses from vomiting	
Gastro-oesophageal reflux	Gastro-oesophageal reflux disease
Surgical causes	Pyloric stenosis
	Malrotation
Central nervous system disease	Raised intracranial pressure
Infection	Urinary tract infection
Metabolic	Inborn errors of metabolism
Increased losses from diarrhoea	
Fat malabsorption	Cystic fibrosis
	Cholestatic liver disease
	Ileal resection
Mucosal abnormality	Coeliac disease
Short gut	Bowel resection (necrotising enterocolitis, gastroschisis, midgut volvulus)
	Congenital short gut
Chronic infection	Inflammatory bowel disease
Defective intracellular lipid transport	Abetalipoproteinaemia
Inadequate lymphatic drainage	Congenital lymphangiectasia
	Acquired secondary to Fontan's procedure
Lactase malabsorption	Hereditary
	Acquired post infection
Sucrose malabsorption	Isomaltase deficiency
Glucose malabsorption	Galactose malabsorption
Protein malabsorption	Protein losing enteropathy
Non-GI losses	Diabetes mellitus
	Renal tubular acidosis
Excessive caloric expenditure	
Chronic infection	HIV, tuberculosis
Respiratory disease	Cystic fibrosis, poorly controlled asthma
Cardiac disease	Congenital cardiac diseases or heart failure

(*continued*)

Inadequate caloric intake	
Chronic inflammation	Juvenile idiopathic arthritis
Malignancy	Leukaemia, lymphoma
Thyroid disease	Hyperthryoidism
Central nervous system causes	Diencephalic syndrome

Eating disorders

Differential diagnosis of eating disorders	Differentiating features
Hyperthyroidism	Tachycardia, sweating, anxious
Crohn's disease	Weight loss, abdominal pain, poor appetite
Depression	Sleep disturbance, irritability
Hypothyroidism (producing amenorrhoea and hypothermia)	Normal appetite, no distorted body image
Avoidance of eating	Usually after an event, e.g. choking, develop a phobia; usually acute onset
Achalasia (severe weight loss)	Desire to eat present but progressive difficulty swallowing
Normal thinness	Evaluate the parents, normal appetite and normal body image

HISTORY

KEY POINTS				
Feeding history	Breast- or bottle-fed Age at weaning onto solids Types of foods Quantity of food consumed Fluid consumption Behaviour during feeds Food aversion Food allergies	**Medical history**	Recurrent infections or fevers Recurrent episodes of vomiting or lethargy	**🚩 Red flags** Recurrent infections Recurrent vomiting Chronic diarrhoea Dyspnoea with feeds Signs of abuse or neglect
Meal patterns	When, where and with whom does the child eat? Distractions at meal time Snacks during day	**Surgical history**	Previous bowel operations	Maternal depression or psychiatric illness
Birth history	Planned pregnancy Gestation Birthweight Complications	**Medications**	Over-the-counter or prescription medications Laxatives* Diuretic use*	Difficult family circumstance

(continued)

KEY POINTS

Maternal history	Depression Psychiatric disorder Eating disorder Nutritional beliefs Relationship with child	**Social history**	Available supports Who lives at home? Who looks after child? Difficulties at home* Financial worries Drug or alcohol use * Choice of clothing to hide body habitus* Exercise practices* Parental responses to weight loss*
Stool pattern	Frequency Consistency Blood Mucus Steatorrhoea	**Growth and development**	Size clothes parents buy for child Reaching milestones Temperament Energy levels
Family history	FTT in siblings Coeliac or inflammatory bowel disease Cystic fibrosis Immune deficiencies Metabolic disease Endocrine disease	**Interventions tried**	How parents have been dealing with child's eating habits Parental approach to mealtime*
Weight loss*	Is weight loss as a result of decreased intake or output?* Has it been voluntary?*	**Menstrual history***	Menarche * Regularity of menstruation * Occurrence of last menstruation*
Dietary history*	Portion size* Food choices* History of dieting* Binge eating*	**Systems review***	Alopecia* Cold intolerance* Vomiting* Abdominal pain* Constipation* Haematemesis* Cold intolerance* Palpitations*
Mental status*	Suicidal ideation*		

Note: *indicates features of eating disorders.

EXAMINATION

All children should have accurate measurement of weight, height and head circumference plotted on an appropriate centile chart including previous measurements.

Failure to thrive features

- Assess overall appearance of child and interaction
- Evidence of weight loss: loose skin folds, lack of subcutaneous fat
- Developmental assessment
- Inspect skin, hair and nails
- Neurological exam: tone and reflexes
- Cardiovascular exam: murmurs or signs of heart failure
- Respiratory exam: distress, wheeze or crepitations
- Gastrointestinal exam: abdominal distension or organomegaly

Observation of parent

- Interaction with child
- Attitude toward child
- Response to discussion on failure to thrive
- Feeding skills

Eating disorder features

- Growth parameters
- Temperature (hypothermia)
- Orthostatic changes in blood pressure and heart rate (taken 2 minutes after lying and standing)
- Dry skin
- Lanugo
- Cold extremities
- Callus on knuckles
- Eroded enamel (posterior aspects of upper teeth)
- Subconjunctival haemorrhages
- Petechiae in the distribution of the superior vena cava

Red flags

- Hypothermia, hypotension and bradycardia
- Heart failure
- Clubbing
- Dysmorphic features
- Developmental delay
- Organomegaly and/or lymphadenopathy
- Poor parent–child interaction

- Withdrawn child with gaze avoidance
- Wearing of bulky clothing*
- Dehydration*(associated electrolyte abnormalities likely to be present)
- Lanugo hair*
- Parotid enlargement*
- Evaluate for acute weight loss*

INVESTIGATIONS

Investigations are not routinely indicated in cases of FTT, unless an organic cause is suggested in the history or examination findings. Therefore, investigations should be targeted and individualised.

If coeliac disease is suspected, what investigations should be performed?
- IgA anti-tissue transglutaminase antibodies *and* serum IgA levels
- Stool culture and sensitivity
- Full blood count (FBC) with differential
- Liver function tests
- Urea and electrolytes
- Urinalysis

If baseline investigations are required, what tests may be requested?
- FBC: may show anaemia due to iron, folate or vitamin B_{12} deficiency, or anaemia of chronic disease
- C-reactive protein, erythrocyte sedimentation rate: raised with infection or inflammation
- Coeliac screen
- Urinalysis and culture: urinary tract infection
- Urea and electrolytes: renal function, dehydration
- Liver function tests: low albumin
- Thyroid function tests: hyperthyroidism
- Stool for fat, faecal elastase and microscopy culture and sensitivity

In adolescents with suspected eating disorder, what tests are required?

All patients should have the following: FBC, urea and electrolytes, bicarbonate, calcium, magnesium, phosphate, glucose, amylase, liver function tests, coagulation profile and erythrocyte sedimentation rate.

Endocrine tests such as thyroid function, luteinising hormone, follicle-stimulating hormone, oestradiol and prolactin should be measured.

A 12-lead electrocardiogram and urinalysis are also required.

MANAGEMENT PLAN: FIVE-STEP APPROACH

1. Clarifying and pitfall avoidance strategies
   a) failure to thrive
   b) eating disorders
2. Nutritional intervention for failure to thrive
3. Feeding behaviour modification for failure to thrive
   a) psychosocial stressors
   b) hospital admission
4. Management of eating disorders
5. Hospitalisation for eating disorders

Clarifying and pitfall avoidance strategies

Failure to thrive

PARENTS

- Failure to thrive and the mother. **Pitfall**: discussing with a mother that her infant in not growing adequately is extremely anxiety provoking; therefore, the doctor requires a plan for investigation or treatment. If breastfeeding, encourage supplementation. The caloric intake per kilogram must be known in all infants and children with FTT.
- Aetiology of FTT. **Rationale**: parents should be advised that investigations should be tailored to the clinical presentation and ad hoc tests will have a low yield.

DOCTOR

- FTT and the short infant or child. **Pitfall**: the child who is short and failing to thrive with normal milestones may have a syndrome, e.g. Russell–Silver's syndrome or cystinosis.
- FTT and organic disease. **Pitfall**: rethink the diagnosis of idiopathic FTT if the infant or child develops symptoms in addition to FTT, e.g. vomiting. Evaluate the child for vomiting with coincidental FTT. Fortunately, most infants and children do not develop additional symptoms. Regular growth monitoring in conjunction with dietetic support is helpful in avoiding this pitfall.

Eating disorders

PARENTS

- Eating disorders and blame. **Pitfall**: parents do not cause eating disorders and should not be blamed. Avoid spending significant time on the 'why' of the problem and focus on the solution ('prescription, not description').
- Parents and their understanding of eating disorders. **Pitfall**: parents need to understand that eating disorders are serious conditions with significant morbidity and mortality. No one develops an eating disorder for secondary gain. Without treatment, eating disorders are unlikely to remit spontaneously.

- Eating disorders affect the decision-making ability of those affected. **Rationale**: the child or adolescent with an eating disorder needs to be guided to the solution by his or her parents and health professionals.
- Weight gain and the family. **Rationale**: parents are responsible for the child or adolescent's weight gain, and weight restoration is the first step toward recovery.
- Parents and meals. **Rationale**: parents must supervise and support the child or adolescent with his or her meals and snacks.
- Food refusal. **Rationale**: the behavioural management approach uses natural consequences to address food refusal. For example, the teenager is not allowed to visit his or her friends until a proper dinner is eaten.
- Parents and therapist. **Rationale**: parent need active support when addressing their teenagers with eating disorders and family-based counselling is effective.

DOCTORS

- Frequency of visits. **Rationale**: in the early weeks visits should occur weekly, with evaluation of height, weight, heart rate and blood pressure at each visit. Deterioration in these parameters allows the decision for hospitalisation to be made in a balanced fashion and not dependent on one parameter only.
- Rapid weight gain. **Pitfall**: teenager may drink water to 'fluid load' themselves, if they are apprehensive about their weight gain. As a rule the 'real' weight gain is associated with an improved eating pattern that can be confirmed by the parents.
- Meeting the parents. **Rationale**: it is useful to meet with the parents to clarify the challenges that they have experienced. Parents need to be encouraged to persist with insisting on adequate nutrition and limit-setting with their child and adolescent.
- Being positive with the patient. **Rationale**: having an eating disorder is both disabling and stressful for the teenager. When progress is being made, acknowledge the gain achieved.

Nutritional intervention for failure to thrive

A high-calorie diet is required to allow for catch-up growth (*see* Evidence 2). Energy intake should be 50% higher than the basal caloric requirements and should be based on their expected, not actual, weight.

> Catch-up growth requirements (kcal/kg/day) = [calories required for age (kcal/kg/day) × ideal weight for age (kg)] / [actual weight (kg)]

A 3-day food diary can be helpful for monitoring intake and identifying how it can be improved. Age-appropriate dietetic advice should be given to parents.

Measures to improve caloric intake include:

- addition of fats to diet, e.g. full fat butter, cheese, cream
- ensuring appropriate milk intake for age

- avoidance of juice and fizzy or sweetened drinks
- at mealtimes, offer solids before liquids
- concentration of formula
- breastfed infants may need fortified breast milk
- avoid junk foods – although they are high in calories, they are low in protein.

Feeding behaviour modification for failure to thrive

Parents should be educated about strategies that can help establish healthy eating behaviours. Concerns about poor weight gain can be extremely stressful for parents; this in turn can create a more stressful environment and continue to negatively affect the child's eating behaviour. A child's eating behaviour is strongly influenced by the family environment, including the parent's own eating behaviours and child feeding practices.

Measures to promote healthy eating behaviours include the following.

- Force-feeding must be avoided; instead, positive reinforcement should be given to children.
- Parents should offer food in a positive and supportive manner and allow the child to determine how much he or she will eat. Children should not be punished for not eating enough and should be encouraged to feed and serve themselves.
- Establish a relaxed and pleasant mealtime routine. The television and other distractions should be minimized. Meals should not be rushed.
- Parents and older siblings should sit together with the child during meals to allow the child to model appropriate behaviour and to help establish a social and supportive environment.
- It is normal for a child to reject food on first exposure. Therefore, continue to offer a variety of foods, in a supportive manner, to improve acceptance.
- Meals and snacks should be offered every 3 hours.

Psychosocial stressors

The family's general practitioner and community public health nurses have a key role to play in helping to address psychosocial stressors that may be contributing to the child's FTT (*see* Evidence 1). Additional support should be offered to families to help them cope with difficulties. Families may need referral to local social services or counselling services.

Hospital admission

Most cases of FTT can be managed on an outpatient basis, with regular follow-up and home visits if feasible. A multidisciplinary approach with input from dietitians, general paediatricians, social workers, speech and language therapist and child psychology is often required for difficult or severe cases.

Hospital admission may be required in:

- severe cases

- for investigation of likely organic FTT
- if there is concern about possible abuse or neglect
- if there is concern about parental behaviour or compliance with treatment.

Management of eating disorders

Once the diagnosis of an eating disorder is made, treatment can begin. The question of location of treatment, whether inpatient or outpatient, comes up for discussion. Current evidence suggests that outpatient treatment is as effective as inpatient treatment (*see* Evidence 3). Parents play an important role in aiding resolution of eating disorders, given the initial presence of denial of a problem by the adolescent, the difficulty encountered in enforcing attendance at counselling appointments and their child's reluctance to gain weight. The development of a therapeutic alliance between therapists and parents is important to ensure that the parents 'stay the course' with their child (*see* Evidence 4).

Hospitalisation for eating disorders

The decision to admit a child or adolescent with an eating disorder to hospital can be difficult and is usually undertaken for medical reasons.

The following criteria favour that decision, especially if the patient is symptomatic:
- significant bradycardia (heart rate <50 beats/minute during the day or <45 beats/minute at night)
- symptomatic hypotension
- dehydration
- acute food refusal
- arrested growth and development
- absolute weight <75% to 80% of ideal body weight.

Once a decision on hospitalisation has been made, then a strict treatment plan needs to be in place that includes:
- strict bed rest (activity only permissible with appropriate weight gain)
- monitoring of vitals, especially blood pressure
- judicious use of fluids
- initial caloric intake should approximate intake pre-hospitalisation – the motto 'start low and go slow' (*see* Evidence 5) is employed when refeeding the hospitalised teenager with an eating disorder.

In adolescents with eating disorders the risk of the refeeding syndrome must be considered, especially if the patient is <70% ideal body weight; monitoring of phosphate, magnesium and potassium is required.

Parents often ask if there are any medications that can improve the eating disorder (*see* Evidence 6); no trials to date have demonstrated an effective treatment.

FOLLOW-UP

- Continue to follow until catch-up growth achieved
- With successful intervention, children's weight should begin to move up the centile chart after 4–8 weeks
- Patients with eating disorders need to be seen weekly until weight gain established
- Monitoring of physiological parameters is required
- Blood work should be done if acute deterioration occurs

WHEN TO REFER?

- Failure to gain weight after 2–3 months despite intervention
- Suspected organic cause
- Concerns about possible abuse or neglect
- Early features of anorexia nervosa
- Early features of bulimia nervosa

CLARIFICATION STATEMENTS FOR PARENTAL MISCONCEPTIONS

'If my baby is not growing, there must be a reason.'

In many cases of FTT, no clear reason is found to explain the failure of growth. Children tend to put on weight at a consistent rate and as they get older parents recognise that they are lighter than their peers but otherwise normal.

'Since my teenager has an eating disorder, she needs to be admitted to hospital!'

Admission to hospital should not be the first response. The eating habits of your teenager need to be modified and this is best done in the home environment with the support of the local child and adolescent mental health team.

'I know my daughter has anorexia nervosa, but if she would just eat, her problems would be solved!'

Putting on weight is the first step in the treatment of anorexia nervosa, but it is not the only step. Teenagers with this condition have a distorted body image and many have difficulties in adult life.

SUMMARY PRACTICE POINTS

- FTT is recognised from growth chart review.
- Assessing the adequacy of caloric intake is essential.
- Force-feeding amplifies feeding difficulties.
- Repeated clinical examination is necessary in infants and children with FTT.
- Evaluate for the psychosocial contribution to the FTT.
- Eating disorders need to be recognised early.
- Parents have to set boundaries and be the monitors of the child or teenager.

EVALUATING THE EVIDENCE

Evidence 1	
Theme E1	*Early intervention programmes in failure to thrive (FTT)*
Question	What is the impact of an early intervention programme in children with FTT?
Design	Randomised controlled trial
Level of evidence	Jadad 4
Setting	Department of paediatrics and psychology, academic medical centre, the United States
Participants	Potential participants were recruited from low-income, urban communities' paediatric primary care practices. Children with FTT had to meet one of two criteria using age- and gender-specific growth charts: sustained weight for age <5th centile or weight for length <10 centile. Children in the average growth (AG) group had to meet two criteria: sustained weight for age and weight for length >10th centile. All eligible children were <25 months of age on commencing the study, and had a gestational age >36 weeks, birthweight ≥2500 g with an absence of congenital problems, disabilities or chronic illness.
Intervention	Children with FTT were randomised to receive the clinical intervention plus home intervention (HI) or clinical intervention only (CO). The AG children received standard primary paediatric care. The intervention consisted of home visits on a weekly basis for 1 year, with a focus on supporting the primary caregiver's personal, emotional and environmental needs, promoting and modelling responsive parent–child interaction and providing problem-solving strategies regarding personal, parenting and child issues.
Outcomes	Primary outcomes were assessed at 8 years of age and evaluated growth, cognitive performance, academic performance, home behaviour and school behaviour.
Main results	One hundred and thirty children with FTT were recruited, with 66 assigned to the HI group and 64 to the CO group – study completion rates were 47 and 49, respectively, at 8 years. One hundred and nineteen children were recruited to the AG group, with 93 completing the study. By 8 years of age children in the AG group were 5.5 cm taller than those in the HI group and 6 cm taller than those in the CO group. Cognition scores were on average one standard deviation below the normative sample across all three groups.

(continued)

Evidence 1	
Theme E1	**Early intervention programmes in failure to thrive (FTT)**
Main results (*cont.*)	In contrast with published standards, 16.3% of the entire sample had internalising behaviours and 27.4% had externalising behaviours above the clinical cut-off points (there were no differences across groups). When positive behaviours at school were considered, children in the HI group had higher scores on the work hard and learning subscales than children in the CO group.
Conclusion	Children with FTT were shorter than their AG peers at 8 years. The home visiting may have attenuated some of the academic difficulties experienced by the CO group possibly by enhancing maternal sensitivity, thereby helping children to build strong work habits that enabled them to benefit from school.
Commentary	Many children with FTT are seen in hospitals and represent a highly selected population; this study avoided selection bias and recruited patients from a disadvantaged community. The matching of groups allows the impact of the HI to be assessed. This population experiences social disadvantage, however, the gain in work habits can be attributed to the home intervention. At the end of the 1-year intervention, mothers were noted to be more children focused and responsive than those in the control group and presumably this continued afterwards. Three part-time lay home visitors who undertook an eight-session training programme supervised by a community-trained nurse undertook the intervention. This strategy would appear to be cost-effective in addressing the needs of vulnerable children. The impact of FTT needs to be considered in terms of both growth and development.
Reference	Black MM, Dubowitz H, Krishnakumar A, *et al.* Early intervention and recovery among children with failure to thrive: follow-up at age 8. *Pediatrics.* 2007; **120**(1): 59–69.

Evidence 2	
Theme E2	**Nutrient-dense formulas (NDFs) and faltering growth**
Question	Does increasing caloric intake address faltering growth?
Design	Randomised controlled trial
Level of evidence	Jadad 3
Setting	Dietetic department, children's hospital, England
Participants	Children attending a children's hospital, weighing 2–8 kg, diagnosed with faltering growth related to cardiac lesions, cystic fibrosis or other organic causes who were fed either orally or enterally were eligible for inclusion. Poor growth was defined as an infant who was less than the 3rd centile for weight and height for age and/or had a weight gain that was less than 50% of that expected over the 1-week period prior to recruitment. The study duration was 6 weeks.
Intervention	Both groups of infants received formulas containing 4.2 kJ (1 kcal) per millilitre. One was a NDF, the other an energy-supplemented formula (ESF) that contained 4 g/100 mL of glucose polymer (Maxijul) and 4 mL/100 mL long-chain fat emulsion (Calogen). For each infant the aim was a caloric intake of 150–200 kcal/kg/day by bottle, nasogastric tube or gastrostomy tube.

(*continued*)

Evidence 2	
Theme E2	*Nutrient-dense formulas (NDFs) and faltering growth*
Outcomes	The primary outcomes were weight gain and biochemical changes.
Main results	Sixty infants, with a median age of 5 weeks, were recruited from three diagnostic groups: cardiac defects (n = 28), cystic fibrosis (n = 7) and infants with organic faltering growth (n = 25) related to intestinal surgery, neurological syndromes and unknown aetiologies. Of the 49 infants randomised, 26 were assigned to the NDF group, with full data on 21 (84.7%) (four dropouts, two poor data collection, one >20% calories from solids, one total parenteral nutrition administered), and 23 to the ESF group, with full data on 16 (69.5%) (seven dropouts, two total parenteral nutrition, one unable to tolerate fat emulsion, one parent request, one feed change, one poor data collection, general practitioner changed formula). The median volume taken of NDF was 140 mL/kg/day and for ESF it was 143 mL/kg/day. The median weight gain for NDF was 7.2 g/kg/day and for ESF it was 7.6 g/kg/day. The NDF group received 42% more protein than the ESF group. Blood urea concentrations fell by 50% in the ESF group as a consequence.
Conclusion	NDFs should be used where possible in treating infants with faltering growth.
Commentary	In this study both groups demonstrated catch-up growth during the study period; however, the NDF group maintained a normal blood urea compared with the ESF group. Blood urea is the major end product of protein catabolism and is formed in the liver and its plasma concentration is dependent on protein intake. In children with faltering growth, determining the aetiology and treatment of the underlying case is important; however, nutritional therapy when used should include an increased intake of all nutrients in a balanced form, where possible.
Reference	Clarke SE, Evans S, Macdonald A, *et al.* Randomized comparison of a nutrient-dense formula with an energy-supplemented formula for infants with faltering growth. *J Hum Nutr Diet.* 2007; **20**(4): 329–39.

Evidence 3	
Theme E3	*Treatment of anorexia nervosa*
Question	Which is more effective: inpatient or outpatient treatment of anorexia nervosa?
Design	Randomised controlled trial
Level of evidence	Jadad 3
Setting	Inpatient and outpatient psychiatric units, England
Participants	Adolescents aged 12–18 years diagnosed with anorexia nervosa who fulfilled the Diagnostic and Statistical Manual of Mental Disorders, Fourth Edition, criteria modified for age as follows: food restriction with or without compensatory behaviours, weight below 85% of that expected within 1 month of assessment, based on age and current height or previous height centile; intense fear of gaining weight or undue influence of weight or shape on self evaluation; primary or secondary amenorrhoea of at least 3 months, or menstruation while on contraceptive pill.

(*continued*)

Evidence 3	
Theme E3	*Treatment of anorexia nervosa*
Intervention	Participants were randomised to receive treatment in (a) inpatient psychiatric units, (b) specialised outpatient units designed for this trial or (c) general community Child and Adolescent Mental Health Services (CAMHS).
Outcomes	Primary outcomes were at 2 years and were defined as follows: good outcome indicated recovery from anorexia nervosa (weight above 85% of expected, return of menstruation, bingeing/purging no greater than once per month). A poor outcome was indicated if the weight was not above the 85% or the young person was still being treated as an inpatient for anorexia nervosa. The intermediate category consisted of those whose weight had risen to within the normal range, but without return of menstruation, with binge/purging at a frequency greater than monthly or considerable residual concerns about weight and shape according to the Morgan-Russell scale A for food intake.
Main results	Three hundred and forty-seven patients were assessed for eligibility, 100 were excluded as they failed to meet diagnosis, 31 refused consent, 46 chose not to participate, and 170 were randomised but three were excluded post randomisation. Fifty-five were randomised to the CAMHS arm, 55 to the specialist unit and 57 to inpatient care. Adherence rates were 69.1% for CAMHS, 74.5% for the specialist unit and 49.1% for inpatient care. Good, intermediate, poor and unknown outcomes (but alive) for CAMHS were 36%, 36%, 26% and 2%, respectively; for specialised outpatients they were 24%, 51%, 22% and 4%, respectively; and for inpatients units they were 33%, 30%, 30% and 7%, respectively.
Conclusion	In patients with anorexia nervosa first-line inpatient care does not offer an advantage over outpatient management.
Commentary	The primary hypothesis of this study was that inpatient care would be more effective than outpatient care and that specialist outpatient units would be more effective than the general CAMHS units. Clinical intuition suggested that this should be the case but the results did not support the hypothesis. Anorexia nervosa is a chronic condition with fewer than one in five recovered in the first year and with a quarter still having anorexia at 2 years of treatment; therefore, access to local resources would appear to be the appropriate option.
Reference	Gowers SG, Clark A, Roberts C, *et al.* Clinical effectiveness of treatments for anorexia nervosa in adolescents: randomised controlled trial. *Br J Psychiatry.* 2007; **191**: 427–35.

Evidence 4	
Theme E4	*Family-based treatment (FBT) in anorexia nervosa (AN)*
Question	What determines the effectiveness of FBT in AN?
Design	Cohort study
Level of evidence	
Setting	Clinical psychology unit, eating disorders unit, academic medical centre, Australia

(*continued*)

Evidence 4	
Theme E4	*Family-based treatment (FBT) in anorexia nervosa (AN)*
Participants	Fifty-nine patients with AN for <3 years were invited to participate after they received inpatient treatment for their condition in a specialist unit, which included nasogastric refeeding, supported meals, individual supportive psychotherapy, behavioural management and treatment of co-morbid psychiatric conditions including the use of psychotropic medications.
Intervention	Participants and their families were invited to attend 20 outpatient family therapy sessions conducted by therapists trained in a manualised version of FBT.
Outcomes	The primary outcome was weight gain expressed as the percentage of ideal body weight (actual weight was expressed as a percentage of the expected weight corresponding to the 50th centile for height, age and gender according to stand-ardised charts) and the relationship to the Core Treatment Objectives Clinicians Ratings Scale and the Working Alliance Inventory results.
Main results	Fifty (84.5%) patients reached at least 85% of ideal body weight and 20 (40.7%) reached 95% ideal body weight by session 20. In the Treatment Objectives Clinicians Ratings Scale, weight gain was significantly predicted by parental con-trol, unity, criticism and externalisation. Sibling support had little impact. Nine (15.25%) patients dropped out and this was predicted by a lack of parental control. The Working Alliance Inventory scores indicated the stronger the mother–therapist alliance, the greater the weight gain.
Conclusion	This intervention, for those with AN, post hospitalisation was effective in the main-tenance of weight gain and the results were influenced by parental control.
Commentary	Eating disorders in adolescents are stressful for the entire family and occur at a time of increasing independence of adolescents from their parents. The support that parents (especially mothers) receive from therapists plays an important part in the successful outcome for the adolescent. Discharge from hospital does not equate to the resolution of the eating disorder and continued follow-up is required.
Reference	Ellison R, Rhodes P, Madden S, *et al.* Do the components of manualized family-based treatment for anorexia nervosa predict weight gain? *Int J Eat Disord.* 2012; **45**(4): 609–14.

Evidence 5	
Theme E5	*Refeeding the patient with anorexia nervosa (AN)*
Question	How should a patient with AN be fed?
Design	Cohort
Level of evidence	
Setting	Department of adolescent medicine, academic medical centre, the United States
Participants	Patients with malnutrition secondary to AN (Diagnostic and Statistical Manual of Mental Disorders, Fourth Edition, Text Revision) with heart rate <50 beats/minute, temperature <36°C or orthostasis were eligible for inclusion. Each participant had their percentage median body mass index (%MBMI) calculated as 50th centile BMI for age and gender.

(*continued*)

Evidence 5	
Theme E5	**Refeeding the patient with anorexia nervosa (AN)**
Intervention	The oral refeeding protocol consisted of three meals and three snacks (with high-energy liquid supplement drinks if needed) initially providing 1200 calories per day but increasing by 200 calories every other day. All participants received supplemental calcium, zinc and an adult multivitamin with minerals once per day. Phosphate supplementation was not routinely prescribed unless the levels were low (0.9 mmol/L normal range 1.2–2.0). Daily weights, vital signs, electrolytes and a 24-hour fluid balance were measured daily. Free water was restricted to 1 L a day and patients were observed eating their meals and for 45 minutes afterwards.
Outcomes	The primary outcome was weight change and clinical outcome for AN patients on a refeeding protocol.
Main results	Thirty-five adolescents with a mean age (SEM) of 16.2 (1.9) years participated in this study. Mean BMI was 16.3 (2.3) kg/m^2 with a range of 11.1–21.8 kg/m^2. Thirty-three (94%) patients commenced a diet of ≤1400 calories. Twenty-nine (83%) patients lost weight initially, with a peak weight loss noted at 2.9 days. The % MBMI increased from 80.1 (11.5) to 84.5 (9.6) over the admission period, which was 16.7 (6.4) days. Five (20%) received phosphate supplementation and there was no evidence of the refeeding syndrome. None of the patients had nasogastric tube placement.
Conclusion	Hospitalised patients with AN initially demonstrated weight loss and slow weight gain with the recommended refeeding programme. Those placed on higher-caloric diets gained weight at a more rapid rate.
Commentary	This study evaluated the impact of refeeding malnourished adolescents with AN, utilising a 'start low and go slow' protocol starting at 1200 and advancing by 200 calories every second day. The goal of hospitalisation is to increase weight gain, but this must be balanced against the development of the hypermetabolic refeeding syndrome, which may be predicted by a fall in serum phosphate. The initial weight may be related to water loading, which AN patients are known to perform prior to clinic visits to enhance weight, but classic starvation studies show that the extracellular fluid compartment expands during starvation and partially masks the true extent of the weight loss. With adequate nutrition the nitrogen balance becomes positive and the extracellular compartment contracts and fluid is lost.
	Given the need to shorten hospitalisation duration, a more aggressive approach to refeeding may need to be adopted, but this will require randomised controlled trials to determine the best mode of refeeding patients with AN.
Reference	Garber AK, Michihata N, Hetnal K, *et al.* A prospective examination of weight gain in hospitalized adolescents with anorexia nervosa on a recommended refeeding protocol. *J Adolesc Health.* 2012; **50**(1): 24–9.

Evidence 6	
Theme E6	*Drug therapy in anorexia nervosa (AN)*
Question	In adolescents with AN, is adjunctive olanzapine effective?
Design	Randomised controlled trial
Level of evidence	Jadad 5
Setting	Department of child and adolescent psychiatry, academic medical centre, the United States
Participants	Patients aged 12–21 years with a diagnosis were eligible for this study.
Intervention	Patients were allocated to receive olanzapine or placebo for a 10-week period, initially commencing at 2.5 mg daily and increasing to 10 mg/day by week 4.
Outcomes	The primary outcome was change in percentage of mean body weight (%MBW) at weeks 0 (baseline), 5 and 10 in adolescents with AN who were treated with olanzapine or placebo while receiving a comprehensive eating disorder treatment programme.
Main results	Of 94 eligible participants, 74 (78.7%) declined to participate, 20 were randomised to the treatment group, with seven completing, and ten were randomised to the placebo group, with eight completing the study. The % MBW for the treatment group was 82.7 ± 4.4 at week 0 and 88.1 ± 8.8 at week 10; in the placebo group the % MBW was 75.7 ± 7.3 at week 0 and 83.5 ± 8.8 at week 10. Side effects evaluated included drowsiness, increased motor activity, rigidity, tremor, dystonia and dyskinesia. There were no differences in the side effect profile in the treatment or placebo groups.
Conclusion	The study did not support the primary hypothesis that olanzapine would enhance weight gain.
Commentary	In this study 78.7% of eligible patients declined to participate, citing a reluctance to gain weight or wanting to gain weight without the aid of medication. Such views are likely to make drug studies difficult to perform in this population. The evidence from adult studies in patients with AN using olanzapine are contradictory but there is a suggestion that it may be more effective in those with AN binge–purge type.
Reference	Kafantaris V, Leigh E, Hertz S, *et al.* A placebo-controlled pilot study of adjunctive olanzapine for adolescents with anorexia nervosa. *J Child Adolesc Psychopharmacol.* 2011; **21**(3): 207–12.

FAILURE TO THRIVE: MULTIPLE-CHOICE QUESTIONS

Q1   Which of the following options for caloric requirements is/are correct?
  a) Premature infants: 120–140 calories/kg/day
  b) 0–6 months of age: 108 calories/kg/day
  c) 1–3 years of age: 102 calories/kg/day
  d) 4–6 years of age: 90 calories/kg/day
  e) 7–10 years of age: 70 calories/kg/day

Q2   Which of the following statements with regard to FTT is/are correct?
  a) Organic causes are found in 5% of cases.
  b) Organic causes are unlikely in a child who looks well on examination.
  c) Neglect is a rare cause of FTT.
  d) Most cases are classified as mild.
  e) Socio-economic disadvantage is not a risk factor.

Q3   In a child with FTT and vomiting, which of the following conditions should be considered?
  a) Inborn error of metabolism
  b) Urinary tract infections
  c) Raised intracranial pressure
  d) Pyloric stenosis
  e) Gastro-oesophageal reflux disease

Q4   Fat malabsorption leading to FTT occurs in which of the following conditions?
  a) Cystic fibrosis
  b) Cholestatic liver disease
  c) Ileal resection
  d) Jejunal resection
  e) Severe IgA deficiency

Q5   FTT with increased energy expenditure occurs in which of the following?
  a) HIV
  b) Tuberculosis
  c) Congenital heart disease
  d) Cystic fibrosis
  e) Cystinosis

Q6   'Red flags' in a child with FTT include which of the following?
  a) Hypothermia
  b) Bradycardia
  c) Poor parent–child interaction
  d) Gaze avoidance by the child
  e) Dysmorphic features

Q7   In the investigation of FTT, which of the following investigations is/are appropriate?
  a) Faecal elastase
  b) Liver function tests
  c) Vitamin D level
  d) Calprotectin level
  e) IgE

Q8 Syndromes that are associated with failure to thrive include which of the following?
a) Russell–Silver's syndrome
b) Turner's syndrome
c) Diencephalic syndrome
d) Down's syndrome
e) Noonan syndrome

Answers

A1	a, b, c, d, e	**A2**	a, b, c, d, e
A3	a, b, c, d, e	**A4**	a, b, c
A5	a, b, c, d	**A6**	a, b, c, d, e
A7	a, b	**A8**	a, b, c, d, e.

SLIDES

1. Bilateral cleft palate
2. Failure to thrive
3. Wrist swelling nutritional rickets

Chapter Fourteen

NOCTURNAL ENURESIS

COMMON SCENARIO

Jonathan is an 8-year-old boy who is brought by his parents who are very worried that Jonathan has never had a dry night since he was born. They feel Jonathan is too old to be still wetting the bed every night and are upset that is now affecting his school life and his ability to stay overnight at friends' houses. They are worried it is their fault or that maybe Jonathan's bladder is not working correctly. Jonathan's father remembers having a similar problem when he was small and finding it very distressing.

LEARNING OBJECTIVES

- Understand the aetiology of enuresis
- Be able to differentiate primary enuresis from secondary causes
- Know the appropriate investigation to undertake
- Know the treatment modalities and their success rates

BACKGROUND

Nocturnal enuresis can be defined as involuntary voiding of urine occurring at night at an age when the majority of children have achieved continence. It is one of the most common problems in general paediatrics and, indeed, general practice and is at times one of the most difficult to manage satisfactorily. It affects approximately 25% of children at age 4 and only 5%–10% of those aged 7. By age 10, only 5% will still wet the bed and the rate of spontaneous resolution is approximately 15% per year throughout the teenage years, leaving a very small percentage still suffering from the condition by age 18. It affects boys more than girls and the prevalence would appear to be similar in most countries with no obvious racial differences.

The terminology used to describe children with voiding problems in the literature can be confusing. The most recent National Institute for Health and Care Excellence (NICE) guidelines have therefore simplified the terminology commonly used.

Suggested terminology	NICE definition
Nocturnal enuresis	Enuresis is intermittent incontinence in discrete episodes when asleep; the term nocturnal is often used for clarity. Bedwetting is synonymous with enuresis and with nocturnal urinary incontinence
Monosymptomatic nocturnal enuresis	Nocturnal enuresis without any daytime urinary symptoms
Non-monosymptomatic nocturnal enuresis	Nocturnal enuresis with associated daytime urinary symptoms
Overactive bladder	Bladder condition where main symptom is urgency and symptoms may include frequency and wetting
Daytime symptoms	Refers to the presence of lower urinary symptoms which include urinary urgency, frequency, poor urinary stream, the need for abdominal straining to void and urinary incontinence

Physiological development of continence

Voiding in early life is not under conscious control and involves uninhibited bladder contraction secondary to bladder filling. It may also be initiated by stimulating activities or exposure to the cold. As the child grows there is progressive maturation of this system, whereby the child becomes aware of bladder filling followed by an ability to ignore detrusor contraction signals. Eventually, the child gains control of sphincter relaxation and urinary continence is achieved. Supportive evidence of this maturation process has been identified in distinct electroencephalographic changes in children at night as they develop control.

Aetiology

Maturational delay

A delay in the natural development of continence as described earlier is felt to be the most common reason for the persistence of nocturnal enuresis. The strength behind this argument lies in the fact that the vast majority of children with nocturnal enuresis will achieve continence with time.

Reduced bladder capacity

Some children have constitutionally small bladders. The normal bladder capacity (in ounces) in children up to 10 years of age can be estimated by adding 2 to the child's age in years. Therefore, they may end up with a full bladder towards the end of the night.

Inability to wake during sleep in response to the need to void

This is a fundamental problem for all children with enuresis. Many parents report that their child is a deep sleeper and cannot be woken. Research involving urodynamic and electroencephalographic studies support the theory that nocturnal enuresis is due to a disorder of brainstem arousal whereby the immature brainstem fails to recognise bladder fullness.

Genetics

It is well known that nocturnal enuresis is a strongly inherited trait. When there is one parent with a history of enuresis, the risk in progeny is 44%. This rises to 77% when both parents have a history of nocturnal enuresis. There is also a twofold increase of incidence in monozygotic twins compared with their dizygotic counterparts. There have been a number of gene loci linked with enuresis including chromosomes 13q, 12q, 5q11 and 22q11. Unfortunately, this knowledge has not led to any new treatments.

Nocturnal polyuria

Urine production normally falls at night to about 50% of daytime levels but in enuretic children, there is nocturnal polyuria due to a lack of the normal nocturnal increase in vasopressin (ADH) secretion. This explains the response of two thirds of children with nocturnal polyuria to desmopressin treatment.

Psychological

Traditionally, psychological issues were thought to account for a large number of cases of nocturnal enuresis. However, these are far more likely to be associated with the development of secondary enuresis and have not been shown to be positively correlated with the presence of primary enuresis.

Underlying medical condition

In certain cases there may be an underlying medical cause for their enuresis particularly if there is a daytime element to it. Spinal dysraphism and polydipsia secondary to either diabetes mellitus or diabetes insipidus are extremely rare differential diagnoses. The prevalence of enuresis in sickle-cell disease is higher than normal and is thought to be due to chronic sickling compromising renal concentrating capacity. Children with obstructive sleep apnoea have an increased incidence of enuresis, which improves with adenotonsillectomy.

HISTORY

As in all cases, it is important that a detailed history is taken. This ensures that a child's general health can be ascertained along with any other warning signs that might suggest pathology. This provides an overview of a child's general health and should include a developmental history. The initial consultation with parent and child should be handled with great compassion and sensitivity, exonerating the child from blame.

KEY POINTS				
Pattern of enuresis	How frequent? How many dry nights a week? What time of the night does wetting usually occur? Any trigger factors? Ever had a dry night?	**Fluid intake**	Caffeine Fizzy drinks Thirst Have fluids been restricted?	**🔍 Red flags** Polydipsia or polyuria Weight loss/poor weight gain Anorexia Developmental concerns
General health and development	Energy levels Weight loss Appetite Developmental concerns	**Impact of enuresis**	Able to have sleepovers? Affected child's self-esteem	Recurrent UTIs Family or personal history of sickle cell disease History suggestive of obstructive sleep apnoea History of tripping
Symptoms of urinary tract infection (UTI)	Frequency Dysuria Fever Offensive urine	**Family history**	Mother, father, first-degree relative with history of enuresis Family history of diabetes	
Daytime symptoms	Urgency Wetting during day Voiding at school	**Past medical history**	UTI Neurological problems	
Bowel habit	Constipation	**Sleep pattern**	Is he or she a deep sleeper? Snoring or apnoeic episodes Does he or she wake after wetting?	
Practical considerations	How close is the toilet to the bedroom? Does he/she share room with sibling?	**Treatments tried**	Any medications tried Star charts or reward systems	

EXAMINATION

All children presenting with nocturnal enuresis should have a full systemic examination, including height and weight measurement.

- Height and weight should be plotted on appropriate centile charts.
- Blood pressure should be checked.
- The back and spine should be examined for any anomalies.
- The ankle jerks should be elicited.
- The abdomen should be palpated for masses, including a palpable bladder.
- The genital area should be inspected for any abnormalities.

Red flags

- Evidence of recent weight loss
- Hypertension
- Spinal abnormalities such as sacral dimple, tuft of hair, naevi or sacral lipoma
- Abnormal neurological examination
- Abnormal genital examination – signs of infection or trauma
- Palpable bladder post voiding

DIFFERENTIAL DIAGNOSIS

Organic causes	Example
Neuropathic conditions	Spinal cord abnormalities
	Neurofibromatosis
Metabolic or endocrine	Diabetes mellitus
	Diabetes insipidus
Anatomic malformations	Renal concentrating defects
Psychogenic causes	Psychogenic polydipsia
Renal	Urinary tract infection
Haematological condition	Sickle-cell disease

INVESTIGATIONS

Should all children have a dipstick urine examination?

Urine dipstick, followed by microscopy and culture if there is any abnormality detected, is an appropriate screening tool. Beyond this, further investigations should be guided by findings on exam or in the history.

Do children with nocturnal enuresis require urodynamic studies?

In general, a thorough physical examination and history are enough to elicit a diagnosis of uncomplicated nocturnal enuresis without the need for extensive investigations. The decision to conduct urodynamic studies or bladder imaging should only be made in special circumstances and under specialist supervision.

Should children with nocturnal enuresis have a psychology assessment?

Most children do not require any further assessment beyond a thorough history and examination. However, it should always be remembered that nocturnal enuresis can be associated with significant psychological morbidity and can have a profound effect on a child's self-esteem.

Are bladder diaries useful in the investigation of nocturnal enuresis?

No studies support the usefulness of bladder diaries in the diagnosis of nocturnal enuresis. However, they can be useful in helping families manage the condition and the response to appropriate treatment.

MANAGEMENT PLAN: THREE-STEP APPROACH

1. Clarifying and pitfall avoidance strategies:
   a) for parents
   b) for the doctor
2. Non-pharmacological treatment:
   a) enuresis alarms
3. Pharmacological treatment:
   a) desmopressin
   b) desmopressin combined with alarm therapy
   c) desmopressin combined with anticholinergic medication

Clarifying and pitfall avoidance strategies

For parents

- Define the problem. **Rationale**: place enuresis in context, i.e. current age of the child, the frequency of the wetting and the trend (if any) towards resolution. Discuss outcome in terms of realistic expectations based on these factors.
- Discern the parental response to the enuresis. **Rationale**: determine what the parents have done to deal with the enuresis. Common strategies include restricting fluids after dinner. Evaluate how effective this strategy has been and how compliant the child has been. Inquire as to their response to the wet bed, whether they scold the child or not, and also what non-verbal messages they impart (e.g. heavy sighing, annoyance). Ask parents how their child responds to a dry night occurring. If the child is very happy, then the inference that he is unhappy with the wet night is not unreasonable. Seek clarity on who strips the bed when the wetting occurs. Discern the social impact of enuresis on the child, e.g. inability to go on sleepovers or camping.
- Explain the inheritance of enuresis to both parent and child. **Rationale**: if the inheritance is explained, the issue of 'blame' can be put in context. The child may feel the wetting is his or her fault when in fact the child has a genetic predisposition to the condition. Children easily understand the concept of inheritance and this will reduce their anxiety level.
- Mechanism of enuresis explained. **Rationale**: it is very useful to use the following storyline. (1) Urine is produce by the kidneys on a continual basis, (2) it is stored in the bladder, (3) as the bladder approaches a nearly full state, messages are sent to the brain that it is time to wake up and go to the toilet, (4) but children with a predisposition to enuresis usually are in a deep sleep and do not wake up, (5) therefore when then bladder is full it empties and as a consequence they wet. If they did not sleep so deeply they would wake up. Uses of drawings are helpful to illustrate this storyline.
- The appropriate response to enuresis. **Rationale**: enuresis can be a frustrating experience for both parents and child. Parents, on understanding the aetiology

of, enuresis need to develop a balanced response and avoid negative feedback to the child. For children under 7 years of age, medications are not generally recommended and for those over 7 they should devise a strategy for stripping the wet bed and ensure they adopt a 'no blame' culture. If an older sibling teases a younger sibling about his or her enuresis then the aetiology and mechanism should be explained by the parents to the older sibling, which usually results in the cessation of teasing.

For the doctor

- Outlining strategies that may be useful to parents. **Pitfall**: most parents and children want resolution of the enuresis. Before suggesting any strategy, assess it in terms of a cost–benefit ratio: how much effort must be employed for what potential gain? Consequently, it is best to use effective time-limited strategies, as adherence is related to ease and perceived effectiveness.
  - Star charts are often recommended but there is limited evidence for their effectiveness.
  - Bladder training exercises. **Rationale**: if the bladder can hold more urine then the chance of wetting is reduced. The volume of urine that the bladder can hold can be derived from the formula 'age + 2 in ounces', e.g. age 7 + 2 = 9 oz (252 mL). Bladder training exercises do increase bladder capacity, but this does not translate into a reduction in night-time wetting frequency (*see* Evidence 1).
  - Night-time lifting of the child to void. **Rationale**: lifting the child to void is frequently used by parents to reduce wetting, especially in those <6 years of age (where medication use is not recommended). It has limited effectiveness (*see* Evidence 2) but because of its labour intensive nature, 30% of parents discontinued its use in the study reviewed (adding weight to the concept that treatment interventions must be acceptable to parents).
- Associated psychological issues in children with enuresis. **Rationale**: The incidence of enuresis is higher in children with ADHD and mild developmental delay. The parental response to enuresis can have a negative effect on the child especially if parents become angry or blame the child for wetting the bed or not trying hard enough to correct the problem.
- Assessing the need for treatment. **Rationale**: in deciding to treat the child with enuresis, assess whether it is the parents or the child or both who want to resolve the issue. Both child and parent must be engaged in the treatment plan to ensure adherence. The child's age must be taken in to account and treatment should commence at 7–8 years of age. Parents, however, may want it to begin sooner.
- Recognising non-primary enuresis. **Pitfall**: enuresis in the obese child (secondary to obstructive sleep apnoea) must be recognised. Treatment of the obstructive sleep apnoea aids the resolution of the enuresis.

Non-pharmacological treatment

Enuresis alarms

Enuresis alarms are powered by battery and the alarm sounds when urine comes into contact with the sensor. There are two different types of alarms currently available: bed alarms, where the sensor pad is placed under a sheet, and body-worn alarms, where the sensor is placed, for example, between two pairs of snugly fitting underpants. The alarms can generate various noises, vibration or sometimes pre-recorded sounds. Studies evaluating alarm devices use a sensor attached to underwear. The alarm works by Pavlovian conditioning. When the child starts to void, the urine completes an electrical circuit that activates the alarm, which helps wake the child. Through repeated awakenings the child learns to inhibit the voiding reflex and/or complete the urination process in the bathroom. Some alarms allow the sound to be varied, which in theory lessens the frequency of the child becoming accustomed to the noise.

These devices are effective in treating enuresis in children with 75% responding initially and long-term response being maintained in 50% (*see* Evidence 3). The paper discussed in Evidence 3 also evaluated the differential response to alarm therapy when it is recommended for children who relapse, having initially responded.

Pharmacological treatment

Desmopressin

Desmopressin or DDAVP is a synthetic antidiuretic hormone analogue used to artificially induce a reduction in urine output during the night. In a physiologically mature system, the antidiuretic hormone is released from the posterior pituitary in a circadian pattern. Desmopressin treatment is effective in children but this is related to adherence to the nightly administration of the medication (*see* Evidence 4). In the study evaluated in Evidence 4, children 5 years and older participated and consequently it is an option in the treatment of young children.

Desmopressin combined with alarm therapy

There are 30%–35% of children who will not respond to single-intervention treatment; consequently, combined therapy is a useful option that improves resolution rates (*see* Evidence 5).

Desmopressin combined with anticholinergic medication

Anticholinergic medications are usually reserved for children with lower tract disease; however, some children with primary enuresis who are refractory to treatment respond to a combination of desmopressin and anticholinergics (*see* Evidence 6). The treatment should only be instituted after the child has been assessed by a consultant with experience in refractory cases of nocturnal enuresis.

FOLLOW-UP

Follow-up is vital, as children require regular outpatient department or general practitioner visits to monitor their progress. Enthusiasm and encouragement is needed, as treatment is often prolonged and may involve cycles of success and failure.

WHEN TO REFER?

- All children with 'red flags' in their history or examination should be referred for further assessment.
- Children who have failed to respond to appropriate treatment interventions, particularly those with daytime symptoms.

CLARIFICATION FOR PARENTAL MISCONCEPTIONS

> *'We have reduced his fluids from 6 p.m. onwards and he is still wetting the bed. He is now 9 years of age. He should be better.'*

The kidney produces urine continuously and when your son reduces his fluid intake he produces less urine, but the primary problem is related to not waking when the bladder is full, as he is in a deep sleep. The focus is to get your child to wake and go to the toilet or use medication instead.

> *'How can I ignore wet sheets on a daily basis? If he took more responsibility he might get better quickly.'*

Children do not develop enuresis by choice and there is a strong genetic predisposition. Parents should agree a no-blame strategy with the child (if old enough) related to stripping the sheets from the bed and placing them in the laundry. Avoiding negative non-verbal communication is essential.

SUMMARY PRACTICE POINTS

- Nocturnal enuresis is a very common problem of childhood.
- It is a diagnosis of exclusion and a thorough medical history and physical examination should be carried out to rule out a pathological cause before treatment options are tried.
- The natural history of the condition is resolution in the vast majority of children.
- Treatment should not be considered until the child is at least 8 years old, unless there is significant stigma attached to the condition.
- Preliminary methods such as motivational techniques, reducing night-time fluids,

and diary keeping will result in an improvement in most children and should be tried for at least 3 months before further methods are used.

- Alarm pads require a highly motivated child and family, and long-term therapy may be required and the risk of relapse is very real.
- Pharmacological therapy is largely limited to desmopressin oral therapy at present. It is highly efficacious and can be used intermittently; however, it does not cause maturation of the continence process and the risk of relapse on cessation of treatment is as high as 70%.

EVALUATING THE EVIDENCE

Evidence 1	
Theme E1	**Bladder capacity and nocturnal enuresis**
Question	Does increasing bladder capacity improve the cure rate of alarm therapy for children with monosymptomatic nocturnal enuresis?
Design	Randomised controlled trial
Level of evidence	Jadad 1
Setting	Academic medical centre, Germany
Participants	One hundred and forty-nine children with monosymptomatic nocturnal enuresis (at least 14 wet nights in the previous 4 weeks)
Intervention	Five groups of children with interventions as follows: • group A – holding exercises plus placebo • group B – holding exercises plus oxybutynin • group C – no holding plus placebo • group D – no holding plus oxybutynin, which was continued for 12 weeks • group E – control group no intervention. At the end of the pretreatment phase, all groups had an enuretic alarm added to the treatment protocol.
Outcomes	A full response was defined as less than one wet night during 28, and lasting cure was defined as a full response after 1 year of follow-up.
Main results	Neither full response nor cure was influenced significantly by increased maximal voided volume achieved in either groups A or B with holding exercises. Overall, full responses ranged between 50% and 73% and overall cure ranged from 50% to 67%.
Conclusion	In monosymptomatic nocturnal enuresis, increasing maximal voided volume does not affect response or cure rates of subsequent alarm treatments.
Commentary	In this paper the results, inclusive of confidence intervals, are outlined as a graph representation clearly indicating the lack of impact of holding exercises in the responsiveness to alarm enuretic therapy despite effectively increasing maximal voided volume of urine. It is a timely reminder of the multiple aetiology of primary nocturnal enuresis.

(continued)

Evidence 1	
Theme E1	***Bladder capacity and nocturnal enuresis***
Reference	Van Hoeck KJ, Bael A, Lax H, *et al.* Improving the cure rate of alarm treatment for monosymptomatic nocturnal enuresis by increasing bladder capacity: a randomized controlled trial in children. *J Urol.* 2008; **179**(3): 1122–6; discussion 1126–7.

Evidence 2	
Theme E2	***Behavioural interventions for enuresis***
Question	Among young children with nocturnal enuresis, are simple behavioural interventions effective in reducing the number of wet nights?
Design	Randomised controlled trial
Level of evidence	Jadad 1
Setting	Academic centre, the Netherlands
Participants	Five hundred and seventy children (aged 4–5 years) with monosymptomatic nocturnal enuresis
Intervention	Lifting the child to the toilet 1½ to 2 hours after falling asleep (with or without a password to assess if the child were awake), or reward (star chart), and a control group with no intervention.
Outcomes	The primary outcome was the percentage of children who achieved the continence criterion of 14 successive dry nights.
Main results	After 6 months, lifting the child to the toilet without the use of a password was the only intervention that resulted in significantly more dry children than the control group (37% versus 21%; absolute risk reduction =16%; number needed to treat = 7).
Conclusion	Lifting the child to urinate without the use of a password leads to more dry nights than with no active treatment in children aged 4–5 years with nocturnal enuresis.
Commentary	Use of enuretic alarm systems and pharmacotherapy is reserved for children older than 7 years of age. Parents of younger children may be anxious to try behavioural approaches. This study offers an alternative strategy for them. While 37% were successful, 30% dropped out of the study; therefore, parents need to be motivated and the child should only wet once per night
Reference	Van Dommelen P, Kamphuis M, van Leerdam FJ, *et al.* The short- and long-term effects of simple behavioural interventions for nocturnal enuresis in young children: a randomized controlled trial. *J Pediatr.* 2009; **154**(5): 662–6.

Evidence 3	
Theme E3	*The use of alarms in enuresis*
Question	In children with primary monosymptomatic nocturnal enuresis, is alarm therapy effective?
Design	Cohort study
Level of evidence	
Setting	Department of urology, academic medical centre, Turkey
Participants	Sixty-two children with previously untreated enuresis (three or more bedwetting episodes per week), were eligible for inclusion. The male to female ratio was 2:1, and the age ranged from 5 to 16 years, with a mean of 9.7 years.
Intervention	An enuretic alarm device (utilising a small electrical moisture sensor clipped to the pyjamas near the urethra) was utilised for 3 months. In patients for whom the treatment had been successful but who experienced a subsequent relapse, the device was reutilised for a further 3 months to determine if the child responded for a second time.
Outcomes	The primary outcome, assessed after 3 months of use of the alarm therapy, was defined in term of wet nights. A response was defined as a maximum of 1 wet night per month. A relapse was defined as an increase in the number of wet nights in a patient who had a response. The secondary outcomes assessed response in those who relapsed after successful treatment with the alarm device.
Main results	After 3 months, 47 (75.8%) patients responded. After discontinuing therapy, 22 (46%) relapsed and these patients reused the alarm treatment for 3 months to once again achieve a response; however, only 13 (59%) of this group responded. When the alarm system ceased in this group of 13, only 6 (42%) remained dry at night. Overall, 31 of 47 patients maintained a full response after the enuretic alarm treatment had been discontinued in long-term follow-up.
Conclusion	Thirty-one (50%) patients responded to enuretic alarms and also maintained the response after extended follow-up.
Commentary	This paper provides sequential data on the relapse rates and subsequent response or lack of response to the reintroduction of enuretic alarm devices. There is no clear explanation as to why response fails to occur on the reintroduction of the alarm device.
	Practitioners need to explain this to parents when commencing enuretic alarm therapy, as they are likely to be disappointed with the failure to re-achieve a response, having done so initially. The differential response to alarm treatment remains unexplained. No data are provided on parental adherence rate or wetting severity that may negatively affect outcomes.
Reference	Tuncel A, Mavituna I, Nalcacioglu V, *et al.* Long-term follow-up of enuretic alarm treatment in enuresis nocturna. *Scand J Urol Nephrol.* 2008; **42**(5): 449–54.

Evidence 4	
Theme E4	**Desmopressin as a treatment for enuresis**
Question	In children over 5 years of age, is desmopressin effective?
Design	An open-label multinational study
Level of evidence	
Setting	Paediatric centres in four countries: Canada, the United Kingdom, Germany and France
Participants	Seven hundred and forty-four children aged 5 years or older with monosymptomatic nocturnal enuresis (more than 6 wet nights a week)
Intervention	After an initial screening period of 2 weeks with no treatment there was a run-in phase of 2 weeks, where a dose of 0.2 mg of desmopressin was administered. Patients who remained wet after this phase had the doses incremented to a maximum of 0.6 mg.
Outcomes	Response to desmopressin in terms of reduced wet nights per week from the screening phase to the last 2 weeks of treatment. Responders were categorised in two groups: >90% and between 50% and 89% dry nights. Non-responders had <50% dry nights.
Main results	At 6 months, 41% of patients had experienced >50% reduction in the mean number of wet nights. Compliance and increased dosage were also associated with response, and more patients experienced >50% reduction of wet nights after 6 months of treatment than earlier in the study.
Conclusion	This study demonstrates that long-term desmopressin treatment in clinical settings is effective while tolerated in patients with primary nocturnal enuresis.
Commentary	This study recruited unselected patients to represent those who would be seen in clinical practice. Response rates to desmopressin varied with age, with 33.5% of 5- to 8-year-olds, 47.5% of 9- to 11-year-olds and 61.6% of those 12 years or older responding, a fact that will interest parents. In children who took >75% of their tablets, 46.2% had >50% dry nights, as opposed to those who took <50% of their tablets, in whom 25% had >50% reduction in wet nights. Side effects attributed to desmopressin included 1% with abdominal pain, 1% with abdominal pain unspecified and 1% with headache.
Reference	Lottmann H, Baydala L, Eggert P, *et al.* Long-term desmopressin response in primary nocturnal enuresis: open-label, multinational study. *Int J Clin Pract.* 2009; **63**(1): 35–45.

Evidence 5	
Theme E5	*Treatment options in enuresis*
Question	What is the efficacy of alarm devices and desmopressin as single and combined therapy in children with monosymptomatic nocturnal enuresis?
Design	Randomised controlled trial
Level of evidence	Jadad 1
Setting	Academic medical centre, Germany
Participants	Forty three children with primary nocturnal enuresis were eligible for inclusion.
Intervention	Two groups: group A was treated initially with desmopressin therapy that was combined with an alarm therapy after 3 months; group B was treated with an alarm therapy treatment that was combined with desmopressin after 3 months.
Outcomes	The number of children who were dry at 6 months (maximum of 2 wet nights per month) and the number who relapsed at 1 year
Main results	After a standardised treatment course for 6 months, 11 of 16 (68%) children in group A and 11 of 14 (78%) children in group B became dry (absolute risk reduction = 10%; number needed to treat =10; favouring alarm therapy). The relapse rate at 1 year was 1(6%) for group A and 0 (0%) for group B. Altogether 22 of 30 (73%) children were dry after combined therapy.
Conclusion	Combined therapy proved effective in treatment of monosymptomatic nocturnal enuresis after 6 months with no statistical differences between the two different orders of treatment.
Commentary	The numbers in this study are small and the results indicate no statistically significant difference between the groups. It suggests that early combined therapy be utilised after initial unsuccessful therapy, regardless of the primary treatment mode.
Reference	Vogt M, Lehnnert T, Till H, *et al.* Evaluation of different modes of combined therapy in children with monosymptomatic nocturnal enuresis. *BJU Int.* 2010; 105(10): 1456–9. Epub 2009 Sep 17.

Evidence 6	
Theme E6	*Combined medical treatments in patients with enuresis*
Question	In children with primary nocturnal enuresis who fail to completely respond to desmopressin, is the addition of an anticholinergic medication effective?
Design	Randomised controlled trial
Level of evidence	Jadad 5
Setting	Department of urology, academic medical centre, the United States
Participants	Children aged 6–17 years, with monosymptomatic nocturnal enuresis, who had experienced treatment failure with desmopressin, at maximal dosage, were eligible for inclusion. Failure was defined as either no response (0%–49% decrease in wet nights per week) or partial response (50%–89% decrease in the number of wet nights per week). Children with any lower tract symptoms and or constipation were excluded.

(*continued*)

Evidence 6	
Theme E6	*Combined medical treatments in patients with enuresis*
Intervention	Patients were randomised to receive desmopressin plus placebo or desmopressin plus long-acting tolterodine (an extended-release anticholinergic medication) for 1 month.
Outcomes	The primary outcome was the enuretic response rate, with a full response defined as no wet nights; response defined as >90% reduction in the number of wet nights; and partial response defined as a 50%–89% reduction number of wet nights.
Main results	Forty-one patients were enrolled; however, seven were excluded for non-compliance. Of the 18 patients in the desmopressin plus tolterodine group, eight (45%) responded, while five (31%) of the desmopressin placebo group responded (absolute risk reduction (ARR) = 14%; number needed to treat (NNT) = 8). 'No response' or 'zero change' was noted in 44% of the placebo group and in 0% of the long-acting tolterodine group (ARR = 44%; NNT = 3).
Conclusion	This study represents the first prospect of a placebo-controlled trial indicating a benefit from an anticholinergic bladder-relaxing therapy for monosymptomatic primary nocturnal enuresis.
Commentary	Anticholinergic therapy is useful in children with lower urinary tract symptoms, and such patients were specifically excluded from this study. The authors did not attempt to define a mechanism to explain the improvement with anticholinergic therapy but speculated that restricted bladder capacity due to overactive bladder at night may be a factor. This strategy may be a useful adjunct to treatment for those parents who do not wish to use an alarm enuretic device; however, combined desmopressin therapy and enuretic alarms should be used in conjunction as the first strategy in combination treatment.
Reference	Austin PF, Ferguson G, Jan Y, *et al.* Combined therapy with desmopressin and an anticholinergic medication for nonresponders to desmopressin for mono-symptomatic nocturnal enuresis: a randomized double-blind placebo-control trial. *Paediatrics.* 2008; 122(5): 1027–32.

ENURESIS: MULTIPLE-CHOICE QUESTIONS

Q1   Which of the following statements are true?
  a) The frequency of enuresis is 25% in 4-year-olds.
  b) The frequency of enuresis is 5% in 10-year-olds.
  c) Enuresis is more common in boys.
  d) Enuresis is less common in obese children than non-obese.
  e) Enuresis is more common in children with hypercalciuria.

Q2   Aetiological factors in enuresis include which of the following?
  a) Small bladder capacity
  b) Maturational delay
  c) Genetic predisposition is 40% if one parent had enuresis

    d) Genetic predisposition is 70% if both parents had enuresis

    e) Deep sleep pattern

Q3 Which of the following statements are true?

    a) Fifteen per cent of children with enuresis have psychological problems according to their parents.

    b) The normal amount of urine produced during the day is 1 mL/kg/hour.

    c) Urine production decreases at night by 50%.

    d) The bladder capacity is derived from the formula 'age plus 2' in ounces.

    e) Nocturnal polyuria is associated with a lack of DDAVP.

Q4 Which of the following conditions are associated with an increased incidence of enuresis?

    a) Sickle-cell disease

    b) Vesicoureteric reflux

    c) Obesity

    d) Diabetes mellitus

    e) Transposition of the great vessels

Q5 Which of the following investigations should be undertaken in a 9-year-old child with enuresis?

    a) Ultrasound of bladder

    b) Urinalysis or urine culture

    c) Urodynamic studies

    d) Serum calcium

    e) Serum creatinine

Q6 Effective treatment strategies for children with enuresis include which of the following?

    a) Fluid restriction after 6 p.m.

    b) Bladder training exercises

    c) Star charts

    d) Lifting to void

    e) Psychotherapy

Q7 With regard to alarm treatment for enuresis, which of the following statements are true?

    a) Alarm treatment works by Pavlovian conditioning.

    b) It can be used in children from 5 years of age onwards.

    c) The initial response rate is 75% after 2 months of treatment.

    d) The success rate long term is 50%.

    e) Alarm therapy is unsuitable for children who have otitis media.

Q8 Which of the following statements relating to the treatment of enuresis is/are correct?

a) Forty per cent of children have a 50% reduction in night-time wetting.
b) The response is age related.
c) Adherence to treatment is high at 85%.
d) Two per cent of children develop hyponatraemia.
e) One per cent of children develop abdominal pain.

Answers

A1	a, b, c	**A2**	a, b, c, d, e
A3	b, c, d, e	**A4**	a, b, c, d
A5	b	**A6**	None of these options is correct
A7	a, b, c, d	**A8**	a, b, e

Chapter Fifteen

DAYTIME WETTING

COMMON SCENARIO

'She started wetting last year in school, which was a surprise because the last time she had a urine infection was when she was 3, although we have had to deal with constipation problems for the past 6 months '

LEARNING OUTCOMES

- Understand the epidemiology and natural history of daytime wetting
- Understand the current definitions of symptoms
- Know the clinical presentations of the common aetiologies
- Develop a systematic approach to assessment
- Develop an approach to treatment

BACKGROUND

Daytime wetting is common in children. In adults its occurrence indicates the presence of underlying pathology. In children it must be assessed in terms of the child's age, presence of a history of urinary tract infections (UTIs), vesicoureteric reflux and constipation. The overall prevalence of daytime wetting among school-age children is 17%; however, more specific data are required when discussing the issue with parents. The natural history of daytime wetting in children has been assessed in a large British cohort. The wetting frequency was classified as infrequent incontinence (wetting fewer than two times a week) or as frequent incontinence defined by the Diagnostic and Statistical Manual of Mental Disorders criteria (wetting more than two times a week). The prevalence rates of infrequent and frequent incontinence at 4.5 years were 13.5% and 1.9%, respectively; at 5.5 years they were 7.8% and 1.5%, respectively; at 6.5 years they were 9.7% and 1.0%; at 7.5 years they were 6.9% and 1.0%; and at 9.5 years they were 4.4% and 0.5%.

Most parents anticipate their child will attain normal bladder control by 4 years of age.

Bladder (detrusor) functioning

The function of the bladder is to store urine prior to its elimination from the body. The bladder fills passively, and then produces a sensation on fullness. Normally this is not associated with any discomfort and does not lead to incontinence. The functioning of the bladder is complex. The trigger to void emanates from the centres rostral to the pons, but the cortex regulates when and where voiding takes place. Parasympathetic fibres mediate contraction of the detrusor smooth muscle and relaxation of the outflow region of the bladder. The bladder contacts in a synchronous fashion with concurrent relaxation of the pelvic floor muscles and urinary sphincters, resulting in the passage of urine.

Daytime wetting is not a discrete clinical entity and several factors must be examined. The association between daytime wetting and previous UTIs is well established, as is the association with vesicoureteric reflux. The exact mechanism that leads to symptom progression is not known, but these two conditions must be explored in every child with daytime wetting.

The association of constipation with daytime wetting is well recognised. This is sometimes referred to as bowel bladder dysfunction. In all children presenting with daytime wetting the presence of constipation must be considered. The dilated rectum may act as a trigger for detrusor overactivity and urgency but the mechanism is unclear. Parents are often surprised when questions are asked relating to possible constipation when their major concern is their child's wetting. A voiding diary that incorporates a stool chart (inclusive of the Bristol stool chart) can be helpful when both the parent and the child are unsure of the stooling pattern. Children who present with wetting but have associated constipation should have the constipation treated first. Using a high-fibre diet as a treatment strategy is often ineffective, as these children often limit their fluid intake to reduce wetting frequency. Therefore, laxatives should be the primary strategy for the treatment of constipation.

Given the confusion that has arisen regarding terminology relating to daytime wetting, standard definitions and specific features are outlined here. There may be overlap between conditions and the doctor should be guided by the clinical history.

Terminology explained	
Frequency: increased frequency is more than eight voids per day; decreased frequency is fewer than three voids per day	**Weak stream** is the observed ejection of urine with a weak force and is relevant from infancy onward
Incontinence is the uncontrollable leakage of urine; it is intermittent or continuous	**Intermittency** is the occurrence of micturition in several discrete bursts rather than in one continuous stream (this is regarded as physiological if not accompanied by straining in those <3 years of age)

(continued)

Terminology explained	
Urgency is the sudden and unexpected urge to void, applied to children at 5 years of age; the attainment of bladder control must have previously occurred	**Holding manoeuvres** are the observed strategies to avoid voiding and these are standing on tiptoes, forcefully crossing the legs or squatting with the heel against the perineum in children who have attained bladder control or who are 5 years of age
Nocturia is the awakening at night to void, applied in a child older than 5 years	**Post micturition dribble** is the involuntary leakage of urine post voiding in children who have attained bladder control or are 5 years of age
Hesitancy is difficulty in initiation of voiding or the requirement for the child to wait a considerable period of time before voiding starts	**Straining** is the application of abdominal pressure to initiate voiding and is relevant at all ages

HISTORY

KEY POINTS				
Voiding habits	Has he or she ever been dry? How often does he or she void? Normal urinary stream Volume of urine passed Continuous dribbling of urine Wetting when cough, laugh or strain Underwear damp or clothes saturated Urgency Dysuria Haematuria	**Fluid intake**	Type of fluids Water, fizzy drinks, caffeine Volume of fluid in 24 hours Excessive thirst	**🔍 Red flags** Never dry during day suggests ectopic ureter or incontinent epispadias Delayed motor milestones suggests neurogenic bladder Polydipsia, high volume of urine with >700 mL on bladder volume and low osmolality suggests diabetes insipidus
Night-time wetting	Onset Ever been dry at night?	**Family history**	Daytime or night-time wetting Stressors in family	
Voiding behaviour	Tend to hold on Cross legs Squatting or squirming to hold urine Void at school Avoid using public toilets	**Bowel habit**	Constipation Soiling Fibre in diet	

(continued)

KEY POINTS				
Neurological problems	Unsteady gait Frequent falls Weakness in legs Numbness or pins and needles	**Treatment tried**	Any medications tried Duration of treatment Star charts or reward systems Bladder training exercises	
Developmental history	Age at which bladder and bowel control achieved Developmental concerns	**Impact on child**	Bullying or teasing at school Bothered by wetting	
Past medical history	UTIs Attention deficit hyperactivity disorder Cerebral palsy Autism Developmental delay	**Hygiene and skin care**	Use of soaps or irritants Girls wipe from back to front or front to back Skin irritation	
Investigations	Urine sample sent to lab for analysis Renal or bladder ultrasound			

EXAMINATION

- Height and weight
- Back: check for cutaneous manifestations of occult spinal dysraphism
- Abdomen: check for palpable stool in LIF
- Check if bladder is palpable; if it is, ask the child to void
- Urological: inspect meatus, labia and vaginal introitus; note any skin excoriation, wetting of underwear and faecal staining
- Neurological: assess lower limb power, sensation and reflexes; in the perianal area, assess anal tone and ensure the corrugators cutis ani reflex is present (anal wink)

🛈 Red flags

- Lump, bumps, hairy tufts on the back
- History of tripping when running (evaluate in clinic if history positive)
- Lax anal tone suggests chronic constipation is present in conjunction with daytime wetting
- Excoriation of skin may suggest polyuric state

DIFFERENTIAL DIAGNOSIS

Causes	Clinical features
Constipation	Daytime wetting may be only complaint; check stooling pattern and assess calibre of the stool.
Overactive bladder and urge incontinence	The most frequent symptom is urgency in this group and many have frequency as well as incontinence. This is a disorder of bladder filling phase and many children will have a specific behavioural response, to suppress the symptom of urgency, e.g. forcefully crossing their legs, squatting with the heel against the perineum or dancing on their tiptoes.
Voiding postponement	These children actively postpone voiding, often in specific situations. Their parents frequently note that they display withholding manoeuvres. They void infrequently and have feelings of urgency. They also may actively reduce their fluid intake.
Underactive bladder	These children have low voiding frequency and need to increase intra-abdominal pressure to initiate, maintain or complete voiding. On uroflow measurement they often produce an interrupted pattern.
Dysfunctional voiding	These children habitually contract the urethral sphincter during voiding. Uroflow measurement indicates a staccato pattern. Recurrent UTIs and constipation are very common in this group of children.
Stress incontinence	This is the leakage of small amounts of urine at exertion or at increased intra-abdominal pressure. It is rare in neurologically normal children. This needs to be differentiated from voiding postponement (where the child fails to get to the toilet on time) and overactive bladder (in which the detrusor muscle may contract with an increase in intra-abdominal pressure).
Vaginal reflux	This occurs in prepubertal toilet-trained girls who experience incontinence in moderate amounts within 10 minutes of normal voiding.
Diabetes insipidus	Rarely will this condition present with daytime wetting, as the symptoms of thirst (for water) with large urinary output leads to an early diagnosis. The specific gravity of the urine is low in the untreated child.
Giggle incontinence	Voiding occurs after an episode of laughter and bladder function is normal.
Renal concentrating defects	Increased volume of urine is a clinical feature – check for underlying vesicoureteric reflux or other renal disease.
Functional polydipsia	Children who drink excessive fluids naturally pass large volumes of urine and some may wet. Recording the fluid intake allows for diagnosis.
Neurogenic bladder from occult spina bifida or tethered cord	Daytime incontinence and tripping on running are clinical features.
Idiopathic hypercalciuria	This may present with frequency, urgency and dysuria, with no evidence of stone formation.
Extraordinary daytime urinary frequency	Children with this condition may void frequently, often twice an hour, rarely wet themselves and only display symptoms during the day.

INVESTIGATIONS

Are radiological investigations required?

Ultrasonography of the kidneys, ureter and bladder is useful in assessing the child with daytime wetting. Key aims are to assess (a) renal length, (b) the presence of a duplex system that may result in an ectopic ureter being recognised, (c) bladder wall thickness, (d) residual volume of urine post voiding, (e) anatomical abnormalities of the bladder, e.g. ureterocoele, and (f) rectal diameter, which can indicate constipation.

Imaging of the spine is indicated if there is a history of tripping and findings on neurological examination.

Is urinalysis and urine culture required?

Every child with daytime wetting requires a urinalysis and urine culture and for many it will be normal. The presence of blood should prompt a urinary calcium to creatinine ratio to exclude idiopathic hypercalciuria, which rarely presents with daytime wetting. If the specific gravity is 1010 it may suggest renal disease and if low, at 1005, a concentrating defect may be present with resulting polyuria. Most children will have a normal urinalysis and urine culture.

Role of urodynamic studies

Uroflow studies measure rate of urinary flow and give data on voided volume, post-residual void and rate and pattern of flow. This process can be regarded as a precursor to full urodynamic investigation, which requires video fluoroscopy (if available). These tests are usually carried out in nephrology or urology clinic settings.

Pre- and post-void bladder ultrasound

Most children with proven lower urinary tract dysfunction who do not respond to treatment will require an ultrasound to be performed. Pre-void views allow assessment of the bladder wall, lower ureteral dilatation and the bladder neck. After voiding, the post-void ultrasound can determine the residual volume of urine (which should be <10% of the expected bladder volume for age. The formula used to obtain the bladder capacity is 'age + 2 in ounces'. The bladder of a 5 year old child can hold (5 + 2) = 7 ounces or 206 ml of urine (1 fluid ounce = 29.5 ml).

MANAGEMENT PLAN: FOUR-STEP APPROACH

1. Clarifying and pitfall avoidance strategies
   a) for parents
   b) for the doctor
2. Voiding diaries
3. Non-pharmacological treatment: urotherapy
   a) timed voiding and voiding postures
   b) optimising fluid intake
   c) treatment of constipation
   d) use of biofeedback
4. Pharmacological treatment

Clarifying and pitfall avoidance strategies

For parents

- Explain normal and abnormal bladder functioning. **Rationale**: parents need to understand how the bladder functions. It is a muscle that stores urine. As the bladder approaches its capacity it signals the brain that it needs to empty. In young infants this occurs reflexly; however, as children grow older they learn to appreciate the sensation that they need to void. This can be voluntarily suppressed for a period of time. If children lose the ability to appreciate these symptoms of bladder fullness, they wet. Relearning this process takes time, and both child and parent must be actively engaged in the process. Indicate clearly to parents that children with constipation can have associated daytime wetting
- Explain age of normal acquisition of daytime continence. **Rationale**: outlining the age of acquisition of daytime continence (*see* Background section) helps to inform parents that this is not a rare problem, but they may perceive it as rare.
- If history is unclear use voiding diary. **Rationale**: daytime wetting is a complex clinical problem with multiple aetiologies. The elucidation of the history can be difficult; parents may not know the answer and the child may be embarrassed and reluctant to engage clinically. Rather than pursuing the history, employ the use of a voiding diary instead (*see* Evidence 1).
- Define the parental response to wetting. **Rationale**: defining the parental response to wetting is important. If delay has occurred in seeking medical attention then ask, why? Many parents are at a loss to understand why wetting occurs when the child had previously been dry.
- Define the school's response to wetting. **Rationale**: most schools are sympathetic to a child with daytime wetting but it is important to know how the child manages in school. Some children, especially infrequent voiders, are reluctant to use the school toilets and as a consequence wet in the late afternoon.

For the doctor

- Classify children with daytime wetting as:
  - new-onset daytime wetting or never dry
  - daytime wetting with previous UTIs
  - daytime wetting with a history of constipation.
- Ensure the criteria outlined in the Differential Diagnosis section are used in coming to a diagnosis.
- If the diagnosis is unclear, use a voiding diary (*see* Evidence 1).
- Use behavioural approaches first. **Pitfall**: patients with daytime wetting are challenging and the correct treatment strategy needs to be put in place. Frequently, to fix the problem, clinicians resort to medication use (*see* Evidence 2), which should be avoided as an initial treatment strategy.
- Associated psychological problems in children with daytime wetting. **Pitfall**:

children with daytime wetting have an increased frequency of psychological problems with double the anticipated frequency of attention deficit hyperactivity disorder; oppositional behaviour and conduct problems are twice as frequent. Failure to recognise these issues is likely to increase treatment failure rates.

Voiding diaries

Bladder diaries involve reporting bladder related events over a 24-hour period. It is generally recommended that a diary be maintained prior to commencing a treatment strategy and also be used to evaluate the response to treatment. For an expert physician dealing with children with daytime wetting, bladder diaries are often unnecessary. For the doctor who is unused to children with daytime wetting, however, they are very useful. The dysfunctional voiding scoring system has been validated and is a useful clinically (*see* Evidence 1).

Non-pharmacological treatment: urotherapy

Urotherapy is the name applied to non-pharmacological and non-surgical interventions to improve or rectify micturition habits. Urotherapy is an essential part of the treatment of daytime wetting and covers a wide array of interventions, which include advice on:

- timed voiding and voiding postures
- optimising fluid intake
- treatment of constipation
- use of biofeedback.

Timed voiding and voiding postures

Explanation: the child voids every 2 hours during waking hours, an alarm watch serves as a prompt (*see* Evidence 3) for this activity. For girls, emphasise correct voiding technique: appropriate posture, feet touching the ground – if this does not occur, use a footstool to support the child's feet and to ensure the abdominal muscles are relaxed.

Explain double voiding. **Rationale**: the concept of double voiding needs to be fully understood by the child (after the child's void, the bladder is emptied 30 seconds later) and often it is best to allow 30 seconds at least between the two voids. Measuring the volume of urine voided on the second void gives an excellent indication of residual urine volumes (>20 mL of urine is abnormal). Timed voiding is very useful for those who are infrequent voiders. Timed voiding results in an 80% improvement in those who have voiding dysfunction or who are infrequent voiders.

Optimising fluid intake

Optimising fluid intake in children with daytime wetting is necessary and many may have reduced their fluid intake in an effort to control symptoms. Ideally children should drink 50 mL/kg per day to a maximum of 2.5 L.

Treatment of constipation

The treatment of constipation is essential (*see* Chapter 12: Constipation in Children).

Use of biofeedback

Biofeedback, if available, is an adjunct to urotherapy and is effective (*see* Evidence 4). With biofeedback the child develops a greater control over the pelvic muscles and increased awareness. Ultimately it allows the child to listen to the urine stream and ensure the intensity follows a bell-shaped curve. More recently, using biofeedback equipment incorporating computer screens, pelvic floor activity can be represented through computer-generated graphics.

Pharmacological treatment

Children with concurrent UTIs need antibiotic treatment.

Anticholinergic medications inhibit detrusor activity and as a consequence there is increased bladder capacity, increased compliance and reduced detrusor overactivity. Oxybutynin is frequently used in children and is beneficial to those with detrusor overactivity, reduced bladder capacity and urgency (*see* Evidence 5). It is prudent to monitor post-void residual urine volume, as incomplete emptying can occur. These children are also predisposed to constipation, and it is prudent that constipation is not present when prescribing it.

Children with daytime wetting who are resistant to treatment because they are unable to sense when their bladders are full or do not recognise that they are commencing to wet, benefit from the use of an enuretic alarm. The child wears the alarm for a 14-day period and the alarm is activated when the child commences to wet. The success rate (based or retrospective analysis) is 35%.

Girls with wetting related to vaginal reflux need to modify their voiding technique to resolve their wetting. This can be achieved by voiding in a straddling position. The girl, while facing the back of the toilet, spreads her labia post voiding which allows for urine drainage from the vagina. Adequate wiping, after each void is necessary. Children with vaginal reflux want the wetting to abate and this provides a useful strategy.

Giggle micturition is usually seen in school-age girls. The usual explanation is that this originates centrally in association with laughter. If it is an isolated finding then a trial of methylphenidate is useful.

Extraordinary daytime frequency does not require treatment, and parents can be reassured it will self-resolve in 4–6 weeks.

FOLLOW-UP

Follow-up is dependent on the primary condition.

WHEN TO REFER?

- Children with daytime wetting occurring more than twice a week
- Wetting that is cyclical in nature (consider constipation)
- Children with tripping
- Parents who are frustrated by their child's wetting

CLARIFICATION STATEMENTS FOR PARENTAL MISCONCEPTIONS

'Will my child outgrow this problem in the next few months?'

Many children with daytime wetting improve with urotherapy and medication; it was previously thought that wetting was only a problem of childhood, but this is not the case. A small percentage of children with wetting persist with this problem into adulthood – an issue that in recent years has attracted more attention from adult urologists.

'How can constipation cause daytime wetting?'

The association between daytime wettings and constipation is recognised but not well understood.

'Do we really need to treat the daytime wetting? Just give her time and she will get better.'

The concept of daytime wetting improving spontaneously is incorrect. If untreated, one-third of children will be symptomatic in their teenage years. Many find ways of coping with their symptoms.

SUMMARY PRACTICE POINTS

- Be clear in use of terminology, e.g. urgency, hesitancy.
- Specifically evaluate for holding manoeuvres.
- Constipation is a cause of daytime wetting.
- If evening wetting, check if infrequent voider.
- If the history is vague, use a voiding diary.
- Do not use medication (anticholinergics) on the first visit, unless you are sure of the diagnosis.
- Children with recurrent UTI present with daytime wetting.

EVALUATING THE EVIDENCE

Evidence 1	
Theme E1	*Diaries and voiding dysfunction*
Question	Can a diary predict the presence of voiding dysfunction?
Design	Clinical prediction rule
Level of evidence	
Setting	Department of urology, academic medical centre, Canada
Participants	Two groups were invited to participate. Group A were thought to have voiding dysfunction (referred to the paediatric urology clinic with symptoms of daytime urinary incontinence, history of abnormal voiding habits or history of urinary tract infections). Group B were an aged-matched cohort recruited from other clinics and with no history of urological complaints.
Intervention	All participants completed the questionnaire, which consisted of qualitative and quantitative questions relating to urinary incontinence, voiding habits, urgency, posturing, bowel habits, and stressful life conditions, e.g. new baby, new home, new school, school problems, abuse (physical, sexual), home problems (divorce/death; accident/injury). The questions were assigned a score from 0 to 3 (0 = almost never; 1 = less than 50% of the time; 2 = about half the time; 3 = almost every time). A 'not applicable' response was available. The total score ranged from 0 to 30.
Outcomes	A receiver operator curve was plotted based on the scores of thee respondents.
Main results	One hundred and four patients aged 3–10 years attended the urology clinic (male to female ratio, 1:3). The median symptom score for group A was 14 and for group B it was 4. The optimum cut-off score for girls was 6 (sensitivity 92.8%, specificity 87.1%) and for boys was 9 (sensitivity 92.8% and specificity 91.3%).
Conclusion	The dysfunctional voiding scoring system provides an accurate and objective grading of voiding behaviours in children.
Commentary	Voiding dysfunction represents 40% of the referrals to paediatric urology clinics; however, for the general practitioner or general paediatrician who sees these children infrequently, this voiding diary is an important ancillary aid and consequently it should be used. The questions asked prompt reflection on potential aetiologies of the wetting and allow an appropriate treatment plan to be formulated. The diary responses reflect the child's experience over the last month. If the history is unclear or confusing, using the diary as a daily log will clarify the symptom complex.
Reference	Farhat W, Bägli DJ, Capolicchio G, *et al.* The dysfunctional voiding scoring system: quantitative standardization of dysfunctional voiding symptoms in children. *J Urol.* 2000; **164**(3 Pt. 2): 1011–15.

Evidence 2	
Theme E2	**Time voiding for daytime wetting**
Question	Is initial timed voiding useful in all children who present with daytime wetting?
Design	Chart review
Level of evidence	
Setting	Department of paediatric urology, academic medical centre, the United States
Participants	Children referred to a paediatric urology service, with daytime wetting, who were initially treated with timed voiding, were eligible for inclusion. Patients were excluded if they did not have daytime wetting, or if neurogenic or anatomical abnormalities were present.
Intervention	Children were asked to void every 2–3 hours during the day. Compliance was assessed through the use of elimination diaries completed by the families.
Outcomes	The follow were the outcome measures recorded (a) no change, (b) slight improvement reflecting a reduction of 10%–50% of wetting frequency or (c) significant improvement >50% reduction in wetting.
Main results	Of 315 patients reviewed, 183 (58.1%) were excluded, as they were treated with oxybutynin, and 57 (18.1%) were already using oxybutynin at their first visit to the clinic. Sixty-three patients were analysed: 51 (81.0%) girls and 12 (19.0%) boys. The mean age was 7.7 ± 2.2 years. At the follow-up visit after 4 months of timed voiding, four (6.3%) were dry, 24 (38.1%) had significant improvement, 23 (36.5%) had slight improvement and 12 (19%) were unchanged.
Conclusion	This retrospective chart review suggests that anticholinergic medications are overused in the first-line treatment of children with daytime wetting. Approximately 45% showed improvement after 4 months of conservative treatment.
Commentary	This is a retrospective review that reports the customs and practices of consultants involved in the care of children with daytime wetting. The recommended approach is the use of timed voiding strategies; however, this was followed in 24% of eligible patients. The use of initial medications as the primary strategy may reflect an attempt to relieve the patients' distress, reduce workload or deal with poorly motivated parents; however, it is at variance with the recommendations to use timed voiding and evaluate for constipation. The use of anticholinergic medication will make constipation worse. No data were reported on adherence or side effects related to anticholinergic medication use.
Reference	Allen HA, Austin CA, Boyt MA, *et al.* Initial trial of timed voiding is warranted for all children with daytime incontinence. *Urology.* 2007; **69**(5): 962–5.

Evidence 3	
Theme E3	*Use of a watch alarm in children with daytime wetting*
Question	How effective is the addition of a timer watch to non-surgical non-pharmacological treatment (urotherapy) in children with daytime wetting with overactive bladders?
Design	Randomised controlled trial
Level of evidence	Jadad 2
Setting	Department of paediatrics, academic medical centre, Denmark
Participants	Children aged 5–14 years with at least one episode of daytime incontinence weekly, voiding frequency of six or more times daily, overactive bladder (urgency), normal urinalysis, normal ultrasound of urinary tract, no indication of bladder underactivity or lower urinary tract obstruction (as assessed by uroflowmetry) and no constipation were eligible for inclusion.
Intervention	Children were allocated to receive either timer-assisted or standard urotherapy (which included the intake of 1200 mL of fluid per day and a requirement to void every 2 hours during the day). The watch provided had seven alarms. Wet days were logged and 48-hour bladder diaries were obtained during weeks 1 and 11.
Outcomes	The primary outcome was the change in the number of wet days from the pre-intervention phase to those at weeks 11–12 post intervention. A 0%–49% reduction in wet days was defined as no response, 50%–89% reduction was defined as partial, ≥90% as a response and complete dryness was defined as a full response.
Main results	Sixty-one children were eligible but two became dry in the run-in phase, so 59 were randomised: 30 to the treatment group, 28 to the control group and one was excluded. The mean ages were 7.48 years in the treatment group and 7.65 years in the control group. In the treatment group, 18 (60%) improved (nine had complete dryness, one was a responder and eight had partial response) and in the control group five (18%) had a partial response (absolute risk reduction = 42%; number needed to treat= 3).
Conclusion	A programmable watch improves adherence to timed voiding regimen in children with daytime wetting.
Commentary	Compliance or adherence to treatment regimens determines their effectiveness. This study indicates that the use of a programmable alarm watch improves outcomes, as it enhances adherence to the programme through the alarm prompt. No correlation to age was noted; therefore, this option could be applied to children as young as 5 years. The authors indicate that children once dry were able to dispense with the alarm watches within months without relapse.
Reference	Hagstroem S, Rittig S, Kamperis K. Timer watch assisted urotherapy in children: a randomized controlled trial. *J Urol.* 2010; **184**(4): 1482–8.

Evidence 4	
Theme E4	*Biofeedback and daytime wetting*
Question	How effective is biofeedback in the treatment of daytime wetting?
Design	Cohort study
Level of evidence	
Setting	Department of urology, academic medical centre, Turkey
Participants	Children with abnormal voiding patterns with increased pelvic floor activity, symptoms of frequency, urgency, daytime urinary incontinence and recurrent urinary tract infections, good motivation and a willingness to undergo biofeedback sessions and follow-up evaluations were eligible for inclusion.
Intervention	Voiding biofeedback was the intervention utilised. Participants had surface electromyography patches placed on the perineum at 3 o'clock and 9 o'clock (to measure electrical activity in the perineal muscles) and another electrode placed on the rectus abdominis muscle. Muscle activity was presented as a column of light on a screen and which varied with relaxation levels. Children were expected to practice the voiding biofeedback techniques at home every day.
Outcomes	The primary outcomes were improvement in symptoms and improvements on urodynamic testing.
Main results	One hundred and eighty-eight patients were enrolled in this study, with 168 completing the programme and assessed at 6 months (20 patients dropped out, four (2.1%) due to perceived technique ineffectiveness, three (1.6%) due to technique related difficulties and 13 (6.9%) due to irregular follow-up). Not all patients had all symptoms and the improvement rates were as follows: daytime wetting (59%), frequency (92.5%), infrequency (66.7%) and urgency (81.4%). The following improvements occurred in the urodynamic studies: staccato voiding (85.2%), flattened voiding (87.8%) and bladder overactivity (80.4%).
Conclusion	Biofeedback was effective in reducing symptoms of voiding dysfunction in children.
Commentary	Voiding biofeedback is increasingly used in the treatment of children with daytime wetting. This is a case series and not a randomised controlled trial; therefore, the treatment effect has to be evaluated with caution. This study reported follow-up at 2 years; however, inferring that the treatment effect was only related to the biofeedback is inappropriate and thus the 6-month figures are reported. The impact of biofeedback would best be assessed through a large randomised controlled trial.
Reference	Yagci S, Kibar Y, Akay O, *et al.* The effect of biofeedback treatment on voiding and urodynamic parameters in children with voiding dysfunction. *J Urol.* 2005; **174**(5): 1994–7; discussion 1997–8.

Evidence 5	
Theme E5	*Drug therapy for daytime wetting*
Question	In children with daytime wetting which is more effective and safer: oxybutynin or tolterodine?
Design	Randomised controlled trial
Level of evidence	Jadad 1
Setting	Academic medical centre, Turkey
Participants	Sixty children aged 3–13 years with daytime wetting were enrolled
Intervention	Tolterodine 1 mg daily or oxybutynin 0.4 mg per kg per day in three divided doses
Outcomes	The primary outcome was the reduction in daytime wetting at six months and number of side effects experienced by the participants.
Main results	Of 30 in the tolterodine group 13 (43.3%) symptoms resolved, 5 (16.7%) significantly improved, 6 (20%) partially improved and 6 (20%) had no response. In the oxybutynin group 11 (36.6%) symptoms resolved, 6 (20%) significantly improved, 5 (16.7%) partially improved and 8 (26.77%) had no response. In the tolterodine group full or significant response occurred in 60% and in the oxybutynin group it was 56.6% (absolute reduced resk (ARR) = 3.4%; number needed to treat (NNT) = 30). Side effects were encountered, 13 (43%) in the tolterodine group and 27 events occurred in 20 (60%) of the oxybutynin group (ARR = 17%; NNH = 6). Eight patients were switched over to tolterodine at the end of the study because of side effects.
Conclusion	From a clinical perspective tolterodine and oxybutynin are effective. The responses are variable. The high frequency of side effects makes oxybutynin less desirable.
Commentary	Despite being prescribed frequently to treat children with daytime wetting there are very few randomised control trials to support oxybutynin use. Newer medications are being used based on data abstracted from adult studies and consequently more randomised controlled trials are required to establish therapeutic efficacy in children and also establish the frequency of side effects.
Reference	Kilic N, Balkan E, Akgoz S, *et al.* Comparison of the effectiveness and side-effects of tolterodine and oxybutynin in children with detrusor instability. *Int J Urol.* 2006; **13**(2): 105–8.

DAYTIME WETTING: MULTIPLE-CHOICE QUESTIONS

Q1   Contributory facts to daytime wetting include which of the following?
   a) History of UTI
   b) Constipation
   c) History of vesicoureteric reflux
   d) Positive family history of enuresis
   e) History of infantile colic

Q2 Which of the following statements with regard to bowel and bladder dysfunction is/are correct?
   a) A dilated rectum may trigger bladder contractions.
   b) Voiding diaries and stools charting are helpful in establishing the diagnosis.
   c) Treatment with a high-fibre diet is effective.
   d) Laxative therapy is effective.
   e) A high fluid intake is ineffective in the treatment of this condition.

Q3 Which of the following statements is/are correct?
   a) Frequency of micturition is more that six voids a day.
   b) Decreased frequency is fewer than three voids a day.
   c) Holding manoeuvres used to avoid voiding include the child squatting with his or her heel against his or her perineum.
   d) Nocturia is defined as a child awakening to void at night after 7 years of age.
   e) Hypercalcaemia causes polyuria.

Q4 Which of the following symptoms and signs suggest significant pathology if present in a 6-year-old with daytime wetting?
   a) The child has never been dry during the day.
   b) The child voids more than 2 mL/kg/hour.
   c) The child wets with laughing.
   d) The child has had a previous UTI.
   e) The child has a family history of deafness.

Q5 Alarm signs in a 6-year-old with daytime wetting include which of the following?
   a) History of tripping when running
   b) The presence of a palpable bladder post voiding
   c) The presence of skin excoriation in the groin region
   d) The presence of a tuft of hair on the lower back
   e) The presence of the corrugator cutis ani reflex

Q6 Features of voiding postponement include which of the following?
   a) Early-morning wetting
   b) The presence of withholding manoeuvres
   c) Infrequent voiding
   d) The presence of urgency
   e) The presence of abdominal pain

Q7 The differential diagnosis of daytime wetting includes which of the following?
   a) Hypercalciuria
   b) Functional polydipsia
   c) Vesicoureteric reflux
   d) Hypokalaemia
   e) Diabetes insipidus

Answers

A1	a, b, c, d	**A2**	a, b, d, e
A3	b, c, e	**A4**	a, b, e
A5	a, b, c, d	**A6**	b, c, d
A7	a, b, c		

Chapter Sixteen

COUGH IN CHILDREN

COMMON SCENARIO

'His coughing is bothering us all especially when it happens at night. We are so stressed that something is wrong, especially when they call from the crèche, that I'm now smoking 10 cigarettes a day – before all of this it was only five.'

LEARNING OBJECTIVES

- Understand the function of cough
- To have a strategy to classify and problem solve cough
- Recognise 'red flags' in the history or examination that require further investigation
- To have a strategy for investigation
- To define treatment plans for the common causes of cough
- Evaluate the available evidence to support your treatment options

BACKGROUND

Cough is a common symptom in children who attend their general practitioners. It is a symptom not a disease and the aetiologies in children are different from adults.

The mechanism of cough is as follows: after an initial rapid inspiration, a forced expiration against a closed glottis occurs, at which time the glottis opens with a simultaneous respiratory effort that involves contracture of the diaphragm and muscles of the abdominal wall, and as a consequence a blast of rapidly moving air expels air and any movable substance from the trachea. Cough is primarily a protective reflex; it enhances mucociliary clearance, aids clearance of excessive secretions and airway debris from the respiratory tract. Cough receptors are located in the larynx to the bronchial tree and the cough reflex is mediated through the vagus nerve in the afferent pathway, to the brainstem with cortical modulation and the motor pathway is to the respiratory muscles. The cough reflex can be sensitised by viral respiratory tract infections, asthma, gastro-oesophageal reflux and through medication, e.g. angiotensin-converting enzyme inhibitors. Children who are less than 5 years of age normally do not expectorate sputum when they cough, which influences the physician's diagnostic approach.

Cough can be classified as acute, acute persistent, chronic, recurrent, post-viral or non-specific in nature. The differential diagnosis of acute cough includes acute respiratory tract infections (both upper and lower), inhaled foreign body, seasonal allergic rhinitis or represents the first presentation of a chronic disease. In acute persistent cough the differential includes the above and post-infectious cough, pertussis-like illnesses, tuberculosis or intrathoracic lesions.

The differential diagnosis of children with chronic cough (>8 weeks) is extensive, but less than 5% of children who present with cough will have symptoms beyond 8 weeks. As a consequence, aetiologies are determined from cohort studies and the results may not be generalisable to all populations. In a prospective cohort study of children referred with cough for greater than 3 weeks (mean, 6 months) under 18 years who were extensively investigated the following diagnoses were made: persistent bacterial bronchitis, 40%; natural resolution, 22%; bronchiectasis, 6%; asthma, 4%; upper airway cough syndrome, 3%; gastro-oesophageal reflux, 3%; habit cough, 1%; idiopathic, 5%; multiple causes, 55%. Forty-three per cent of households had smokers, 62% had cough under 1 year and 89% of coughs were described as wet. In children who present with chronic cough two aetiologies will be found in 50% of patients.

In this chapter we have chosen to address the symptom of cough as acute, chronic in a well child and chronic in an unwell child. This offers a pragmatic approach that reflects the clinical presentation of these children. The definitions of acute, acute persistent, chronic, recurrent, post-viral and non-specific cough are given, which is consistent with terms that are used in the literature.

Terminology	Definition
Acute cough	Cough present for less than 3 weeks
Acute persistent cough	Acute persistent cough present for 3–8 weeks
Chronic cough	Cough present for more than 8 weeks
Recurrent cough	More than two episodes in 1 year in the absence of upper respiratory tract infections (URTIs)
Post-viral cough	Cough that starts with a URTI but persists longer than 3 weeks
Non-specific cough	Dry cough with no other symptoms and a normal chest X-ray

HISTORY

KEY POINTS					
Characteristics of cough	Duration Sputum production Haemoptysis Cough always the same Wet, dry, barking or spasmodic Diurnal variation Seasonal variation Relationship to feeds	**Past history**	Atopic disease Gastro-oesophageal reflux Aspiration Tracheo-oesophageal repair	**🔍 Red flags** Cough from birth Choking episode Persistent wet coughing and the absence of URTIs Wet cough with diarrhoea Poor weight gain Feeding difficulties
Associated symptoms	URTI symptoms (fever, runny nose, wheeze) Postnatal drip (sneezing, itch, worse when lying down) Post-tussive vomiting Wheeze, shortness of breath	**Birth history**	Prematurity complications Ventilation	
Onset	Following URTI Following choking episode Present since birth/early infancy	**Family history**	Atopy (allergic rhinitis, asthma, eczema, allergies) Cystic fibrosis Immune deficiency	
Triggers	Asthma triggers (cold air, morning occurrence, exercise induced) Viral trigger	**Impact**	Number of school days lost	
Treatments	Hospitalisation required Antibiotics Inhalers – use of spacers and volumatics Over-the-counter medications Response to medication Duration of treatment Reason discontinued	**Social history**	Crèche attendance Smokers in house Tuberculosis exposure	
Investigations	Chest X-rays Pulmonary function tests Bloods Sputum cultures	**Immunisation history**	Are immunisations up to date	
General health and development	Diarrhoea Weigh loss Developmental concerns Difficulty feeding			

EXAMINATION

- Height and weight should be plotted on an appropriate centile chart.
- Heart rate and respiratory rate should be recorded and compared to age-specific norms.
- Ear, nose and throat examination, looking specifically for presence of tonsils, nasal polyps, deviation of nasal septum, inflamed turbinates.
- Signs of atopy: Dennie–Morgan's folds, eczema (check flexures for evidence of dry excoriated skin, lichenification).
- Fingers and toes should be examined for signs of clubbing.
- Chest examination should look for evidence of deformity, hyperinflation, signs of respiratory distress and auscultation for bronchial breath sounds, differential air entry, crepitations (if still present after cough) or wheeze.

ⓠ Red flags

- Child looks unwell
- Growth failure
- Presence of finger clubbing
- Absence of tonsils
- Hyperinflated chest
- Chest deformity
- Persistent wet cough on examination
- Spontaneous production of sputum
- Fixed crackles post coughing
- Respiratory distress

DIFFERENTIAL DIAGNOSIS

The differential diagnosis of cough is extensive, and therefore a useful approach is to consider whether the cough is acute or chronic, and whether the child appears well or unwell.

Acute cough	Features	
URTI	Wet cough	Fever
	Coryza	Irritability
Croup – viral	Barking cough (like seal)	Preceding URTI
	Stridor	Fever
	Hoarseness	
Croup – spasmodic	Barking cough (like seal)	Acute onset
	No preceding URTI	

(continued)

Foreign body aspiration	Cough No preceding URTI	History of choking episode
Chronic rhinitis (upper airway cough syndrome (first episode))	Cough Throat-clearing noises Itchy eyes	Sneezing, runny nose Conjunctivitis
Lower respiratory tract infection Pneumonia (*see* Chapter 4: The Child with a Fever)	Cough initially dry but change to wet character Fever Anorexia	Signs of respiratory distress Focal findings on physical examination
Chronic cough (well child)	**Cough characteristics and other features**	
Post-viral cough	Cough day and night, regarded as troublesome with sleep disturbance	History of URTI
Pertussis or pertussis-like illness (parapertussis, adenovirus)	Troublesome spasmodic cough Initial URTI Unvaccinated children at high risk Dyspnoeic after prolonged spasm, vomit post bout of coughing	Whoop audible on inspiration, apnoea in infants. Evaluate for residual atelectasis post illness
Cough variant asthma	Isolated cough (no wheeze) Personal or family history of atopy	Worse at night and early morning Cough after exercise Response to asthma medication
Chronic rhinitis	Cough Throat clearing noises Sensation of 'something dripping into throat' Worse at night or when lying down	Personal or family history of atopy Sneezing, runny nose Dennie–Morgan's folds
Recurrent URTI	Wet cough Clear history of URTI and lower respiratory tract infection occurring in sequence without periods of resolution	Crèche attendance with increased exposure to viral illnesses Overcrowding
Psychogenic cough	Bizarre honking, dry cough Absent at night or when child distracted	Child not distressed despite prolonged coughing

(continued)

Chronic cough (unwell child or with chronic condition)	Cough characteristics and other features	
Cystic fibrosis	Wet cough persistent, recurrent episodes of 'bronchiolitis' Clubbing Diarrhoea Fixed focal post-tussive crepitations on examination in established disease	Failure to thrive despite excellent appetite Screening for disease detects 90% of those who would develop clinically active disease in first year of life
Protracted bacterial bronchitis	Persistent wet cough	*See* Commentary evidence, p. 310
Foreign body	Wet cough, may be diagnosed as having non-responsive asthma	History of choking episode (may be forgotten so ask specifically to aid recollection)
Tuberculosis	Wet cough Progressive cough	Weight loss
Recurrent aspiration	Wet cough Acute onset Respiratory distress Feeding difficulties	Underlying risk factors Neuromuscular disorder or neurodevelopmental delay Oesophageal stricture Achalasia
Primary ciliary disorders	Wet chronic cough Recurrent sinusitis	Situs inversus (50%)
Non-cystic fibrosis bronchiectasis	Wet cough	Episodic recurrent episodes of cough treated as pneumonia
Immune-deficiency states	Wet cough Absence of tonsils Recurrent pneumonias	Respond to antibiotics (but symptoms recur)
Gastro-oesophageal reflux disease	Posseting or regurgitation Haematemesis <1 year of age Poor weight gain Unsettled, crying with feeds	Apnoea or cyanosis Stridor Wheezing History of aspiration or recurrent lower respiratory tract infection

INVESTIGATIONS

Is a chest X-ray needed?

In the majority of children with chronic cough an X-ray is warranted. Bilateral hyperinflated lung fields can be seen in asthma, while unilateral hyperinflation suggests inhaled foreign bodies. If reported as normal it does not exclude bronchiectasis. Be guided by the clinical history. A history of repeated pneumonias on X-rays should prompt detailed investigations, which may include computed tomography scan.

Should allergy testing be undertaken?

In a child with an atopic background, skin prick testing or IgE and radioallergosorbent testing can be useful.

Should spirometry be performed?

In children over 5 years, spirometry (inclusive of bronchodilator responsiveness) is helpful. However, the presence of bronchial hyper-reactivity does not automatically imply that a child with isolated cough will respond to bronchodilator therapy.

Should a sputum culture be obtained?

A child less than 5 years will not normally produce sputum. However, if sputum is produced it should be sent for culture and sensitivity. In children with chronic cough, the growth of *Staphylococcus aureus* or a *Pseudomonas* species should prompt consideration of further diagnostic tests to exclude cystic fibrosis.

Should a Mantoux test be done on a routine basis?

A Mantoux should not be done routinely. In a child with a progressive wet cough or chest X-ray features suggestive of tuberculosis, a Mantoux should be performed. Obtaining a morning gastric aspirate for culture and sensitivity should be done.

Should a sweat test be performed?

Routine performance of a sweat test is not required. Screening for cystic fibrosis (if carried out) will identify 85%–90% of affected children. If symptoms of a chronic wet cough persist after treatment with antibiotics a sweat test should be performed, but the child should be evaluated by a paediatrician.

MANAGEMENT PLAN: TWO-STEP APPROACH

1. Clarifying and pitfall avoidance strategies
2. Treatment options and specific therapies:
   a) over-the-counter medications
   b) asthma therapy
   c) treatment of upper airway cough syndrome
   d) antibiotic treatment
   e) gastro-oesophageal reflux treatment
   f) treatment of habit cough

Clarifying and pitfall avoidance strategies

When dealing with the parents of a child who presents with cough, the following strategy is useful.

- Explain that cough is a symptom and not a disease
- Determine the impact of the cough on the family life. **Rationale**: cough if it occurs at night may lead to sleep deprivation for parents and affect their coping skills and influence their desire for treatment.
- Ascertain the parents' beliefs on the cough aetiology. **Rationale**: parents' views may be incorrect, e.g. smoking and its impact on cough.
- Explain to parents that coughing occurs in well children (*see* Evidence 1). **Rationale**: parents vary in their ability to cope with cough and the sleeplessness that occurs with it.
- Explain the physiological role of cough in airway clearance. **Rationale**: parents, once they understand the function of cough, are likely to accept watchful waiting.
- Ensure that the parents have kept a recording of the cough and a cough diary (if it is persistent). **Rationale**: having a record of the cough, timing, and frequency will aid in the clinical diagnosis and in the assessment of clinical significance.
- Evaluate for factors that can aggravate the cough, for example tobacco smoke.
- Prior to embarking on a treatment option build a case to support the treatment option and avoid using multiple treatments at the one time, e.g. inhaled steroids and antibiotic treatment. **Rationale**: cough will only respond to the correct treatment, multiple treatments will confuse the parent as to the underlying diagnosis.
- Acute cough is the most frequent reason parents consult their family doctor and knowledge of the correct natural history is essential (*see* Evidence 2). **Rationale**: an ability to predict the resolution rates of acute cough will gain the parents' trust and they are more likely to accept watchful waiting.
- Outline the natural history of the cough if watchful waiting is being pursued.
- In children with cough the importance of the history and physical examination cannot be underestimated and if necessary should be undertaken a second time if symptoms persist (*see* Evidence 3). **Rationale**: an ability to discern the important elements of the history and physical examination allows the more sinister symptoms and signs of cough to be interpreted.

Treatment options and specific therapies

Over-the-counter medications

Parents whose children have upper and lower respiratory tract infections may choose to use over-the-counter medications for symptom control. There is little evidence to support their efficacy and in general they are not superior to placebo. Cough suppression therapy with dextromethorpan or codeine have been associated with morbidity and is not recommended. Recently honey has been shown to be beneficial in children with URTI and can be used (*see* Evidence 4).

Asthma therapy

An empiric trial of inhaled corticosteroids is useful in children with isolated dry cough. If possible establish the presence of bronchial hyper-reactivity through pulmonary function testing if the child is old enough. A dose of fluticasone at 200–400 µg or equivalent is appropriate. Proper inhaler technique needs to be evaluated with a spacer device. An objective assessment measure of symptom control should be used. Treatment should be continued for at least 6–12 weeks – fortunately, most patients respond to 4 weeks of treatment.

Treatment of upper airway cough syndrome

In children with upper airway cough syndrome nasal steroids are the most effective treatment (*see* Evidence 5). Antihistamines offer some symptomatic control but are not as effective as they are in the adult population. Prior to commencing treatment, proper technique must be assessed. The spray nozzle should be directed laterally and not medially into the nose. If the spray is directed medially little benefit will accrue to the patient. The patient must avoid sniffing immediately afterwards, as the spray will be swallowed. Improvement usually occurs within 2–4 weeks if the aetiology is upper airway cough syndrome. Monitoring by the parents of the cough and associated symptoms is essential. Currently sublingual immunotherapy is being evaluated in children and adolescents with promising results (*see* Evidence 6).

Antibiotic treatment

Antibiotic treatment is not warranted in those with viral related URTIs. If patients present with persistent purulent nasal discharge then a course of antibiotics is useful. In children who present with pertussis a course of erythromycin is warranted. Children who present with moist coughs, in whom a diagnosis of protracted bacterial bronchitis is made, benefit from a course of amoxicillin and clavulanate (*see* Evidence 7). Children with bronchiectasis should be placed on a prophylactic macrolide antibiotic three times per week to reduce their risk of respiratory exacerbations.

In patients with cystic fibrosis the respiratory management consists of physiotherapy to improve mucociliary clearance. Medications that aid this process include pulmozyme and hypertonic saline 7%, which need to be used on a daily basis. Sputum cultures may grow *Pseudomonas* species mucoid or non-mucoid or else *S. aureus*. If the initial sputum grows *Pseudomonas* then intravenous antibiotics will be required for 2 weeks. Subsequently, to reduce *Pseudomonas* load, the use of nebulised tobramycin or colomycin is effective. Currently children are also placed on Zithromax 10 mg/kg three times per week. (For pneumonia treatment *see* Chapter 4: The Child with a Fever.)

Gastro-oesophageal reflux treatment

The presentation of isolated cough related to gastro-oesophageal reflux disease is uncommon. A trial of a proton pump inhibitor is warranted but the effectiveness of such treatment is unknown.

Treatment of habit cough

The absence of nocturnal coughing in this condition comes as a relief to the parents however the frequency of the cough during the day may cause significant distress. Self-hypnosis and biofeedback have been recommended as treatment options. Another option in the acute phase is to ask the child to use a clicker each time he or she coughs and to monitor this hourly with the aim of reducing the number of coughs from hour to hour. For some patients sipping ice cold water can be helpful in reducing the number of coughing episodes.

FOLLOW-UP

Depends on primary condition

WHEN TO REFER?

- Acute cough indicators, especially if choking episodes
- Cough that has a changing character
- Moist cough persisting beyond 3 weeks
- Cough productive of sputum
- Cough with abnormal examination, e.g. clubbing or chest deformity
- Cough with weight loss
- Cough that is progressive in nature

CLARIFICATION STATEMENTS FOR PARENTAL MISCONCEPTIONS

'My pharmacist has a lot of cough treatments, surely they all can't be useless?'

Cough is only a symptom and not a diagnosis; cough suppressants do not treat the underlying cause. In addition they have a number of side effects especially if incorrect doses are given. Studies have indicated that they are no better than placebo treatments.

'We smoke outside, what's the problem?'

Cigarette smoke makes coughing worse. Smoking outside the home is not a solution, as the smoke is still present on clothes and hair, and on entering the home it diffuses into the atmosphere where your child breathes it in.

'Does the cough mean that his immune system is weakened?'

No. The vast majority of children with cough have self-limited viral infections, which will resolve spontaneously if given time.

SUMMARY PRACTICE POINTS

- Classify the cough into a pattern.
- If unable to assess quality of cough ask parent to record the cough.
- Remember multiple aetiologies probable (ask if cough always the same).
- Re-evaluate after each intervention.
- Discourage use of over-the-counter cough preparations.
- Explain that asthma is unlikely to present only with cough in the absence of risk factors.
- Do not use multiple treatment options at the same time unless multiple aetiologies for cough present.
- Maintain a system for monitoring the significance of the cough.
- Nocturnal coughing can lead to sleep deprivation in children.
- When treating cough, use one strategy at a time unless other aetiologies are present.

EVALUATING THE EVIDENCE

Evidence 1	
Theme E1	*Normal cough frequency in children*
Question	What is the normal cough frequency in children who are well?
Design	Cohort study
Level of evidence	
Setting	Department of paediatrics, academic medical centre, England
Participants	Children aged 8–12 years, who were well, with no personal or family history of asthma (in first-degree relatives), and who had never been prescribed anti-asthma medication were eligible for enrolment.
Intervention	Participants used the RBC-7 device for recording cough over a 24-hour period. The RBC-7 device is worn around the waist and has three electrocardiogram leads connected to the chest, three electromyographic (EMG) leads and a microphone. The microphone and the EMG leads record the cough. An accelerometer applied to the waist indicates activity levels. The RBC-7 records 10 seconds of data every 15 minutes, which allows removal of the device to be detected. The results were visually displayed on a computer screen for analysis.
Outcomes	The primary outcome was the cough frequency over a 24-hour period in normal children. An episode of coughing was defined as a period of cough EMG peaks with less than 2 seconds of baseline activity between the peaks and a prolonged coughing bout as one with at least 10 EMG peaks.
Main results	Forty-four children were recruited but only 41 completed the study. The three excluded had upper respiratory tract infections. The mean number of coughing episodes was 11.3 per 24 hours (range 1–34). Only two (5%) children coughed at night and only five (11%) had prolonged bouts of coughing.

(continued)

Evidence 1	
Theme E1	*Normal cough frequency in children*
Conclusion	The frequency of coughing in normal children ranges from 1 to 34 episodes per 24 hours, with a mean of 11.3. Nocturnal coughing occurred in 5% of children.
Commentary	Children with cough make frequent visits to their family doctors and paediatrician. This study is important as normal children were assessed who were at low risk of asthma, the authors used objective assessment methods to evaluate the presence of coughing and have provided normative data that are clinically useful. The absence of cough at night is expected and if present the aetiology should be sought. Being able to put cough in context in terms of daily frequency needs to be part of the discussion with parents. The RBC-7 device, if available, is potentially helpful in children who have a history of cough but in whom the diagnosis is uncertain, as it provides objective data.
Reference	Munyard P, Bush A. How much coughing is normal? *Arch Dis Child.* 1996; **74**(6): 531–4.

Evidence 2	
Theme E2	*The duration of acute cough in children*
Question	What is the duration of acute cough in children?
Design	Cohort study
Level of evidence	
Setting	Primary care practices, England
Participants	Participants were consecutive children aged 0–4 years attending primary practices, who had had a cough for 28 days or less, without asthma (identified clinically or defined as a medical recommendation for preventive or regular reliever treatment) or any other chronic disease were eligible for enrolment.
Intervention	Parents and clinicians were asked to predict the duration of cough. Parents were telephoned on a weekly basis and they also completed an initial questionnaire (validated for age). The questionnaire, using a Likert scoring system, assessed cough, shortness of breath, fever, general well-being on a daily basis and for 2 days after the cough resolved.
Outcomes	The primary outcome was to determine the post-consultation duration of the cough, and to compare clinician and parent predictions of cough duration.
Main results	Eight hundred and forty-three children were screened and 256 (88%) of 290 were recruited, with follow-up data available on 228 (89%). Fifty per cent had recovered at 10 days, 75% at 16 days and 90% at 25 days. Cough resolution at <7 days was 30%: the parent estimate was 29% but the clinician prediction was 55%–60%. Resolution at <14 days was 70%: parent prediction 70%, clinician prediction >90%. Sleeplessness resolved in 25% at 4 days, in 50% at 7 days, in 75% at 12 days and in 90% at 22 days.
Conclusion	When counselling parents of children with acute cough, clinicians need to know the resolution rates. Clinicians are more likely to overestimate the rates of resolution than parents.

(continued)

Evidence 2	
Theme E2	*The duration of acute cough in children*
Commentary	The presence of cough in young children is not regarded as trivial by parents. In primary care settings, laboratory investigations are less likely to be done than in the hospital setting. This study serves to reassure parents that the presence of prolonged symptoms does not imply the presence of serious disease. Also, providing resolution rates at the beginning of the consultation is likely to promote realistic expectations on the part of parents and reduce the re-consultation rate and further reassure that antibiotics are unnecessary. Informing parents about the impact of acute cough on sleep is prudent as, if informed at the initial consultation, they are more likely to delay re-consultation and wait for natural symptom resolution.
Reference	Hay AD, Wilson A, Fahey T, *et al.* The duration of acute cough in pre-school children presenting to primary care: a prospective cohort study. *Fam Pract.* 2003; **20**(6): 696–705.

Evidence 3	
Theme E3	*History and examination in a child with chronic cough*
Question	What is the utility of symptoms and signs in children with chronic cough in the predicting the aetiology?
Design	Prospective cohort study
Level of evidence	
Setting	Department of respiratory medicine, children's hospital, Australia
Participants	Participants were children with chronic cough (>3 weeks) referred to a tertiary care centre.
Intervention	All patients had a standard history that evaluated duration and character of the cough, past history of dyspnoea, wheeze, haemoptysis, swallowing difficulties, failure to thrive, allergies, recurrent respiratory tract infections, smoke exposure, upper airway problems including snoring, family history of atopy and asthma. All children had a complete clinical examination. While all children had chest X-rays and pulmonary function tests (>6 years) done, a more extensive array of tests were done to determine a diagnosis including bronchoscopy, bronchoalveolar lavage, computed tomography of the chest (50%), sweat testing and gene mutation for cystic fibrosis, immunoglobulin levels, mycoplasma and pertussis titres.
Outcomes	The primary outcome was the ability of the signs and symptoms to predict the specific aetiology of the chronic cough, classified as non-specific cough (habit cough, gastro-oesophageal reflux, upper airway cough syndrome, or children with spontaneous resolution of their cough) or specific cough (bronchiectasis, protracted bacterial bronchitis, bronchiolitis obliterans, aspiration lung disease, eosinophilic lung disease, tuberculosis, pertussis or mycoplasma infections).
Main results	Of the 100 children enrolled, the mean age was 2.8 years and the mean duration of cough was 6 months. For specific cough the best predictor was chronic moist daily cough; sensitivity 96%, specificity 26%, positive predictive value (PPV) 74% and negative predictive value 73%.

(*continued*)

Evidence 3	
Theme E3	*History and examination in a child with chronic cough*
Main results (*cont.*)	The PPV of historical features were cough >6 months 74%, exertional dyspnoea 70%, chronic dyspnoea (parent indicated child was short of breath or aware of increased respiratory rate during coughing) 83%, recurrent pneumonia 71% and haemoptysis 83%. The value of physical examination and investigation for predicting a cause of specific cough (PPV %) was chest examination 84%, any abnormality on chest X-ray 79%, major abnormality on chest X-ray 87% and spirometry 75%.
Conclusion	The presence of a daily moist cough is a useful marker in predicting a specific cause of cough. The presence of findings on clinical examination and the presence of chest X-ray abnormalities are useful in predicting whether the child has specific cough aetiology.
Commentary	In this study, patients underwent extensive investigation to discern the aetiology of their chronic cough. The importance of clarifying the character of the cough is essential and if the parents cannot describe cough then recording on a mobile phone is useful. The aetiology of chronic cough is variable. In a study by Marchant *et al.* (2006) of 108 patients at a tertiary centre in Australia, aetiologies were persistent bacterial bronchitis 40%, bronchiectasis 6%, asthma 4%, upper airway cough syndrome 3%, habit 1%, idiopathic 5%, multiple causes 55% or children with natural resolution of their cough 22%. In a study by Khoshoo *et al.* (2009) of 40 patients at a pulmonary clinic in America, aetiologies were gastro-oesophageal reflux 28%, upper airway cough syndrome 23%, asthma 13%, idiopathic 10%, infection 5%, aspiration 3%, multiple causes 20%. In a study by Asilsoy *et al.* (2008) of 108 patients in a tertiary centre in Turkey, aetiologies were asthma 25%, persistent bacterial bronchitis 23%, upper airway cough syndrome 20%, gastro-oesophageal reflux 5%, bronchiectasis 3%, tuberculosis/mycoplasma 2%, congenital malformation 1%, multiple causes 19% or children with natural resolution of their cough 2%.
References	Marchant JM, Masters IB, Taylor SM, et al. Utility of signs and symptoms of chronic cough in predicting specific cause in children. *Thorax.* 2006; **61**(8): 694–8.
	Marchant JM, Masters IB, Taylor SM, *et al.* Evaluation and outcome of young children with chronic cough. *Chest.* 2006; **129**(5): 1132–41.
	Khoshoo V, Edell D, Mohnot S, *et al.* Associated factors in children with chronic cough. *Chest.* 2009; 136: 811–15.
	Asiloy S, Bayram E, Agin H, *et al.* Evaluation of chronic cough in children. *Chest.* 2008: 134: 1122–8.

Evidence 4

Theme E4	*Treatment of upper respiratory tract infections (URTIs)*
Question	Is honey effective in the treatment of URTI in children?
Design	Randomised controlled trial
Level of evidence	Jadad 5
Setting	Ambulatory care settings, Israel
Participants	Children aged 1–6 years with a history of cough attributed to URTI were eligible for inclusion. URTI was defined as the presence of cough and rhinorrhoea for ≤7 days. Parents completed a five-question questionnaire (three questions related to the child's cough, one to each on the impact of the cough on the child's and parents' sleep) which used a 7-point Likert scale (0 = not at all; 6 = extremely). Children with a Likert score of 3 or higher on two of the three cough-related questions and 3 or higher on the sleep questions were eligible.
Intervention	The pre-intervention questionnaire was completed on day 1 and children were then assigned to one of three different types of honey groups (eucalyptus, citrus, labiatae) or placebo (silan date extract). The treatment 10 g of honey or placebo was given 30 minutes before the child's bedtime. The post-intervention questionnaire was completed the following day.
Outcomes	The primary outcome was the change in cough frequency
Main results	Of the 435 assessed for eligibility, 300 were enrolled, 75 to the eucalyptus group [11 lost to follow-up, 64 (85%) completed study], 75 to citrus honey [13 lost to follow-up, 62 (82.6%) completed study], 75 to the labiatae honey [two lost to follow-up, 73 (97.3%) completed study] and 75 to placebo [four lost to follow-up, 71 (94.6%) completed study]. The mean cough score and percentage improvement post intervention for eucalyptus honey group was 3.7 and 45.9%, for the citrus honey group it was 3.8 and 52.6%, for the labiatae honey group it was 3.7 and 48.6%, and the placebo group it was 3.6 and 27.7%. [Eucalyptus absolute risk reduction (ARR) = 18.2%, number needed to treat (NNT) = 6; citrus ARR = 24.9%, NNT = 5; labiatae ARR = 20.9%, NNT = 5]. If the composite scores were used for assessment the NNTs would be eucalyptus 5, citrus 5 and labiatae 6.
Conclusion	The use of honey resulted in a reduction of symptoms compared with placebo.
Commentary	Cough related to URTI is generally self-limited; however, parents often wish for active intervention. While there is a multitude of over-the-counter preparations, their lack of proven effectiveness and their potential side effects have resulted in a lack of endorsement of their use by the medical community. This study offers an alternate treatment option. The researchers used only one dose of honey and restricted it to children beyond 1 year of age. Honey should not be used in children 1 year or younger, because of the risk of infantile botulism, and its frequent use can lead to dental caries. The impact of the natural resolution of symptoms on placebo response and the treatment impact of the honey was not assessed in this study (a no-intervention group would have been required).
Reference	Cohen HA, Rozen J, Kristal H, *et al.* Effect of honey on nocturnal cough and sleep quality: a double-blind, randomized, placebo-controlled study. *Pediatrics.* 2012; **130**(3): 465–71.

Evidence 5	
Theme E5	**Nasal steroids for chronic rhinitis**
Question	How effective are nasal steroids for chronic rhinitis?
Design	Randomised controlled trial
Level of evidence	Jadad 5
Setting	Department of paediatrics, general hospital, England
Participants	Children with perennial rhinitis were eligible to enter the study. All participants had at a least one positive skin prick test to common allergens (house dust mite being the most common).
Intervention	Participants received flunisolide (in an aqueous propylene glycol solution) or placebo (aqueous propylene glycol) for a 1-month period and then entered the crossover phase for another month. Sprays were administered three times per day.
Outcomes	The primary outcome was the overall control of symptoms ranked as total, good, minor, none or worse. Diary cards were maintained on a weekly basis assessing sneezing, stuffy nose, runny nose and nose blowing symptoms. Symptoms were ranked as none (0), mild (1), moderate (2), or severe (3).
Main results	Of the 27 patients enrolled, with an age range of 7–16 years (mean 7.4 years), 26 completed the study. In the treatment group 13 (50%) had a total or good response compared to 3 (11.5%) in the placebo group (absolute risk reduction = 38.5%; number needed to treat= 3). Five patients (19%) in the treatment group had no effect or were worse, compared with 20 (77%) in the placebo group. Symptoms scores improves were much improved in the treatment group as compared with placebo.
Conclusion	Nasal steroids are effective in the treatment of perennial rhinitis.
Commentary	There are few randomised controlled trials assessing the effectiveness of steroid nasal sprays in the treatment of perennial rhinitis. Currently these sprays are the treatment of choice for symptomatic children. When utilising these sprays parents must be counselled and advised on their correct use. These sprays when inserted into the nostril must be aimed laterally and not medially to ensure they are effective.
Reference	Sarsfield JK, Thomson GE. Flunisolide nasal spray for perennial rhinitis in children. *Br Med J.* 1979; **2**(6182): 95–7.

Evidence 6

Theme E6	*Immunotherapy and chronic rhinitis*
Question	What is the impact of sublingual immunotherapy (SLIT) tablets in children with rhinoconjunctivitis?
Design	Randomised controlled trial
Level of evidence	Jadad 5
Setting	Twenty-nine paediatric centres in Germany, Spain, Poland, Denmark and France
Participants	Children and adolescents aged 5–17 years with a history of moderate to severe allergic rhinoconjunctivitis for at least 2 years, confirmed by means of a positive skin prick test result (wheal >3 mm), a timothy grass pollen-specific IgE level ≥0.7 kU/L and a retrospective rhinoconjunctivitis total symptom score (RTSS) of 12/18 were eligible for inclusion.
Intervention	Patients received SLIT tablets containing freeze-dried allergen extract of five grass pollens (orchard, meadow, perennial rye, sweet vernal and timothy grass) at a dose of 300 IR or placebo. Tablets, both active and placebo, dissolve within 2 minutes and allergens are captured by oral dendritic cells within 30–60 minutes. Treatment began 4 months before the expected onset of the pollen season.
Outcomes	The primary outcome was the reduction in the RTSS and rescue medication use at the end of the grass pollen season.
Main results	Of the 320 children screened, 278 were randomised, 139 to the intervention group, with 131 (94.2%) completing the study, and 139 to the placebo group, with 135 (97.1%) completing the study. The RTSS score in the placebo group was 4.51 ± 2.93 and 3.25 ± 2.86 in the intervention group (absolute risk reduction (ARR) = 28%; number needed to treat (NNT) = 4). The mean proportion of days rescue medication was taken in the treatment group was 35.4% and in the placebo group was 46.5% (ARR = 11.1%; NNT = 9). Adverse events that lead to withdrawal occurred in nine participants (seven in the treatment group: one episode of chest pain, one episode of oral blistering, three episodes of oral pruritis, one episode of mouth oedema and one episode of vomiting).
Conclusion	SLIT tablets were effective in reducing symptom scores and rescue medication in children and adolescents with grass pollen-related rhinoconjunctivitis.
Commentary	The RTSS consists of the six most common symptoms of pollinosis: sneezing, rhinorrhoea, nasal pruritis, nasal itching, ocular pruritis and watery eyes. A scoring system of 0–3 is used, where 0 is no symptoms, 1 is mild symptoms (symptoms clearly present but minimal awareness, easily tolerated), 2 is moderate symptoms (definite awareness of bothersome but tolerable symptoms) and 3 is severe symptoms (symptoms hard to tolerate and/or cause interference with activities of daily living, sleeping or both). Children with rhinoconjunctivitis experience significant symptoms and as yet there is no uniformly effective treatment. Subcutaneous immunotherapy is available but the need for injections makes it inconvenient and there is the risk of serious adverse effects; consequently sublingual immunotherapy is preferable. With the increasing incidence of rhinitis, a definitive treatment rather than a symptomatic treatment is required.
Reference	Wahn U, Tabar A, Kuna P, *et al*. SLIT Study Group. Efficacy and safety of 5-grass-pollen sublingual immunotherapy tablets in pediatric allergic rhinoconjunctivitis. *J Allergy Clin Immunol*. 2009; **123**(1): 160–6.

Evidence 7	
Theme E7	*Chronic cough and antibiotic treatment*
Question	In children with a chronic wet cough is antibiotic treatment effective?
Design	Randomised controlled trial
Level of evidence	Jadad 3
Setting	Department of paediatrics, children's hospital, Australia
Participants	Children (aged 6 month to 6 years) with a history of chronic cough (>3 weeks) that was observed to be moist by a doctor were eligible for inclusion. Those with a suspected underlying lung disease or developmental delay were excluded.
Intervention	Participants received either amoxicillin-clavulanate 22.5 mg/kg dose twice daily or placebo and completed a cough diary. The cough scoring system used was the verbal category descriptive score, where on a daily basis cough is scored as follows: 0 = no cough, 1 = cough for one or two short periods only, 2 = cough for more than two short periods, 3 = frequent coughing but does not interfere with school or other activities, 4 = frequent coughing that interferes with school and other activities, 5 = cannot perform most activities.
Outcomes	The primary outcome was cough resolution which was defined as a 75% reduction in the baseline cough score at the end of the trial or cessation of the coughing for a minimum of 3 days within the trial period. Baseline cough scores were assessed in the 2 days prior to randomisation.
Main results	Of the 55 children who were eligible, 50 were randomised, 25 to each group. Twelve (48%) children in the amoxicillin-clavulanate group and four (16%) in the placebo group achieved cough resolution (absolute risk reduction = 32%; number needed to treat = 4) (95% confidence interval: 2–27). One child in the treatment group developed vomiting and ceased participation in the study. Thirty-seven (74%) participants had bronchoscopy with bronchoalveolar lavage (BAL) performed (19 in the treatment group and 18 in the placebo group). BAL microbiology identified bacteria in 30 (81%). The bacteria identified were *Haemophilus influenzae* (n = 14, 38%), *Streptococcus pneumoniae* (n = 9, 24%) and *Moraxella catarrhalis* (n = 7, 19%).
Conclusion	In children with chronic wet cough a 2-week course of amoxicillin-clavulanate will result in resolution of symptoms in a significant number.
Commentary	Children in this study who had positive microbiology on BAL were presumed to have persistent bacterial bronchitis (PBB). In general children with PBB are under 6 years of age, have a wet cough that is worse when changing posture, just after lying down in bed or first thing in the morning. Sometimes they cough so much they appear short of breath. PBB aetiology has been linked to the production of biofilms by bacteria, which allow them substantial protection against standard courses of antibiotic therapy. If children with PBB experience an associated viral illness the cough worsens and gradually returns to the mean. Despite persisting coughing these children do not look unwell and on examination are not hyperinflated and do not wheeze. The diagnosis should be prompted by the history and the response to antibiotic treatment. PBB has remained largely unrecognised and is often misdiagnosed as asthma. Treatment of children with amoxicillin-clavulanate is the treatment of choice. (Craven and Everard, 2013)

(continued)

Evidence 7	
Theme E7	*Chronic cough and antibiotic treatment*
References	Marchant J, Masters IB, Champion A, *et al*. Randomised controlled clinical trial of amoxycillin clavulanate in children with chronic wet cough. *Thorax*. 2012; **67**(8): 689–93.
	Craven V, Everard ML. Protracted bacterial bronchitis: reinventing an old disease. *Arch Dis Child*. 2013; **98**(1): 72–6.

COUGH: MULTIPLE-CHOICE QUESTIONS

Q1 Which of the following statements is/are true?
   a) Cough is a protective reflex.
   b) Cough improves mucociliary clearance.
   c) Children with cough expectorate sputum at 3 years of age.
   d) The cough reflex is mediated by the vagus nerve.
   e) The cough reflex can be sensitised by ACE inhibitors.

Q2 Features of pertussis include which of the following?
   a) Apnoea in infancy
   b) Coughing spasms triggered by feeding
   c) Frequent vomiting
   d) Atelectasis on chest X-ray
   e) An audible whoop on expiration

Q3 Features of cystic fibrosis include which of the following?
   a) Failure to thrive
   b) Poor appetite
   c) Finger clubbing but not toe clubbing
   d) Hepatomegaly
   e) Nasal polyps

Q4 Features of upper airway cough syndrome include which of the following?
   a) Morning sneezing
   b) Throat clearing
   c) Rhinorrhoea
   d) Eczema
   e) Stridor

Q5 Red flags for cough include which of the following?
   a) Recurrent hiccoughs
   b) Cough from birth
   c) A dry cough in the absence of URTIs
   d) Constipation
   e) Post-tussive vomiting

Q6 Treatment for upper airway cough syndrome includes which of the following?
a) Oral steroids
b) Nasal steroids
c) Oral antihistamines
d) Subcutaneous immunotherapy
e) Sublingual immunotherapy

Q7 Effective treatment for URTIs includes which of the following?
a) Antibiotics
b) Nasal steroids
c) Over-the-counter cough medications
d) Honey
e) Codeine drops

Q8 Which of the following statements is/are correct?
a) Parents are better than doctors in predicting acute cough duration.
b) Acute cough-related sleeplessness resolves for 60% after 4 days.
c) Acute cough resolves in 50% by 6 days.
d) Forty per cent of children with acute cough require antibiotic treatment.
e) Ninety per cent of children with acute cough have no symptoms at 10 days.

Q9 Causes of chronic cough include which of the following?
a) Bronchiectasis
b) Mycoplasma pneumonia
c) Recurrent aspiration
d) Pulmonary stenosis
e) IgG subclass deficiency

Q10 Which of the following statements is/are correct?
a) Habit (psychogenic) cough is rare in children.
b) Habit (psychogenic) cough occurs at night.
c) Erythromycin prophylaxis is useful in cystic fibrosis.
d) Hypertonic saline 3% is used to treat cystic fibrosis.
e) Chronic persistent bronchitis occurs in children.

Answers

A1	a, b, d, e	A2	a, b, c, d
A3	a, c, d, e	A4	a, b, c
A5	b, e	A6	a, b, c, d, e
A7	d	A8	a
A9	a, b, c	A10	c, e

SLIDE

1. Pertussis (subconjunctival haemorrhage)

Chapter Seventeen

THE CHILD WITH WHEEZE

COMMON SCENARIO

'My 2-year-old son has wheeze, persisting for 1 week, after an upper respiratory tract infection. He has had two previous head colds without wheezing being present and I wonder if this could be the beginning of asthma!'

LEARNING OBJECTIVES

- Recognise asthma phenotypes
- Recognise the presentations of asthma
- Define an investigative plan for a child with wheeze
- Define a treatment plan by severity of symptoms
- Understand the reasons why intensification of asthma treatment may fail

BACKGROUND

Wheezing in infants and children is a common clinical presentation to the primary care physician and the general paediatrician. Wheeze is an indicator of intrathoracic airway obstruction. It has a musical quality. Wheeze, when related to diffuse small airway obstruction, is expiratory in nature but with increasing severity of airway obstruction it is heard both in inspiration and expiration. The pitch of the wheeze changes with the degree of obstruction, the higher the pitch the more severe the obstruction. In diffuse diseases the wheezing is heard all over the chest but if unilateral in location it suggests bronchomalacia, foreign body or external compression of the bronchus by an enlarged lymph node, as occurs in tuberculosis.

Despite wheeze being an extremely common symptom our understanding is still evolving. Common conditions which feature wheeze as a significant symptom include bronchiolitis, acute viral (transient) wheeze, and atopic asthma.

In infancy bronchiolitis is the leading cause of hospitalisation during the winter months with wheeze, and usually affects infants <9 months of age. It is usually defined as a viral episode of respiratory distress characterised by corzya, cough with tachypnoea, wheezing and crepitations on examination. The usual aetiology is respiratory syncytial virus infection, but other viruses including parainfluenza, adenovirus and rhinoviruses are implicated. Recurrent episodes of bronchiolitis increase the risk of non-atopic wheezing, which abates by 12 years of age.

Infants with acute viral wheeze tend to be older than those with bronchiolitis but there is an overlap in age. These children are mostly non-atopic and have not been sensitised to allergens and their wheeze is induced by a viral illness. Their airways are smaller than average, which may be related to in utero exposure to smoking. These children's wheeze abates as they get older but the airway abnormalities persist.

Some children who wheeze have parents who were themselves treated for asthma; the child often has eczema or chronic rhinitis. Parents report that the child wheezes in response to viral illnesses, exercise and coming into contact with allergens. These children have normal lung functions in infancy but demonstrate bronchial hyperreactivity (BHR) on pulmonary function tests at 6 years of age. BHR is the airways response to metacholine challenge tests and a reduction in FEV1 (the volume exhaled during the first second of a forced expiration) of 12% or greater is indicative of asthma.

For parents of a child who wheezes, their primary questions are (a) does my child have asthma and (b) will my child outgrow his symptoms? Several epidemiological studies have attempted to answer these questions and a single yes or no answer is not available. However, to assess asthma risk in children several indices have been developed. Currently the modified Asthma Predictive Index is most useful. The components include (a) a history of at least four episodes or more of wheezing with at least one being diagnosed by a physician, (b) the child must meet at least one of the major criteria and two of the three minor criteria (major criteria: parental history of asthma, physician-diagnosed atopic dermatitis, allergic sensitisation to one or more aero allergen; minor criteria: allergic sensitisation to milk, egg, or peanut, wheezing unrelated to viral illness, and serum eosinophil ≥4%). The percentage of children with a positive index who have asthma at 13 years is 51.5%, and for those with a negative index the percentage with asthma at 13 years is 15.8%. Clearly the value of the index is in predicting those who will not have asthma.

The child who presents with wheeze related to a foreign inhalation will not have a remembered history in 20% of cases. The presences of recurrent pneumonias, recurrent wheeze which is not responsive to treatment or the presence of unilateral wheeze should alert the doctor to this potential aetiology. Chest X-ray in inspiration and expiration are often not practicable and a computed tomography scan of the thorax should be performed. Bronchoscopy is required to retrieve the foreign body.

HISTORY

KEY POINTS				
Wheeze	Does it sound like a whistling noise? Distinguish from a transmitted sound which is both audible and palpable	**Associated symptoms**	Cough, respiratory distress	**🔍 Red flags** Choking episode Food triggers of wheeze Wheezing with failure to thrive Wheezing non-responsive to bronchodilator treatment
When is the wheeze noticed?	With exercise or afterwards With feeds or afterwards Is it seasonal in occurrence?	**Past medical history**	Upper respiratory tract infection Eczema Chronic rhinitis Episodes of bronchiolitis Food allergies Congenital heart disease Gastro-oesophageal reflux, recurrent aspiration, stricture from corrosive ingestion	
What are the triggers of the wheeze?	Upper respiratory tract infections, exercise, allergen exposure, dust, grasses, pollens, foods: milk, egg, peanut	**Drug history**	Beta blockers	
Progression of the wheeze	Inspiratory, expiratory or both Severity of wheeze	**Family history**	Smoking inside or outside the home Family history of asthma Housing conditions – presence of dampness Heating, open fire, kerosene heaters	
Response of wheeze to medication	Response to bronchodilator treatment, oral steroids, inhaled steroids as assessed by parents and doctor	**Neonatal history**	Prematurity Bronchopulmonary dysplasia	

(continued)

KEY POINTS			
Use of spacer devices	All children who use a metered-dose inhaler should use a spacer device to ensure adequate delivery of medication	**Developmental history**	Cerebral palsy Developmental delay
Wheeze with cough and fever	Suggests Mycoplasma pneumonia	**Systemic review gastrointestinal tract**	History of choking, foreign body aspiration presents with wheeze if acute episode is missed
Other respiratory symptoms	Evaluate for breathlessness, chest tightness and cough	**Psychosocial history**	Days absent from crèche or school Number of times parent or guardian has been contacted by crèche or school regarding symptoms of wheeze
Healthcare utilisation	Visits to family doctor and emergency departments		

EXAMINATION

- Height and weight
- Separate wheeze from transmitted sounds, stridor
- Respiratory rate, pulse rate
- Hyperinflation
- Retractions
- Air entry pitch of wheeze high, medium or low
- Wheeze expiratory, inspiratory, or both
- Check for liver edge (pushed down due to lung hyperinflation)
- Dennie–Morgan's folds (which are indicative of chronic rhinitis)

Red flags

- Failure to thrive
- Hyperinflation
- Chest deformity
- Harrison's sulcus
- Wheeze on minimal exertion (tracheal obstruction)

DIFFERENTIAL DIAGNOSIS

	Wheeze	Other features
Transmitted sounds	Non-true wheeze	Sounds are both audible and palpable
Acute viral wheeze	Episodic wheeze	Upper respiratory tract infection precedes onset of wheeze
Bronchiolitis	Wheeze in winter months	Age under 1 year, cough and dyspnoea common features, crackles with wheeze on examination
Mycoplasma pneumonia	Wheeze in 30%	Fever, cough, malaise, often 5 years or older. Can aggravate asthma
Missed foreign body aspiration	Episodic wheeze	In 80% there is a history of choking. Inspiratory and expiratory chest X-ray aid diagnosis. May present with 'asthma' non-responsive to treatment
Aspiration pneumonia	Wheezing in relation to feed	Assess risk conditions, e.g. gastro-oesophageal reflux, achalasia, cerebral palsy, developmental delay
Food allergy	Wheezing post ingestion of suspect food (strong temporal relationship)	Check for associated features of anaphylaxis
Tracheomalacia	Wheeze often persisting	Have associated chronic cough due to lower respiratory infections
Vocal cord dysfunction	Wheezing	Dyspnoea, refractory to bronchodilator treatment
Cystic fibrosis	Wheeze (rarely a significant symptom unless allergic bronchopulmonary aspergillosis present)	Respiratory symptoms in children with cystic fibrosis include cough, sputum production. Check for clubbing and hyperinflated chest
Immotile cilia syndrome	Wheeze described but rare to present with isolated wheeze	Recurrent otitis media and purulent rhinorrhoea, cough a prominent feature

INVESTIGATIONS

Full blood count with differential

The percentage of eosinophils (>4%) is the most useful information gleaned from the full blood count.

Chest X-ray

In the child with asthma, a chest X-ray contributes little to the diagnosis, unless the child has atypical features or one of the red flags described earlier.

Pulmonary function tests

Pulmonary function tests are useful in evaluating children with wheeze; unfortunately, they must be older than 4–5 years of age. The FEV1 reflects obstruction to airflow and is used in assessing asthma. The use of the ratio of residual volume to total lung capacity may be a superior measure of air trapping but is not currently used. For children under 5, impedance ossillometry and measuring residual volume techniques are available but have not translated into clinical use.

A reduction in FEV1 with metacholine challenge or improvement with a bronchodilator suggests a diagnosis of asthma.

The measurement of peak expiratory flow rate can also be used to assess asthma; an improvement of ≥20% with a bronchodilator suggests bronchial hyper-reactivity.

Fractional excretion of nitric oxide

Fractional excretion of nitric oxide is not a sensitive indicator of current asthma control

Allergy testing

Allergies that children experience are often evident from the history. Many parents will want allergy testing performed. Skin testing is useful but usually only confirms what the history has indicated; however, in asthma that is uncontrolled, they can be helpful. Blood testing, for allergies, is expensive and if undertaken should be done prudently.

MANAGEMENT PLAN: SIX-STEP APPROACH

1. Clarifying and pitfall avoidance strategies
2. Acute asthma
3. Education:
   a) environmental control
   b) smoking cessation
   c) inhaler technique and spacer devices
4. Medication strategies in asthma management
   a) medication usage
   b) intensification strategy (pitfall avoidance)
5. Monitoring asthma control
6. Management of bronchiolitis

Clarifying and pitfall avoidance strategies

- Asthma diagnosis. **Pitfall:** there is no specific test that can be used to diagnose asthma in the young child. It is best to talk in terms of probabilities (high, medium and low). Re-emphasise this approach on repeated discussions and explain to parents that the diagnosis will evolve over time.

- Asthma types. **Rationale**: it is best to discuss the clinical symptom complexes, e.g. acute viral wheeze, atopic asthma, exercise-related asthma. This puts the symptoms in a context to which the parent can relate.
- Assessing wheeze. **Pitfall**: clinically make a distinction between a wheeze and a transmitted sound. Wheeze is initially an expiratory musical sound that is audible, whereas a transmitted sound is inspiratory in timing but is both audible and palpable.
- When assessing wheeze use a specific system. **Rationale**: wheeze is only one element of respiratory distress; therefore, learning a score that assesses respiratory distress allows the recognition of improvement or deterioration.
- Clarifying medication adherence. **Pitfall**: when assessing medication adherence, ask how often parents forget to administer the medication.
- Assess how parents view the diagnosis of asthma. **Rationale**: for some nationalities the diagnosis of asthma is regarded as extremely serious; therefore, it is best to clarify the severity of the diagnosis and the expected outcomes from the treatment regimens.
- Remember that all wheeze is not asthma, and that not all asthma is wheeze.
- Have an awareness of the relative effectiveness of treatment. **Rationale**: how effective are (a) oral steroids in acute viral wheeze (*see* Evidence 1) and (b) newer treatments of acute asthma (*see* Evidence 2).

Acute asthma

(*See* Chapter 3: First Response)

Education

Asthma is a chronic condition and as such parents and children (when old enough) are responsible for trigger avoidance, the recognition and treatment of acute symptoms and for the administration of maintenance therapy. Physicians must be actively aware of these goals, if they wish to have a positive impact on patient care (*see* Evidence 3).

Environmental control

Parents are keen to modify the environment to reduce asthma symptoms and lessen the need for medication usage. The impact of environment modification is modest at best. Parents whose child is allergic to house dust mite may choose to use a barrier bed-covering system and use high-temperature washing of bed linen. The removal of soft toys from the bedroom is helpful. The value of removing carpets is uncertain but is frequently chosen by parents. The bedroom should be well ventilated except if the child has pollen and grass allergies. Pet allergies to cats and dogs occur frequently. These pets should not be allowed in the child's bedroom and if possible should remain outside the home. If a pet triggers the child's asthma symptoms then it is prudent to remove the animal from the home. If grasses trigger the child's symptoms then the child should be indoors when the grass is being cut.

Smoking cessation

Smoking aggravates asthma-related symptoms and its cessation is strongly recommended for parents of asthmatic children. Smoking negates the impact of preventer medications and bronchodilator therapy. Parents may be reluctant to discontinue smoking; however, they must be counselled and advised to do so. If parents successfully discontinue smoking it may be possible to reduce their child's medication usage or in some cases discontinue it all together.

Inhaler technique and spacer devices

The assumption that medication administration once demonstrated to the patient does not need to be reviewed is false. Children should have their inhaler technique reviewed on a yearly basis, especially if their asthma has become difficult to treat after a period of stability. Children using metered-dose inhalers should utilise spacer devices to enhance medication delivery. Although bulky, the parents need to be instructed in their importance. Once the child is over 7 years of age the delivery system can be changed to a turbohaler system, thus avoiding the use of a spacer extension.

Small numbers of patient use nebulisers to deliver their asthma medications. Metered-dose inhalers with spacer devices are equivalent to nebulisers in the delivery of medications.

Medication strategies in asthma management

Medication usage

Medication usage in asthma is incremented in a stepwise approach.

FOR CHILDREN LESS THAN 5 YEARS

- Mild intermittent symptoms: use short-acting bronchodilator; symptoms should occur less than twice per week.
- Regular preventer: initially commence inhaled steroids at a low dose (200 µg/day) or use a leukotriene inhibitor.
- Initial add-on therapy: combine inhaled steroids with a leukotriene inhibitor.
- Persistent poor control: refer to a paediatrician.

CHILDREN OLDER THAN 5 YEARS

- Mild intermittent symptoms: use bronchodilator for symptoms of wheeze twice a week or less.
- Regular preventer: use inhaled steroids at a dose of 200 µg/day. In children with asthma, ongoing inhaled steroids are recommended (*see* Evidence 4); however, parents may not prefer this option and seek to use higher-dose intermittent steroids. This option should be explored in those cases (*see* Evidence 5).

- Initial add-on therapy: add a long-acting beta agonist (LABA) and assess control. If it is good, then continue (*see* Evidence 6):
  - if inadequate, increase the inhaled steroids to 400 µg/day; if stable, continue
  - if inadequate, add a leukotriene inhibitor
- Persistent poor control: increase the dose of inhaled corticosteroids to 800 µg/day and refer to a paediatrician.
- Continuous or frequent steroid use: this reflects the most severe form of asthma and these patients need to be carefully monitored.

Intensification strategy (pitfall avoidance)

When intensifying asthma care, ensure the following **pitfalls** have been avoided.

- Parents are adhering to the treatment regime; occasionally it is necessary to check that prescriptions are being filled.
- Check inhaler technique.
- Ensure the absence of cigarette smoking in the home; ask specifically if parents are smoking outside the house (this is not a suitable smoke avoidance strategy).
- Review the home environment, check for potential triggers e.g. poor heating systems, excessive dampness.
- Review the diagnosis – is it really asthma?
- Consider the presence of a co-morbid condition, e.g. gastro-oesophageal reflux, upper airway cough syndrome, food allergies.
- Assess asthma symptoms objectively through peak flow meter readings. These should be undertaken at least twice a day.
- Ensure that the parents and child have a written rescue plan, to enact if the child should develop an acute asthma attack.

Children with exercise-induced asthma should take a short-acting beta agonist prior to exercise to ameliorate their asthma-related symptoms.

Monitoring asthma control

Chronic conditions such as asthma need to be monitored on an ongoing basis. Peak flow meters are useful especially in children with poor symptom recognition. Readings should be obtained and recorded every morning and evening. A drop of 20% in the peak expiratory flow rate suggests worsening symptoms. Reviewing these readings at each doctor visit aids adherence.

- The Childhood Asthma Control Test is a validated tool to assess asthma control in 4- to 11-year-olds. It assesses symptoms within a 4-week window and is useful to use in conjunction with clinical assessment.
- Asthma Action Plans: the provision of action plans for children with asthma is essential but not utilised universally. The benefits are clear in aiding asthma control.

Management of bronchiolitis

The primary drug in the treatment of bronchiolitis is oxygen, which improves the infant symptomatically. Oxygen is best administered by soft nasal prongs, which reduce irritation to the nose. If the infant is unable to feed, nasogastric feeding is preferred. The value of bronchodilator treatment is transient and there is no role for steroid treatment. Hypertonic saline is effective in the treatment of moderate to severe bronchiolitis (*see* Evidence 7), and its use is recommended.

FOLLOW-UP

- This is dependent on asthma severity.
- Patients with asthma, on maintenance treatment, should be assessed on a 6-monthly basis, with a view to stepping down their treatment if they are stable.

WHEN TO REFER?

- Multi-trigger asthma children
- Children who have recurrent episodes of bronchiolitis (three or more in a year)
- Children who receive two or more courses of oral steroids in a 6-month period or on a high dose of inhaled steroids
- Parent who are 'in denial' about the diagnosis
- Children with abnormal physical examination (impaired growth or chest deformity)
- Children with nocturnal wheezing
- Wheeze that does not respond to bronchodilator therapy

CLARIFICATION STATEMENTS FOR PARENTAL MISCONCEPTIONS

'I know my child is wheezy because I can feel it.'

Not all audible sounds are wheezes. Transmitted sounds are both palpable and audible because the inspiratory sound is transmitted through the airways and therefore palpable. Wheeze in most cases is an expiratory sound and non-palpable.

'We smoke outside, surely that will do.'

The child with asthma needs to avoid negative impact of cigarette smoke as it aggravates asthma-related symptoms. Parents should discontinue smoking. Even if they smoke outside, there is still smoke present on their clothes when they return into the house.

'I am concerned that my child will become dependent on his inhaler.'

In asthma, the aim is to normalise the child's life in terms of activity and to balance this against medication use. If he has symptoms that are asthma related and they are not controlled, the quality of your child's life will be affected; therefore, it is best to think in terms of a normal life with the assistance of medications rather than the presence of symptoms and no medication use. What do you think?

SUMMARY PRACTICE POINTS

- The asthma predictive index has a high negative predictive value.
- The best predictor of future asthma exacerbation is the degree of current control achieved by the patient.
- Classify and clarify the patient's asthma state.
- When assessing control use specific questions, for example: do you use your blue inhaler on a daily basis, or, how often do you forget to take your preventer medications?
- Screening questionnaires (the Asthma Control Test and the Asthma Control Questionnaire) are useful to aid assess of the asthma patient.
- Normal lung function does not always mean good asthma control.
- Inhaled corticosteroids help with both symptom and exacerbation control but they do not alter the natural history or progression of asthma.

EVALUATING THE EVIDENCE

Evidence 1	
Theme E1	*Oral steroids for acute viral wheeze*
Question	How effective is oral prednisolone in preschool children with acute virus-induced wheezing?
Design	Randomised controlled trial
Level of evidence	Jadad 5
Setting	Emergency departments of three academic medical centres, England
Participants	Children aged 10–60 months were eligible if they presented to hospital with an attack of wheezing judged by the physician to have been triggered by an upper respiratory tract infection. Initially children were treated with 10 puffs of albuterol, administered through a metered-dose inhaler and volumatic mask, or nebulised albuterol (2.5 mg if the child was <3 years of age and 5 mg if the child was ≥3 years of age).
Intervention	Participants in this study were randomised to receive oral prednisolone (10 mg/day for 5 days if <24 months and 20 mg/day for 5 days if ≥24 months) or placebo for acute viral wheeze in addition to bronchodilator therapy.

(*continued*)

Evidence 1	
Theme E1	**Oral steroids for acute viral wheeze**
Outcomes	The primary outcome was duration of hospitalisation which was divided into two periods: the time from enrolment to the time of actual discharge from the hospital and the time from enrolment to the time the patient was deemed 'fit for discharge', since actual discharge may have been influenced by non-clinical factors. Secondary outcomes included the Preschool Respiratory Assessment Measure (PRAM) scores at baseline, 4, 12, and 24 hours.
Main results	One thousand, one hundred and eighty patients were assessed for eligibility, 480 were not enrolled, 318 declined and 162 did not meet the criteria, but 700 underwent randomisation and initial data are available on 687: 343 in the prednisolone group and 344 in the placebo group. The median time to discharge in the prednisolone group was 10.1 hours and in the placebo group 12.0. There is no difference in the primary outcome measure. The PRAM scores for at 4, 12 and 24 hours for placebo were 2.74 ± 2.3, 2.28 ± 2.03 and 1.58 ± 1.64, respectively, and for prednisolone were 2.48 ± 2.2, 2.49 ± 1.98 and 1.52 ± 1.75, respectively.
Conclusion	In children with acute viral wheeze who do not have classic atopic asthma, oral steroids are not beneficial.
Commentary	This study indicates that in children with acute viral wheeze who do not have classic atopic asthma, oral steroids are ineffective. For 81.4% of the placebo group and 78.8% of the oral steroid group it was their first hospital presentation, potentially indicative of significant wheeze and respiratory distress. The PRAM scores in this study are in the mild to moderate range, however each child received a high dose of albuterol prior to the performance of the PRAM scoring and consequently the maximal wheezing severity was underestimated. The short hospitalisation durations of 13.9 hours (placebo group) and 11 hours (prednisolone group) are surprising but clearly reflect the practices of the host institution. The components of the PRAM score are outlined in Chapter 3: First Response.
Reference	Panickar J, Lakhanpaul M, Lambert PC, *et al.* Oral prednisolone for preschool children with virus-induced wheezing. *N Engl J Med.* 2009; **360**(4): 329–38.

Evidence 2	
Theme E2	**Hypertonic saline for acute wheezing in preschool children**
Question	Is hypertonic saline effective in children aged 2 to 5 with acute wheezing?
Design	Randomised controlled trial
Level of evidence	Jadad 5
Setting	Department of paediatrics, academic medical centre, Israel
Participants	Children, aged 1 to 6 years, with acute wheezing and a clinical score ≥ 6, were eligible for inclusion.
Intervention	Initially all eligible wheezy patients received 5 mg of nebulised albuterol and after this the clinical score was assessed. Those with a clinical score over 6 were randomised to the treatment group and received two nebulised doses of hypertonic saline 4 mL with 2.5 mg of albuterol at 20-minute intervals.

(*continued*)

Evidence 2	
Theme E2	*Hypertonic saline for acute wheezing in preschool children*
Intervention (*cont.*)	The control group received two nebulised doses of 0.9% sodium chloride with 2.5 mg of albuterol, also 20 minutes apart.
Outcomes	The primary outcome was the admission rate and the duration of hospitalisation.
Main results	Sixty-one patients were assessed for eligibility but 20 were excluded (three for not meeting criteria and 20 refused), 41 were randomised, 16 to the treatment group and 24 to the control group. The admission rate for the treatment group was 62.2% and for the control group was 92% (absolute risk reduction = 29.8%; number needed to treat = 4). The length of stay was reduced by 1 day in the treatment group, a mean of 2 days, versus 3 days in the control group. Twelve (75%) of the treatment group and 21 (84%) of the control group had previously wheezed. Eleven (68.8%) of the treatment group and 13 (52%) of the control group had parents who smoked.
Conclusion	The use of hypertonic saline in children with acute wheezing reduces admission rates and the length of hospitalisation.
Commentary	The outcome from this study suggests (if replicated) that hypertonic saline is effective in the treatment of acute wheeze. Approximately 30% of patients when approached refused to participate. The high rate of smoking in the studied population may make the results less generalisable.
Reference	Ater D, Shai H, Bar BE, *et al.* Hypertonic saline and acute wheezing in preschool children. *Pediatrics.* 2012; **129**(6): e1397–403.

Evidence 3	
Theme E3	*The gap between best practice and asthma clinical care*
Question	Can asthma outcome be improved through education of primary care physicians?
Design	Randomised controlled trial
Level of evidence	5
Setting	Primary care practices, metropolitan area, Australia
Participants	Family practitioners and families with asthmatic children aged 2–14 years, from two regions of a metropolitan city, were eligible to participate.
Intervention	General practitioners (GPs) in the intervention group received the Practitioner Asthma Communication and Education (PACE) Australia programme, which comprises two 3-hour educational sessions focusing on communication and education strategies to facilitate quality asthma care. The programme has five themes: assessment of the pattern of asthma; appropriate use of asthma medications; provision of a written asthma action plan (WAAP); doctor–patient communication; and patient education. The program was enhanced through the use of video vignettes. GPs in the control group were offered the PACE programme at the end of the study period.
Outcomes	The primary outcome measure was the percentage of patients who were provided with a WAAP (in the study period of 12 months).

(*continued*)

Evidence 3	
Theme E3	*The gap between best practice and asthma clinical care*
Main results	Among the GPs, 183 registered interest, 150 were randomised, 78 to the intervention group, of whom 57 (73%) completed the study, and 72 to the control group, of whom 49 (68%) completed the study. Among the patient group 1290 were invited to participate, of whom 235 registered interest and 221 were randomised; 111 to the intervention group with 106 (95.5%) completing the study and 110 to the control group with a 107 (97%) completing the study. At baseline assessment WAAPs were provided to 45% of the intervention group and 45% of the control group; at 12 months the intervention group WAAP percentage was 75 and the control, 54% [absolute risk reduction (ARR) = 23% (95% confidence interval (CI): 11–36); number needed to treat (NNT) = 5]. Other GP behaviours also changed, such as asking parents to demonstrate use of devices [intervention group 50%, control group 39%, ARR = 11% (95% CI: −2% to 11%); NNT = 9], and prescribing spacer devices >90% of the time [intervention group 69%, control group 40%; ARR = 29% (95% CI: 16–42); NNT = 4].
Conclusion	The PACE Australia programme improved GPs' asthma management practices and led to improved patient outcomes.
Commentary	The PACE programme attempts to change physician behaviour to reflect best practice in the treatment of asthma through matching treatment with asthma pattern, correct use of medication with appropriate devices and providing WAAPs for children. This process was aided by enhancing the doctor's communication skills. While successful from the doctor's perspective, the failure to recruit large numbers of families (235 of 1290 or 18.2%) suggest that more emphasis must be placed on parents to engage with studies that will ultimately improve their children's outcomes.
Reference	Shah S, Sawyer SM, Toelle BG, *et al.* Improving paediatric asthma outcomes in primary health care: a randomised controlled trial. *Med J Aust.* 2011; **195**(7): 405–9.

Evidence 4	
Theme E4	*The use of inhaled corticosteroids in wheezy preschool children*
Question	Is ciclesonide effective in wheezy preschool children with a positive asthma predictive index?
Design	Randomised controlled trial
Level of evidence	Jadad 5
Setting	Seventy-seven centres in nine countries (Brazil, Germany, Hungary, India, the Netherlands, South Africa, Spain and Switzerland)
Participants	Children aged 2–6 years were eligible if they had a documented clinical history of asthma (defined as three or more episodes of wheezing, or troublesome recurrent symptoms, and/or episodes of wheezing, as reported by parents) for greater than 6 months plus a stringent asthma predictive index (*see* Commentary) or a positive test for atopy. Those with episodic viral wheeze were excluded.

(*continued*)

Evidence 4	
Theme E4	*The use of inhaled corticosteroids in wheezy preschool children*
Intervention	Ciclesonide at a dose of 40, 80 or 120 µg or placebo after a 2- to 4-week wash-out phase where only inhaled salbutamol was used on demand, were evaluated. Medication was administered through a spacer device but for those aged 2–3 a spacer device with mask was used. A night-time and daytime symptom score diary ranging from 0 (no symptom) to 4 (very bad symptoms: awake most of the night, or unable to carry out daily activities as usual) was completed by parents. The maximum score was 8. In the last week of the washout phase children with a symptom score of ≥1 on ≥4 days or those who had used rescue medication on ≥4 days were eligible for enrolment as they were symptomatic during their baseline phase.
Outcomes	The primary outcome was the (time to) severe wheezing which required systemic steroids as judged by the treating physician at which time they were withdrawn from the study.
Main results	Of the 1164 patients enrolled, 994 were randomised, 248 to ciclesonide 40 µg, 246 to ciclesonide 80 µg, 253 to ciclesonide 120 µg and 247 to placebo. The mean age was 4 years in each group. Severe wheezing occurred in 25 (10.2%) of the placebo group, as compared with 11 (4.4%), 18 (7.3%) and 17 (6.7%) in the ciclesonide 40, 80 and 120 µg groups, respectively (absolute risk reduction (ARR) = 5.8%, 2.9%, 3.5%; number needed to treat (NNT) = 17, 34, 29).
Conclusion	Ciclesonide had a modest effect in reducing wheezing rates in those children with a positive asthma predictive index.
Commentary	This large study included a population at high risk of wheeze. The difference between exacerbation rates in the placebo group (10.2%) and the pooled ciclesonide group (6.2%) (ARR = 4%; NNT = 25) suggest that the parents of those patients with significant disease chose not to enter this study with a 25% chance of assignment to the placebo group. This study used the Asthma Predictive Index (API), which was derived from the Tucson cohort study. It has recently been modified and endorsed by the US National Asthma Education and Prevention Program's *Expert Panel Report 3*. This modified API has three major criteria (parental history of asthma, clinician-diagnosed atopic dermatitis and allergic sensitisation to at least one aeroallergen) and three minor criteria (allergic sensitisation to milk, egg or peanut; wheezing unrelated to colds; and blood eosinophils ≥4%). The API may well have a role in defining children who respond to inhaled steroids. Those children who do not have the any of the API criteria are at low risk of developing persistent asthma.
Reference	Brand PLP, Garcia-Garcia ML, Morison A, *et al.* Ciclesonide in wheezy preschool children with a positive asthma predictive index or atopy. *Respir Med.* 2011; 105: 1588–95.

Evidence 5	
Theme E5	*Inhaled steroids for children with recurrent wheezing*
Question	In children with recurrent wheeze, which is more effective: daily or intermittent budesonide?
Design	Randomised controlled trial
Level of evidence	Jadad 5
Setting	Departments of paediatrics, academic medical centres, the United States
Participants	Children aged 12–53 months were eligible if they met the following criteria: during the previous year they had at least four episodes of wheezing (or three episodes of wheezing and controller use for ≥ 3 months), positive values on the modified Asthma Predictive Index, at least one episode requiring systemic glucocorticoids, urgent or emergency care or hospitalisation, and during a 2-week run-in period, they had fewer than 3 days/week of albuterol use and fewer than 2 nights with awakening.
Intervention	Children were randomly assigned to receive a budesonide inhalation suspension for 1 year as either an intermittent high dose regimen (1 mg twice daily for 7 days, starting early during a predefined respiratory tract illness) or a daily low dose regimen (0.5 mg nightly) with corresponding placebos.
Outcomes	The primary outcome was the frequency of exacerbations requiring oral glucocorticoids therapy.
Main results	Of the 450 children enrolled, 172 were excluded in the run-in (54 had excessive asthma symptoms). Of the 278 randomised, 139 were assigned to the intermittent regimen, with 113 (87.5%) completing the study, and 139 were assigned to the daily regimen group, with 100 (71.9%) completing the study. The number of prednisolone courses/person/year for asthma in the intermittent regimen was 0.95 and 0.97 for the daily regimen (no difference). The annualised days of treatment and cumulative dosage for budesonide was 24 days and 46 mg for the intermittent group, and 337 days and 150 mg for the daily group. No adverse effects were noted in terms of height, weight and head circumference between the two groups.
Conclusion	A daily low-dose regimen of budesonide was not superior to an intermittent high-dose regimen in reducing asthma exacerbations.
Commentary	The Global Initiative for Asthma guidelines recommend daily controller treatment for children with intermittent wheezing, a history suggestive of asthma, and at least three wheezing episodes in the previous year. This paper offers an alternate strategy for children and their parents, which many will choose to accept. Central to its success is the clear recognition and initiation of treatment at the onset of an upper respiratory tract infection. The used of nebulised budesonide suspension in an era of metered-dose inhaler therapy with a spacer device suggest that the study needs to be replicated to ensure equivalence.
Reference	Zeiger RS, Mauger D, Bacharier LB, *et al.* Daily or intermittent budesonide in preschool children with recurrent wheezing. *N Engl J Med.* 2011; **365**(21): 1990–2001.

Evidence 6	
Theme E6	*Options for treatment when asthma is uncontrolled on low-dose inhaled steroids (ICSs)*
Question	What is the impact of step-up therapy for children with uncontrolled asthma while receiving ICSs?
Design	Randomised controlled trial
Level of evidence	Jadad 5
Setting	Paediatric asthma care centres, the United States
Participants	Children and adolescents aged 6–17 years with mild to moderate asthma diagnosed by a physician using the National Asthma Education and Prevention Program, with an ability to perform spirometry and an FEV1 (the volume exhaled during the first second of a forced expiration) of >60%, whose asthma was uncontrolled, were eligible for entry. Uncontrolled asthma was defined as one of the following for more than 2 days per week on average during a 2-week period: diary-reported symptoms (cough rated as moderate or severe or wheezing rated mild, moderate or severe), rescue use of an inhaled bronchodilator with two or more per day, or peak flows under 80% of predetermined reference value.
Intervention	Patients entered a three-period crossover trial for a total of 48 weeks. During each 16-week period they received 250 µg of fluticosone twice daily (step-up inhaled corticosteroid therapy), fluticosone 100 µg plus 50 µg of a long-acting beta-agonist twice-daily step-up (LABA step-up) or fluticosone 100 µg plus 5 or 10 mg of leukotriene-receptor antagonist montelukast (LTRA step-up therapy). The initial 4 weeks of the last two 16-week periods were considered to be active washout phases from the previous period. Written action plans were provided to determine when oral steroids were to be used.
Outcomes	The primary outcome was a composite of three outcomes (the need for oral steroids for exacerbations, asthma control days and FEV1) to determine a differential response of 25%.
Main results	Four hundred and eighty patients were enrolled but 298 were excluded in the run-in phase; consequently, 182 underwent randomisation, of whom 157 (86%) completed all three periods and 165 (91%) completed two phases. One hundred and sixty-one (98%) patients had a differential response to treatment. The proportion of patients who had a better response to LABA was higher than those who had a better response to LTRA (52% versus 34%) (absolute risk reduction (ARR) = 18%; number needed to treat (NNT) = 6). When LABA and ICS step-up were compared the percentages were 54% versus 32% (ARR = 22; NNT = 5). The responses to LTRA and ICS were similar. A total of 120 courses of prednisolone were prescribed, 30 in the LABA group, 47 in the ICS group and 43 in the LTRA group, indicating that the step-up therapy on its own is not always successful. A total of 25 treatment failures occurred, three patients were hospitalised and 22 required a second course of oral steroids.
Conclusion	In children with uncontrolled asthma, LABA step-up provided a better differential response than ICS step-up or LTRA step-up. However, many children responded to ICS step-up or LTRA step-up, indicating the need to regularly assess treatment strategies for asthma.

(continued)

Evidence 6	
Theme E6	*Options for treatment when asthma is uncontrolled on low-dose inhaled steroids (ICSs)*
Commentary	This study suggests that there is a ceiling effect in the use of ICS therapy. The use of LABA provided the best response to address exacerbations of asthma; however, baseline characteristics did not predict the response to treatment rate. The use of LABA alone is not recommended as a treatment strategy. The Childhood Asthma Control Test for 4- to 11-year-olds and the Asthma Control Test for 12- to 17-year-olds helped to predict patients who responded to LABA. The Childhood Asthma Control Test is a seven-item scale that assesses asthma using a four-item pictorial scale, score range 0–3, related to asthma symptoms today, with exercise, cough-related to asthma and night-time wakening. Three items with a scale of 0–5 assess the number of asthma symptoms days, the frequency of wheeze and the frequency of nocturnal symptoms in the last 4 weeks. Scores ≤19 suggest poor control.
Reference	Lemanske RF Jr, Mauger DT, Sorkness CA, *et al.* Step-up therapy for children with uncontrolled asthma receiving inhaled corticosteroids. *N Engl J Med.* 2010; **362**(11): 975–85.

Evidence 7	
Theme E7	*The use of hypertonic saline in bronchiolitis*
Question	How effective is nebulised hypertonic saline in children with moderate to severe bronchiolitis?
Design	Randomised controlled trial
Level of evidence	Jadad 5
Setting	Department of paediatrics, academic medical centre, China
Participants	Children admitted to hospital with moderate to severe bronchiolitis were eligible for enrolment. Prior to randomisation all patients were categorised as having moderate to severe bronchiolitis based on a 12-point severity scale, with 0–3 assigned to the following parameters: respiratory rate, presence of and nature of wheezing, retractions and overall condition. Score 0–12. Scores 0–4.9 were rated as mild, 5–8.9 as moderate and 9–12 as severe.
Intervention	Participants received nebulised 3% hypertonic saline (HS) or 0.9% sodium chloride to treat their clinical symptoms.
Outcomes	The primary outcome was length of hospitalisation.
Main results	One hundred and thirty-five patients were eligible, but nine refused to participate and 126 were randomised, 64 to the HS group, with seven discharged within 12 hours after enrolment and 57 completing the whole study, and 62 randomised to the normal saline (NS, sodium chloride) group, with seven discharged within 12 hours and 55 completing the whole study. The average age of the HS group was 5.9 ± 4.1 months and length of stay was 4.8 ± 1.2 days; for the NS group the average age was 5.8 ± 4.3 months and length of stay was 6.4 ± 1.4 days. The clinical scores for the HS group and the NS group were 5.7 and 7.3, respectively, on day 1. No adverse effects were recorded from the administration of HS.

(continued)

Evidence 7	
Theme E7	*The use of hypertonic saline in bronchiolitis*
Main results (*cont.*)	Respiratory syncytial virus was detected in 40 (72.7%) of the HS group and in 42 (73.7%) of the NS group.
Conclusion	The use of HS resulted in a reduction of 1.6 days in children admitted to hospital with moderate to severe bronchiolitis.
Commentary	This is a large study that addresses the use of HS in the treatment of moderate to severe bronchiolitis where there is an absence of bronchodilator therapy. While the length of stay was reduced by 1.5 days, the duration of wheezing and the time to alleviation of cough was also shorter. No data were provided on readmission rate or on oxygen requirements of infants. The majority of the patients were positive for respiratory syncytial virus infection, which depletes the mucous layer water content, damages the airway surface liquid epithelium and reduces the height of the periciliary liquid and clearance of mucus. In vitro HS increase airway surface thickness; decreases epithelial oedema improves mucus elasticity and viscosity and accelerates the transport of mucus.
Reference	Luo Z, Fu Z, Liu E, et al. Nebulized hypertonic saline treatment in hospitalized children with moderate to severe viral bronchiolitis. *Clin Microbiol Infect.* 2011; **17**(12): 1829–33.

WHEEZE: MULTIPLE-CHOICE QUESTIONS

Q1 Which of the following statements is/are correct?
   a) Wheeze reflects intrathoracic airway obstruction.
   b) Wheeze has a musical quality.
   c) Wheeze is initially an expiratory sound.
   d) The pitch of the wheeze indicates the degree of airway obstruction.
   e) Unilateral wheeze suggests bronchomalacia.

Q2 With regard to bronchiolitis, which of the following statements is/are true?
   a) Wheeze and crepitations are found on clinical examination.
   b) Typically, patients are under 6 months of age.
   c) Bronchiolitis typically commences with an upper respiratory tract infection.
   d) Respiratory syncytial virus causes 50% of cases.
   e) Oxygen is the primary treatment.

Q3 With regard to acute viral wheeze, which of the following statements is/are correct?
   a) It usually occurs in atopic patients.
   b) Children are usually sensitised to aero allergens.
   c) Smoking in pregnancy is a risk factor.
   d) The airways of affected children are smaller than normal.
   e) Children respond to oral steroid therapy promptly.

Q4 Which of the following statements are true with regard to asthma?
a) A positive family of asthma history is a risk factor.
b) Wheeze is triggered by upper respiratory tract infections.
c) Bronchial hyper-reactivity is present in 60% of asthmatic children.
d) Cold air can trigger asthma symptoms.
e) Atopic eczema is a risk factor for asthma.

Q5 Major criteria for the Asthma Predictive Index include which of the following?
a) Two episodes of wheeze, one of which was diagnosed by a doctor
b) Allergic sensitisation to aeroallergens (more than one)
c) Egg or peanut allergy
d) The presence of atopic dermatitis
e) Presence of smoking in the home

Q6 Minor features of the Asthma Predictive Index include which of the following?
a) Wheeze unrelated to viral illnesses
b) Smoking in the home
c) An eosinophil count of >4%
d) Positive family history of asthma
e) Allergic sensitisation to milk, egg or peanut

Q7 Which of the following are true with regard to foreign body aspiration?
a) Twenty per cent do not remember a choking episode occurring.
b) Clinical presentation includes wheeze not responsive to treatment.
c) Chest X-ray on inspiration and expiration is the investigation of choice in a 5-year-old.
d) Bronchoscopy is the treatment of choice.
e) Recurrent pneumonia is a recognised clinical presentation.

Q8 Clinical 'red flags' in a child with wheeze include which of the following?
a) A history of choking
b) Wheeze that is associated with food ingestion
c) Wheeze with failure to thrive
d) A history of abdominal pain
e) Wheeze that is not responsive to bronchodilators

Q9 Which of the following statements is/are true?
a) Transmitted sounds are audible but not palpable.
b) Thirty per cent of mycoplasma respiratory infections are associated with wheeze.
c) Vocal cord dysfunction responds to nebulised steroid treatment.
d) Wheeze is common with pulmonary exacerbation in cystic fibrosis.
e) Aspiration pneumonia occurs in children with cerebral palsy.

Q10 Which of the following statements with regard to immotile cilia syndrome are correct?

a) Otitis media is common.

b) Dextrocardia is present in 75%–80% of cases.

c) Purulent rhinorrhoea is a frequent clinical finding.

d) Clinical diagnosis is usually made by 3 years of age.

e) Wheeze is rare.

Q11 Which of the following statements is/are true with regard to pulmonary function tests?

a) Children often need to be 5 years or older to perform standard spirometry.

b) The FEV1 is a commonly used measure to assess lung function in asthmatics.

c) The ratio of residual volume to total lung capacity is a good measure of air trapping but it is not commonly used.

d) A change of FEV1 by 20% is required to demonstrate the presence of bronchial reactivity.

e) Pulmonary function tests are required to make a diagnosis of asthma in a child over 6 years of age.

Answers

A1	a, b, c, d, e	**A2**	a, c, d, e
A3	c, d	**A4**	a, b, d, e
A5	b, d	**A6**	a, c, e
A7	a, b, d, e	**A8**	a, b, c, e
A9	b, e	**A10**	a, c, e
A11	a, b, c		

SLIDE

1. Pectus excavatum

Chapter Eighteen

THE CHILD WITH SUSPECTED CONGENITAL HEART DISEASE

COMMON SCENARIO

'She was unwell last month with an infection. When we went to the general practitioner she said she heard a murmur. A neighbour's child had a murmur and needed surgery. I'm worried sick she might have a hole in her heart or need an operation.'

LEARNING OBJECTIVES

- To understand common congenital heart lesions and how they present
- To be able to distinguish an innocent murmur from a significant cardiac murmur
- To be able to assess a child's cardiac status and perform a detailed cardiac examination
- To understand the management of cardiac defects

BACKGROUND

Congenital heart defects are anatomical malformations of the heart and/or great vessels. Eight per 1000 live children are born with congenital heart disease (CHD). The presentation of CHD can vary, from the asymptomatic child presenting with a murmur, to the infant or child who presents acutely unwell with cyanosis or heart failure.

Murmurs are a common clinical finding and the leading cause of referral to paediatric cardiologists. Up to 50% of normal children may have a murmur at any one time, but without any underlying pathology. In the newborn period, a murmur is noted in 0.6%–77%, depending on the age of the child at examination, the clinical experience of the examiner and the cohort of patients reviewed. However, 50% of children with CHD do not have a murmur in the immediate postnatal period.

The majority of cases are multifactorial, with genetic and environmental factors having a role to play. The incidence of CHD is significantly increased by a positive family history. If a single sibling had CHD, the risk is 2%; if two siblings had CHD, the risk is increased to 4%; and if a parent had CHD, the risk is 5%. CHD is associated with a variety of chromosomal disorders and syndromes. Thirty per cent of neonates with chromosomal abnormalities have CHD. Between 6% and 10% of patients with CHD have associated chromosomal abnormalities.

Common syndromes include:

- *Down's syndrome* – 40% of children have CHD, of those with CHD atrioventricular septal defects (AVSDs) occur in 40% of cases; additional associated defects include atrial septal defects (ASDs), ventricular septal defects (VSDs) and tetralogy of Fallot
- *Turner's syndrome* – associated with coarctation of the aorta and aortic stenosis
- *Noonan's syndrome* – associated with pulmonary stenosis and VSDs
- *Marfan's syndrome* – associated with aortic root dilatation
- *DiGeorge's syndrome* – associated with interrupted aortic arch, truncus arteriosus, pulmonary atresia, tetralogy of Fallot
- *Williams's syndrome* – associated with supravalvular aortic stenosis (AS) and pulmonary artery stenosis.
- *Edward's syndrome* –associated VSD and coarctation of the aorta

The consumption of alcohol in pregnancy and the use of certain drugs is associated with an increased risk of cardiac defects. Drugs include anti-epileptics (Valproic acid carbamazepine, phenytoin), lithium, amphetamine and warfarin.

Congenital heart defects are classified into three types based on their haemodynamic effect: left-to-right shunts, obstructive lesions and cyanotic lesions.

Symptoms of heart failure in early infancy include poor feeding, recurrent infections, shortness of breath, sweating, easy fatigability, failure to thrive and irritability. Older children may present with dyspnoea on exertion, decreased exercise tolerance, poor weight gain, oedema, palpitations and chest pain.

Frequency of types of congenital heart disease	
VSD	30%
Patent ductus arteriosus (PDA)	12%
ASD	7%
Pulmonary stenosis	7%
Aortic stenosis	5%
Coarctation of the aorta	5%
Tetralogy of Fallot	5%
Transposition of the great arteries (TGA)	5%
Truncus arteriosus	2%

INNOCENT MURMURS

The commonest murmur heard in children is the functional, innocent or physiological heart murmur. These all relate to a structurally normal heart but can cause great concern within the family. There are many different types, depending on the possible site of their origin. Innocent murmurs are typically louder in the presence of fever or anaemia. They never have a diastolic component, are asymptomatic and do not produce thrills.

They should:

- be soft (low intensity)
- be systolic
- be asymptomatic (no cardiac signs or symptoms)
- be localised
- have a musical, buzzing quality
- vary with posture and/or respiration.

Types of innocent murmurs	
Peripheral pulmonary artery stenosis murmur	This is frequently seen in preterm neonates, is a physiological finding and disappears after a few weeks of age, never causing symptoms. It is a systolic murmur best heard bilaterally in the mid-axillary line.
Still's murmur	This is the most common innocent murmur. It is typically found in children 3–8 years of age. It is vibratory in nature and is found at the mid-left sternal edge. It may be caused by turbulence around a myocardial muscle in the left ventricle. It decreases on standing and upon performance of the Valsalva manoeuvre.
Venous hum	This is commonly heard in the neck and beneath the clavicles. It is a pansystolic murmur (the only innocent murmur with a diastolic component). It is best heard when the child is sitting and disappears when the child is supine or if the ipsilateral jugular vein is compressed. If the child's head is turned to the contralateral side, the murmur intensifies.
Pulmonary flow murmur	This is a soft blowing systolic murmur audible at the left upper sternal border in older children.
Carotid bruit	This is a systolic murmur 2/6 intensity, audible above the clavicles along the carotid artery.

LEFT-TO-RIGHT SHUNTS (ACYANOTIC)

Newborns who have severe left-to-right shunts (VSD, PDA, ASD) never present with heart failure in the first few days of life. The pulmonary vascular resistance has not fallen by this age, limiting any left-to-right shunt and hence symptoms. The symptoms and signs, however, do become more apparent over the first few weeks of life, reaching a maximum at about 3 months of age when the pulmonary vascular resistance is at its lowest.

Ventricular septal defect

A VSD is a developmental defect in the interventricular septum resulting in communication between the two ventricles. The two main factors that determine the magnitude of the left-to-right shunt are the size of the defect and the pulmonary vascular resistance. The defect may be described as membranous, muscular, subpulmonary or as an ASD. Infants with a moderate to large VSD present at 6–8 weeks of age (when the pulmonary vascular resistance has fallen significantly) with symptoms and signs of congestive heart failure. An infant or child with a small VSD may be asymptomatic with normal growth. Examination may reveal an active precordium with a right ventricular heave, a harsh loud pansystolic murmur with a possible thrill maximal at the left lower sternal border. With very large defects, an unimpressive ejection murmur may only be heard with a loud P2.

Atrial septal defect

An ASD is a developmental defect in the interatrial septum resulting in communication between the two atria. The defect may be described as an ostium secundum (defect in the centre of the atrial septum), ostium primum (defect in the lower end of the septum) or sinus venosum (defect high in the septum near the junction of the right atrium and superior vena cava). ASDs are usually asymptomatic in childhood or can present with exertional dyspnoea or mild fatigue. If an ostium primum defect is present, it may present in early infancy with heart failure. Examination reveals an ejection systolic murmur in the pulmonary area and a widely split and fixed second heart sound.

Patent ductus arteriosus

The ductus arteriosis connects the descending aorta (distal to the origin of the left subclavian artery) to the left pulmonary artery. In the foetus, the duct allows blood to flow from the pulmonary artery into the aorta, thereby bypassing the lungs and allowing oxygenation in the placenta. A PDA is defined as persistence of the ductus arteriosus beyond 1 month of age. The ductus arteriosus normally closes in the first 72 hours after birth. Failure of the duct to close is common in premature infants with up to 50% of preterm infants under 1500 g having a PDA. Small PDAs are usually asymptomatic, whereas a large PDA causes recurrent lower respiratory infections, failure to thrive and heart failure. Examination reveals a continuous machinery murmur below the left clavicle, a hyperdynamic precordium and bounding peripheral pulses.

OBSTRUCTIVE LESIONS

Coarctation of the aorta

Coarctation of the aorta is caused by a narrowing in the aortic arch. There are three types: (1) preductal (narrowing proximal or before the ductus arteriosus; a PDA will allow blood to flow from the pulmonary artery into the descending aorta), (2) post-ductal (narrowing distal or after the ductus arteriosus; blood will not be able to flow to the kidneys or lower limbs) and (3) periductal (narrowing at the level of the ductus; blood flow through the PDA may be in both directions). Presentation depends on the level of narrowing. Infants with *preductal narrowing* present as acutely unwell in the newborn period once the duct closes, with diminished pulses in the upper limbs and absent pulses in the lower limbs. Children with *postductal narrowing* are usually asymptomatic, with normal growth and development. They may have symptoms of hypertension or lower limb hypoperfusion, such as intermittent claudication. Femoral pulses may be weak with radiofemoral delay. A consistent difference of pressure of 15–20 mmHg between the right arm and right leg should prompt investigation for coarctation. Usually no murmur is heard. In *periductal narrowing*, the presentation is varied.

Hypoplastic left heart syndrome

There is significant hypoplasia of the left side of the heart. The systemic circulation is duct dependent and maintained by the right ventricle. There are varying degrees of hypoplasia, or atresia of the aorta and mitral valves. It is frequently associated with coarctation of the aorta. Ideally the diagnosis is made antenatally. When the ductus arteriosus closes, infants present with circulatory collapse, absent femoral and brachial pulses and signs of heart failure with severe metabolic acidosis.

Interrupted aortic arch

Interrupted aortic arch is the absence or discontinuation of a portion of the aortic arch. There are three described types.
1. Type A: the interruption occurs distal to the left subclavian artery.
2. Type B: the interruption occurs between the left carotid artery and the left subclavian artery.
3. Type C: the interruption occurs between the innominate artery and the left carotid artery.

Aortic stenosis

Aortic stenosis results from the abnormal formation of the aortic valve during foetal cardiac development. It results in obstruction to the flow of blood from the left ventricle into the aorta. Stenosis may be at, below or above the aortic valve. The majority of children with valvular AS are asymptomatic. Others may present with dyspnoea, exertional fatigue, chest pain or syncope. Critical AS presents in the newborn period with circulatory collapse. Examination may reveal a prominent apex with a forceful character, a soft A2 with an apical ejection click, and ejection systolic murmur at the left upper sternal edge and a praecordial and carotid artery thrill.

Pulmonary stenosis

Pulmonary stenosis results from the abnormal formation of the pulmonary valve during foetal cardiac development. It results in obstruction to the flow of blood from the right ventricle into the pulmonary artery. Stenosis may be at, below or above the level of the pulmonary valve. It is associated with Noonan's and Alagille's syndromes. Presentation depends on the severity of stenosis. Children may be asymptomatic or present with cyanosis and signs and symptoms of congestive cardiac failure.

CYANOTIC CONGENITAL HEART DEFECTS

In cyanotic congenital heart defects, systemic venous blood bypasses the pulmonary circulation and gets shunted from the right to the left side of the heart. The most important causes of cyanotic CHD are commonly referred to as the 5Ts:
1. tetralogy of Fallot
2. transposition of the great arteries (TGA)
3. tricuspid atresia
4. total anomalous pulmonary venous circulation
5. truncus arteriosus.

Tetralogy of Fallot

The four primary components are a VSD, subvalvular pulmonary stenosis, overriding aorta and right ventricular hypertrophy. Symptoms depend on the degree of right ventricular outflow tract obstruction. Infants can present with cyanosis and hypercyanotic spells or can be relatively asymptomatic with the finding of an incidental murmur and associated clubbing.

Hypercyanotic spells occur as a result of spasm of the right ventricular outflow tract. They commonly occur after crying or increased exertion and are self-aggravating, i.e. the more upset the infant becomes, the more cyanotic they get. If severe and left untreated they can lead to death. Examination may reveal central cyanosis, clubbing and a harsh long ejection systolic murmur at the upper sternal edge and a single second heart sound.

Transposition of the great arteries

The aorta arises from the right ventricle and the pulmonary artery from the left ventricle. Two parallel circulations exist and this is incompatible with life postnatally unless there is communication at atrial, ventricular or ductal level. Defects can be classified as simple or complex. In simple or D-TGA, the aorta and pulmonary arteries arise from inappropriate ventricles. There are three forms of complex TGA: (1) TGA with VSD, (2) TGA with ventricular septal aneurysm and mild pulmonary stenosis and (3) TGA with VSD and severe pulmonary stenosis. Presentation depends on the type of TGA. Infants with simple TGA present with severe cyanosis, with little or no associated respiratory distress, as soon as the ductus closes. Typically there is no murmur and a single S2. Children with a TGA and VSD present with congestive heart failure due to increase pulmonary blood flow related to the VSD. When pulmonary stenosis is present and mild, children present similarly; however, when stenosis is severe, children present with cyanosis and dyspnoea.

Tricuspid atresia

Tricuspid atresia results from abnormal formation of the tricuspid valve during foetal cardiac development. This usually presents with severe cyanosis and tachypnoea from birth. Examination reveals cyanosis, a systolic murmur at the lower left sternal border and a single second heart sound.

Ebstein's anomaly

The tricuspid valve is malpositioned. The condition is associated with maternal lithium ingestion. Children may be asymptomatic or present with cyanosis or in supraventricular tachycardia. Examination may reveal a soft long systolic murmur and a split S1.

Total anomalous pulmonary venous drainage

Instead of draining into the left atrium, the four pulmonary veins drain abnormally into the right atrium. As a result, oxygenated and deoxygenated blood mix causing mixed venous blood to circulate around the body. There are four types, depending on the site of drainage.
1. **Supracardiac**: pulmonary veins drain into the superior vena cava.
2. **Cardiac**: pulmonary veins drain into the right atrium or coronary sinus. Supracardiac and cardiac types are usually non-obstructive and present with signs and symptoms of congestive heart failure. Cyanosis is usually mild.
3. **Infracardiac**: pulmonary veins drain into the portal vein or the inferior vena cava. This is almost always obstructive and presents in the newborn period with marked cyanosis and collapse. A murmur is usually not present.
4. **Mixed**: a combination of these types.

Truncus arteriosus

Truncus arteriosus occurs when only one artery arises from the heart and forms both the aorta and the pulmonary artery. It is commonly associated with 22q11 deletion. It is commonly associated with a VSD and an abnormal truncal valve. If there is no associated pulmonary stenosis, signs of congestive cardiac failure develop early. If there is severe pulmonary stenosis or atresia, infants become cynotic once the ductus arteriosis closes, with right-to-left shunting. Examination may reveal a continuous ejection systolic murmur and a single second heart sound.

HISTORY

KEY POINTS FOR CHILDREN <1 YEAR OF AGE				
Birth history	Gestation Birthweight Murmur noted at birth Oxygen saturations recorded	**Medical and surgical history**	Previous hospital admissions Recurrent chest infections	**🛇 Red flags** Recurrent chest infections Failure to thrive History of breathlessness
Maternal history	Medication use during pregnancy Infections Antenatal scan findings Diabetes Alcohol intake IVF	**Growth and development**	Poor weight gain Delayed motor milestones Easy fatigablity Irritability	
Family history	Murmurs Chromosomal malformations Syndromes	**Systems review**	Cyanotic or 'blue' episodes Breath-holding episodes Cold hands and feet Sweating	
Feeding	Breathlessness with feeds Early stopping of feeds	**Vaccinations**	Routine vaccinations Palivizumab	

EXAMINATION

All children should have their height and weight plotted on an appropriate centile chart.

- Look for dysmorphic features
- Look for signs of respiratory distress
- Check oxygen saturation
- Assess pulses
- Check blood pressure
- Examine for surgical chest scars and clubbing
- Feel for thrills, heaves and locate the apex beat
- Listen to the heart sounds, additional sounds or murmurs

❶ Red flags

- Cyanosis
- Dysmorphic features
- Absent or reduced pulses
- Hepatomegaly
- Respiratory distress
- Clubbing
- Poor perfusion (delayed capillary refill, cool extremities, weak pulses)
- Hypertension

Surgical chest scars	Likely procedure
Right lateral thoracotomy	Right modified Blalock–Taussig shunt
Left lateral thoracotomy	Left modified Blalock–Taussig shunt
	Coarctation of the aorta repair
	Pulmonary artery banding
Median sternotomy scar	Open heart surgery
	Cardiopulmonary bypass
	Proximal aortic arch repair

INVESTIGATIONS

When should pulse oximetry be performed?

All newborn infants should have pulse oximetry performed prior to discharge from the maternity hospital (*see* Evidence 1). Pulse oximetry screening offers an effective, accurate and reliable means for maximising detection of cyanotic CHD in asymptomatic newborns. A level ≥95% is taken as normal.

Is a chest X-ray useful in distinguishing innocent from pathological murmurs?

No, but chest X-rays can give useful information about heart size and pulmonary vascular markings and response to heart failure treatment.
- Oligaemic lung fields can be seen in tetralogy of Fallot and Ebstein's anomaly
- Plethoric lung fields can be seen with left-to-right shunts

In the newborn period, the cardiac silhouette shows:
- 'egg on side' appearance in transposition of the great vessels
- 'boot shape' appearance in tetralogy of Fallot
- 'box shape or wall-to-wall heart' appearance in Ebstein's anomaly
- 'snowman in a snowstorm' in total anomalous pulmonary venous connection.

Is a hyperoxia test useful in the investigation of cardiac disease in the newborn period?

A hyperoxic test can be very helpful In the evaluation of cyanosis in the newborn period. It differentiates between cardiac and respiratory causes of cyanosis. The infant breathes 100% oxygen via face mask for 15 minutes. If the post-ductal arterial blood gas oxygen concentration rises above 33 kPa, then cyanotic CHD is extremely unlikely.

(continued)

INVESTIGATIONS (*cont.*)

What information can be obtained from an electrocardiogram?

An electrocardiogram is not diagnostic, but it can provide useful additional information and is considered by many to be an essential component of the cardiac examination. Electrocardiography should not be used as a screening test for CHD.

- Superior axis (−0 to −180°): AVSD, tricuspid atresia, Ebstein's anomaly, Noonan's syndrome, AVSD and tetralogy of Fallot
- Long PR interval: AVSD
- Right ventricular hypertrophy: large VSD, AVSD, Tetralogy of Fallot, pulmonary stenosis
- Left ventricular hypertrophy: aortic stenosis, coarctation of the aorta, PDA, VSD

When should an echocardiogram (ECHO) be performed?

All children with suspected CHD should have an ECHO performed under the supervision of a paediatric cardiologist. An ECHO provides information about cardiac anatomy and defects, the presence of shunting, ventricular function and size.

What information is provided by cardiac catheterisation?

Cardiac catheterisation provides good definition of vascular anatomy and enables assessment of haemodynamics. However, the procedure is invasive and exposes children to ionising radiation. Diagnostic catheterisation is not indicated in the routine preoperative evaluation of most congenital defects. Therefore, diagnostic cardiac catheterisation is used in circumstances in which the anatomy is still ill-defined after non-invasive measures, including cardiac magnetic resonance imaging, have been used.

Normal pressures and saturations:
- right atrium, 4 mmHg, 65%
- right ventricle, 25/4 mmHg, 65%
- pulmonary artery, 25/15 mmHg, 65%
- left atrium, 6 mmHg, 99%
- left ventricle, 75/6 mmHg (age dependent) 98%
- aorta, 75/50 (age dependent) 97%.

MANAGEMENT PLAN: TWO-STEP APPROACH

1. Clarifying and pitfall avoidance strategies:
   a) parents
   b) doctor
2. Medical management of specific conditions

Clarifying and pitfall avoidance strategies

Parents

- Parental anxiety and cardiac murmurs. **Rationale:** many parents are anxious when their child is diagnosed with a cardiac murmur. Determine whether it is innocent or indicative of a cardiac defect. Put in place an action plan for diagnosis if unsure.
- Language use and murmurs. **Rationale:** parents are not medically trained and do not have detailed knowledge of anatomy; therefore, terms such as 'a hole in the

heart' may be understood as exactly that. Don't assume that parents know what this colloquial term means (use the phrase 'connection between the pumping chambers of the heart'). If the child has a major heart defect, the breaking bad news strategy should be used (see Chapter 2: Communication) and specific pitfalls related to cardiology avoided (see Evidence 2).

- Explaining what is a murmur. **Rationale**: for innocent murmurs indicate that the circulating blood causes minor vibrations that generate the noise that is audible as a murmur.
- Teaching parents about congenital heart disease. **Rationale**: parents of children with cyanotic heart disease will need to be educated on (a) the warning signs of clinical deterioration, (b) when to contact their doctor, (c) accurate medication administration and (d) feeding regimens, especially if nasogastric feeding is being used. For infants, feeding is their equivalent of exercise and if they are feeding poorly it may indicate early cardiac failure or an associated illness.
- Supporting parents of children with CHD. **Rationale**: parents of children will need to liaise with their cardiac centre, usually through the cardiology clinical nurse specialist.

Doctor

- Communicating with parents. **Pitfall**: children with CHD (see Evidence 2).
- Newborn assessment with oximetry. **Rationale**: see Evidence 1.
- Chest pain in children. **Rationale**: chest pain is common in children and parents will be concerned that it is cardiac in origin. This is rarely the case (see Evidence 3).
- Problem-solving organic murmurs. **Pitfall**: missing organic heart disease is a challenge for the doctor but useful strategies are available (see Evidence 4).
- Innocent murmurs. **Pitfall**: during clinical examination it should be possible to determine if the murmur is innocent utilising change in posture; however, if the murmur never changes, do not assume that it is innocent just because the child has no symptoms.
- Recognising congestive heart failure early. **Pitfall**: difficulty feeding, feeding slower than usual or fast breathing with respiratory distress are early features of congestive cardiac failure. Always count the respiratory rate and pulse rate.
- Value of palivizumab in children with cyanotic CHD. **Rationale**: children with cyanotic CHD benefit from palivizumab administration (see Evidence 5).
- Antibiotic prophylaxis. **Rationale**: this will be dependent on the cardiac lesion.
- Monitor growth. **Rationale**: height and weight need to be monitored on an ongoing basis.
- Awareness of learning disabilities. **Rationale**: while outcomes in surgery are improving, there needs to be an increased awareness of the disabilities that may occur in children with complex CHD (see Evidence 6).

Medical management of specific conditions

Medical management of congenital heart defects is directed toward prevention of heart failure, prevention of pulmonary vascular disease and optimisation of growth and development. Heart failure treatment options include diuretics, angiotensin-converting enzyme inhibitors, angiotensin receptor blockers, aldosterone antagonists, digoxin and propranolol. In severe heart failure inotropic support (dopamine, dobutamine, adrenalin and milrinone) may be required. Growth and calorific intake should be closely monitored. High-calorie supplements are often required, with some children needing continuous or intermittent nasogastric or percutaneous endoscopic gastrostomy feeds.

To maintain patency of the ductus arteriosus in the newborn period, intravenous prostaglandin is administered and titrated according to affect.

Ventricular septal defect

A significant number of small VSDs close spontaneously in the first 2 years, and 80% of muscular VSDs close spontaneously. If a VSD occurs with associated heart failure, then high-caloric feeds and diuretics (frusemide and spironolactone) are indicated. Surgical closure is indicated for large VSD where medical treatment has failed or if there is evolving pulmonary hypertension. The prognosis for VSDs is excellent.

Atrial septal defect

Eighty per cent of small secundum defects (3–8 mm) close spontaneously by 18 months of age. If closure is required, the majority is achieved by patch repair. Isolated ostium primum ASD requires elective surgical repair (because of valve involvement) between 2 and 5 years of age. Sinus venosum defects require surgical repair because of anomalous pulmonary veins. An AVSD requires initial nutritional and diuretic therapy and corrective surgery at around 4 months of age. Mitral regurgitation or complete heart block is a post-operative sequela in 5%–10% of cases.

Patent ductus arteriosus

A very small PDA may close spontaneously and require no treatment. For preterm infants with PDA, initial therapy is fluid restriction and prostaglandin synthetase inhibitors such as indomethacin or ibuprofen. These agents achieve closure in 60% of cases. If the duct persists and the child is symptomatic, surgical ligation is indicated. Older children with PDA have a transcatheter occlusion.

Pulmonary stenosis

Many cases require no treatment but do require close follow-up to detect signs of progression. Children with moderate to severe stenosis require treatment, which can be performed electively. Balloon dilatation is the treatment of choice in all age groups when the gradient across the pulmonary valve reaches 60 mmHg. Re-stenosis may occur, requiring further dilatation.

Aortic stenosis

Strenuous activity should be avoided in moderate to severe aortic stenosis. Serial echocardiography to monitor progress is reasonable if asymptomatic. A Doppler gradient of over 70 mmHg is a commonly used threshold for intervention. Options include balloon valvuloplasty, valvotomy or valve replacement.

Coarctation of the aorta

If presenting in the neonatal or post-neonatal period, urgent cardiology referral is indicated. Infusion of prostaglandin E2 should be commenced to maintain ductal patency. Surgical repair involves either a subclavian flap repair or resection with an end-to-end anastomosis. Lifelong blood pressure monitoring is required to detect re-coarctation or residual stenosis. Options include further surgical repair, balloon angioplasty or the insertion of an endovascular stent.

Tetralogy of Fallot

Hypercyanotic spells require immediate treatment with oxygen. The infant should be placed in the knee-to-chest position to push blood from the inferior vena cava into the right ventricle and out of the pulmonary artery. Morphine sulphate is given to relieve pain and fear and propranolol is given to relax the spasm. Corrective surgery is usually performed at 6 months of age; however, some children may require an initial Blalock–Taussig shunt to increase pulmonary blood flow. During surgery the VSD is closed and the right ventricular outflow tract is reconstructed and the aorta is redirected into the left ventricle. One-year survival is over 98%.

Transposition of the great arteries

Children who present with cyanosis and circulatory collapse need immediate resuscitation, correction of metabolic acidosis and commencement of prostaglandins. Balloon atrial septostomy may also be required. Arterial switch operation is usually undertaken in the first 2 weeks of life and this procedure has a 98% 1-year survival.

Total anomalous pulmonary venous drainage

Surgical intervention is required for all types of TAPVD. The basic concept of TAPVD repair is to redirect pulmonary venous blood flow into the left atrium. The mortality rate is 10%–15%.

Truncus arteriosus

Early surgery is indicated to prevent pulmonary vascular disease. Surgical repair involves separating the pulmonary arteries from the main truncus, closing the VSD with a patch and creating a conduit between the right ventricle and the pulmonary artery. The mortality rate is 10%. The conduit will have to be replaced during childhood as the child grows.

Tricuspid atresia

Prostaglandin E2 infusion and balloon atrial septostomy are performed if severe cyanosis in the newborn period. A Blalock–Taussig shunt is then performed, followed later by a Fontan procedure (redirection of blood flow from the inferior vena cava to the right pulmonary artery with then functionally a univentricular heart).

Hypoplastic left heart syndrome

In cases where an antenatal diagnosis has been made, to maintain patency of the ductus arteriosus, prostaglandin should be commenced immediately after birth. Where an antenatal diagnosis has not been made, neonates presenting with circulatory collapse should be resuscitated and commenced on prostaglandins. Surgical management of hypoplastic left heart syndrome involves three stages. The Norwood procedure is performed in the newborn period. The right ventricle is converted into the main ventricle for both the pulmonary and systemic circulation. A Blalock–Taussig shunt or Sano shunt is created to shunt blood to the pulmonary circulation. If coarctation is present, it is corrected. Post Norwood, children's oxygen saturations are usually 70%–80%. Aspirin is given to prevent stent thrombosis. Children have a 75% survival rate at this time. At 3–5 months of age, a Glenn procedure is performed when circulation through the lungs no longer requires high ventricular pressure. The shunt is taken down and the superior vena cava is connected directly to the pulmonary circulation. The final stage takes place 18–36 months after the Glenn. The inferior vena cava is connected to the pulmonary circulation. At this stage, all deoxygenated blood flows passively into the lungs, so there is no mixing of oxygenated and deoxygenated blood.

FOLLOW-UP

- Innocent murmurs do not require follow-up.
- Children with CHD will require review depending on the lesion type.

WHEN TO REFER?

- Red flags in the history or examination
- Cyanosis
- Urgent referral in the newborn period for children at risk of haemodynamic compromise
- Timely referral of children with suspected CHD based on the underlying suspected defect, risk of potential haemodynamic compromise, mortality and morbidity

CLARIFICATION STATEMENTS FOR PARENTAL MISCONCEPTIONS

'I understand that the murmur is innocent, but I really think he needs further tests to make sure that there isn't a problem.'

If the murmur has been reviewed by a paediatrician and deemed to be innocent and if no red flag symptoms or signs are evident then it is reasonable to observe. The vast majority of murmurs heard in healthy asymptomatic children are innocent.

'If he didn't have a murmur or any signs at birth, how can it be called a congenital defect?'

Many children with CHD do not have signs or symptoms at birth. This does not mean that the defect was not present. Children develop symptoms over time as their circulation develops and adapts to life outside of the womb.

'What do you mean by a hole in the heart? Is blood flowing out of this hole?'

This term is use to indicate a connection between the two pumping chambers of the heart, which are usually separate. It is a poor choice of words especially if discussion is taking place in the absence of a diagram of the heart.

SUMMARY PRACTICE POINTS

- With the exception of the venous hum, murmurs are all systolic in timing.
- Innocent murmurs are louder with fever.
- Pansystolic murmurs are organic in aetiology.
- Very large VSDs may have a soft murmur (often weight gain is poor).
- Recurrent infection with a murmur should prompt referral.
- Carefully record respiratory rates in children with murmurs.
- All newborns require pulse oximetry prior to discharge from hospital.
- Children with CHD have a high incidence of learning difficulties.
- Chest pain is rarely attributed to heart disease in children.

EVALUATING THE EVIDENCE

Evidence 1	
Theme E1	*Detection of congenital heart disease*
Question	How effective is pulse oximetry in detecting critical congenital heart disease?
Design	Cohort study
Level of evidence	
Setting	Six maternity units, England
Participants	Asymptomatic infants born at >34 weeks' gestation were eligible for inclusion, including babies in whom a mid-trimester ultrasonography suggested congenital heart disease.
Intervention	Pulse oximetry assessments were undertaken on the upper and lower limbs on all asymptomatic infants; repeat testing was done when the physical examination was unremarkable. Criteria for abnormal results included oxygen saturations <95% in either extremity or a difference of 2% between the two. The reference standard was echocardiography for all infants who had abnormal results. Echocardiography results were classified as normal, not significant, significant, serious and critical.
Outcomes	The primary outcome was the sensitivity and specificity of pulse oximetry in the detection of critical congenital heart defects (causing death or requiring invasive intervention before 28 days) or major congenital heart disease (causing death or requiring invasive intervention within 12 months of age).
Main results	Of the 20055 babies screened, 53 had major congenital heart disease (24 critical), giving a prevalence of 2.6 per 1000 live births. The sensitivity of pulse oximetry was 75% (95% confidence interval (CI): 53.3–90.2) for critical cases and 49.06% (95% CI: 35.06–63.2) for all major congenital heart defects. If the 35 cases already suspected from antenatal assessment were excluded, the sensitivity was reduced to 58.33% (95% CI: 27.67–84.83) for critical cases and to 28.75% (95% CI: 14.64–46.3) for all major defects. The false positive results occurred in 169 (0.8%) and the specificity was 99.16% (95% CI: 99.02–99.28). Of the false positive results, six had significant congenital heart disease and 40 others required medical intervention.
Conclusion	Pulse oximetry is a safe test, easy to use and adds to existing screening tests for congenital heart disease. It identifies cases that are missed with antenatal ultrasonography thus allowing for earlier intervention.
Commentary	In the newborn period the cardiovascular system undergoes adaptive changes. The symptoms of potentially serious cardiac disease may be absent and examination may be normal. Pulse oximetry offers a useful method to aid detection of infants with potentially serious congenital heart disease. The authors of this study utilised a 2% difference in oxygen saturations as being clinically relevant; others studies that have used a 3% difference reduced the false positive rate to 0.17%. The five-scale characterisation of results is clinically useful.
Reference	Ewer AK, Middleton LJ, Furmston AT, *et al.* Pulse oximetry screening for congenital heart defects in newborn infants (PulseOx): a test accuracy study. *Lancet.* 2011; **378**(9793): 785–94.

Evidence 2	
Theme E2	*Breaking bad news about infants with congenital heart disease*
Question	How do paediatric cardiologists (PCs) communicate the diagnosis of congenital heart disease (CHD) to parents?
Design	Online survey
Level of evidence	
Setting	Community-based survey
Participants	Parents of children with CHD were eligible for inclusion (provided they were members of online support groups).
Intervention	Parents or guardians completed an 82-question survey relating to quantitative and qualitative questions regarding the parents' experience at the time of the diagnosis of CHD.
Outcomes	The primary outcome was the parental recall of 'their breaking bad news experience'.
Main results	Of the 1001 responses received, 31 did not meet the eligibility criteria and 129 were incomplete, so 841 responses were analysed. At the time of the survey the subjects with CHD ranged in age from <1 year to >30 years; however, 63% were younger than 6 years. Seventy-three respondents reported their child had died and in 66% of cases this was related to hypoplastic left heart syndrome. The most commonly reported diagnoses were hypoplastic left heart syndrome (25%), tetralogy of Fallot (12%), transposition of the great vessels (9%) and ventricular septal defect (5%). In their first PC consultation parents received the following information: treatment options (75%), written information (63%), survival data (29%), Internet resources (29%), outcome data for different centres (16%) and support group information (14%). Approximately 25% would have liked more information at the time of diagnosis. The biggest stressors for parents related to uncertainty about the future for their child (87%). Specific issues raised included use of the word 'rare' by the PC to the parents. This was interpreted by 27% as 'few or no others alive with this condition' and by 25% as 1 per 1 000 000. Twenty-six per cent of parents requested a second opinion; this was inversely related to the parents' perception of the PC's compassion. They were also influenced if (a) they were not optimistic about their child's prognosis, (b) if they felt pressured to terminate the pregnancy and (c) if told their child's condition was rare.
Conclusion	Parental perceptions are influenced by the demeanour and counselling approach adopted by the PC when outlining the diagnosis of CHD to parents. From this initial experience their perceptions and decision management strategies are shaped.
Commentary	This study is based on parental recall of receiving a diagnosis of CHD in their child. This is a seismic event that changes their lives, and delivering such news must be done in a sensitive fashion. The parents' perception of the event will influence their future actions with regard to management. Data provided from this study that specific words, e.g. 'rare', caused anxiety, and physician characteristics were important. Breaking bad news is part of paediatric practice; however, utilising a 'log of lessons' concept should be employed, where the team reviews potential pitfalls before discussions with the parents take place.

(continued)

Evidence 2	
Theme E2	*Breaking bad news about infants with congenital heart disease*
Commentary *(cont.)*	This log then becomes the basis for teaching the skill to new trainees and reducing the distress experienced by families.
Reference	Hilton-Kamm D, Sklansky M, Chang RK. How not to tell parents about their child's new diagnosis of congenital heart disease: an Internet survey of 841 parents. *Pediatr Cardiol.* Epub 2013 Aug 8.

Evidence 3	
Theme E3	*Chest pain (CP) outcome in children and adolescents*
Question	What is the outcome for children and adolescents who develop CP?
Design	Cohort study
Level of evidence	
Setting	Department of cardiology, children's hospital, the United States
Participants	The medical records of children >6 years of age with an International Classification of Diseases-9 code CP, attending a children's hospital over a 10-year period, were reviewed.
Intervention	This was an observational study to determine the outcome of children and adolescents with CP over a median period of 4 years.
Outcomes	The primary outcome was deaths related to cardiac aetiologies. The secondary outcomes related to the clinical history at presentation and the aetiologies of CP.
Main results	Of the 3700 patients reviewed, the median age was 13.4 years. Symptoms at presentation included pain on exertion (33%), palpitations (22%), dyspnoea (16%), dizziness (11%) and syncope (1.3%). Abnormal physical findings were few and included ejection clicks (1.4%) and pectus excavatum (1.1%). Ventricular hypertrophy was found in (2.5%). Thirty-eight per cent of patients had echocardiography, with an anomaly rate of 0.8%. Twenty-seven patients had cardiovascular magnetic resonance imaging, with two being abnormal. The aetiology of the CP was musculoskeletal (36%), pulmonary (7%), gastrointestinal (3%), anxiety (1%), cardiac (1%) and unknown (52%). Of the 37 cardiac aetiologies, 14 had supraventricular tachycardia, 10 had pericarditis, 4 had myocarditis, 3 had anomalous right coronary artery, 2 had cardio inhibitory syncope and 1 each had dilated cardiomyopathy, ectopic atrial tachycardia, and non-sustained ventricular tachycardia. There were three deaths: two from suicide and one from fatal retroperitoneal haemorrhage. All three had normal cardiac evaluations. Eighteen per cent of children had attended the emergency department with CP.
Conclusion	CP in children and adolescents rarely has a cardiac cause and of those discharged from the clinic, none had died after 4 years of follow up.
Commentary	This large study adds weight to the view that CP rarely has a cardiac cause discerned, but is a significant cause of parental anxiety and leads to extensive investigation. Children or adolescents who have exertional dyspnoea, concerning medical or family histories, abnormal cardiac examinations or abnormal electrocardiograms should be investigated further.

(continued)

Evidence 3	
Theme E3	*Chest pain (CP) outcome in children and adolescents*
Commentary (*cont.*)	Cardiac sudden death has an incidence of 0.6–6.2/100 000 and these are related to hypertrophic obstructive cardiomyopathy, coronary artery anomalies or from arrhythmias.
Reference	Saleeb SF, Li WY, Warren SZ, *et al.* Effectiveness of screening for life-threatening chest pain in children. *Pediatrics.* 2011; 128(5): e1062–8.

Evidence 4	
Theme E4	*Assessing cardiac murmurs*
Question	Do general paediatricians accurately assess cardiac murmurs in children?
Design	Cohort study
Level of evidence	
Setting	Outpatient department, academic medical centre, Canada
Participants	General paediatricians were invited to evaluate a mixed population of children with cardiac murmurs both innocent and organic. Patients included had either an innocent murmur or a simple asymptomatic cardiac lesion as assessed by a consultant cardiologist and confirmed by echocardiography.
Intervention	The paediatricians performed a clinical assessment, limited to praecordial palpation and auscultation, on five to nine patients and recorded their assessments on standardised collection sheets. Afterward, they received a formal didactic teaching session on clinical skills to assess cardiac murmurs in the outpatient department.
Outcomes	The primary outcome was the sensitivity and specificity in differentiating cardiac murmurs and was calculated for each paediatrician. For patients evaluated by the same paediatrician, inter-rater reliability agreement was calculated.
Main results	Thirty (80%) of the office-based paediatricians contacted agreed to participate in the study. Thirty-seven children were assessed: 21 innocent murmurs and 16 asymptomatic cardiac lesions, which included ventricular septal defect (5), pulmonary valve stenosis (4), aortic valve stenosis (3), sub-aortic stenosis (2), bicuspid aortic valve (1) and mitral valve regurgitation (1). Correct classification was achieved for 142 (74%) of observations. The mean sensitivity was 82 (standard deviation: 24%) and mean specificity was 72 (standard deviation: 24%). The confidence in diagnosis was as follows: 2% entirely confident, 18% very confident, 45% confident, 32% unsure and 4% very unsure. The inter-rater reliability was poor (kappa statistic of 0.05), which indicates the significant disagreement in the clinical assessments that occurred between paediatricians.
Conclusion	The diagnostic accuracy of clinical assessment of heart murmurs, by office-based paediatricians, is suboptimal, and educational strategies are required to remedy this situation.
Commentary	The results are concerning, as it implies that 18% of patients with an organic murmur will be misdiagnosed and 28% of those with innocent murmurs would be referred for cardiac assessment. The challenge for the paediatrician is to diagnose children with organic disease.

(*continued*)

Evidence 4	
Theme E4	***Assessing cardiac murmurs***
Commentary (*cont.*)	The following data are useful for that assessment: pansystolic murmur (odds ratio (OR) = 54), grade 3 murmur (OR = 4.8), murmur heard best at left upper border (OR = 4.2), harsh quality of murmur (OR = 2.4), abnormal second sound (OR = 4.1) and early midsystolic click (OR = 8.4).
Reference	Haney I, Ipp M, Feldman W, *et al.* Accuracy of clinical assessment of heart murmurs by office based (general practice) paediatricians. *Arch Dis Child.* 1999; **81**(5): 409–12.

Evidence 5	
Theme E5	***Palivizumab in congenital heart disease (CHD)***
Question	How effective is palivizumab in the reduction of hospitalisation of children with CHD with respiratory syncytial virus (RSV) infection?
Design	Randomised controlled trial
Level of evidence	Jadad 5
Setting	Multi-centre trial, the United States, Canada, Sweden, Germany, Poland, France, the United Kingdom
Participants	Children, <24 months of age, with documented CHD (either partially treated or unoperated) were eligible for inclusion. Children with unstable cardiac or respiratory status, including cardiac defects so severe that survival was not expected, or for whom cardiac transplantation was planned, were excluded.
Intervention	Children were randomised (1:1) to receive either palivizumab (15 mg/kg) or an equal volume of placebo by intramuscular injection every 30 days for a total of five doses.
Outcomes	The primary outcome was antigen-confirmed RSV hospitalisation.
Main results	A total of 1287 children were randomised, 639 to the palivizumab group and 648 to the placebo group. Overall 90.3% of the children in the palivizumab group and 91.8% of those in the placebo group received all five planned injections. Sixty-three (9.7%) of the placebo group and 34 (5.3%) of the palivizumab group were hospitalised because of RSV infection (absolute risk reduction (ARR) = 4.4%; number needed to treat (NNT) = 23). The number of intensive care admissions was 24 (3.7%) for the placebo group and 13 (2.0%) for the Palivizumab group (ARR = 1.7%; NNT = 58). Twenty-one (3.3%) of the palivizumab group and 27 (4.2%) of the placebo group died. No deaths were attributed to the palivizumab.
Conclusion	Palivizumab was safe, was tolerated in children with CHD and effective in reducing the frequency of RSV infection in a high-risk population (relative risk reduction = 45%).
Commentary	For the practising paediatrician having a treatment that reduces the rate of admission from 9.3% to 5.3% (45% reduction) is significant both in terms of improved patient health and reduction in acute healthcare costs.

(*continued*)

Evidence 5	
Theme E5	***Palivizumab in congenital heart disease (CHD)***
Commentary (*cont.*)	Palivizumab is safe and effective. Indications for palivizumab include 1) haemo-dynamically significant congenital heart disease, 2) chronic lung disease, 3) premature infants ≤ 28 weeks and 6 days gestation and 4) infants with a significant congenital anomaly of the airway or neuromuscular conditions that compromise the handling of respiratory secretions. Other indications may be added to this list with time.
Reference	Feltes TF, Cabalka AK, Meissner HC, *et al.*; Cardiac Synagis Study Group. Palivizumab prophylaxis reduces hospitalization due to respiratory syncytial virus in young children with hemodynamically significant congenital heart disease. *J Pediatr.* 2003; **143**(4): 532–40.

Evidence 6	
Theme E6	***Outcome of congenital heart disease***
Question	What is the outcome for neonates with complete transposition of the great arteries (TGA)?
Design	Prospective cohort study
Level of evidence	
Setting	Centres attached to the Congenital Heart Surgeons' Society Data Center, Toronto, Canada
Participants	Neonates younger than 15 days and admitted with TGA to one of the 24 Congenital Heart Surgeons' Society Data Centres were eligible for enrolment.
Intervention	Treatment was not assigned or randomised but was selected by the physician caring for the infant. Options available were (a) arterial switch, (b) atrial repair (either Senning or Mustard repair) or (c) Rastelli repair.
Outcomes	The primary outcomes were long-term survival, re-intervention rates, re-operations, pacemaker implantation, functional assessment and psychosocial deficits.
Main results	Twenty-four institutions entered 829 patients (TGA (n = 631), TGA with ventricular septal defect (TGA+VSD) (n = 167), TGA+VSD+pulmonary stenosis (n = 30) and TGA+pulmonary stenosis (n = 1)). Repair was by arterial switch (n = 516), atrial repair (Senning = 175; Mustard = 110) or Rastelli (n = 28). Survival rates were 85% at 6 months and 81% at 15 years. One hundred and sixty-seven had a re-intervention. Seventy-six per cent, at 15 years were asymptomatic (class 1), 22% had mild limitation of activity or on one medication (class 11) and 2% had moderate symptoms or on more than one medication. However, 31% reported their children to have learning disabilities, 13% reported behavioural problems, 12% reported hyperactivity and 3% reported cerebral palsy.
Conclusion	Survival after surgery for TGA is good and most children had a functional outcome that is commensurate to their peers. The adverse neurodevelopment outcome needs to be addressed.
Commentary	This study does not reflect current practice, as today neonates with a simple TGA or TGA+VSD are managed by arterial switch.

(*continued*)

Evidence 6	
Theme E6	*Outcome of congenital heart disease*
Commentary (*cont.*)	This study was undertaken in an era of transition from the atrial switch and its associated learning curve. While children will do well from a cardiac perspective the general paediatrician needs to be aware of the high risk of learning disabilities in these children, and in conjunction with the school services, should ensure that appropriate educational resources are provided.
Reference	Williams WG, McCrindle BW, Ashburn DA, et al.; Congenital Heart Surgeons' Society. Outcomes of 829 neonates with complete transposition of the great areteries 12–17 years after repair. *Eur J Cardiothorac Surg.* 2003; **24**(1): 1–9; discussion 9–10.

HEART DISEASE: MULTIPLE-CHOICE QUESTIONS

Q1 Which of the following statements is/are correct?
   a) In Down's syndrome, 40%–50% have congenital heart disease.
   b) Turner's syndrome is associated with coarctation of the aorta.
   c) Noonan's syndrome is associated with tetralogy of Fallot.
   d) Foetal alcohol syndrome is associated with VSDs.
   e) Williams's syndrome is associated with supravalvular stenosis.

Q2 Which of the following are features of Still's murmur?
   a) Most common between 2 and 5 years of age
   b) Increases in intensity on standing
   c) Located at the upper sternal border
   d) Associated with a thrill in 10% of children
   e) Vibratory in quality

Q3 Which of the following statements regarding a venous hum are correct?
   a) Heard at the apex
   b) Heard inferior to the clavicles
   c) It is a pansystolic murmur
   d) Best heard with the child sitting
   e) Best heard when the child is standing

Q4 Which of the following statements relating to a VSD is/are true?
   a) Very large VSDs have loud murmurs.
   b) Small VSDs have loud murmurs.
   c) VSDs become prominent when pulmonary vascular resistance rises.
   d) Small VSDs are associated with normal height but reduced weight gain.
   e) VSDs usually have pansystolic murmurs.

Q5   Which of the following statements relating to a PDA is/are correct?
   a) The patent ductus normally closes by 8 hours after birth.
   b) Failure of the PDA to close occurs in more than 25% of 1500 g infants.
   c) In a PDA a machinery murmur is audible below the right clavicle.
   d) Failure of the PDA to close can lead to failure to thrive.
   e) Peripheral pulses are bounding in an infant with a PDA.

Q6   Which of the following statements relating to AS is/are correct?
   a) The vast majority of children with AS are asymptomatic.
   b) Chest pain is a recognised presentation of AS.
   c) The second sound in AS is soft.
   d) Ejection clicks at the apex are heard in AS.
   e) Ten per cent of children with AS present with cyanosis and fatigue.

Q7   Features of tetralogy of Fallot include which of the following?
   a) VSD
   b) Left ventricular hypertrophy
   c) Subvalvular aortic stenosis
   d) Overriding aorta
   e) Clubbing

Q8   Features of TGA include which of the following?
   a) Cyanosis
   b) Loud pansystolic murmur
   c) Loud second heart sound
   d) Soft second heart sound
   e) Congestive heart failure

Q9   Which of the following is/are correct in regard to cardiac silhouettes?
   a) 'Egg on its side' is a feature of TGA
   b) 'Boot shape' appearance in tetralogy of Fallot
   c) 'Snowman' in total anomalous pulmonary venous drainage
   d) 'Box shape' appearance in Ebstein's anomaly
   e) 'Rosary' appearance in coarctation of the aorta

Q10 Features of organic murmurs include which of the following?
   a) Pansystolic murmurs
   b) Diastolic murmur
   c) Reduced femoral pulses
   d) Active praecordium
   e) Cyanosis

Answers

A1	a, b, d, e	**A2**	e
A3	b, c, d	**A4**	b, e
A5	b, e	**A6**	a, b, c, d
A7	a, d, e	**A8**	a, d, e
A9	a, b, c, d	**A10**	a, b, c, d, e

SLIDE

1. Edward's syndrome

Chapter Nineteen

RECURRENT HEADACHES IN CHILDREN

COMMON SCENARIO

'She's 11, and over the past 3 months she's started to have these headaches. Maybe two or three times a week and they're always quite bad. She's missed about 6 days of school by now, which is a pity because she's doing really well. She's always top of the class and into everything that's going: gymnastics, dance and guitar. Her aunt had a brain haemorrhage last year and we're very worried.'

LEARNING OBJECTIVES

- Know the potential aetiologies of recurrent headaches
- Understand the diagnostic criteria for migraine, migraine with aura and tension headache
- Understand the 'red flags' in the history and physical examination and their clinical significance
- Know the indications for headache neuroimaging
- Be able treat acute migraine
- Understand the principles of chronic migraine treatment

BACKGROUND

Most recurrent headaches in children and adolescents are due to either migraine or tension headaches. As adult definitions of migraine do not always apply in children, there may be a continuum between migraine and tension headaches. In most cases, a careful history taking and examination can rule out any potentially serious underlying pathology. Reassurance is extremely important. Treatment should focus on lifestyle modification, the identification and removal of trigger factors and simple analgesia. Investigations such as electroencephalography and computed tomography (CT) or magnetic resonance imaging (MRI) are rarely indicated.

DIFFERENTIAL DIAGNOSIS

Differential diagnosis of recurrent headache	Features
Migraine	Migraine with aura
	Migraine without aura
	Migraine syndromes
Headache	Tension headache
	Cluster headaches
	Chronic daily headaches
Ophthalmological (refraction errors)	Refraction errors
Raised intracranial pressure	Hydrocephalus and blocked shunt
	Brain tumours or space-occupying lesion
	Post-traumatic
	Idiopathic intracranial hypertension
Infections	Meningitis
	Sinusitis
	Otitis media
Vascular	Intracranial bleed
	Venous sinus thrombosis
Secondary to drugs/toxins	Carbon monoxide
	Analgesia
	Caffeine
	Marijuana and cocaine

Migraine and its variants

Migraine affects 3%–10% of children. Twenty per cent may experience their first attack prior to 5 years of age. The incidence increases steadily with age, affecting boys and girls equally before puberty, and girls more commonly thereafter. Migraine is characterised by episodes of head pain that is always throbbing and frequently unilateral frontal or temporal in position. Pallor is a prominent feature and the child may be described as being 'ghostly pale'. Most children with significant migraine stop what they are doing and go to a darkened room, lie down and fall asleep. The headache is often gone on awakening. Headache due to migraine lasts over 3 hours and <72 hours (*status migrainous* is >72 hours in duration and needs emergency management). Acute migraine is of relatively sudden onset, and can occur with or without a prodrome – also known as aura.

In *migraine without aura* (or common migraine), attacks are associated with nausea, vomiting or sensitivity to light, sound or movement. Up to 15% of patients suffer from *migraine with aura* (or classic migraine). In these patients migraine is preceded by transient focal neurologic symptoms, which are commonly visual (scotoma, fortification spectra) and resolve with the onset of head pain. Some children experience derealisation phenomena such as macropsia-micropsia – this is also known as 'Alice in Wonderland syndrome'.

There are various types of migraine syndromes described. When the neurological symptoms and signs associated with migraine appear after the headache onset (Horner's syndrome, hemifield deficits), this is referred to as transformation migraine. In ophthalmoplegic migraine there is often ptosis and a divergent squint, which may last for over 24 hours. Hemiplegic migraine is rare and often familial. The hemiplegia state may outlast the headache, but rarely lasts more than 6–12 hours. Basilar migraine is characterized by dizziness and vertigo as predominant features. It is relatively short-lived and may occasionally be associated with bilateral transient visual loss.

Triggers

Triggers for migraine include stress, fasting, sleep deprivation and extremes of activity. Food triggers may sometimes be identified and it may be useful to keep a record of what is eaten just prior to a headache to see if a consistent pattern emerges. Common triggers include nuts, caffeine (including cola drinks), citrus fruits, spiced meats, monosodium glutamate, chocolate and blue cheese. Exercise, especially if associated with competitive sports, may precipitate migraine in some children. Oestrogens and androgens are likely to be responsible for the change in the incidence of migraine seen at, or around puberty.

Outcome of childhood migraine

There are very few long-term studies but it appears that the outcome seems to be better in boys than in girls. Outcome seems to be worse if headaches start before the age of 6 years. Many children with migraine will follow family patterns and thus genetic factors appear important. Migraine does tend to decrease in frequency and severity with age but this may not occur until early middle age has been reached.

Tension headaches

Tension headaches are the other main cause of headache in childhood. Typically they are a response to stress. Tension headaches have a number of characteristics. They tend to be bilateral; they vary in severity and have a pressing or tightening quality. Scalp pain needs to be elicited in the history, suggested by pain on brushing hair and so forth. The triggers for tension headaches may include school bullying, excess extra-curricular activities after school, marital discord, unemployment, death in the family or moving home. Often the family doctor is best equipped to elucidate these triggers. Suggested strategies to reduce tension headaches include:

- look for and correct the cause of stress
- avoid frequent analgesia if possible
- encourage normal school attendance
- clearly explain the non-serious nature of tension headaches to the child
- relaxation exercises, physiotherapy and hypnosis may be helpful.

Brain tumours

Although much feared, brain tumours are relatively infrequent occurrences in child-hood, with an incidence of 3 per 100 000. Children with brain tumours usually have symptoms other than headache alone. Infra-tentorial tumours may present in the absence of headache, with difficulty in walking, confusion, hyperreflexia, cranial nerve palsies and head tilt. Supra-tentorial tumours presenting with a headache may have associated diplopia, poor academic performance, seizures, focal hyperaesthesia of a limb or speech impairment.

It is traditionally taught that the headache of raised intracranial pressure that awakens the child from sleep, is maximal in the morning and improves during the day. While such a history should always trigger concern, the lack of this pattern does not exclude raised intracranial pressure. A progressive headache pattern, indicated by an increased frequency and severity of headaches, suggests serious brain patho-logy. Children with brain tumours may present with a story of initial mild headaches increasing in a crescendo fashion to severe and frequent headaches. The reverse is also true in that headaches recurring over a period longer than 6 months in the absence of other neurological symptoms are rarely due to a brain tumour. The one exception to this rule is a craniopharyngioma, in which there are usually other clues, such as short stature, delayed puberty and visual field defects.

Idiopathic intracranial hypertension

Idiopathic intracranial hypertension is the clinical syndrome of raised intracranial pressure, in the absence of space-occupying or vascular lesions, without enlargement of the cerebral ventricles and for which no causative factor can be identified. It was previously known as benign intracranial hypertension; however, it is now recognised as a malignant phenomenon as it can rapidly lead to irreversible blindness. Idiopathic intracranial hypertension may present with a severe frontal headache that interferes with normal daily activities. The headache may increase in intensity on bending over and is often more frequent in the morning. The patient may also complain of intermit-tent darkening of parts or the whole of their visual fields (transient visual obscuration). Neurological examination is abnormal including papilloedema and optic atrophy on fundoscopy, and at times a sixth nerve palsy. Neuroimaging is normal. Diagnosis is based on history and exam including formal visual field assessment, and lumbar punc-ture demonstrating high opening pressure. Associated factors are obesity, steroids withdrawal, hormonal contraceptive use, some antimicrobial agents, vitamin A, and also venous sinus stenosis. Prompt referral to a tertiary centre is warranted. Treatment options include carbonic anhydrase inhibitors, loop diuretics, fenestration of the optic nerve, high volume lumbar puncture and cerebrospinal fluid shunting.

Sinusitis

Ethmoid and frontal sinusitis may be associated with headache in older children. The headache is usually throbbing, dull and made worse when the child bends over or coughs. Percussion of the sinuses may elicit tenderness. Sinus radiographs and ear, nose and throat referral may be organised.

Hydrocephalus and shunt blockage

In those children with known hydrocephalus who have a ventriculo-peritoneal shunt in situ, shunt malfunction (mechanical or infection) needs to be considered. These headaches are often associated with vomiting, altered consciousness or signs of raised intracranial pressure.

TERMINOLOGY EXPLAINED

Headache studies frequently utilise the International Headache Society's criteria – these are provided for migraine with and without aura and tension headaches in children. The use of these criteria is important to standardise patient recruitment for headache-related studies and to enhance the generalisability of the results.

International Headache Society criteria for paediatric migraine without aura

The diagnostic criteria are as follows.
a) At least five attacks fulfilling the criteria b–d
b) Headache attacks lasting 1–72 hours
c) Headache has at least two of the following characteristics:
1. unilateral location, maybe bilateral, frontotemporal (not occipital)
2. pulsating quality
3. moderate or severe pain intensity
4. aggravation by, or causing avoidance of, routine physical activity (e.g. walking or climbing stairs)
d) During the headache, at least one of the following:
1. nausea and or vomiting
2. photophobia and phonophobia, which may be inferred from behaviour
e) Not attributed to any other disorder

International Headache Society criteria for paediatric migraine with aura

The diagnostic criteria are as follows.
a) At least two attacks fulfilling criteria b–d
b) Aura consists of at least one of the following but no motor weakness:
1. fully reversible visual symptoms including positive features (e.g. flickering lights, spots, lines) and/or negative features (i.e. loss of vision)
2. fully reversible sensory symptoms including positive features (i.e. pins and needles) and/or negative features (i.e. numbness)
3. fully reversible dysphasic speech disturbance
c) At least two of the following:
1. homonymous visual symptoms and/or unilateral sensory symptoms

2. at least one aura symptom develops gradually over 5 minutes and/or different aura symptoms occur in succession over 5 minutes
3. each symptom lasts between 5 and 60 minutes

d) Headache fulfilling criteria b–d for migraine without aura

The migraine with aura begins during the aura or follows the aura within 60 minutes.

International Headache Society criteria for episodic tension-type headache

a) At least 10 episodes fulfilling criteria b–d 2–4
b) Headaches lasting 30 minutes to 7 days
c) Two or more of the following:
1. pressing or tightening quality
2. mild to moderate severity
3. bilateral location
4. not aggravated by routine activity
d) Both of the following:
1. no nausea or vomiting
2. phonophobia or photophobia is absent

HISTORY

A detailed history should be taken from all children presenting with recurrent headaches. This ensures that a child's general health can be ascertained along with any other warning signs that might suggest underlying pathology. Careful history taking and examination and follow-up with a headache diary are key to the proper evaluation of headaches. The history should be elicited from the child initially with parents offering their input afterwards. The history should clarify if all the headaches are the same or if the child is experiencing several types of headaches, e.g. migraine and tension headaches.

KEY POINTS				
Types of headaches	How many types of headaches do you suffer from?			**Q Red flags** Increase in severity or frequency of headaches
Description of headache	Localisation Duration Radiation Relieving factors Aggravating factors	**Precipitants of headache (temporal relationship)**	Particular food Lighting Stress Intense exercise	Behavioural change Frequent or persistent vomiting

(continued)

KEY POINTS				
Associated features	Aura (if child cannot describe the aura, he or she may be able to draw it) Blurred vision Nausea or vomiting Marked pallor Photophobia Seizures	**Relief of headaches**	What medications have been tried? How soon after the headache does the child take analgesia? Do they need to lie down to relieve the headache? Have any dietary changes been made?	**𝗤 Red flags** Persistent early morning headache or headache that wakes child from sleep Excessive analgesia usage Child <4 years of age and those with poor communication skills
Length of symptoms	How long have headaches been present? Have they become more severe? Are they occurring more frequently?	**Impact on life**	Number of school days lost Change in academic performance Change in behaviour Extracurricular activities	
Timing of headaches	Evening or early morning School days or weekends	**Family history**	Migraine Travel sickness Vertigo Epilepsy	
Home environment	Recent changes or stresses in the home	**General health**	Appetite, energy, recent weight loss Previous illnesses	

EXAMINATION

- Measurement of head circumference
- Height and weight percentiles
- Blood pressure measurement
- Skin lesions or birth marks
- Cranial nerve examination, including extraocular movements, fundoscopy, visual acuity and visual fields
- Full neurological examination including gait assessment
- Check for sinus tenderness or pain with head movement

Red flags

- Macrocephaly
- Short stature
- Hypertension
- Signs of raised intracranial pressure
- Neuro-cutaneous signs
- Abnormal neurological examination or visual examination

INVESTIGATIONS

Is it appropriate to perform neuroimaging in order to reassure parents?

Up to 30% of CT/MRI brain scans performed are for parental reassurance. Apart from resource and radiation exposure implications, it is important to stress to parents that early investigation and the finding of a normal CT/MRI scan may give a false sense of reassurance and potentially delay rescanning if the headache characteristics change. It is important to stress to parents that CT brain scans are equivalent in radiation exposure to some 80 chest X-rays and therefore CT should not be performed for reassurance only.

What is the most important diagnostic tool?

The most important diagnostic tool to help determine the cause of headaches is the headache diary. Parents should be asked to keep a diary of the events leading up to the onset of the headache. This can help determine if a specific trigger can be avoided to prevent future headaches.

When is neuroimaging indicated?

In a previously healthy child with headache, criteria for requesting neuroimaging include:
- an accompanying change in personality
- abnormal neurological or visual examination
- frequent or persistent vomiting
- crescendo pattern of headaches
- signs of raised intracranial pressure
- focal and generalised seizures
- nocturnal headache occurrence.

MANAGEMENT PLAN: THREE-STEP APPROACH

1. Clarifying and pitfall avoidance strategies
   a) parents and child
   b) for the doctor
2. Non-pharmacological treatment of headaches:
   a) models of care
   b) cognitive behavioural therapy
   c) self-hypnosis

3. Pharmacological treatment of headaches:
    a) migraine prophylaxis
    b) migraine treatment

Clarifying and pitfall avoidance strategies
Parents and child

- Clarify the parental response to the headache and their perception on headache aetiology. **Rationale**: their response will determine the intensity of the interventions necessary. Previous parental experiences with headache will influence how they view the occurrence of headache in their child.
- Clarify the child or adolescent's response to the headaches. **Rationale**: his or her response to the headaches will determine the intensity of interventions necessary. Encourage the child to be a detective by assessing what triggers or intensifies or improves the pain. Prior to answering these questions, encourage the child to think about the answer. If he or she does not know or is unsure, then a headache diary is useful.
- The vague headache history in children. **Pitfall**: prior to dismissing the history ensure that a headache diary has been kept for at least 3 months. The elements of the headache diary include frequency, duration, intensity, potential triggers and response to medication of the headaches. Be especially cautious in the child under 4 years of age or those children with communication difficulties, as they will be unable to describe their headache; their behaviour or how they hold their head may indicate the presence of headache.
- Headache and the risk of brain tumours. **Rationale**: the parents will have this as a concern. Brain tumours presenting with headaches and the indication for CT of the brain should be clarified as part of every consultation for chronic headache (*see* Clarification statements for parental misconceptions).

For the doctor

- The best first question to ask a child with headache is: *are all the headaches the same?* **Rationale**: this will allow both mixed-pattern headaches (combination of migraine and tension headache) and progressive headaches to be recognised.
- Obtain the history from the child or adolescent. **Rationale**: while parents may want to give the history seek it from the patient. Children aged 7 years and older are often able to give a clear history.
- If the history is unclear, utilise a headache diary. **Rationale**: headache diaries clarify the history.
- Defining the presence of an aura. **Rationale**: children may have difficulties in explaining the 'aura' experience however getting them to draw it is often very effective.
- Define the impact of headache in terms of school loss. **Rationale**: school loss is frequent but the focus with the parent is to determine what does the child do when

absent from school, e.g. does the child go to bed to sleep? Or does he or she watch television? This approach allows the concept of secondary gain to be introduced and often parents will recognise it.

- Ask if the parents can tell if their child has a headache without asking him or her. **Rationale**: with tension headaches children often look well and the headache abates if the child is distracted.
- Define the headache pattern. **Rationale**: classify the headaches as (a) acute, (b) acute recurrent, (c) chronic persistent or (d) chronic progressive. This approach allows for ease in determining therapeutic plans.
- Ensure the impact of medication has been assessed. **Rationale**: if excessive analgesia is ingested then rebound headache may well be occurring. This occurs in adolescents.
- Diet and migraine. **Rationale**: diet and its role in migraine must be part of a full therapeutic approach including normal sleep pattern, absence of fasting and stress reduction techniques. The foods implicated in migraine, are significant for a small percentage of migraineurs and include cheese, chocolate, tinned fruit and monosodium glutamate in Chinese food. If dietary measures are used the following approach should be used: assess frequency of migraine (e.g. one a month), eliminate one food for 3 months and reintroduce it after 3 months for 3 months and determine if any impact (N = 1 study).
- Be clear to indicate sinister headache feature and the indication for neuroimaging. **Rationale**: indications for neuroimaging include (a) headaches that wake the child from sleep, (b) headaches that occur on wakening from sleep, (c) headaches that are associated with confusion or disorientation, (d) headaches that are persistent under 4 years of age, (e) migraine headaches that change in character, (f) persistent vomiting on awakening, (g) papilloedema, (h) optic atrophy, (i) new-onset nystagmus and (j) visual field reduction.
- Be aware of pitfalls in the central nervous system examination. **Rationale**: detailed neurological examination can be time consuming, but the minimum examination should include the following: optic fundus, eye movements, walking and pronator drift.
- Give practical solutions and tools to the child with headache, having made a diagnosis. **Rationale**: empowerment of child and adolescent with headaches should be the goal.

Non-pharmacological treatment of headaches

Models of care

The most common headaches in children and adolescents are migraine and tension headaches. Once a diagnosis has been made specific education pertaining to mechanism, triggering factors and their avoidance must be established. Whether a specific educational module should be established or reliance placed on the doctor to provide the information is uncertain (*see* Evidence 1). Evidence suggests that parents may be well informed regarding headaches in children and adolescence.

At each clinic visit review the headache frequency and intensity. If no changes or improvement have occurred log the headache frequency using a headache diary especially recording the headache intensity (using a visual analogue scale), headache duration and triggers, as headache recall, over a period of months is not reliable. In headaches, where the anticipated outcome does not occur, the doctor should have a low threshold in reconsidering the diagnosis.

Cognitive behavioural therapy

There are two elements to cognitive behavioural therapy: (1) cognitive, how you think, and (2) behavioural, how you respond. Cognitive behavioural therapy addresses the here and now. It has proved very successful as an adjunct to the reduction of headache frequency in children and adolescents. It is well accepted by adolescents, as it provides a specific strategy for them to address their headaches (*see* Evidence 2).

Self-hypnosis

Self-hypnosis is an effective strategy to aid children and adolescents in dealing with headaches. The technique must be practised on a regular basis (daily initially) to ensure the child or adolescent becomes competent in the technique.

Pharmacological treatment of headaches

Migraine prophylaxis

Some patients, especially those with frequent or severe migraine, benefit from prophylactic treatment. Topiramate is effective in the prophylaxis of migraine (*see* Evidence 4). Propanolol and pizotifen are used, but there is an absence of high-quality trials to support their use.

Migraine treatment

The use of analgesia early in the course of migraine has long been known to be effective in acute migraine. Patients should be encouraged to focus on early recognition of symptoms and implement their treatment plan. Analgesia, lying down in their bedroom with curtains drawn, and the avoidance of noise are helpful. Migraine headaches normally abate if the child sleeps. In studies of acute migraine, both triptans and ibuprofen are effective (*see* Evidence 5); however, the high placebo response rate in migraine is unexplained. Sumatriptan therapy plus naproxen sodium in combination has also been shown to be effective in the treatment of migraine in adolescents (*see* Evidence 6). More important, the issue of placebo responders were addressed in the study outlined in Evidence 6.

All patients with a chronic headache should (a) know their diagnosis, (b) understand the triggers and have a specific approach to them and (c) institute their acute headache action plan in a timely fashion (with success rate monitoring). If patients are taking excessive analgesia, they may be experiencing rebound headache but more important, their diagnosis and treatment strategy should be re-evaluated.

FOLLOW-UP

All children with recurrent headache require close follow-up. Children without alarming signs or symptoms who do not need immediate specialist referral should be followed up. Parents should be asked to keep a headache diary. Ongoing education about lifestyle modification and avoidance of trigger factors should continue.

WHEN TO REFER?

- Children who fit the criteria for neuroimaging
- Children with migraine not responding to simple analgesia or requiring prophylactic treatment
- Any child with an abnormal neurological or fundoscopic examination
- Children in whom the headache pattern changes

CLARIFICATION STATEMENTS FOR PARENTAL MISCONCEPTIONS

> *'Her migraine headaches must be food related.'*

Triggers for migraine are multifactorial and if the child or adolescent has a strong temporal relationship between food ingestion and a migraine, then this supports the hypothesis of cause and effect. However, the converse must be proven; avoidance of the trigger must result in an absence or at least a marked reduction in migraine frequency. Headache diaries are valuable in these situations.

> *'She's started getting regular headaches and they've examined her. Now they tell me that everything is normal, but I won't be happy unless they do a brain scan. Why not be absolutely sure?'*

It is hard to be reassured when fears loom large. However, if she has had a full neurological examination and nothing has shown, doctors will not rush to scan or take X-rays. A CT brain scan will beam as much radiation as 80 chest X-rays and can also give a false sense of security. If a CT brain is done early there may not be willingness to repeat the scan again if the headaches start to change. If there is cause for concern, it will show up in the examination and headache pattern. Up to 30% of CT brain scans happen purely to reassure parents, and not because they are needed. A scan is usually advised if a child was previously healthy, now has a headache and has any of these symptoms:

- a personality change
- a neurological and visual examination that is not normal
- frequent vomiting
- a persistent headache that happens when he or she wakes up, or one that wakes the patient from sleep
- persistent vomiting when he or she wakes from sleep
- in a patient with migraine where the pattern changes
- an electroencephalogram (brainwave test) showing focal seizures or focal changes.

'What do you mean the headaches are aggravated by stress? She is a child.'

Children's symptoms of stress may be manifested through headaches, abdominal pain or school avoidance. If the child was aware of the trigger then the stress could be addressed. Parents need to be detectives to discern what the potential triggers are. In the school situation, bullying and learning difficulties should be addressed.

SUMMARY PRACTICE POINTS
- Always review a child with simple headaches 4–6 weeks post initial consultation to see the pattern of headaches using a diary.
- Get expert opinion on any headache with focal features or rapidly changing pattern.
- Assess trigger factors for both migraine and tension headaches.
- The use of neuroimaging for parental reassurance only is unwise.
- Skull and sinus radiographs are generally unhelpful in children with headaches.
- Prompt analgesia and retiring to a quiet, dark room is effective in treating many migraine attacks.
- Sumatriptan may be used selectively in children with severe attacks.
- Migraine prophylaxis is rarely required in childhood but may improve school and social performance when needed.

EVALUATING THE EVIDENCE

Evidence 1	
Theme E1	*Non-pharmacological intervention for headache*
Question	What is the impact of a multidisciplinary approach to headache treatment as opposed to the traditional clinic model (TCM)?
Design	Randomised controlled trial
Level of evidence	Jadad 3
Setting	Paediatric neurology clinic, academic medical centre, the United States
Participants	Participants were children and adolescents 10–18 years of age, in good health, with a history of recurrent primary headaches for a minimum of 2 months.
Intervention	The TCM was a consultation with a paediatric neurologist only. The headache clinic model (HCM) was a 1-hour group psycho-educational session, in a group setting with patients and parents in attendance, divided into two 30-minute sessions, after which they had their neurology consultation. The first half of the educational session, delivered by a neurology nurse, related to headache aetiology (inclusive aggravating factors such as stress), potential investigations and treatment options. The second session, delivered by a psychologist, focused on lifestyle issues, methods of stress reduction inclusive of cognitive behavioural methods and adherence to treatment regimens.
Outcomes	Primary outcomes included difference in headache-related knowledge and reduction in headache-related disability between the two groups, as measured by the Pediatric Migraine Disability Assessment and the Functional Disability Inventory at baseline and at 6 months.
Main results	One hundred and fourteen patients were eligible for enrolment but 33 were excluded, nine did not meet inclusion criteria and 24 declined to participate. Forty were randomised to the TCM and 41 to the HCM. The interval between referral and consultation was 17 days. The aetiology of headaches in the TCM group was migraine, eight (20%); episodic tension, three (7%); mixed-pattern, 23 (58%); and chronic daily, six (15%). In the TCM HCM group the headache aetiology was migraine, 18 (43%); episodic tension, 3 (7%); mixed-pattern, 14 (35%); and chronic daily, 6 (22%). Neuroimaging was performed in 22 (55%) of the TCM group and in 28 (59%) of the HCM group. The headache knowledge pre-test score increased from 14.2 to 15.9 in the TCM group and from 14.0 to 17.7 in the HCM group. A reduction of at least 50% in disability occurred in 63.6% of the TCM group as compared with 54.5% of the HCM group (absolute risk reduction = 8.9%; number needed to treat = 12). Satisfaction levels with both interventions were high (27 out of a possible 30).
Conclusion	Both models provided satisfactory results. The use of the Pediatric Migraine Disability Assessment may have resulted in a bias, as the results show migraineurs were more represented in the TCM group. The time spent in direct patient contact was 30 minutes by the neurologist and given the score of the headache knowledge test the parents must have been well informed.
Commentary	Studies on headaches have indicated a very high placebo effect. The reasons for this are unknown. Both groups of patients were satisfied with the interventions provided in this study.

(*continued*)

Evidence 1	
Theme E1	**Non-pharmacological intervention for headache**
Commentary (*cont.*)	The physician contact time was 27 minutes in the HCM group and 31 minutes in the TCM group and both groups had a high percentage of imaging (55% in the TCM group and 59% in the HCM group). The level of intervention may not be generalisable to a busy general paediatric clinic, but it would appear prudent to develop a headache educational module to bridge the deficit – if it is present in one's clinical practice – given the frequency of headaches in children and adolescents.
Reference	Abram HS, Buckloh LM, Shilling LM, *et al.* A randomized, controlled trial of a neurological and psychoeducational group appointment model for pediatric headaches. *Childrens Health Care.* 2007; **36**(3): 249–65.

Evidence 2	
Theme E2	**Non-pharmacological interventions for headache**
Question	What is the effect of cognitive behavioural therapy (CBT) and applied relaxation (AR) in adolescents with headaches?
Design	Randomised controlled trial
Level of evidence	Jadad 3
Setting	Community setting, Germany
Participants	Participants were children and adolescents aged 10–18 years of age with primary headaches (migraine, tension-type headaches or combined headache), diagnosed by a physician with an occurrence frequency at least two headaches per month. Participants were required to have access to a computer and to read and write German. Patients taking prophylactic medications or receiving psychotherapeutic treatment were excluded.
Intervention	CBT and AR were compared with educational intervention (EDU) accessed online. Each group had the same frequency of e-mail contact with their therapists. The CBT modules online, conducted over 6 weeks, focused on education relating to headaches, stress management and the teaching of progressive relaxation techniques, stress management techniques, enhancing proactive strategies and problem-solving. The AR group focused on self-relaxation, cue-controlled relaxation and differential relaxation. The instructions for CBT and AR were also provided on a CD to the participants as an added aid. The EDU group received education on headaches and these participants were in regular e-mail contact.
Outcomes	The primary outcome was a reduction by 50% (responder rate) in the headache frequency post treatment measured at 6 months and was compared to baseline frequency (pre-intervention phase) using a 4-week diary. The headache frequency, intensity (using a visual analogue score from 0 for no pain to 10 for severe pain) and duration in hours were recorded.
Main results	Eighty-seven patients reported interest in participating in this study, nine did not meet the criteria and ten did not participate. Of the 68 randomised, three did not start the study. Of the 65 who participated, 24 were randomised to CBT, 22 to AR and 19 to EDU.

(continued)

Evidence 2	
Theme E2	***Non-pharmacological interventions for headache***
Main results (*cont.*)	Four in the CBT group dropped out, as two had no motivation, one had migraine when reading and one had no computer. Only 41 participants completed the 6-month follow-up assessment; however, full data sets were not available on all patients. Migraine occurred in 16 (66%) of the CBT group, 13 (60%) of the AR group and 10 (53%) of the EDU group. The mean duration of headaches was 3.6 years in the CBT group, 2.9 years in the AR group and 2 years in the EDU group. At post treatment, 19% (3/16) of the EDU group responded, compared with 63% (10/16) of the CBT group (absolute risk reduction (ARR) = 46%; number needed to treat (NNT) = 3) and 32% (6/19) of the AR group (ARR = 13%; NNT = 8). However, at the 6-month follow-up, 55% (5/9) of the EDU group had responded, compared with 63% (7/11) of the CBT group (ARR = 8%; NNT = 9) and 56% (9/16) of the AR group (ARR = 3%; NNT = 34).
Conclusion	All three groups studied had similar favourable outcomes at the 6-month follow-up.
Commentary	This online programme for children and adolescents with headache was well accepted by participants, with its focus on coping strategies and information; however, the absence of full data is disappointing and would need to be addressed in future studies. While not a primary outcome, both the CBT group and the AR group coped more effectively with their headaches when they occurred, and such strategies are important to improve functioning in the child or adolescent and as an empowerment aid. At the 6-month follow-up (primary outcome) all groups were similar, emphasising the importance of appropriate education for those headache sufferers. Information given to headache sufferers must be accurate and relevant if it is to be effective. The impact of the e-therapists (seven graduate students of clinical psychology) was not explored but they may have an important support role to play in this type of online intervention.
Reference	Trautmann E, Kröner-Herwig B. A randomized controlled trial of Internet-based self-help training for recurrent headache in childhood and adolescence. *Behav Res Ther.* 2010; 48(1): 28–37.

Evidence 3	
Theme E3	***Treatment options in migraine: propranolol or hypnosis?***
Question	Which is more effective as prophylactic treatment of migraine: propranolol or self-hypnosis?
Design	Randomised controlled trial
Level of evidence	Jadad 1
Setting	Outpatient department, academic medical centre, the United States
Participants	Participants were children aged 6–12 years of age with classic migraine, defined as paroxysmal headache associated with all of the following: (a) unilateral head pain; (b) nausea/vomiting; (c) visual aura (scotoma, visual field defects) or other transitory neurologic disturbance (sensory or motor); and (d) a history of migraine in one of the parents or siblings.

(*continued*)

Evidence 3	
Theme E3	*Treatment options in migraine: propranolol or hypnosis?*
Participants (*cont.*)	Children had to have had a minimum of four headaches per month in the preceding 4 months, with normal neurological examination at the beginning and end of the study, a normal IQ and normal computed tomography brain scan if the electroencephalogram was abnormal.
Intervention	After a 4-week baseline assessment of headache, patients entered a 1-week run-in phase followed by a 10-week placebo or propranolol treatment phase, which was followed by a 1-week washout phase. This 12-week intervention was replicated in phase 2 but all children were taught self-hypnosis. Therefore, three groups were analysed: (1) placebo plus self-hypnosis, (2) propranolol plus placebo plus self-hypnosis and (3) placebo plus propranolol plus self-hypnosis. A headache intensity score was calculated with a point each for analgesia use, vomiting, sleeping to relieve the pain, missed school, and headache duration for 3–5 hours. Two points were scored if the headache lasted longer than 6 hours.
Outcomes	The primary outcome was the reduction in headache frequency attributable to propranolol and self hypnosis compared to placebo.
Main results	Thirty-three patients were enrolled, with 28 completing the study (two dropouts occurred with the drug component phase and three did not attend enough hypnosis sessions). The mean number of headaches in the 3-month study period was as follows: placebo group, 13.3; propranolol, 14.9; self-hypnosis, 5.8. There was a 56% reduction in headache frequency with self-hypnosis (absolute risk reduction = 56%; number needed to treat = 2). The headache intensity scores were 2.4 for placebo, 2.4 for propranolol and 2.3 for self-hypnosis, indicating no change in the clinical intensity of the headaches.
Conclusion	Self-hypnosis reduced the frequency of the migraine headaches but not the severity; whereas propranolol neither reduced the frequency or the severity of the migraine.
Commentary	In children with migraine headache prevention is the goal. This study, though small, emphasised the benefits that can accrue from self-hypnosis in children. This technique must be used on a daily basis to be effective and as such adherence issues arise. Self-hypnosis involved practising progressive relaxation techniques, and then learning from a menu of options exercises in self-regulation of pain. This process empowers the child, a key concept in self-management. The failure of propranolol to produce a therapeutic response is surprising, given its use in clinical practice. To date all studies on propranolol have been small and a large trial is required to define its role in migraine prophylaxis.
Reference	Olness K, MacDonald JT, Uden DL. Comparison of self-hypnosis and propranolol in the treatment of juvenile classic migraine. *Pediatrics.* 1987; **79**(4): 593–7.

Evidence 4

Theme E4	*Migraine drug prophylaxis*
Question	What is the effectiveness of topiramate in adolescent migraine?
Design	Randomised controlled trial
Level of evidence	Jadad 5
Setting	Academic medical centres, the United States and Belgium
Participants	Adolescents 12–17 years of age with migraine for more than 6 months, as defined by International Headache Society criteria. Patients experienced 3–12 migraine episodes on no more than 14 days per month in the 3 months prior to enrolment and preventive therapy was warranted in these patients because of symptom frequency. Excluded patients were those unable to clearly distinguish migraine from non-migraine headache, overusers of acute migraine treatment and those with a body mass index $>40\,kg/m^2$.
Intervention	This study commenced with a 9-week pre-treatment phase comprising a 1-week screening period, a 4-week washout of disallowed migraine preventive medications and a 4-week prospective baseline period. This was followed by a 16-week double-blind treatment phase with an exit/taper phase lasting up to 6 weeks. Patients were randomised to receive topiramate 50 mg/day, topiramate 100 mg/day or placebo.
Outcomes	The primary outcome was the percentage reduction in the monthly migraine attack rate over the last 12 weeks of the double-blind phase compared with the prospective baseline phase.
Main results	One hundred and six patients were randomised, 103 entered the double-blind phase, and 85 completed the double-blind phase: 26 in the placebo group, 29 in the topiramate 50 mg group and 30 in the topiramate 100 mg group. The percentage reduction in the monthly migraine rates were placebo, 44.4%; topiramate 50 mg/day, 44.6% (absolute risk reduction (ARR) = 0.2%; number needed to treat (NNT) = 500); topiramate 100 mg/day, 72.2% (ARR = 27.8%; NNT = 4). At least 50% of the topiramate 100 mg/day group were migraine free in the last 4 weeks of the double-blind phase. Side effects of topiramate include weight loss and dizziness.
Conclusion	Topiramate 100 mg/day was effective in the prevention of paediatric migraine and was well tolerated.
Commentary	This study indicates a high response to placebo therapy which is well recognised in both the adult and paediatric literature. The reduction in the headache burden is a central component of migraine management. The use of topiramate has a definite role in conjunction with bio-behavioural interventions and other preventive measures. Adolescents with migraine and other headaches have significant co-morbidities inclusive of epilepsy (odds ratio (OR) = 2), persistent nightmares (OR = 2.3), motion sickness (OR = 1.6), abdominal complaints (OR = 2.4), asthma (OR = 2.2) (Lateef *et al.*, 2012). Such conditions may well require pharmacological treatments that need to be taken into account when determining treatment options.
References	Lewis D, Winner P, Saper J, *et al.* Randomized, double-blind, placebo-controlled study to evaluate the efficacy and safety of topiramate for migraine prevention in pediatric subjects 12 to 17 years of age. *Pediatrics.* 2009; **123**(3): 924–34.
	Lateef TM, Cui L, Nelson KB, *et al.* Physical comorbidity of migraine and other headaches in US adolescents. *J Pediatr.* 2012; **161**(2): 308–13.

Evidence 5	
Theme E5	*The acute treatment of migraine*
Question	In acute migraine, which is more effective: zolmitriptan or ibuprofen?
Design	Randomised controlled trial
Level of evidence	Jadad 4
Setting	Tertiary care setting, Germany
Participants	Children and adolescents aged 6–18 years with migraine, diagnosed utilising the International Headache Society criteria, were eligible for inclusion.
Intervention	The study drugs were used for three sequential headaches. These were zol-mitriptan 2.5 mg, ibuprofen 200 mg for children under 12 years, ibuprofen 400 mg for adolescents and placebo. Medications were taken when the pain was moderate or severe. The order of drugs was randomised.
Outcomes	Outcome was pain relief (defined as no or mild headache after moderate to severe headache) at 2 hours.
Main results	Thirty-two patients enrolled (male to female ratio, 1:1.3) but three dropped out. Twenty-nine completed the study, and mean age was 13.9 plus or minus −2.8 years. The mean headache attack frequency was 2.6 ± 1.5 per month and the mean duration of untreated headache was 22 ± 16 hours. Measure of pain present at 2 hours was placebo, 72%; zolmitriptan, 38% (absolute risk reduction (ARR) = 34%; number needed to treat (NNT) = 3); ibuprofen, 31% (ARR = 41%; NNT = 3).
Conclusion	Zolmitriptan and ibuprofen are both effective in the treatment of acute migraine.
Commentary	Studies in migraine treatment usually show a high placebo response rate but this was not evident in this study; however, the selected patients would appear to represent the severe end of the migraine spectrum, with mean headache duration of 22 hours. The response rate to triptans is assumed to increase with age. This study did not attempt to evaluate as an a priori a subgroup analysis based on age, but a post hoc analysis of children under 13 years of age indicated an ARR of 37% (NNT = 3) for zolmitriptan. This finding needs to be evaluated prospectively.
Reference	Evers S, Rahmann A, Kraemer C, *et al.* Treatment of childhood migraine attacks with oral zolmitriptan and ibuprofen. *Neurology.* 2006; **67**(3): 497–9.

Evidence 6	
Theme E6	*The treatment of acute migraine in adolescents*
Question	How effective is the combination of sumatriptan and naproxen sodium (suma/nap) in adolescent migraine?
Design	Randomised controlled trial
Level of evidence	Jadad 5
Setting	Primary care, specialist and research centres with an interest in paediatric migraine treatment in the United States

(*continued*)

Evidence 6	
Theme E6	**_The treatment of acute migraine in adolescents_**
Participants	Subjects were eligible if they were aged 12–17 years at screening, had more than a 6-month history of two to eight migraines per month (with or without aura, as defined by International Headache Society criteria), typically lasting longer than 3 hours with moderate to severe headache pain.
Intervention	Patients who had moderate to severe headache after 2 hours having received a placebo (single blind) medication were eligible (placebo non-responders) for enrolment in the double-blind phase. In this phase, subjects treated one moderate to severe migraine with suma/nap 10/60 mg, 30/180 mg or 85/500 mg, or placebo. All tablets looked identical.
Outcomes	The primary outcome was the percentage of subjects pain free at 2 hours post treatment attack. 'Pain free' was defined as the absence of headache pain post treatment from moderate or severe at baseline, without previous use of rescue medication. An important secondary end point was pain freedom maintained from 2–24 hours without use of rescue medication.
Main results	Of the 976 patients screened, 683 entered the first phase of the study, and of these, 61 (9%) were placebo responders. A total of 589 were randomised to one of the four groups.
	The percentage of patients with pain at 2 hours were as follows:
	• placebo, 90%
	• suma/nap 10/60 mg, 71% (absolute risk reduction (ARR) = 19%; number needed to treat (NNT) = 5)
	• suma/nap 30/180 mg, 73% (ARR = 17%; NNT = 6)
	• suma/nap 85/500 mg, 76% (ARR = 14%; NNT = 8).
	Three (<1%) patients experienced hot flashes and three (<1%) experienced muscle tightness in the neck and jaws. These side effects occurred in those using the two higher drug dosages.
	In the secondary outcome measures, failure to achieve pain-free status at 2–24 hours was as follows:
	• placebo, 91%
	• suma/nap 10/60 mg, 76% (ARR = 15%; NNT = 7)
	• suma/nap 30/180 mg, 75% (ARR = 16%; NNT = 6)
	• suma/nap 85/500 mg, 77% (ARR = 14%; NNT = 8).
Conclusion	All doses of suma/nap were well tolerated and similarly effective in the treatment of acute adolescent migraine as compared with placebo.
Commentary	This study limited the impact of placebo responders through its single blind run-in phase and recruited patients with significant migraine (headaches >3 hours). The treatment results were similar, with a trend favouring the suma/nap 10/60 mg dosage. The side effects experienced reflect triptans sensations.
Reference	Derosier FJ, Lewis D, Hershey AD, _et al._ Randomized trial of sumatriptan and naproxen sodium combination in adolescent migraine. _Pediatrics._ 2012; **129**(6): e1411–20.

HEADACHE: MULTIPLE-CHOICE QUESTIONS

Q1 Which of the following statements is/are correct regarding paediatric migraine?
a) The headache is frequently unilateral in location.
b) Pallor is a frequent clinical finding.
c) It commences <5 years in 8% of paediatric patients.
d) The headache pain is dull in character.
e) Tinnitus occurs in 2% of patients with migraine.

Q2 Which of the following statements about paediatric migraine is/are correct?
a) Migraine is improved by sleep.
b) The headache duration is 3–72 hours.
c) The headache is made worse by walking.
d) The aura occurs prior to the migraine headache.
e) Soft music helps to relieve the headache.

Q3 Potential triggers of migraine headache in children include which of the following?
a) Sleep deprivation
b) Stress
c) Extremes of physical activity
d) Foods – cheese, chocolate
e) Topiramate

Q4 Which of the following statements is/are true with regard to children with tension headache?
a) Stress is a major trigger.
b) Analgesia is effective if given early.
c) Self-hypnosis is effective.
d) The child is unable to watch television.
e) Parents can recognise the child is in pain.

Q5 Which of the following statements with regard to brain tumours in children is/are true?
a) The incidence is 3/100 000.
b) Nausea without vomiting is a feature.
c) Short stature is a recognised presentation.
d) Diplopia occurs in supratentorial tumours.
e) Fifteen per cent present with disturbed sleep.

Q6 Which of the following statements about idiopathic intracranial hypertension is/are true?
a) The headache is frontal in location.
b) Pain is increased with forward bending.
c) Obesity is a risk factor.

d) If untreated, it leads to blindness.

e) Transient visual obscurations are a feature.

Q7 Indications for neuroimaging in a child with headache include which of the following?

a) Personality change

b) Headache at night

c) Classic migraine if <5 years

d) Focal neurological signs

e) Crescendo pattern headache

Q8 Which of the followings statements is/are true regarding analgesia therapy for headaches?

a) Analgesia, in migraine headache, should be administered at the start of the aura.

b) Analgesia usage in migraine should be avoided if nausea is present.

c) Twenty-five per cent of patients with a migraine headache who use ibuprofen are headache free at 2 hours post ingestion.

d) Excessive analgesia usage can cause a rebound headache.

e) Analgesia is effective in 75% of tension headaches.

Q9 Which of the following statements concerning paediatric migraine therapy is/ are correct?

a) There is a high placebo response rate.

b) Topiramate is an effective prophylactic therapy.

c) Self-hypnosis is superior to propranolol in clinical trials.

d) Cognitive behavioural therapy is not effective in chronic headaches.

e) The triptans are contraindicated because of cardiac toxicity.

Answers

A1	a, b	A2	a, b, c, d
A3	a, b, c, d	A4	a, c
A5	a, c, d	A6	a, b, c, d, e
A7	a, b, d, e	A8	a, b, e
A9	a, b, c		

Chapter Twenty

SEIZURES

COMMON SCENARIO

'She has always been excellent at school and in the past I received great feedback on her performance at parent–teacher meetings. However, in the last few months, her school reports have been concerning. The teacher thinks she is daydreaming constantly and now that I think about it, I've noticed the same at home. All of a sudden she just stops and stares and I can't get her attention. It only lasts for a few seconds, but it is becoming more obvious and I'm not sure if I'm overreacting.'

LEARNING OBJECTIVES

- Understand the classification of seizures
- Recognise common epilepsy syndromes
- Perform a focussed seizure history and examination
- Explain what investigations are indicated in the investigation of seizures
- Know when to start, how to select and when to discontinue anti-epileptic medication
- Evaluate the available evidence to support your treatment options

BACKGROUND

Epilepsy is one of the commonest chronic neurological conditions in childhood. Population-based studies indicate that up to the age of 15 years, 2% of children have at least one unprovoked seizure, with 1% having repeated seizures. The annual incidence of childhood-onset epilepsy in developed countries is 60 per 100 000. The incidence is threefold higher in the first year of life.

Convulsions are defined as intermittent stereotyped involuntary muscle contractions, ether sustained (i.e. tonic) or interrupted (i.e. clonic). Epileptic seizures are defined as a transient clinical event that result from abnormal and excessive activity of cerebral neurons, resulting in paroxysmal disorganization of one or several brain functions. The clinical events can be extremely diverse. Epilepsy is defined as a group of conditions, in which unprovoked epileptic seizures occur repetitively.

The pathology of epilepsy is extremely diverse. In recent years, knowledge on childhood epilepsy has markedly improved with magnetic resonance imaging (MRI) and molecular genetics. The two most common types of brain pathological malformations in childhood epilepsy are developmental cortical malformation and mesial temporal sclerosis. Genetic factors are paramount in childhood epilepsy. The mode of inheritance can be monogenetic, and mutations in the same gene can result in different phenotypes. However, most of the idiopathic epilepsies follow a polygenic mode of inheritance. If one parent has epilepsy then the overall risk of epilepsy in their offspring is 4% and this rises to 10% if both parents are affected. Children of epileptic mothers are more likely to develop epilepsy than children of epileptic fathers. For siblings of an affected child the risk of epilepsy is 4%.

In 2010, the International League Against Epilepsy published new guidelines on the *Revised Terminology and Concepts for Organization of the Epilepsies*.

Focal seizures are conceptualised as originating at some point within networks limited to one hemisphere. They may evolve into bilateral convulsive seizures. Seizures are characterised according to one or more of the following features:

- aura
- motor
- autonomic
- awareness/responsiveness: altered or retained.

Generalised seizures are conceptualised as originating at some point within and rapidly engaging bilaterally distributed networks.

Generalised seizure types	
Clonic	Rhythmic movements of muscles
Tonic	Sudden increase in body tone
Tonic–clonic	Rhythmic movements and increased body tone
Myoclonic	Sudden and rapid body jerks
Atonic	Sudden loss of body tone
Absence	Brief loss of consciousness with no change in body tone

Causes of seizure	
Genetic	Genetic defect directly contributes to the epilepsy and seizures are the core symptom of the disorder
Structural-metabolic	Seizures are caused by a structural or metabolic disorder of the brain
Unknown	The cause is unknown and might be genetic, structural or metabolic

FEBRILE CONVULSIONS

Febrile convulsions affect about 3% of neurologically normal children aged between 6 months to 5 years of age. Seizures occur during an acute febrile illness without signs or symptoms of meningitis or encephalitis. Seizures usually occur in the early course of a febrile illness. Common infections include viral upper respiratory tract infections, tonsillitis, otitis media, viral exanthems (human herpesvirus 6) and fevers associated with immunisation. Human herpesvirus 6 is a recognised cause of febrile convulsions. Febrile convulsions are divided into simple and complex. Simple seizures are generalised tonic–clonic, last <15 minutes and do not recur in the same illness. Complex seizures have focal components, are prolonged or recur within a 24-hour period. The majority of febrile convulsions are simple and warrant no neurological investigations. The recurrence risk after a single febrile convulsion is approximately 33%. Risk factors for recurrence include first seizure at less than 15 months of age, parent or sibling with febrile seizures or epilepsy, febrile seizure occurrence at low temperatures and a short interval between the fever and seizure. Febrile seizures are extremely frightening for parents, who may fear that their child is dying during the seizure. Reassurance, education and written instructions for the management of febrile illness and possible further febrile convulsions are essential. Routine laboratory investigations or neuroimaging are not required. No preventive treatment is required; however, rectal diazepam can be used at onset of a febrile seizure if there is a history of previous prolonged febrile convulsions. About 3% of children will develop epilepsy, particularly if seizures are recurrent. If the child has not been neurologically normal prior to the febrile seizure then clinical follow-up is required, as the risk of epilepsy is higher than the general population and technically the seizure that such children experience with fever may not be benign.

FOCAL SEIZURES

The clinical features of focal seizures reflect the cortical origin of the seizures. Temporal lobe epilepsy seizures affect language and memory, processing or emotions. A typical aura may involve a funny epigastric feeling, confusion, a feeling of déjà vu, gustatory hallucinations, fear or anxiety. Frontal lobe epilepsy is often undiagnosed or misdiagnosed as a sleep or psychiatric disorder. Seizures are usually brief, stereotypic, nocturnal and frequent. Clinical features are diverse and include hyper-motor behaviours, bicycling automatism and vocalisations. Parietal lobe epilepsy is uncommon and difficult to categorise. Paraesthesia (numbness or pins and needles), a feeling of crawling or itching, pain, sexual sensations and disturbance of body image are recognised symptoms associated with a parietal lobe aura. Occipital lobe epilepsy occur less frequently and commonly presents with visual symptoms including hallucinations, visual field defects and light flickering or flashing.

COMMON EPILEPSY SYNDROMES

An epilepsy syndrome is determined by the seizure type, age of onset, electroencephalogram (EEG) findings and neurological and non-neurological signs.

Benign childhood epilepsy with centrotemporal spikes, benign rolandic epilepsy, benign partial epilepsy of childhood

Benign childhood epilepsy with centrotemporal spikes accounts for up to 20% of childhood epilepsies. Age of onset is almost always between 3 and 13 years. In 20%–30% of cases there is a positive family history. It usually consists of partial seizures affecting the mouth, face and speech. Both daytime and night-time seizures may occur although in most children the seizures occur during sleep only (80% of cases). In nocturnal seizures clonic movements of the mouth, drooling and gurgling sounds are often followed by generalised tonic–clonic convulsions. Seizures rarely generalise during the daytime. Symptoms include feeling of tingling on one side of the mouth involving the tongue, lips and inside of cheek, twitching of the corner of the mouth, unilateral jerking of the face, speech arrest, drooling, numbness of face or mouth and guttural sounds.

Seizures characteristically occur while the patient is asleep or on awakening, and are no longer than 30–60 seconds. EEG shows typical biphasic centrotemporal spikes with a horizontal dipole, easily brought on by sleep.

Anti-epileptic drug (AED) treatment is rarely indicated. About 10%–20% of children only ever have one seizure, with 20% of children having frequent seizures. Avoidance of sleep deprivation and ensuring that the child has a good sleep routine is important. However if they are associated with frequent secondary generalisation, AED treatment is indicated. The prognosis is excellent with most children outgrowing their seizures by age 15.

Childhood absence epilepsy

Childhood absence epilepsy is a form of idiopathic generalised epilepsy and account for more than 10% of childhood epilepsy. A family history is often present. Seizures start between the ages of 4 and 10 years, with a peak incidence at 4–7 years. Typical absence seizures are characterised by sudden impairment of consciousness, the child stares blankly and is non-responsive. There may be minor motor phenomena, including jerking of eyelids or subtle hands automatism. Episodes are brief, typically lasting 10 seconds. The child has no recollection of the event and there is no post-ictal phase, with the child quickly resuming normal activities. Up to 100 seizures can occur a day, with typically 20 seizures occurring daily. School performance may be adversely affected. Absence seizures must be distinguished from focal seizures. Focal seizures are often longer in duration, may be associated with an aura, have more complex automatisms and are followed by a post-ictal phase.

EEG shows characteristic 3 Hz spike and slow wave discharges. Hyperventilation is an efficient precipitant of typical absence and can be safely performed during an EEG.

First-line drug treatment includes sodium valproate or ethosuximide, with lamotrigine as second line. Carbamazepine, vigabatrin and tiagabine are contraindicated in the treatment of absence seizures. The prognosis for typical childhood absence epilepsy is excellent, with most children becoming seizure free before 12 years of age. Ten per cent of children with absence seizures develop generalised epilepsy in adolescence.

Juvenile absence epilepsy

The onset of juvenile absence epilepsy occurs later than childhood absence epilepsy, typically between 10 and 17 years of age. It accounts for approximately 10% of epilepsy in childhood. In one third of cases there is a family history. The seizures occur less frequently, limited to 1 or just a few daily seizures. Other seizure types, particularly generalised tonic–clonic seizures are more common, more common upon wakening and are often the reason for the epilepsy being brought to medical attention. EEG shows faster generalised spike and wave discharges. Treatment options are similar to childhood absence epilepsy and are generally well controlled in 80% of cases. Avoidance of sleep deprivation and limiting alcohol intake should be addressed. Treatment may be lifelong in cases.

Juvenile myoclonic epilepsy

Juvenile myoclonic epilepsy, also known as Janz's syndrome, is one of the most common epilepsy syndromes. Approximately 5% of people with epilepsy have juvenile myoclonic epilepsy. The seizures typically begin in early adolescence and persist into adulthood. The seizures are characterised by early-morning jerks of the head, neck and upper limbs that usually occur shortly after waking. Myoclonic jerks are characterised by brief, bilateral, usually symmetrical synchronous muscle contractions. Seizures can be triggered by sleep deprivation, stress, menstruation, photic stimulation or alcohol consumption. Other seizure types can also occur, including generalised tonic–clonic and absence seizures. Typical EEG features are 3 Hz spike and wave discharges. Juvenile myoclonic epilepsy is inherited; however, the exact mode of inheritance is unclear. In 50% of cases there may be a positive family history.

All patients require lifelong treatment. Although the condition is described as benign, patients are at risk for generalised tonic–clonic seizures. Precipitating factors such as sleep deprivation and alcohol consumption should be avoided. The drug of choice is sodium valproate, which has an 80% success rate. However, in children of childbearing age, valproate is contraindicated because of the risk of foetal malformations; therefore, levetiracetam or lamotrigine are alternative first line AEDs. Carbamazepine may worsen myoclonic jerks.

West's syndrome

West's syndrome encompasses a triad of infantile spasms, developmental delay or regression, and hypsarrhythmic EEG pattern. The onset is infancy, generally between 3 and 6 months of life. Infantile spasms are clusters of brisk flexion–extension of the neck with abduction–adduction of the upper limbs. After a cluster, the patient is often exhausted or distressed. Clusters recur several times a day. The repetitive character of the spasms is an important diagnostic clue, especially in those infants where the spasms are very subtle in expression and often misjudged for normal baby movements. Developmental delay often occurs before the onset of the spasms. Lack of interest in the surroundings with loss of visual attention is a key feature. Hypsarrhythmia is characterised by a chaotic succession of very high-amplitude slow waves, intermixed with multifocal and asynchronous spikes and sharp waves.

Seizure control is difficult to achieve. Corticosteroids/adrenocorticotropic hormone and vigabatrin have been proven to be effective treatments. Video EEG is essential to monitor response to drugs. Seizures persist in about half of patients. The aetiology of West's syndrome includes cerebral malformations, central nervous system infections and trauma, perinatal and postnatal complications, inborn errors of metabolism. In 10% of cases no cause is found. 20% of children with West's syndrome evolve into Lennox–Gastaut's syndrome.

Lennox–Gastaut's syndrome

Lennox–Gastaut's syndrome is a severe childhood-onset epilepsy and accounts for approximately 5% of childhood epilepsy. The onset is usually before 4 years of age. Although multiple seizure types are associated with Lennox–Gastaut's syndrome, tonic seizures are the typical seizure type. Similarly to West's syndrome, the aetiology of Lennox–Gastaut's syndrome includes cerebral malformations, birth trauma, central nervous system infection and trauma, inborn errors of metabolism and tuberous sclerosis. In 30% of cases no cause is found. Learning difficulties, developmental delay or regression and behavioural problems are common. The EEG shows paroxysms of fast activity and generalised slow spike and wave discharges. Seizures are often difficult to control despite multiple AED treatment. Long-term prognosis is unfavourable.

HISTORY

Events leading up to seizure	Child well/unwell Any warning signs Aura Provoking factor Time of day What was the child doing? Awake or asleep	**Family history**	Seizures Febrile seizures Developmental delay Metabolic diseases	**❶ Red flags** A febrile seizures <6 months of age Seizure in a child with development delay Seizures not responsive to standard treatment History of poor adherence to treatment regime or aversion to medication use
The seizure	Duration Description of seizure – sequence of events Limb involvement Eye rolling or flickering or deviation Facial twitching Stiffening Incontinence Tongue biting Colour change Level of consciousness Able to stop movement or distract from staring episode	**General health**	Energy levels Appetite Weight loss	
Post seizure	Tired Recall of event Weakness How long did it take to return to normal/baseline?	**Development**	Milestones achieved Delayed milestones Regression in development Behavioural concerns/changes	
History of previous episodes	Description of events Frequency Change in episodes Video recording of events	**Medical or surgical**	Head trauma Meningitis/encephalitis	
Birth history	Gestation Resuscitation required NICU admission Cooling at birth	**Social history**	Difficulties at school Additional resource hours or extra tuition required	
Identified triggers	Sleep deprivation Alcohol Stress Menstruation Photosensitivity			

EXAMINATION

- Measure and plot height, weight and head circumference on an appropriate centile chart
- Full neurological examination including fundoscopy
- Skin examination for neurocutaneous stigmata (e.g. café au lait macules)
- Blood pressure measurement
- Developmental stage: gross motor, fine motor, language and hearing, social skills

---

❶ Red flags

- Macrocephaly or microcephaly
- Focal neurological signs
- Neurocutaneous stigmata
- Signs of raised intracranial pressure (hypertension, bradycardia, sixth nerve palsy, papilloedema)
- Dysmorphic features
- Meningism or decreased level of consciousness

DIFFERENTIAL DIAGNOSIS

Accurately diagnosing epilepsy can be challenging, as there is a wide variety of paroxysmal events that can be misdiagnosed as epileptic in nature. Misdiagnoses are common and clinicians should have an understanding of the differential diagnoses; the implications of inappropriate medication and the psychological impact of the diagnosis. A careful history, examination and review of parental videos (if available) should enable clinicians to confidently determine whether an episode is epileptic in nature.

Cause	Clinical features
Benign neonatal sleep myoclonus	Rhythmical jerks of the limbs, generalised or focal, occur in brief or prolonged clusters, which could last up to 15 minutes. The trunk and the face remain unaffected. The jerks cease on wakening and can be induced by rocking the crib while the neonate is asleep. The myoclonus resolves after a few weeks and rarely after several months.
Shuddering	Shuddering attacks are benign events of infancy. They consist of rapid shivering of the head, shoulder, and occasionally the trunk, usually lasting not more than a few seconds. Frequency can be up to numerous episodes a day. The pathophysiology of shuddering attacks is unknown, although a relationship to essential tremor has been postulated

(continued)

Cause	Clinical features
Reflex-anoxic seizures	Seizures result from temporary asystole of reflex origins. These especially occur in the second year of life and may be precipitated by unexpected bump to the head or a fall. The child goes pale, loses muscle tone and consciousness, and might present with body stiffening, limb jerking and eye deviation. The episode resolves within a minute and consciousness resumes.
Breath-holding spells	Breath-holding spells occur in approximately 5% of children below the age of 5 years. They are preceded by the child vigorously crying due to frustration, anger or pain, and followed by holding their breath in expiration. The child goes cyanotic, loses consciousness and becomes limp, followed by a quick recovery.
Gastro-oesophageal reflux	Gastro-oesophageal reflux presents in children with change in posture, colour, breathing and heart rate. Sandifer's syndrome is associated with hiatus hernia and involves spasmodic torsional dystonia with arching of the back and rigid opisthotonic posturing. Typically observed from infancy to early childhood, children with mental impairment or cerebral palsy may experience it into adolescence.
Cardiogenic syncope	Syncope of cardiac origin may resemble convulsive seizures. Causes include structural heart defects and rhythmic disturbances, commonly the *long QT syndrome*. The QTc interval is prolonged in most cases; however, prolonged electrocardiogram (ECG) recording may be warranted. Appropriate management can prevent sudden death. Important clinical features distinguishing syncope from seizure include light-headedness, nausea, chest pain, palpitations or low pulse, pallor and sweating. Syncope can occur after a long period of standing, or after exercise. A family history may be present.
Sleep disorders	Sleep disorders are very common, with an overall incidence of 20% to 30% of children. These include *pavor nocturnus* (night terrors), nightmares, somnambulism (sleep walking) and narcolepsy. Night terrors are often familial. They usually occur in the first hours of sleep during non-rapid eye movement sleep. Typically the child screams while sitting in bed terrified and wide-eyed. Any attempts at waking up the child are ineffective until they go back to sleep. The child has no recollection of the event.
	These episodes can be confused with frontal lobe epilepsy (FLE). Patients with FLE can experience nocturnal events such as paroxysmal awakening, nocturnal dystonia, and episodic nocturnal wandering, in addition to asymmetric tonic seizures from the supplementary motor area. First-line treatment of FLE is carbamazepine or oxcarbazepine.
Psychogenic non-epileptic seizures	These are frequent in adolescents and can occur in children as young as 5 years old. They are commonly observed in children with epilepsy and can be misjudged as refractory seizures. Attacks can mimic generalised tonic–clonic seizures; important distinguishing features include more rhythmic and coordinated movements, a quick recovery, recollection of the event and precipitation by observation.
Migraine	Migraine auras can be often misdiagnosed as focal epileptic seizures, especially in children with a concurrent diagnosis of epilepsy. Photosensitivity, visual phenomena, clouding of consciousness, nausea and vomiting are all features of migraine and generally have a much slower course than in epilepsy. A careful history of trigger factors should be explored.

INVESTIGATIONS

When should an EEG be performed?

The decision to perform an EEG after a first seizure should be considered as it may help determine recurrence risk (an abnormal EEG doubles the risk of further seizures), make a syndromic diagnosis and identify precipitating factors. It is important to recognise that up to 40% of children with seizures will have a normal EEG. The sensitivity of the EEG is just over 50% after a single event and 70% after multiple events. An EEG can help determine whether epilepsy is focal or generalised in nature or syndromic. It can help guide therapeutic decisions and help predict prognosis.

When should an MRI be performed?

MRI is not indicated in febrile seizure and benign epilepsy syndromes such as childhood and juvenile absence epilepsy, benign focal epilepsy of childhood and juvenile myoclonic epilepsy.

MRI is indicated in children who have an abnormal or focal neurological examination, in focal seizures and should be considered in children with refractory epilepsy and neonatal or infant onset epilepsy.

Should an ECG be performed?

All children with a convulsive seizure should have a 12 lead ECG recorded with calculation of the corrected QT interval

Should children with prolonged febrile convulsion have an EEG performed?

An EEG is not indicated in children with recurrent or prolonged febrile convulsions, as the yield of abnormality is low.

When is a sleep-deprived EEG indicated?

A sleep-deprived EEG may be helpful in children with recurrent seizures and a normal awake or standard EEG. In addition, it may be useful diagnosing syndromes such as benign rolandic epilepsy with centrotemporal spikes.

When is a video EEG recording indicated?

If there is uncertainty whether events are epileptic, a video EEG can be useful.

Should levels of AEDs be routinely monitored?

Routine monitoring of AEDs is not indicated. It can be useful in children with difficult to control epilepsy, status epilepticus, concerns regarding compliance or suspected toxicity.

MANAGEMENT PLAN: FIVE-STEP APPROACH

1. Clarifying and pitfall avoidance strategies:
   a) parent and child
   b) doctor
2. Anti-epileptic drugs
3. Ketogenic diet
4. Surgery for epilepsy
5. Vagal nerve stimulation

The aim of epilepsy treatment is to achieve complete seizure freedom without any adverse effects on growth or development. The most important first step is to ensure that the episodes are in fact epileptic, to determine what the seizure type is and what the epilepsy syndrome is.

Clarifying and pitfall avoidance strategies

Parent and child

- Clarifying the diagnosis. **Rationale**: the diagnosis of epilepsy (seizure type and epileptic syndrome) must be clarified for the child and parents. While many parents conceptualise epilepsy as tonic–clonic seizures this is not the case. There are many epileptic syndromes where the diagnosis evolves over a period of time because the seizures are initially subtle in nature.
- Parental response to epilepsy. **Rationale**: parents on witnessing their child's first seizure often believe their child is dying and consequently they require the pathopysiology of the seizures to be explained, while ensuring that they are able to provide first aid measures to their child in the acute setting.
- Deciding on therapy. **Rationale**: the choice of medication, probable success rate and side effect profile needs to be explained to the parent (*see* Evidence 1).
- Seizure triggers for epilepsy. **Rationale**: the most common trigger is not taking the prescribed anti seizure medication; for some children and adolescents sleep deprivation and stress are triggers. Very rarely, flickering lights may trigger a seizure.
- Epilepsy and the school. **Rationale**: thirty per cent of children with epilepsy fail to achieve their academic potential. Parents, once aware of this, can take proactive measures to have their child assessed if academic achievement is suboptimal.
- Co-morbidities affecting the child with epilepsy. **Pitfall**: ensure parents are aware of the co-morbidities associated with epilepsy, which include migraine (associated with rolandic and occipital epilepsy), attention deficit hyperactivity disorder, depression and anxiety.
- Prevention of febrile seizures. **Rationale**: parents, whose child has had a febrile seizure, will wish to reduce the risk; however, antipyretic therapy is not superior to placebo **and** not every febrile episode will result in a seizure (*see* Evidence 2).

Doctor

- Deciding on specialist input. **Rationale**: the decision to seek specialist input will be influenced by several factors: (a) seizure type, (b) associated co-morbidities in the child and (c) ability to reassure parents.
- Medication side effect profile. **Pitfall**: failing to advise parents about potential side effects is likely to reduce adherence to the treatment regimen. Newer medications are used in children, based on extrapolation from adult data in the absence of rigorous paediatric trials and consequently unforeseen side effects may occur.
- Breakthrough seizures. **Pitfall**: if a child has a breakthrough seizure, analyse why this has occurred: (a) medication not incremented with weight gain, (b) intercurrent illness present or (c) additional medication required. If a child presents with

a breakthrough seizure it is appropriate to increment the dose of medication by 10%–12% pending serum levels. For parents break through seizures are anxiety provoking.

● Acute seizure treatment. *See* Evidence 7, 8: Chapter 3: First Response.

● The first seizure. **Pitfall**: one unprovoked generalised seizure is not an indication for medication. Await the occurrence of a second seizure, but instruct the parents in first aid measures to reduce their stress but ensure the child has had a proper neurological examination and the 'red flag' issues are addressed.

Anti-epileptic drugs

AEDs work by decreasing excitation or enhancing inhibition of electrical activity in the brain. They alter electrical activity in neurons by affecting sodium, potassium, calcium or chloride channels or alter chemical transmission between neurones by affecting neurotransmitters such as GABA and glutamate. Parents and children should receive written information about the prescribed AED, potential side effects, drug dosing, escalation and monitoring.

In general, when commencing AEDs, start with a low dose and gradually increase up to maintenance dose. Where possible, aim for seizure control with one AED. When polytherapy is needed, select AEDs with different mechanisms of action.

Sodium valproate is the first line treatment for children with generalised tonic–clonic seizures. However, it should not be prescribed to females of childbearing age, because of the risk of foetal malformation. If unsuitable, lamotrigine can be prescribed as an alternative. Lamotrigine can cause serious skin rashes including Stevens–Johnson syndrome, so it should be introduced slowly.

Sodium valproate is the first-line treatment for children with myoclonic seizures. It is particularly useful for the treatment of juvenile myoclonic epilepsy. If unsuitable or ineffective, levetiracetam or topiramate can be prescribed. Carbamazepine, phenytoin and lamotrigine should not be used for the treatment of myoclonic seizures.

Ethosuximide and sodium valproate are first line treatments for absence seizures (*see* Evidence 3). If tonic–clonic seizures are likely, sodium valproate should be prescribed. If unsuitable or ineffective, lamotrigine can be prescribed.

Sodium valproate should be prescribed as first line treatment for tonic and atonic seizures, if unsuitable or not effective, lamotrigine can be tried.

For children with infantile spasms, prednisolone or vigabatrin should be prescribed as first-line treatment (*see* Evidence 4). If the child has tuberous sclerosis, vigabatrin should be prescribed as first line.

For focal epilepsy, carbamazepine and lamotrigine are prescribed as first-line treatment, alternative first-line treatments include levetiracetam, oxcarbazepine and sodium valproate.

In children who have remained seizure free with AEDs for 2 years, the decision to withdraw AEDs can be considered. The decision to discontinue AEDs should be made on an individual basis taking into consideration the likelihood of remaining seizure free after withdrawal, the risks and benefits of withdrawal and the presence of factors predictive of high recurrence. There is no general consensus on these risk factors; however multiple seizure types, previous polytherapy and abnormalities in the post withdrawal EEG are associated with a high risk of recurrence. Drugs should be withdrawn slowly and no more than one drug should be withdrawn at any one time.

Refractory epilepsy is defined as inadequate control of seizures despite optimal treatment with conventional medication. Approximately 25%–30% of children will continue to experience seizures that are resistant to AEDs.

Ketogenic diet

The ketogenic diet is a high-fat, low carbohydrate diet that has been used in the treatment of epilepsy for over 80 years. The usual fat to carbohydrate ratio is 3:1 or 4:1. Ketones provide an alternative fuel for the brain. However the mechanism of effect of ketosis on seizures is not fully understood. Postulated theories include the stabilising effect of ketone bodies and the effect of the resultant acidosis on modifying the seizure threshold. A trained dietitian needs to oversee and monitor all children on a ketogenic diet to ensure that it is nutritionally adequate with an appropriate amount of vitamins, minerals and trace elements. Epilepsy resistant to AEDs may be considered for a ketogenic diet. The ketogenic diet has been shown to be efficacious in reducing the frequency of seizures in children with refractory epilepsy (*see* Evidence 5).

Epilepsy surgery

In recent years there has been a resurgence of interest in surgical treatment for treatment resistant focal epilepsy if debilitating seizures occur despite appropriate medication and the benefit of surgical resection outweighs the risk of resecting the epileptic area of the cortex. Resective surgery of an epileptogenic focus can be curative in 40%–80% of cases. The primary aim is to accurately localise and excise the epileptogenic region without causing cognitive or neurological deficit. Ictal and inter-ictal EEGs aid localisation in conjunction with MRI. All children, prior to surgical intervention, require neuropsychological assessment

Indications include:
- medically intractable seizures
- where surgical intervention might be curative, e.g. focal lesions.

Types of epilepsy surgery:
- temporal lobe resection for mesial temporal sclerosis – the most commonly performed surgery
- extra-temporal resection – less common, majority frontal lobe
- multiple subpial resections – alternative to cortical resection
- lesionectomy
- corpus callosotomy – offered as a alternative to hemispherectomy in patients with

a severely damaged hemisphere but motor, sensory or visual function would be valuable to preserve

• hemispherectomy.

Vagal nerve stimulation

Vagal nerve stimulation is used in drug-resistant epilepsy where surgical resection is not an option. A small device is surgically implanted under the skin and connected to the left vagus nerve. The device stimulates the vagus nerve to aid reduction in the frequency of seizures. Its effects are thought to be mediated through the thalamus. Ideal candidates for this treatment are those whose cognitive and motor ability allow them to activate the vagal nerve stimulation to prevent the seizure occurring. Small studies show a reduction in seizure frequency of 40%–90% in 40%–60% of treated patients. Side effects include hoarseness and throat discomfort which are mild and transient. Gastro-oesophageal reflux and obstructive apnoea, if present, become worse.

WHEN TO REFER?

• All children with first afebrile seizures need to be assessed by a paediatrician.
• Referral to a Paediatric Neurologist should be considered for:
    ○ children with recurrent seizures
    ○ patients with seizures and development delay
    ○ children who require more than 1 anticonvulsant medication for seizure control
• Follow up of child with seizures should be undertaken by a Consultant Paediatrician or Paediatric Neurologist

CLARIFICATION STATEMENTS FOR PARENTAL MISCONCEPTIONS

'Can playing video games induce seizure?'

Playing video games is not contra indicated in children with seizures. It is best to avoid perpetuating myths around epilepsy as children wish to integrate normal activities into their lifestyle.

'Will he outgrow his epilepsy?'

The prognosis for epilepsy is dependent on the seizure type and the presence of an epileptic syndrome. Normally a child or adolescent needs to be free of seizures for at least 2 years before medication can be weaned.

'Are there any diets that can help my child's epilepsy, as I don't want him on medication?'

There are no diets (except the ketogenic diet) which can reduce your child's seizure frequency. Adherence to the medication protocol is essential to reduce the seizure frequency.

SUMMARY PRACTICE POINTS

- Two per cent of children will have at least one unprovoked seizure.
- Febrile seizures only occur from 6 months to 5 years.
- Children with febrile seizures are by definition neurologically normal.
- Temporal lobe seizures affect language, memory and emotional responses.
- Benign rolandic epilepsy does not require treatment.
- Absence seizures are frequently missed. As the duration is 10 seconds, take a video of the child over a period of time to capture the seizure event.
- Infantile spasms are subtle at presentation; the repetitive nature of the movements is the best clue. Parents often will take a video of these movements and this aids the diagnosis in conjunction with the increasing frequency.
- An EEG is not indicated on the presentation of a first seizure unless associated risk factors are present.
- One-quarter of parents will be unhappy with AED treatment, therefore (a) monitor for side effects and (b) taper treatment for effectiveness while attempting to minimise side effects.

EVALUATING THE EVIDENCE

Evidence 1	
Theme E1	*Satisfaction with anti-epilepsy drugs (AEDs)*
Question	What are the satisfaction levels of patients with AEDs?
Design	Multicentre, open, observational, prospective study
Level of evidence	
Setting	Departments of child psychiatry and neurology, multiple academic medical centres, Italy
Participants	Children were eligible for inclusion if they were aged 3–17 years, with definite epilepsy (two or more unprovoked seizures), who were being initiated on drug treatment (for the first time) or changing drug treatment due to lack of efficacy or the occurrence of side effects.
Intervention	Satisfaction was assessed using the Hedonic Visual scale or through direct questioning (depending on the patients age). Quality of life (QoL) was assessed utilising an adolescent quality of life questionnaire and a caregiver QoL questionnaire.
Outcomes	The primary outcomes were satisfaction and quality of life ratings.

(continued)

Evidence 1	
Theme E1	*Satisfaction with anti-epilepsy drugs (AEDs)*
Main results	A total of 330 patients were invited to participate, and 324 were enrolled in the study, with 317 attending the 1-month follow-up visit and 293 completing the 3-month follow-up visit. Of the 24 dropouts, three had adverse events, three had poor compliance, two withdrew consent, three had uncontrolled seizures, ten were lost to follow-up, one changed address and two changed physicians. Two hundred and twenty-two (75.8%) patients were satisfied with their AEDs and 71 (24.2%) were not.
Conclusion	About one in four of children and adolescents are dissatisfied with their treatment with AEDs. The dissatisfaction is related to the chronicity of the epilepsy, adverse events (requiring medication change) and caregivers/parents with poor quality of life.
Commentary	Epilepsy is a chronic condition and the impact on parents may be more significant than on the child. The anxiety experienced by mothers may lead to depressive symptoms and parents report sleep problems and tiredness related to their child's epilepsy. One interesting aspect of this study is the modest (18.1%) change in satisfaction or dissatisfaction over the study period despite the presence of an active surveillance for side effects. The impact of associated co-morbid states in the reported study [present in 84 (25.9%) patients and for 46 (14.2%) the co-morbidities were nervous system related] may have modified family viewpoints. Parents may well be influenced by the initial choice of AED and therefore the most appropriate AED should be used, though a therapeutic response cannot be guaranteed.
Reference	Beghi E, Messina P, Pupillo E, *et al.* TASCA Study Group. Satisfaction with antiepileptic drugs in children and adolescents with newly diagnosed and chronic epilepsy. *Epilepsy Res.* 2012; **100**(1–2): 142–51.

Evidence 2	
Theme E2	*The prevention of febrile seizure recurrence with antipyretics*
Question	Can antipyretics at their maximal recommended dose prevent the recurrence of febrile seizures?
Design	Randomised controlled trial
Level of evidence	Jadad 3
Setting	Paediatric departments of five general hospitals, Finland
Participants	Previously well children who experienced one febrile seizure were eligible to participate.
Intervention	Children were initially allocated to receive rectal diclofenac or placebo rectally (to ensure rapid absorption) and after 8 hours were allocated to oral placebo, acetaminophen (dose 15 mg/kg) or ibuprofen (10 mg/kg) up to four times a day for temperatures >38°C. For temperatures >40°C open-label acetaminophen was administered.
Outcomes	The primary outcome measure was the recurrence of febrile seizures.

(*continued*)

Evidence 2

Theme E2	The prevention of febrile seizure recurrence with antipyretics
Main results	A total of 231 children were enrolled (age 4 months to 4 years), 63 (27.3%) had experienced a complex seizure, and 27 (111.6%) had more than 1 seizure in a 24-hour period. Two hundred and thirty-one children were randomised, 117 to rectal diclofenac and 114 to rectal placebo. In the second randomisation 76 patients received ibuprofen (41 diclofenac, and 35 placebo), 77 received acetaminophen (39 diclofenac, 38 placebo) and 78 received placebo (44 diclofenac and 34 placebo). Children experienced 851 febrile episodes with 54 (23.4%) of children having a febrile seizure; of these, 46 of 197 (23.4%) had received antipyretics and 8 of 34 (23.5%) had only received placebo (absolute risk reduction = 0.01%; number needed to treat = 1000)
Conclusion	Antipyretics are ineffective in the prevention of febrile seizures in children
Commentary	Parents when witnessing a febrile convulsion are scared and frightened and as a consequence may become fearful of a recurrence of seizures when the child develops a fever. The use of antipyretic medication is ineffective in the prevention of febrile seizures and physicians should focus their effort on education with regard to the benign nature of the febrile convulsion and correct first aid measures.
Reference	Strengell T, Uhari M, Tarkka R, et al. Antipyretic agents for preventing recurrences of febrile seizures: randomized controlled trial. Arch Pediatr Adolesc Med. 2009; 63(9): 799–804.

Evidence 3

Theme E3	Treatment for absence seizures
Question	In the treatment of absence seizures, which is more effective: ethosuximide (ESM), valproic acid (VPA) or lamotrigine (LAM) as first-line drug therapy?
Design	Randomised controlled trial
Level of evidence	Jadad 5
Setting	The primary outcome was the freedom from treatment failure after 16 weeks of therapy. The secondary outcome was attentional dysfunction measured by the Conners' Continuous Performance Test.
Participants	Children were eligible for inclusion if they fulfilled the following: a diagnosis of childhood absence epilepsy based on the International League Against Epilepsy criteria, bilateral synchronous spike–wave discharges (2.7–5 Hz) that occurred on a normal background, and the recording of a least one electro clinical seizure lasting 3 seconds or more on a 1-hour video EEG.
Intervention	Patients were randomised to receive ESM, VPA or LAM.
Outcomes	Assess the effectiveness of ethosuximide, valproic acid and lamotrigine in the treatment of childhood absence epilepsy.
Main results	Of the 453 children randomised, 156 were assigned to ESM, 149 to LAM and 148 to VPA. At 16 weeks the success rates were VPA, 58%; ESM, 53%; and LAM, 29%. [(VPA-LAM, absolute risk reduction (ARR) = 29%; number needed to treat (NNT) = 4), (ESM-LAM, ARR = 24%; NNT = 5)]

(continued)

Evidence 3

Theme E3	Treatment for absence seizures
Conclusion	In the treatment of absence seizures ESM and VPA are effective.
Commentary	While VPA had the highest treatment success rate, the dose utilised is higher than those used in clinical practice and consequently ESM is the preferred first choice. The clinical value of the Conners' Continuous Performance Test is questionable and sequential assessment would be required to assess if the medications resulted in clinically relevant evidence of hyperactive behaviour in children.
Reference	Glauser TA, Cnaan A, Shinnar S, *et al*. Childhood Absence Epilepsy Study Group. Ethosuximide, valproic acid, and lamotrigine in childhood absence epilepsy. *N Engl J Med*. 2010; **362**(9): 790–9.

Evidence 4

Theme E4	The treatment options in infantile spasms
Question	Which is more effective, hormonal treatments or vigabatrin, in the treatment of infantile spasms?
Design	Randomised controlled trial
Level of evidence	Jadad 3
Setting	Department of paediatric neurology, multiple academic medical centres, England
Participants	Infants already enrolled in the United Kingdom Infantile Spasms Study (UKISS) trial with a mean age of 4 years were evaluated.
Intervention	Participants in the original study were randomised to hormonal treatments (prednisolone or tetracosactide depot) or vigabatrin. In this current study participants were followed up by telephone using the Vineland Adaptive Behaviour Scales and an epilepsy questionnaire.
Outcomes	The primary outcomes were the clinical and developmental states of the study participants as assessed by VABS and epilepsy questionnaire.
Main results	Of the 107 original children enrolled, complete follow-up was available on 77, of whom 39 had a proven aetiology for their infantile spasms, 37 had no aetiology determined and one had not been thoroughly investigated. Of the 30 infants not assessed, 9 had died, 14 declined and 7 were lost to follow-up. The median VABS score for all infants (39) on hormonal treatment was 60, but for those with no proven aetiology (21) it was 96, and for those with a proven aetiology (18) it was 45. The median VABS score for all (38) the vigabatrin group was 50, for those with no aetiology identified (16) it was 63 and for those with a proven aetiology (21) it was 50. When followed-up at 4 years in the hormonal treatment group and no aetiology identified 4 had epilepsy (4 of 21) and those with a proven aetiology 18, 13 (72%) had epilepsy. In the vigabatrin group (37) and no aetiology identified group (16), 9 (56%) had epilepsy, and in the proven aetiology group (21), 11(52%) had epilepsy.
Conclusion	Children with infantile spasms and no aetiology defined, treated with hormonal therapy have a better outcome than those treated with vigabatrin.

(*continued*)

Evidence 4	
Theme E4	**The treatment options in infantile spasms**
Commentary	Previously these authors reported that hormonal treatment was superior to vigabatrin in the cessation of infantile spasms on days 13–14 post treatment allocation (hormonal seizure cessation, 73%; vigabatrin, 54%; absolute risk reduction = 19%; number needed to treat = 6). The outcome measure used was the VABS, which assesses adaptive behaviour in four domains: communication, living skills, socialisation and motor functioning. Children with a known aetiology for their infantile spasms (periventricular leucomalacia, hypoxic ischaemic encephalopathy, Down's syndrome or tuberous sclerosis) had a poorer outcome than those without a known aetiology, an important point to consider with parents when discussing prognosis. The death rate in infantile spasms, 9 (8%), indicates the seriousness of this condition, which needs to be discussed with parents when they ask about prognosis.
Reference	Darke K, Edwards SW, Hancock E, *et al.* Trial steering committee on behalf of participating investigators. Developmental and epilepsy outcomes at age 4 years in the UKISS trial comparing hormonal treatments to vigabatrin for infantile spasms: a multi-centre randomised trial. *Arch Dis Child.* 2010; **95**(5): 382–6.

Evidence 5	
Theme E5	**Ketogenic diet and childhood epilepsy**
Question	How effective is a ketogenic diet in children with drug-resistant epilepsy?
Design	Randomised controlled trial
Level of evidence	Jadad 1
Setting	Department of paediatric neurology, academic medical centre, England
Participants	Children aged 2–16 years with daily, or more than seven seizures per week, who had not responded to at least two anti-epileptic drugs, and who had not previously been treated with a ketogenic diet were eligible for inclusion.
Intervention	Children were randomly assigned to receive either the classical or medium chain triglyceride (MCT) version of the ketogenic diet for 3 months in addition to their anti-epileptic medications or just their anti-epileptic medications. Seizure frequency in the month before the study commenced served as baseline seizure frequency.
Outcomes	The primary outcome was the reduction in seizure frequency.
Main results	One hundred and fifty patients were assessed for eligibility and 145 were enrolled. Seventy-three were randomised to the diet group [37 to the classic diet and 36 to the ketogenic diet (MCT)], of whom eight did not receive the diet (five changed their minds, one had seizures improve, two had change of diagnosis), 65 received the diet and 54 were included in the final analysis (ten discontinued the diet, six had poor tolerance, three had parents who were unhappy with diet, one had seizures increase, one had inadequate data). Of the 72 in the control group, 64 participated in the control period (eight did not participate, five changed their mind, one died, one had seizures improve and one had a change of diagnosis), 49 were included in the final analysis (15 had inadequate data recordings).

(*continued*)

Evidence 5	
Theme E5	**Ketogenic diet and childhood epilepsy**
Main results (*cont.*)	The reduction in seizure frequency was 62% from baseline in the ketogenic diet group but an increase to 162% in the control group. Three children had markedly increased number of seizures and if these three were excluded, the increase in seizures would be 12%. The reduction in seizures by 50% in the ketogenic diet group was 38% and in the control group was 6% (absolute risk reduction = 32%; number needed to treat = 3). The reduction of seizures by 90% in the ketogenic diet group was 7% and in the control group was 0%. Side effects of the ketogenic diet were vomiting 24%, diarrhoea 13%, abdominal pain 9%, constipation 33%, lack of energy 24% and hunger 22%. Of those with constipation, 24% required laxative treatment.
Conclusion	Ketogenic diet is useful in those children with treatment intractable epilepsy.
Commentary	Ketogenic diets have been used in treatment of drug-resistant epilepsies; however, the mechanism of action is not known. In this study 57 children had focal seizure and 78 had generalised seizures. Of the ten others, seven had severe myoclonic epilepsy and three were diagnosed as neurodegenerative diseases. The ratio of fat to carbohydrate is 3:1 or 4:1. The use of MCT has increased the ketogenic potential, which means that less fat is required in the MCT diet and therefore more carbohydrate can be used. Implementing ketogenic diets is labour intensive for dietitians and parents – therefore, the withdrawal of 10 (15%) of families is not surprising.
Reference	Neal EG, Chaffe H, Schwartz RH, *et al*. The ketogenic diet for the treatment of childhood epilepsy: a randomised controlled trial. *Lancet Neurol.* 2008; **7**(6): 500–6.

SEIZURE: MULTIPLE-CHOICE QUESTIONS

Q1 Which of the following statements regarding epilepsy is/are correct?
a) Two per cent of children have an unprovoked seizure.
b) The incidence of epilepsy is 1%.
c) Epilepsy incidence is highest in children 4–8 years of age.
d) Lateral temporal sclerosis is a common malformation that causes epilepsy.
e) If one parent has epilepsy the risk to the child is 20%.

Q2 Which of the following statements is/are correct with regard to febrile seizures?
a) Three per cent of normal children are affected.
b) Fifteen per cent of neurologically abnormal children are affected.
c) Human herpesvirus 6 is a common trigger.
d) Three per cent of children with febrile seizures will develop epilepsy.
e) Infants less than 6 months account for 10% of cases.

Q3 Factors that increase the risk of febrile seizure recurrence include which of the following?
a) First seizure less than 6 months
b) First seizure less than 15 months

c) Positive family history of febrile seizures
d) Seizure occurrence at high temperatures
e) Developmental delay

Q4 Which of the following statements is/are correct with regard to benign childhood epilepsy with centrotemporal spikes?
a) It accounts for 20% of childhood epilepsies.
b) It occurs between ages 3 and 13.
c) Eighty per cent occur in the evenings.
d) Common symptoms include tingling on one side of the face.
e) Family history is positive in 60% of cases.

Q5 Which of the following are correct with regard to childhood absence seizures?
a) They account for 10% of childhood epilepsies.
b) Seizures occur between 2 and 5 years of age.
c) Seizures typically last 1–2 seconds.
d) Typically children have 100 seizures per day.
e) Ten per cent develop generalised epilepsy.

Q6 Effective treatment for absence epilepsy includes which of the following?
a) Carbamazepine
b) Vigabatrin
c) Ethosuximide
d) Sodium valproate
e) Tiagabine for refractory absence seizures

Q7 Which of the following statements relating to juvenile myoclonic epilepsy (Janz's
syndrome) is/are correct?
a) Two per cent of adolescents with epilepsy have Janz's syndrome.
b) Typically, early-morning jerking occurs in the head and neck region.
c) Important triggers are sleep deprivation.
d) Sodium valproate is effective therapy for 80%.
e) Carbamazepine is second line treatment and effective in 60%.

Q8 Which of the following is/are correct with regard to Lennox–Gastaut's syndrome?
a) The aetiology is tuberous sclerosis in 25%.
b) Tonic seizures are typical.
c) In 30% no aetiology is discerned.
d) Carbamazepine is effective in 25% of patients to control seizures.
e) Long-term prognosis is unfavourable.

Q9 Which of the following is/are correct with regard to reflex anoxic seizures?
a) Seizures result from profound bradycardia.
b) The triggering event is often mild.
c) The child is pale in 15% of cases during the event.

d) The peak incidence is from 3 to 4 years of age.

e) Rectal diazepam is only required to treat 5% of children.

Q10 Which of the following statements pertaining to the EEG is/are correct?

a) An abnormal EEG increases the risk of epilepsy tenfold.

b) Up to 40% of children with an afebrile seizure will have a normal EEG.

c) An EEG can determine whether a seizure is focal, generalised or syndromic.

d) An EEG should be done on all children with their first seizure.

e) A sleep-deprived EEG should be undertaken in those children with focal seizures.

Answers

A1	a, b, e		**A2**	a, c, d
A3	b, c		**A4**	a, b, d
A5	a, e		**A6**	c, d
A7	b, c, d		**A8**	b, c, e
A9	a, b		**A10**	b, c

Chapter Twenty-one

SLEEP PROBLEMS IN CHILDREN

COMMON SCENARIO

'He's just 3 and has started waking during the night. It can happen up to three or four times in the one night. He keeps appearing at our bedroom door and sometimes I'm so tired that I just take him into our bed. I don't know what's waking him but it can take up to 20 minutes to get him back to sleep.'

LEARNING OBJECTIVES
- Understand normal sleeping patterns in childhood
- Describe the four main sleep-related problems in childhood
- Recognise 'red flags' in the history or examination that require investigation
- Discuss treatment options for children with disordered sleep

BACKGROUND

Sleep is a complex physiological process that is essential for life. The average child spends almost half of his or her life asleep. Sleep disturbance and inadequate sleep have negative effects on a child's cognitive development, mood regulation, behaviour and overall quality of life and family functioning. Sleep is broadly classified into two types: REM (rapid eye movement) sleep and non-REM sleep. Non-REM is further divided into four stages. Sleep architecture refers to how we progress through the five stages of sleep during the night.

There are four main sleep-related problems.
1. Dyssomnias: disorders of initiating and maintaining sleep
2. Hypersomnias: excessive sleepiness
3. Parasomnias: abnormal activity or behaviour during sleep
4. Sleep disordered breathing

The prevalence of behavioural sleep problems is high, with up to 20% of 5-year-olds experiencing moderate or severe sleep problems.

Normal sleep patterns and variations of normal in childhood

A newborn infant has a 4-hour sleep rhythm whereby he or she will awaken every 4 hours. During childhood this rhythm is gradually replaced by the adult pattern of 16 hours wakefulness followed by 8 hours' sleep. Through the preschool years, there is an organisation of the sleep–wake cycle into periods such as morning awake, afternoon nap, afternoon awake and night-time sleep. This pattern of sleeping in preschool children ensures that the young child settles to sleep early in the evening (perhaps as early as 7 p.m.). Over a 24-hour period, they tend to sleep up to 12 hours per day. However, they may resist this because of separation anxiety or if they are not tired enough to sleep due to a late nap or simply if they want to play with their parents or siblings. A school-age child sleeps about 10 hours per day. After a good night's sleep, he or she should feel rested, refreshed and full of energy.

Many parents lie down with or remain near their child until they fall asleep. This practice does not allow the child to learn how to settle to sleep. Parents, early on, should be encouraged to put their baby down to settle in the cot when drowsy but not asleep. Parents need to be calm, supportive and set limits over calls for drinks or to come out of the bedroom. During the night, infants or toddlers may wake up, open their eyes, lift their heads and move their limbs. If they are not touched most of them will fall back to sleep again unless disturbed by an anxious well-meaning parent. Therefore, most young children will awaken periodically during the night and, if they initially fall asleep in their cot or bed they tend to fall asleep again easily. Children who are put to bed already asleep have more night time awakenings than those children put to bed awake.

One of the most widely used sleep screening tools is the BEARS instrument:

B: Bedtime problems
E: Excessive daytime sleepiness
A: Awakening during the night
R: Regularity and duration of sleep
S: Snoring

The BEARS instrument can provide a useful framework for identifying sleep problems in childhood.

DYSSOMNIAS OR DISORDERS OF INITIATING AND MAINTAINING SLEEP

Dyssomnias are by far the most common sleep disorders in childhood. Bedtime resistance and night-time awakenings are one of the most common behavioural problems affecting toddlers and preschool children reported by parents.

From the age of 18 months, toddlers often have problems initiating and maintaining sleep. Toddlers often associate sleep with a particular blanket, rag or favourite teddy and simply will not go to sleep without them. Parents may have frantic searches to ensure a missing favourite teddy or rag is found. All are part of the sleep ritual. Most of the night rituals are discarded after 3–4 years of age. Very young children may wake a number of times each night but usually settle themselves down to sleep without parental intervention. By 1 year of age, 60%–70% of children are able to self-soothe. Some children, however, either cannot or will not settle themselves at night. The key problem is that they fail to develop self-soothing skills. The toddler learns to associate parental presence with sleep and becomes dependent on the parent's presence to fall asleep. Therefore the bedtime routine and parental reaction to night awakenings can perpetuate the problem, if they do not allow the child to initiate sleep and settle back to sleep on their own. Children with attention deficit hyperactivity disorder (ADHD) have twice the rate of sleep-related behavioural problems when compared with children without ADHD.

HYPERSOMNIAS

Hypersomnia is a term used to describe excessive daytime sleepiness. The commonest disorders presenting with hypersomnias are:

- narcolepsy
- idiopathic hypersomnia
- recurrent hypersomnia.

Narcolepsy

Narcolepsy is a chronic neurological disorder of rapid eye movement sleep characterised by excessive daytime sleepiness, cataplexy (sudden and transient loss of muscle tone often triggered by emotion), hypnogogic or hypnopompic hallucinations (vivid, dreamlike experiences that occur while falling asleep or upon awakening), sleep paralysis and sleep fragmentation. Many symptoms of narcolepsy can occur in patients who are sleep deprived. However, only cataplexy is unique to narcolepsy and indicates that the cause is due to a lack of the hypothalamic neuropeptide hypocretin. Hypocretin is involved in the regulation of the activity of norepinephrine, serotonin, histamine and acetylcholine cell groups. There is a strong association with HLA 0602. There are several reports of an association between the H1N1 2009 vaccine and the development of narcolepsy.

Idiopathic hypersomnia

Idiopathic hypersomnia is a condition associated with hypersomnia but it does not meet the diagnostic laboratory criteria for narcolepsy.

Recurrent hypersomnia

Recurrent hypersomnia or Kleine–Levin's syndrome is a rare disease characterised by recurrent episodes of hypersomnia with associated behavioural or cognitive disturbances, hyperphagia and hypersexuality. It affects adolescent males more than females. Patients are asymptomatic between episodes.

PARASOMNIAS

Parasomnias are disruptive sleep disorders that can occur during arousals from REM sleep or during partial arousal from non-REM sleep. They are characterized by abnormal polysomnography. There is often a positive family history. Common trigger factors include sleep deprivation, stress, unfamiliar surroundings and fevers.

The parasomnias include:

- nightmares
- night terrors
- sleepwalking and sleep-talking
- rhythmic movement disorder.

Nightmares

A child who has a nightmare will typically awake crying. Dreams can cause fear, terror or anxiety in the child who may be agitated and distressed. They usually occur in the second half of the night when REM predominates. An older child may be able to vividly describe the dream. When the parent comes into his or her room the child is easily comforted but finds it difficult to get back to sleep. Risk factors include life stressors, sleep deprivation, anxiety and medications that alter REM sleep.

Night terrors

Night terrors affect 1 in 20 children and occur when the child passes from non-REM to REM sleep. The child is typically found by the parents sitting up or standing with dilated pupils, confused and frightened, with a wide-eyed stare and shouting incoherently. There may be associated diaphoresis and tachycardia. Parental attempts to soothe the child are typically rejected. The child will resist efforts to comfort them unless they awaken completely. Night terrors typically last 15 minutes, after which the child usually lies down and falls back asleep. They have no recollection of the event the next day.

Sleepwalking and sleep-talking

Sleepwalking (somnambulism), like night terrors, typically occurs in the first third of the night when the child goes from non-REM to REM sleep. Sleepwalking is often a familial trait and it is most prevalent between the ages of 10 and 12. At least one episode of sleepwalking or sleep-talking (somniloquy) has been reported in up to 30% of children. The child may wander aimlessly and talk incoherently. A typical episode lasts 5–15 minutes. The main component of treatment is to ensure a safe environment for the child.

Rhythmic movement disorder

Rhythmic movement disorder is characterised by repetitive, stereotyped movements of the head, trunk or limbs occurring in sleep. It is commoner in infants and toddlers and is usually transient and self-limiting.

SLEEP-DISORDERED BREATHING

Sleep-disordered breathing has a continuum of severity from partial obstruction of the airway producing snoring, to increased upper airway resistance syndrome, to continuous episodes of complete upper airway resistance or obstructive sleep apnoea (OSA).

Obstructive sleep apnoea

OSA affects 1%–3% of children. OSA is a respiratory disorder characterised by intermittent partial or complete airway obstruction during sleep that may impair gas exchange and interfere with normal sleep architecture.

Increased risk of OSA is associated with:
- Down's syndrome
- neuromuscular disease
- craniofacial abnormality
- achondroplasia
- mucopolysaccharidosis
- Prader–Willi's syndrome
- obesity
- positive family history.

OSA should be suspected in a child with nocturnal snoring, witnessed episodes of brief apnoea or laboured breathing and frequent nocturnal arousals.

Complications of OSA include:
- behavioural problems
- deficits in learning, memory and vocabulary
- excessive daytime sleepiness
- cardiovascular consequences: pulmonary hypertension
- negative impact on quality of life
- failure to thrive.

CHRONIC INSOMNIA IN CHILDREN

Parents frequently complain that their children have difficulty with achieving normal sleep patterns. Some of these children will have an underlying neurodevelopmental disorder such as ADHD, autism or autism spectrum disorder. Other children however may have non-specific neurodevelopmental disorders that affect language and cognition. For this group of children difficulties with sleep initiation, sleep maintenance or both are voiced by parents. Contributing factors towards these difficulties include the child's disability (e.g. blindness), medications especially anti-epileptic medications, or maladaptive parental responses. The insomnia may contribute to daytime sleepiness and behavioural difficulties.

HISTORY

KEY POINTS				
Bedtime problems	Problems getting to sleep Normal sleep time Number of hours of sleep a night Night-time routine to get ready for bed Watch TV/read a book Favourite teddy takes to bed	**Associated symptoms**	Headaches Poor weight gain Episodes of collapse Enuresis Shortness of breath on exertion Syncope	**🔍 Red flags** Cataplexy Apnoeas Behavioural disturbance Decline in academic performance Significant impact on family life Poor weight gain
Daytime sleepiness	Difficulty with waking up in morning Need for naps during day Excessive tiredness Feel get enough sleep	**Parental reaction**	How they respond when their child does not want to go to sleep or wakes in the night Time taken to get back to sleep	
Night-time awakening	Wake during night Difficult to get back to sleep Nightmares Sleepwalking Sleep-talking	**Social history**	Academic performance Participation in extracurricular activities	
During the night	Snoring Difficulty breathing Gasping for air Cessation of breathing Abnormal movements	**Family history**	OSA Sleepwalking Impact of sleep disturbance on family	
Daytime behaviour	Hyperactivity Behavioural problems Learning or concentration difficulties	**Past medical history**	Recurrent tonsillitis	
Sleeping arrangements	Child in own room Sleeps in parent's bed			

EXAMINATION

- All children should have their height, weight and head circumference plotted on an appropriate centile chart
- Examination is usually normal
- Ear, nose and throat: assess pharyngeal shape, tonsillar size and nasal patency
- Presence of craniofacial abnormality

- Cardiovascular examination: prominent right ventricular impulse, loud P2 (second heart sound)

 Red flags

- Failure to thrive
- Obesity
- Dysmorphic features
- Craniofacial abnormalities
- Signs of pulmonary hypertension
- Marked tonsillar enlargement

INVESTIGATIONS

What is the gold standard investigation for children with sleep disordered breathing?

Polysomnography is the gold standard investigation, which provides comprehensive non-invasive monitoring of cardiorespiratory function and sleep. However, it is expensive, labour intensive and not widely available.

Parameters monitored include:
- electroencephalogram
- electrooculogram
- electromyogram
- electrocardiogram
- chest and abdominal movements
- airflow
- oxygen saturations
- carbon dioxide levels
- video monitoring.

An apnoea-hypopnoea index (AHI) is used to determine the severity of OSA. The AHI is calculated by dividing the total number of apnoeas or hypopnoeas by the total duration of sleep in hours.
- Normal AHI index is <1.4
- Abnormal AHI index is >1.4
- Severe OSA is an AHI index of >10

In suspected narcolepsy, what investigations should be performed?

- Polysomnography and multiple sleep latency test
- Cerebrospinal fluid hypocretin levels: levels of <110 pg/mL are diagnostic of narcolepsy with cataplexy
- HLA genotype testing for DQB1 0602

MANAGEMENT PLAN: SIX-STEP APPROACH

1. Clarifying and pitfall avoidance strategies:
   a) parents
   b) doctor
2. Treatment of disorders of initiating and maintaining sleep
3. Treatment of narcolepsy:
   a) pharmacological treatment of excessive daytime sleepiness and cataplexy
   b) behavioural interventions
4. Parasomnia treatment
5. Treatment of obstructive sleep apnoea
6. Melatonin use in children for chronic insomnia

Clarifying and pitfall avoidance strategies

Parents

- Explain the normal sleep patterns of infants and children. **Rationale**: parents, to address sleep-related problems, will need to know the normal sleep duration for infants and child and be familiar with sleep hygiene principles, which include:
  - establishing a fixed time for going to sleep
  - setting out a fixed routine pre-sleep, such as brushing teeth, getting changed into nightclothes and reading a bedtime story
  - a consistent parental approach to bedtime so the child receives consistent messages
  - avoidance of television, video games and computer games prior to bedtime
  - ensuring the child goes to bed awake – parents can sit adjacent to the bed and gradually move back
  - avoiding caffeine drinks.
- Parental inaction on sleep hygiene. **Pitfall**: failure to assess the reasons for inaction will result in a poor outcome. It is best to have the parents describe what they do, and assist them by providing a checklist as outlined in the previous point. Success is dependent on parental consistency.
- Explaining infant and child **unlearning process** of inappropriate sleep habits. **Rationale**: sleep interventions take time to have a successful outcome. Evaluate, with parents the duration of their child's sleep difficulty and explain that the unlearning process will take time and patience will be required.
- Parents and rules. **Pitfall**: discuss with parents their style of parenting. Parents vary in their style of parenting and may not be predisposed to ensuring a structured process is enacted, thus the reduced success rate.
- Assess parental sleep deprivation. **Rationale and Pitfall**: failure to assess the presence of sleep deprivation may lead to treatment failure; parents who are sleep deprived experience mood disturbances and have impaired coping skills.
- Evaluate burden sharing in dealing with the sleepless infant and child. **Rationale**:

who gets out of bed to deal with the crying infant or child? Frequently it is the mother; however, to reduce the impact of sleep deprivation, both parents need to share responsibility.

- Assess the impact of crying on the parents. **Rationale**: assess how they feel when their child is crying, and why do they think it is happening?
- Co-sleeping and secondary gain. **Rationale**: some parents will bring their child into their bed if he or she is crying, to obtain a good night's sleep. This may solve the sleep disruption but when they attempt to relocate the child to his or her room, a further set of difficulties may ensue.

Doctor

- Assessing sleep patterns. **Pitfall**: to discern a child's sleep pattern prospectively, assess it using a graphic representation (e.g. each line on a page represents 1 hour of sleep and the 24 hours represent a day. It is useful to log the timed feeding schedule and also the duration of crying). Parents' narratives related to sleep are subject to recall bias.
- Assess if it is more than a sleep issue. **Rationale**: children with impaired temperaments often have disturbed sleep. Consider the possibility of (a) cow's milk protein allergy, (b) chronic infections, (c) early signs of developmental delay, if irritable, and (d) a syndrome that is associated with sleep difficulties.
- Assess coping skills of the parents. **Rationale**: if parents have impaired coping skills they may wish for sedation as a treatment strategy. This is rarely indicated.
- Natural history of sleep disturbances. **Rationale**: longitudinal studies on sleep-related difficulties in children suggest that they are recurrent (*see* Evidence 1).
- Differentiating parasomnias from nocturnal seizures. **Pitfall**: the key feature to differentiate parasomnias from seizures lies in the duration of the event. Parasomnias last 2–20 minutes, whereas seizures last 20–30 seconds. Typically the seizure will be abrupt arousal, hypermotor behaviour and thrashing whereas the parasomnia child will demonstrate inconsolable crying.

Treatment of disorders of initiating and maintaining sleep

Behavioural or cognitive behavioural therapies are the most appropriate first line interventions for disorders of initiating and maintaining sleep. Behavioural therapy is designed to target disabling, unproductive or maladaptive behaviours. A behavioural intervention is applied to bring about change in how an individual responds to a particular object or event. It is based on learning theory and postulates that most human behaviour is learned through the interaction between an individual and his or her environment. Conditioning is pairing a reinforce measure with a behaviour to weaken or strengthen it. Children are more likely to learn and retain behaviours that are positively reinforced and less likely to learn or retain behaviours for which they receive no reward. In infants with limited language capacity, behavioural interventions are most commonly used.

Perhaps the best known behavioural intervention in children with behavioural sleep problems is graduated extinction (*see* Evidence 2) to treat infants with night-time awakenings. Parents are instructed to gradually increase their response time to their babies crying or 'progressive waiting'. This method, although highly effective, can be extremely challenging for some parents, as they will not be able to tolerate listening to their child crying without intervening, but explaining the process will encourage parents to use this process.

Cognitive therapy is designed to target unhelpful and/or irrational beliefs, attitudes or thoughts. A cognitive behavioural intervention uses both cognitive and behavioural methods to bring about change and is the most widely used intervention in children. Children with night-time fears benefit from this approach (*see* Evidence 3).

Treatment of narcolepsy
Pharmacological treatment of excessive daytime sleepiness and cataplexy
Excessive daytime treatment options include central nervous system stimulants such as methylphenidate, and dextroamphetamine, modafinil and sodium oxybate (*see* Evidence 4). Cataplexy treatment options include tricyclic antidepressants and select-ive serotonin reuptake inhibitors.

Behavioural interventions
Behavioural interventions include scheduling naps during the day, ensuring good sleep hygiene and appropriate exercise.

Parasomnia treatment
The time of occurrence of parasomnias is predictable; it can be assessed from a sleep log. Anticipatory wakening can be used to extinguish the parasomnias. This involves awakening the child every night, for 5–7 nights, 20 minutes before the expected time of the event occurs. The child should be fully alert for 5 minutes prior to returning to sleep. Anticipatory awakening is effective in 60% of cases. It is favoured by parents because no medication is required.

Treatment of obstructive sleep apnoea
Treatment of OSA depends on the underlying cause and includes surgical and non-surgical management.
- Adenotonsillectomy: post-operatively, polysomnography parameters improve by 75–100%. OSA is cured in 60%–80% of cases. Behavioural and health consequences improve within a month. Continued improvement in growth, quality of life, behav-iour, right ventricular function, neurocognition and academic performance.
- Non-invasive ventilation is indicated if (a) adenotonsillectomy is contraindicated, (b) there is minimal adenotonsillar hypertrophy, (c) OSA persists despite ade-notonsillectomy, and (d) if there is a strong parental preference for a non-surgical approach.

- Weight loss, in patients who are obese, may reduce symptoms sufficiently that further intervention is not required. Progressive weight loss is more likely to be sustained rather than rapid weight loss.

Melatonin use in children for chronic insomnia

Children with chronic insomnia related to neurodevelopmental disability benefit from treatment with melatonin (*see* Evidence 5); however, appropriate sleep hygiene strategies need to be employed.

FOLLOW-UP

- Regular specialist follow-up is required in all cases of narcolepsy to monitor response to treatment, recognise potential medication side effects and evaluate how the child and family are adapting to the disease.
- If behavioural sleep disturbance is causing significant distress to the family, follow-up and reassurance is needed to assess response to behavioural interventions and offer continued support.
- Children with OSA require follow-up to assess response to treatment.

WHEN TO REFER?

- Suspected narcolepsy, intermittent or recurrent hypersomnia
- Suspected OSA
- Uncertainty about the diagnosis
- Suspected underlying medical condition

CLARIFICATION FOR PARENTAL MISCONCEPTIONS

> '*I am unhappy with letting my baby cry alone in his room and 5 minutes is a long time to wait when I feel he is distressed. What else can be done?*'

Yes, 5 minutes is a long time to wait. You can reduce the time to 2 minutes if you like. Some parents place a chair in the room so the child can see them but they do not talk to the child. Every second night they move the chair closer to the door and eventually remove it from the room.

> '*When my child wakes up at night I usually pick him up for a cuddle to reassure him. What's the problem?*'

Unfortunately picking the child up and comforting him or her establishes another pattern, which the child learns as 'normal'. If your child is crying and standing up, avoid lifting the child out of the bed but soothe him or her by gently stroking the nape of the neck.

'My child likes to go to bed with a bottle. What's wrong with this?'

Your child may become a trained night feeder and will wake to try and find the bottle, when he or she fails to find it crying will occur. A practical solution for trained night feeders is to reduce the volume of fluid by one ounce every third night. This gradual reduction is frequently successful and parents should offer the child a drink prior to going to bed instead.

'What about some sedation for his insomnia? His grandmother takes pills to help her sleep.'

Sedating children to enhance their sleep is ineffective and not recommended. Melatonin is used in selective children with chronic insomnia.

SUMMARY PRACTICE POINTS

- Very young children frequently awake at night, but usually settle.
- Failure to develop self-soothing skills underlies many sleep awakenings.
- Consider cow's milk protein intolerance, occult infection if child is described as irritable and has sleep problems.
- Use sleep logs to assess sleep patterns.
- Give a handout on components of good sleep hygiene.
- Timing of parasomnias should be predictable.
- In children with daytime sleepiness, think of OSA (obese, dysmorphic).

EVALUATING THE EVIDENCE

Evidence 1	
Theme E1	*Sleep difficulties in children – the natural history*
Question	What is the outcome for infants who have sleep problems?
Design	Longitudinal cohort study
Level of evidence	
Setting	Community clinic, Australia
Participants	Mothers who had 3 years previously participated in a randomised controlled trial with their infants (aged 8–10 months) who had sleeping difficulties were surveyed by post to request participation in this study 3 years later.
Intervention	Participants completed a series of surveys to assess infant sleep problems (standardised maternal questionnaire), maternal well being (Edinburgh Postnatal Depression Scale, EPDS), child behaviour problems (Child Behavior Checklist for ages 1.5–5 years) marital satisfaction (Dyadic Adjustment Scale) and family functioning scale (General Functioning scale, McMaster Assessment Device).
Outcomes	The survey evaluated the presence and severity of sleep-related difficulties, maternal stress levels and maternal depression levels.
Main results	One hundred and fourteen (73%) mothers responded of whom 36 (32%) reported a current sleep problem with half rating it ≥4 out of a seven-point scale, with half of these children having 3 or more disturbed nights' sleep per week. For 14 (12%) the sleep problem had persisted from the infant study. Forty-seven per cent reported their child developed a recurrence of sleep difficulties since completing the study 3 years prior. EPDS scores differed between those mothers whose children had sleep problems and those without (median 8 versus 5). Factors that were associated with the development of sleep problems were the occurrence of nocturnal awakenings and the requirement of an adult to nurse the child to sleep.
Conclusion	The persistence of, or recurrence of sleep-related difficulties is common in the preschool years.
Commentary	This study, from a middle-class population, gives important data on the natural resolution (or not) of sleep difficulties in children. Its prospective nature gives reliable data on the persistence of, or the development of sleep problems in children. The mothers involved had the benefit of involvement in a previous randomised controlled trial, where infants with sleep difficulties were randomised to receive written information about sleep or behavioural management, and used this information to define sleep strategies for their child. Mothers of children with sleep problems had higher scores on depression scales and functioned less well during the day, which is related to sleep deprivation from the multiple awakenings of their child.
Reference	Lam P, Hiscock H, Wake M. Outcomes of infant sleep problems: a longitudinal study of sleep, behavior, and maternal well-being. *Pediatrics*. 2003; **111**(3): e203–7.

Evidence 2	
Theme E2	*How to treat night-time awakening in children*
Question	In extinguishing sleep problems is written information enough?
Design	Randomised controlled trial
Level of evidence	Jadad 2
Setting	Community clinics, Sweden
Participants	Children with sleep problems were invited to participate. Those with cow's milk allergy were excluded. Mothers maintained sleep diaries for a 1-week baseline and 1 week post intervention, which recorded:
	• the time the child was put to bed
	• the duration of protests before going to sleep in the evenings
	• the time it took to fall asleep
	• number and duration of night awakenings, signalled by the child
	• total sleep time at night.
Intervention	Behavioural extinction programme with advice and support or written information only were compared. The programme has two interventions. First the child is taught to fall asleep alone in the evening only. The parents leave the room and give the child brief verbal contact every fifth minute as long as the protests continue. If the child wakes during the night, comfort is provided by the parent. Once the child learns to fall asleep during the evening, the same process is applied to night-time awakenings. The Advice and Support Group (ASG) received a 1-hour consultation with detailed explanations to aid problem-solving their child self-initiating sleep behaviours in the evening, with follow-up telephone support. Two weeks later they had a 30-minute consultation to address the night-time awakenings. The Written Information Group (WIG) only received written information.
Outcomes	The primary outcomes were the protest times on being put to bed and the number of awakenings per night at baseline and at 1 month.
Main results	Seventy-six children were eligible and 67 were randomised (39 ASG, 28 WIG), with a mean age of 9.8 (range 4–30) months. The protest times for the ASG and WIG at baseline were 29 ± 154.5 minutes and 30 ± 19.8 minutes, respectively, and at 1 month were 3.1 ± 3.4 minutes and 2.8 ± 2.1 minutes, respectively. The night-time awakenings in the ASG and WIG were 4.6 ± 1.8 and 4.2 ± 2.1, respectively, at baseline and 1.7 ± 1.6 and 1.3 ± 1.2, respectively, at follow-up. There was no difference in outcome between the groups. The vast majority of parents in both groups found the changes in the settling routine easy to establish.
Conclusion	Both interventions were successful in extinguishing the sleep-related difficulties.
Commentary	Extinction procedures involve putting the child to bed at a designated time and then systematically ignoring him or her until a set time the next morning. A major drawback with this method is low parental acceptance and compliance. Graduated extinction was used in this study. Key elements included:
	• recognising that the child needs to register the environment when falling asleep and should not be put to bed asleep
	• the parent leaving the room allows the registration to occur but he or she can briefly appear at 5–10 minutes

(continued)

Evidence 2	
Theme E2	*How to treat night-time awakening in children*
Commentary (*cont.*)	• difficulties encountered can include the child's protests, misinterpretation of the crying and separation anxiety • parents can aid the child by giving a clear message by speaking calmly, not confusing the child by offering physical comfort, encouraging the use of a transitional object (not a pacifier).
Reference	Eckerberg B. Treatment of sleep problems in families with small children: is written information enough? *Acta Paediatr.* 2002; **91**(8): 952–9.

Evidence 3	
Theme E3	*The treatment of night-time fears (NFs)*
Question	What is the impact of brief interventions in NFs?
Design	Randomised controlled trial
Level of evidence	Jadad 1
Setting	Child psychology department, academic medical centre, Israel
Participants	At baseline the domains of NF, behaviour problems and sleep disruptions were assessed.
Intervention	Children were randomised into two groups: the Huggy-Puppy intervention, which is based on providing children a puppy toy with a request to take care of the toy, and a revised version of the Huggy-Puppy intervention, which is based on providing the same toy with a cover story that the toy will serve as protector. Graduate students related the cover stories to the children and parent and actively encouraged their engagement – this was assessed using the Doll Attachment Scale. Parents completed the Brief Child Sleep Questionnaire (BCSQ), the family background information questionnaire and completed daily sleep logs and utilised the actigraph, which is a miniature wristwatch-like device that records movement over a prolonged period of time.
Outcomes	The primary outcomes were reduction in NFs, reduction in dependency scores, sleep improvement, from baseline and at 6 months.
Main results	One hundred and nine children (64 boys and 45 girls; mean age 58.9 ± 8 months) with severe NF participated. Seventy-three families completed the study. NF score for parents and children was 5.5 ± 1.1 and 4.8 ± 1.6, respectively, at baseline and 2.1 ± 2.0 and 2.3 ± 2.1, respectively, post intervention. Dependency scores for parents and children were 4.9 ± 1.7 and 2.0 ± 1.7, respectively, at baseline and 2.1 ± 2.1 and 1.4 ± 1.6, respectively, post intervention. The number of night-time awakenings at baseline was 2.5 ± 1.8 and this changed to 1.6 ± 0.9 post intervention. The total time awake at baseline was 23 ± 30.4 minutes versus 9.7 ± 17.7 minutes post intervention.
Conclusion	Both interventions were effective in reducing NF in children. However, 17 families in the Huggy-Puppy intervention group and 12 in the revised Huggy-Puppy intervention group received further supplemental cognitive behavioural therapy for the NFs.

(*continued*)

Evidence 3	
Theme E3	*The treatment of night-time fears (NFs)*
Commentary	Behavioural treatments are effective in the therapy of night-time fears. Children are susceptible to night-time fears and for children aged 4–12 years the causes are, unknown (26.7%) fear of intruders (23.3%), imaginary creatures (16.5%), frightening dreams (12.5%), environmental threats (9.1%), animals (7.4%), frightening thoughts (4.5%). Children use a variety of coping strategies, sometimes multiple, which included seeking support from parents (44.2%), avoidance (29.5%), distraction (27.1%), trying to sleep (24%), active control (11.6%) and clinging to the stuffed toy (5.4%). These NFs are associated with a moderate amount of anxiety, which must be addressed. Cognitive behavioural therapy and self hypnosis are also useful strategies to reduce anxiety
Reference	Kushnir J, Sadeh A. Assessment of brief interventions for nighttime fears in preschool children. *Eur J Pediatr*. 2012; **171**(1): 67–75.

Evidence 4	
Theme E4	*The treatment of childhood narcolepsy*
Question	What treatments are effective in treatment of children with narcolepsy–cataplexy?
Design	Retrospective cohort study
Level of evidence	
Setting	Department of psychiatry and behavioural sciences, academic medical centre, the United States
Participants	The charts of children and adolescents with a major complaint of excessive daytime sleepiness and cataplexy (all meeting the International Classification of Sleep Disorders-2 for narcolepsy with cataplexy) were included in the review. All participants had primary narcolepsy.
Intervention	Standard treatment for narcolepsy was offered. Prospective data on medication response was collected in 78% of patients.
Outcomes	Patients were contacted in follow-up to determine their outcome and response to medication
Main results	Narcolepsy onset prior to puberty occurred in 53%, around puberty in 29% and after puberty in 18%. Clinical features experienced by the group were similar except for sleep paralysis, which increased in frequency with age. Excessive weight gain within 6 months of the onset of narcolepsy was noted. The medication use and frequency were as follows: (a) modafinil (84%), (b) sodium oxybate (79%), (c) venlafaxine (68%). Medications such as methylphenidate, tricyclic antidepressants and selective serotonin reuptake inhibitors, while utilised by patients, were not continued. Most children and adolescents required two medications to control their symptoms. The main side effect noted was irritability, which was noted in all medications ranging from 38% to 69%. Weight loss occurred in 20% of children using sodium oxybate but not with modafinil.
Conclusion	Patients with narcolepsy–cataplexy tolerate medications that are currently used in adults with the same condition.

(continued)

Evidence 4

Theme E4	The treatment of childhood narcolepsy
Commentary	This is a retrospective study but gives insights into potential treatment options of narcolepsy–cataplexy. The prevalence of narcolepsy in the United States is 0.05%. Children often evolve into narcolepsy first, with initial symptoms of excessive daytime sleepiness. The mechanism of modafinil is unknown but it is a novel wakefulness-promoting agent. Sodium oxybate improves both daytime sleepiness and cataplexy. The combination of modafinil and sodium oxybate results in patient alertness returning to almost normal.
Reference	Aran A, Einen M, Plazzi G, *et al*. Clinical and therapeutic aspects of childhood narcolepsy-cataplexy: a retrospective study of 51 children. *Sleep*. 2010; **33**(11): 1457–64.

Evidence 5

Theme E5	The role of melatonin in children with chronic insomnia
Question	How effective is melatonin in children with chronic-onset sleep insomnia?
Design	Randomised controlled trial
Level of evidence	Jadad 5
Setting	Department of neurology, academic medical centre, the Netherlands
Participants	Children aged 6–12 years with a 1-year history of chronic sleep onset insomnia were eligible for the study.
Intervention	Participants received melatonin 5 mg or placebo after a 1-week baseline assessment followed by a 4-week treatment phase. Continuation beyond the 1-month study phase was at the parent's discretion.
Outcomes	The primary outcome measures were the lights-off time advance, sleep onset (measured by diary and actigraph) and wake-up time.
Main results	In the melatonin group lights-off time advanced 34 (range 6–63) minutes, actigraph sleep onset 75 (range 36–114) minutes and sleep increased by 41 (range 19–62) minutes. Eighteen months later 13 of the 38 children who could be contacted had discontinued the melatonin as their sleep problem had resolved and in one child because there was no improvement.
Conclusion	Melatonin was effective in modifying the sleep pattern of children with chronic-onset sleep insomnia compared with placebo.
Commentary	Melatonin is a pineal gland hormone and its release is stimulated by light. Evidence suggests that it is useful in treating sleep onset insomnia and delayed sleep phase syndrome, which is seen in children with visual impairment, cerebral palsy, attention deficit hyperactivity disorder and autism. There are several melatonin preparations. Standard release melatonin is indicated in children with sleep initiation difficulties. The usual dose is 3 mg given 30–60 minutes before bedtime. The dose may be increased if there is no response at 14 days.

(continued)

Evidence 5	
Theme E5	*The role of melatonin in children with chronic insomnia*
Commentary (*cont.*)	Those children who have problems with sleep maintenance or early morning awakening should be prescribed controlled or modified-release melatonin usually 2 mg. Melatonin may worsen seizure control, thus children with epilepsy who use it should be monitored for increase seizure activity.
Reference	Smits MG, Nagtegaal EE, van der Heijden J, *et al.* Melatonin for chronic sleep onset insomnia in children: a randomized placebo-controlled trial. *J Child Neurol.* 2001; **16**(2): 86–92.

SLEEP: MULTIPLE-CHOICE QUESTIONS

Q1 Conditions associated with OSA include which of the following?
a) Down's syndrome
b) Achondroplasia
c) Obesity
d) Neuromuscular disease
e) Prader–Willi's syndrome

Q2 Complications of OSA include which of the following?
a) Memory problems
b) Behaviour problems
c) Pulmonary hypertension
d) Daytime somnolence
e) Increased appetite

Q3 Which of the following statements is/are correct?
a) Sleepwalking typically occurs in 10- to 12-year-olds.
b) Sleepwalking has a family predisposition.
c) Sleepwalking children are able to perform complicated tasks.
d) Ten per cent of sleepwalking children have temporal lobe epilepsy.
e) Sedating antihistamines are the treatment of choice.

Q4 Which of the following statements is/are true of night terrors?
a) They affect 5% of children.
b) Children have no recall of the event.
c) Children fall back to sleep with ease.
d) Children are frequently standing up when their parents enter the room.
e) Often have dilated pupils.

Q5 Which of the following statements is/are true of nightmares?
a) Children awake crying.
b) They are easily comforted.

c) They have difficulty getting back to sleep.

d) They occur in REM sleep.

e) Children have full recall in the morning.

Q6 Which of the following is/are features of narcolepsy?

a) Early-morning awakening

b) Excessive daytime sleepiness

c) Cataplexy

d) Hypnogogic hallucinations

e) Vertigo

Q7 Which of the following is/are true of polysomnography?

a) Is the gold standard for OSA assessment.

b) Nocturnal oximetry is a good screening test to perform prior to polysomnography.

c) The apnoea/hypoxia index is derived from polysomnography.

d) Concurrent electroencephalogram recording are made.

e) Concurrent electrocardiogram recordings are made.

Q8 Which of the following is/are true of narcolepsy?

a) HLA typing is available to aid diagnosis.

b) Cerebrospinal fluid hypocretin levels are low.

c) Secretin stimulation test aids diagnosis in atypical cases.

d) Methylphenidate is used for treatment.

e) Polysomnography is required for diagnosis.

Answers

A1	a, b, c, d, e	**A2**	a, b, c, d
A3	a, b, c	**A4**	a, b, c, d, e
A5	a, b, c, d, e	**A6**	b, c, d
A7	a, c, d, e	**A8**	a, b, c, d, e

Chapter Twenty-two

THE CHILD WITH
DEVELOPMENTAL DELAY

COMMON SCENARIO

'We weren't overly worried initially – our daughter was a late walker and she's top of her gymnastic class now. We thought Sam was the same but he just doesn't seem to be making progress.'

LEARNING OBJECTIVES

- Understand normal childhood development and variations of normal development
- Recognise 'red flags' in the history or examination that need further investigation
- Understand the causes of global developmental delay and developmental regression
- Understand the features of autism and its early warning symptoms and signs
- Explain what investigations are indicated in the investigation of global developmental delay
- Appreciate the multidisciplinary approach to managing a child with developmental delay

BACKGROUND

There is a great deal of variation in the age at which different children (even within the same family) achieve the same developmental skills. A good understanding of normal developmental milestones and variations is crucial in order to recognise (a) deviations from normal development, (b) 'red flags' that require investigation and treatment, to enable opportunities for early intervention and guide prognosis, and (c) the child's developmental potential. Some causes of developmental delay are genetic and may have important implications for the family and planning of future pregnancies. Developmental delay is defined as delay in the attainment of developmental milestones at the expected age. It is estimated that 5%–10% of children have developmental disabilities. Any parental concerns about delayed development or regression in skills should be taken seriously. Parental concerns about a child's developmental status are a strong predictor of actual developmental delay. Developmental milestones are the cornerstone of the developmental history and allow the identification of delay or regression and allow confirmation and reassurance of normal development or variations of normal.

The table presented in this section highlights important developmental stages in the first 5 years of life. Some general points to remember are as follows.

- Development of motor skills are attained rapidly during the first year of life.
- Hand preference should not be obvious before 18 months of age.
- Acquisition of speech is mainly in the second year of life.
- More advanced social skills are attained in the third and fourth years of life.

The developmental examination is divided into four areas:

1. gross motor
2. fine motor and vision
3. speech and hearing
4. social skills.

Patterns of developmental delays:

- delay – achieve milestones but at a slower rate
- dissociation – delay in one milestone but not in another
- deviancy – achieve milestones out of sequence
- regression – loss of previously attained milestones.

Developmental delay may be:

- static (genetic disorders, structural brain anomalies)
- acute (brain injury, meningitis, encephalitis)
- progressive (inherited metabolic disorders).

Developmental screening involves:

- consistently enquiring about and documenting a child's developmental progress
- making accurate observations about a child's developmental progress
- actively listening to and addressing parents' concerns about their child's development
- identifying potential risk factors for developmental delay
- validated screening tools can be used to enhance surveillance.

Age (Red flags)	Gross motor	Vision and fine motor	Hearing and speech	Personal and social
6 weeks (*Red flag*: no smiling by 10 weeks)	Symmetrical limb movement Ventral – head in line with body briefly Supine – fencing posture Automatic stepping and walking	Fixes and follows to 90° Turns to light Grasp reflex	Cries and coos Startles to noise	Smiles
3 months (*Red flag*: lack of head control at 3 months)	Moves limbs vigorously No head lag Prone – lifts upper chest up	Fixes and follows to 180° Plays with own hands Holds rattle placed in hand Object held in midline	Quietens to mothers voice Turns to sound	Laughs and squeals
6 months (*Red flags*: persisting primary reflexes; hand preference)	Sits without support Lifts chest up on extended arms Grasps feet Rolls front to back	Palmar grasp Transfers object Shakes rattle Mouths object	Turns to quiet sound Says vowels and syllables	Laughs and screams Not shy
9 months	Tripod sits – rights self if pushed and can reach for toy steadily Pulls to standing Stands holding on Forward parachute Crawling	Reaches for small objects Points with index finger Early pincer grasp Looks for fallen object (object permanence)	Distraction hearing test Says 'mama', 'dada' non-specifically	Chews biscuit Stranger anxiety Plays peek-a-boo Understands 'no' and 'bye-bye'
12 months (*Red flags*: not sitting, no pincer grasp, no tuneful babble, no pointing or other gestures)	Cruises around furniture Walks if held, may take a few steps unsupported	Neat pincer grasp Bangs cubes together Gives toy to parent	Knows name Understands simple commands Says few words <20% of speech understood by strangers	Drinks from cup Finger feeds Waves bye-bye Finds hidden object

(*continued*)

Age (Red flags)	Gross motor	Vision and fine motor	Hearing and speech	Personal and social
15 months	Broad-based gait Kneels Pushes wheeled toy	Sees small objects Tower of two bricks To and fro scribble	Two to six words Communicates wishes and obeys commands	Uses cup and spoon
18 months (*Red flags*: not walking, fewer than six words, not comprehending single commands)	Steady purposeful walk Runs, squats Walks carrying toy Pushes/pulls Creeps downstairs	Circular scribble Points to picture in book Turns pages of book Hand preference	Six to twenty words	Points to named body parts Feeds independently Domestic mimicry Symbolic plays alone Takes off shoes and socks
2 years (*Red flags*: absence of symbolic play; at 2½ years, no two- to three-word sentences)	Kicks ball Walks up and down stairs holding on	Tower of six bricks Copies vertical line	Two- to three-word sentences 60%–70% of speech understood by strangers Uses pivotal grammar Uses question words	Feeds with fork and spoon Begins toilet-training Temper tantrums
3 years	Walks up stairs 1 foot per step, down with 2 Walks on tip-toes Throws ball Pedals tricycle Stands on 1 foot for 2 seconds	Tower of nine bricks Builds train and bridge with bricks if shown Copies circle	Gives first and last name Uses plurals and past tense 80%–90% of speech understood by strangers Knows sex Recognises colours	Washes hands and brushes teeth Make-believe play Likes hearing and telling stories
4 years	Walks up and down stairs one foot per step Hops	Builds steps of bricks Copies cross Draws man	Counts to 10 or more Asks questions Tells stories	Able to undress
5 years (*Red flag*: difficulty telling simple story)	Skips Catches ball Runs on toes	Copies triangle	Asks 'how' and 'when' questions Uses grammatical speech	Uses knife and fork Able to put on clothes and to do up large buttons

SPEECH AND LANGUAGE DELAY

Speech refers to the mechanics of oral communication and language refers to understanding, processing and production of communication. Speech delay can be isolated or can occur with delays in other developmental domains. Speech and language delay is the commonest developmental disability in children. Isolated delay in speech and language is characteristic of autism spectrum disorder or hearing loss. Risk factors for hearing impairment include positive family history, prematurity, treatment with aminoglycosides in the newborn period, unconjugated hyperbilirubinaemia, facial or aural malformations, postnatal meningitis and chemotherapy. To recognise speech delay an understanding of normal speech development is needed. Understanding language generally precedes expression and use. It is more common in boys than girls. In approximately 60% of cases it improves spontaneously by 3 years of age.

Differential diagnosis	Features
Mental retardation	Delayed comprehension, delayed use of gestures, global delay
Hearing loss	Can cause profound speech delay, conductive or sensorineural, may be syndromic or chromosomal, history of intrauterine infection
Autism	Speech delay, other features include ritualistic behaviour, poor eye contact, lack of empathy, more common in boys, echolalia
Psychosocial deprivation	Warning signs in history, poor social circumstances
Expressive language delay	Problems producing speech, difficulty finding words to express themselves, comprehension and IQ normal, use gestures to communicate, shorter, less complex sentences
Receptive language delay	Poor comprehension of language
Maturational language delay	More common in boys, often family history, normal speech by school age
Bilingualism	Can delay language skills, usually proficient in both by 5 years
Elective mutism	Selective, often speak to friends and parents but not at school, often shy or withdrawn
Cerebral palsy	Associated hearing loss, decreased IQ, muscle incoordination
Phonological disorders	Problems with pronunciation of words

Causes of hearing impairment	
Congenital	
Genetic syndromes	Treacher Collins syndrome
	Waardenburg's syndrome
	Alport's syndrome
	Pendred's syndrome
Congenital infections	Rubella
Malformations	Goldenhar's syndrome

(continued)

Causes of hearing impairment
Acquired
Drugs: aminoglycosides, cisplatin
Unconjugated hyperbilirubinaemia causing kernicterus
Meningoencephalitis
Trauma
Chronic suppurative otitis media
DIDMOAD: Diabetes insipidus, diabetes mellitus, optic atrophy, deafness

AUTISM

The diagnostic criteria for autism are currently under revision. Typically a child will be diagnosed between 2 and 4 years of age. Recognition of autism is increasing among the general public and while a general practitioner will not be expected to make a diagnosis of autism, early recognition of potential symptoms and signs is the goal. All healthcare professionals need to be aware of the 'red flags' that are associated with autism, thereby preventing false parental reassurance. These include:

- the development of a plateau or regression in development, in particular language or social skills, but progression of physical development
- speech and language delay (e.g. no words by 2 years of age) or the use of repetitive words
- poor eye contact
- failure to recognise his or her name
- failure to engage physically with parent (does not like to be cuddled)
- poor engagement with parent in activities
- lack of interactive or functional play; does not use toys as they should be used; may focus on one part of toy
- not interested in other children
- resistance to changing routines
- usually develops unusual movements, such as hand flapping, twisting, rocking, spinning, toe walking.

GLOBAL DEVELOPMENTAL DELAY

Global developmental delay (GDD) has been defined by the American Academy of Neurology and the Child Neurology Society as performance at least two standard deviations below the mean, using standardised norm-referenced age-appropriate and developmentally appropriate criteria, in at least two domains. It is one of the commonest reasons for referral to paediatric neurologists. Global developmental delay (GDD) is the preferred term for significant deficits in learning skills and adaptation in children age five years or younger. The term 'intellectual disability' is applied to children older than 5 years of age, when IQ testing is more reliable and is characterised by significant limitations both in intellectual functioning (reasoning, learning, problem-solving) and in adaptive behaviour, which covers a range of everyday social and practical skills, with onset before 18 years of age. The terms 'global developmental delay' and 'intellectual disability' are not interchangeable. A child with GDD will not necessarily test in the intellectually disabled range when older. Global developmental delay affects 1%–3% of children under 5 years of age.

The *degree* of developmental delay can be divided into:
- mild – functional <33% below expected norm
- moderate – functional 34%–66% below expected norm
- severe – functional >66% below expected norm.

The causes of developmental delay are vast; however, key points in the history or examination may point to an underlying cause.

Causes of global developmental delay	
Chromosomal abnormalities	Down's syndrome, translocations, microdeletions, Williams's syndrome, DiGeorge's syndrome, Angelman's syndrome
Structural brain abnormalities	Neuronal migration disorders
Metabolic disorders	Amino acid disorders, carbohydrate metabolism disorders, lysosomal storage disorders, fatty acid oxidation disorders, urea cycle defects, peroxisomal disorders, mitochondrial disorders
Acquired brain injury	Meningitis, encephalitis, head trauma, asphyxia, near drowning, intoxication
Environmental	Psychosocial deprivation
Cerebral palsy	Spastic, ataxic, dsykinetic and mixed
	Prenatal, perinatal or postnatal insult
Non-chromosomal syndromes	Fragile X, neurofibromatosis, tuberous sclerosis
Prematurity	Less than 37 weeks' gestation
Endocrine	Hypothyroidism

Common syndromes causing developmental delay	
Down's syndrome	Dysmorphic features: upslanting palpebral fissures, flat nasal bridge, epicanthic folds, brachycephaly, single palmar crease, sandal toe gap, congenital heart disease, hypotonia
Prader–Willi's syndrome	Hypotonia, feeding difficulties, failure to thrive in infancy, short stature, small hands and feet, almond-shaped palpebral fissures, fair hair, narrow bifrontal diameter, obesity in childhood

(*continued*)

Common syndromes causing developmental delay	
Angelman's syndrome	Normal at birth, feeding problems, developmental delay by 6–12 months, most children non-verbal, epilepsy by 2–3 years, microcephaly, ataxia, happy demeanour, wide smiling mouth, described as 'laughing puppet', sleep disturbance
DiGeorge's syndrome (22q deletion)	Cleft palate, short stature, congenital heart disease, aplasia or hypoplasia of thymus, recurrent infections, failure to thrive
Williams's syndrome (microdeletion chromosome 7)	Dysmorphic facial features (wide mouth, flat nasal bridge, full cheeks and lip), wide mouth, bulbous nose, widely spaced teeth, congenital heart disease, overfriendly personality, hypercalcaemia
Fragile X (mutation of FMR gene on X chromosome)	Hyperextensible joints, long face, prominent ears, dental crowding, macroorchidism post puberty, mitral valve prolapse, language delay

INBORN ERRORS OF METABOLISM

Inborn errors of metabolism are the cause of developmental delay in only a small percentage of cases (1%–5%); however, they are important to identify as some may be treatable and improve the outcome for the child. The incidence of inborn errors of metabolism varies between populations and is a rare cause of isolated developmental delay. The term metabolic refers to all biochemical processes and pathways in the body. There are over 200 metabolic disorders that can cause developmental delay.

Inborn errors of metabolism can be divided into three groups.

1. Disorders that disrupt the synthesis or catabolism of complex molecules. Symptoms are permanent, progressive, independent of intercurrent events and food intake. *Examples*: peroxisomal disorders, lysosomal disorders and disorders of intracellular transport and processing.
2. Disorders that lead to an acute or progressive accumulation of toxic compounds due to a metabolic block. *Examples*: amino acid disorders, organic acidurias, urea cycle defects, galactosaemia.
3. Disorders due to deficiencies in energy production or utilisation within the liver, heart, muscle or brain. *Examples*: mitochondrial disorders, fatty acid oxidation disorders, congenital lactic acidaemias, gluconeogenesis defects.

When to consider an inborn error of metabolism:
- recurrent vomiting, poor feeding, failure to thrive in infancy
- intermittent episodes of lethargy, vomiting, acidosis or decreased level of consciousness
- developmental regression
- illness out of proportion to precipitating cause
- unanticipated symptoms during infection, fever or fasting
- symptoms on weaning
- familial consanguinity

- neonatal or early infant death
- organomegaly
- dysmorphic features
- cataracts, corneal opacities, pigmentary retinopathy
- chronic muscle pain and weakness
- unusual body odours
- renal stones and tubular disease
- cardiomyopathy.

Categories of inborn errors of metabolism:
- amino acid disorders – phenylketonuria, homocystinuria, maple syrup urine disease, tyrosinaemia
- carbohydrate metabolism disorders – glycogen storage diseases, galactosaemia, fructose intolerance, fructose 1, 6 diphospate deficiency
- lysosomal storage disorders – Tay–Sachs's disease, Niemann–Pick's disease, Gaucher's disease
- fatty acid oxidation disorders
- urea cycle defects
- peroxisomal disorders
- mitochondrial disorders.

THE FLOPPY INFANT

A hypotonic infant is commonly referred to as a 'floppy infant'. Hypotonia implies decreased muscle resistance to passive movement. On examination, the infant may have a 'frog leg' and/or 'jug handle' posture. The traction test, ventral and vertical suspension should be performed. Three simple observations can help determine if the hypotonia is central or peripheral in nature.
1. Are there dysmorphic features? If present, then likely central cause.
2. Does the infant fix and follow? if not, then likely central cause.
3. Are the deep tendon reflexes normal? If increased, central cause likely; if decreased, peripheral cause likely.

Causes of floppy infant	
Central hyptotonia	Brain malformation
	Chromosomal disorder
	Cerebral palsy
	Inborn errors of metabolism
	Degenerative central nervous system disease
	Spinal cord disease
	Systemic disease
Peripheral hypotonia	Spinal muscular atrophy
	Neuropathy
	Myasthenia gravis
	Congenital myotonic dystrophy
	Congenital muscular dystrophy
	Inborn errors of metabolism
	Joint laxity disorder

CEREBRAL PALSY

Cerebral palsy is a disorder of movement and posture due to a non-progressive lesion in the developing brain.

Types of cerebral palsy:

- spastic (80%–90%): hemiplegic, diplegic or quadraplegic
- ataxic (<5%): hypotonia, intention tremor
- dyskinetic (5%–10%): dystonia, athetosis, choreoathetosis
- mixed.

Cerebral palsy can be due to prenatal, perinatal or postnatal insult or unknown cause. It is associated with epilepsy (50%), visual problems (40%), hearing and speech and language problems (10%), learning and behavioural difficulties. Hemiplegia can present with asymmetric hand movement, persistence of primitive grasp reflex, early hand preference, absent parachute response and hypertonicity.

DEVELOPMENTAL REGRESSION

Regression or progressive intellectual and neurological deterioration occurs in children who have progressive deterioration in developmental skills for more than 3 months, with loss of already attained intellectual or developmental abilities and the development of abnormal neurological signs. The differential diagnosis for the cause of developmental regression is broad. Regression makes inborn errors of metabolism more likely. A useful approach is to consider whether there is white or grey matter disease, as this can help narrow the differential. Grey matter disease tends to present with early dementia and seizures and white matter disease presents with early spasticity and motor decline. An overview of possible causes of neurodegeneration is presented in the table here.

Causes of developmental regression	
Grey matter diseases without visceromegaly	
Tay–Sach's disease	Cherry-red macula, seizures
Rett's syndrome	Rett's syndrome is a progressive neurodegenerative disorder
	Females affected, develop normally up to 6–12 months of age, gradually loose speech and purposeful hand use
	Acquired microcephaly, associated with epilepsy, autism, ataxia, with stereotypic hand movements (wringing) and intermittent hyperventilation
	80% of patients are positive for MECP2 mutation on the X chromosome
Neuronal ceroid lipofuscinosis (Batten's form)	5–10 years, retinal degeneration, optic atrophy, seizures
Menkes' kinky hair disease	Hypertonia, irritability, seizures, abnormal hair
Grey matter diseases with visceromegaly	
GM1 gangliosidoses	Lysosomal storage disorder
	Infantile, juvenile and adult type
	Macular cherry-red spot
Sandhoff's disease	<6 months, seizures, blindness, macrocephaly
Niemann–Pick's disease	Accumulation of sphingomyelin, under 1 year, cherry-red spot macula
Sialidosis	Lysosomal neuramidase deficiency, types 1 and 2, intractable myoclonic seizures, cherry-red spots on macula, coarse features, corneal clouding
Mucopolysaccharidosis	Coarse features, hepatosplenomegaly types 1, 2, 3, 4
Gaucher's disease	Infantile and juvenile form, opisthotonus
White matter disease: leukodystrophies are inherited white matter diseases due to abnormalities in myelin production or maintenance involving the brain, spinal cord and peripheral nerves	
Adrenoleukodystophy	Males, X-linked
	Behavioural and cognitive decline
Alexander's disease	Macrocephaly, hypotonia
Canavan's disease	Macrocephaly, early hypotonia, optic atrophy, later spasticity
Pelizaeus–Merzbacher's disease	Nystagmus, early hypotonia, later spasticity, ataxia, peripheral neuropathy
Krabbe's disease	Infantile, late infantile, juvenile and adult forms
	Myelin loss, presence of globoid bodies in white matter
	Infantile form: excessive irritability, developmental regression, feeding difficulties, seizures, optic atrophy

(continued)

Causes of developmental regression	
Metachromatic leukodystrophy	Late infancy, hypotonia, absent deep tendon reflexes optic atrophy, decorticate posturing, gait disturbance
Aicardi–Goutières syndrome	Encephalopathy, seizures, sterile pyrexias, calcification
Leigh's disease (white matter)	Presents in first year of life, regression, failure to thrive, feeding difficulties, hypotonia, seizures, myoclonic jerks
Cockayne's syndrome	Autosomal recessive failure to thrive, microcephaly, photosensitivity, premature aging, hearing and eye abnormalities
Pantothenate kinase-associated neurodegeneration (Hallervorden–Spatz's disease)	Late childhood, increasing rigidity, choreoathetoid movements, dystonia, retinal degeneration

HISTORY

KEY POINTS				
Parental concerns	Are you worried about your child's development?	**Family history**	Developmental delay Metabolic conditions Epilepsy Genetic problems Cosanguity Early childhood deaths/sudden infant death syndrome	**Q Red Flags** Failures to achieve expected milestones for specific ages Loss of acquired milestones Family history of developmental delay Hand preference
Maternal and prenatal history	Infections in pregnancy Previous miscarriage Infertility Medications, drugs, alcohol Medical conditions Foetal movements Maternal phenylketonuria HELLP syndrome/acute fatty liver of pregnancy	**Medical and surgical history**	Seizures Meningitis Head trauma Recurrent ear infections History of hypoglycaemia Acutely unwell with mild illness	

(continued)

KEY POINTS				
Birth history	Gestation Birthweight Resuscitation required Ventilation Seizures Jaundice (phototherapy or exchange transfusion) Infection Treated with gentamicin	**Social history**	School performance Language(s) spoken in home Requirement for special needs assistant Resource hours at school Early intervention services Teachers' concerns Interaction with other children	
Newborn period	Poor feeding Poor suck Poor weight gain Irritability Recurrent vomiting	**Behaviour**	Self-injurious behaviour Psychiatric behaviour	
Developmental milestones	Age at attainment of key milestones Regression or loss of skills Hand preference Ataxia Balance problems, frequent falls, clumsiness			

EXAMINATION

All children should have their height, weight and head circumference plotted on an appropriate centile chart.

- Dysmorphic features
- Assessment of gait
- Assess tone, reflexes, power, coordination and sensation
- Examine cranial nerves and fundi
- Cerebellar exam
- Gowers's sign
- Skin exam for neurocutaneous stigmata
- Examine for hepatosplenomegaly
- Cardiac exam: cardiomyopathy

🔔 Red flags

- Significant microcephaly or macrocephaly
- Persistent primitive reflexes after 6–12 months of age (asymmetrical tonic neck reflex and Moro reflex)
- Abnormal limb tone and reflexes
- Thumb adduction and fisting
- Abnormal gait pattern
- Dysmorphic features
- Neurocutaneous stigmata
- Involuntary movements

DIFFERENTIAL DIAGNOSIS

Helpful clues to a diagnosis	Distinguishing features
Hepatomegaly	Lysosomal storage disease
	Glycogen storage disease
Delayed closure of anterior fontanelle	Peroxisomal disorders
Coarse features	Lysosomal storage disease
	Mucopolysaccaridosis
Cardiomyopathy	Fatty acid oxidation disorders
	Mitochondrial disorders
	Lysosomal storage disorders
Prolonged failure to thrive	Fatty acid oxidation disorder
Microcephaly	Smith–Lemli–Opitz's syndrome
	Grey matter disease
	Maternal phenylketonuria
	Cerebral palsy
	Cornelia de Lange syndrome
	GLUT 1 deficiency
Poor feeding and obesity	Prader–Willi's syndrome
Optic atrophy	White matter disease
Hypogonadism	Prader–Willi's syndrome
Macroorchidism	Fragile X syndrome
Macrocephaly	Canavan's disease
	Tay–Sachs's disease
	Glutaric aciduria type 1
	Mucopolysaccharidosis
	L-2 hydroxyglutaric aciduria

(continued)

Helpful clues to a diagnosis	Distinguishing features
Dystonia	Neurotransmitter disease
	Mitochondrial disorders
	Glutaric aciduria type 1
	Wilson's disease
Maple syrup urine	Maple syrup urine disease
Sweaty feet smell	Isovaleric aciduria
Thickened, coarse skin	Mucopolysaccharidosis
	Refsum's disease
Coarse hair	Mucopolysaccharidosis
Kinky hair	Menkes' disease
Cataracts	Peroxisomal disorders
	Homocystinuria
	Galactosaemia
Corneal clouding	Hurler's syndrome
Cherry-red spots on macula	Gangliosidosis (Tay–Sachs's disease, Niemann–Pick's disease, Sandhoff's disease)
	Sialidosis type 1

INVESTIGATIONS

In children with GDD, the yield from investigations looking to determine the underlying cause is highly variable (10%–80%). There are no universally agreed guidelines for the investigation of children with developmental delay. A detailed history and full examination are important in helping to guide and direct investigations.

What genetic investigations are required?

Chromosomal karyotype analysis is recommended in all newborns with problems in development, as at this age it is important to exclude translocation cases of trisomies 13, 18 and 21.

Chromosomal karyotype analysis – should be first-line testing if:
- identification of chromosomal syndromes such as suspected trisomy, e.g. Down's syndrome, sex chromosome abnormalities
- a family history of chromosomal rearrangement
- a maternal history of multiple miscarriages
- array comparative genomic hybridisation (CGH) is unavailable
- a result is required within 10 days.

Chromosomal microarray CGH analysis (aCGH) has a significantly higher yield than karyotyping in children with GDD and has replaced chromosomal karyotyping as first-line genetic testing for unexplained developmental delay.

(continued)

INVESTIGATIONS (*cont.*)

Advantages of array CGH:

- detects any DNA imbalance including extra or missing chromosomes and loss or gain of chromosome material much more precisely than karyotyping
- detects chromosome imbalances when there are no clues to what the chromosome anomaly might be and so would not be detected by performing specific genetic tests (such as FISH)
- reveals which specific genes are included in the deletion or duplication
- useful to further define breakpoints in imbalances that are already known.

Limitations of array CGH:

- will not identify balanced chromosome rearrangements such as balanced translocations and inversions, as these do not result in any loss or gain of chromosome material
- will not detect some types of polyploidy such as triploidy; a standard karyotype is still available and would be undertaken when needed
- will detect some but not all cases of mosaicism
- will not detect point mutations
- may identify chromosome changes, known as copy number variants, which are changes in the general population and are often completely harmless; however, a copy number variant can affect health or development and can make interpreting an array CGH difficult so the parents may need to be tested to help interpret the results.

What radiological investigations are helpful?

In children with significant delay, magnetic resonance imaging findings are positive in 30%–60% of cases. The yield is higher if any of the following features are present:

- abnormal head size
- abnormal neurological signs (cranial nerve abnormalities, cerebral palsy, neurocutaneous signs)
- dysmorphic features
- severe visual impairment (optic atrophy, nystagmus)
- associated seizures.

What is the role of audiometry assessment?

All children with delayed speech and language should have a formal audiometry assessment.

When are metabolic investigations indicated in a child with GDD?

In approximately 1% of cases of GDD, routine metabolic screening will be positive, so the yield is low. The results of universal newborn screening should be reviewed. Metabolic investigations should be selective and targeted.

Metabolic investigations are therefore reserved for cases in which:

- high clinical suspicion (coarse features, organomegaly)
- positive family history
- parental consanguinity
- developmental regression
- there are at-risk populations (e.g. travelling community)
- there is history of episodic decompensation.

(*continued*)

INVESTIGATIONS (*cont.*)

If indicated:
- creatine kinase
- full blood count
- urea, sodium, potassium, calcium
- liver function tests
- thyroid-stimulating hormone and free T4
- lactate
- ammonia
- urate
- amino acids
- biotinidase
- urine amino acids
- urine organic acids
- urine glycosaminoglycans.

Should children with GDD be investigated for fragile X syndrome?

Indicated if following features are present with developmental delay:
- head circumference is normal or large
- child is non-dysmorphic and no evidence of malformations
- family history of learning disability
- if aCGH is normal.

Fragile X is very unlikely to be positive if the child has malformations or if the child has microcephaly.

What is the role of an electroencephalogram (EEG) in the evaluation of GDD?

An EEG should not be routinely performed, but it is useful if there are associated seizures, significant language impairment or suspected neurodegenerative disorders – then an EEG is indicated.

How is autism diagnosed?

The 'gold standard' tools for the diagnosis of autism are the Autism Diagnostic Interview – Revised and the Autism Diagnostic Observation Schedule. Both of these were created from operationalising the Diagnostic and Statistical Manual of Mental Disorders, Fourth Edition, criteria for autism. Autism is a clinical diagnosis.

Investigation	Disease in which abnormal result may be found
Calcium	DiGeorge's syndrome
	Williams's syndrome
	Pseudohypoparathyroidism
Creatine kinase	Muscular dystrophy
	Fatty acid oxidation disorders
Lactate	Erroneous
	Gluconegenetic disorders
	Disorders of pyruvate metabolism
	Mitochondrial disorders
	Biotin responsive disorders
	Fatty acid oxidation disorder
	Organic acidaemias
Ammonia	Urea cycle defects
	Organic acidaemias
	Liver dysfunction
Uric acid	Increased: glycogen storage disorder
	Purine disorder, Lesch–Nyhan's syndrome
	Decreased: molybdenum cofactor deficiency
Urea	Urea cycle disorders
Hypoglycaemia	Fatty acid oxidation disorders
	Mitochondrial disorders
	Organic acidaemias
	Glycogen storage disorders
	Gluconeogenesis disorders
Abnormal liver function tests	Tyrosinaemia
	Urea cycle defects
	Fatty acid oxidation defect
	Mitochondrial disorders
	Galactosaemia
	Peroxisomal disorders
Respiratory alkalosis	Urea cycle defect
Urinary ketones	Elevated in organic acidaemias
Metabolic acidosis (increased anion gap)	Organic acidaemias
White cell enzymes	Lysosomal storage disorders
Acylcarnitines	Fatty acid oxidation disorders
Very long chain fatty acids	Peroxisomal disorders
MECP2 analysis	Rett's syndrome
7-dehydrocholesterol	Smith–Lemli–Opitz's syndrome
Urine glycosaminoglycans	Mucopolysaccharidosis

MANAGEMENT PLAN: FOUR-STEP APPROACH

1. Clarifying and pitfall avoidance strategies
2. Early intervention services
3. Autism and autism spectrum disorder
4. Inborn errors of metabolism

Clarifying and pitfall avoidance strategies

- Listen to parental concern about their child. **Rationale**: parents are often intuitive about their children and their concerns need to be assessed. Utilising formal assessment tools is recommended in clinical practice to validate concerns, as opposed to global assessment (*see* Evidence 1).
- Be able to put the developmental delay in context, in terms of frequency and origin. Examples include autism spectrum disorder 1.6/100 children, intellectual disability (mild) 1/100, intellectual disability (moderate to severe) 3–5/1000, cerebral palsy 2/1000, hearing impairment requiring a hearing aid 1–2/1000, blindness/severe visual impairment 3/10 000.
- Define a prognosis if possible. **Rationale**: most parents will want to know what the future holds and while in an individual case it may not be possible to specify, normally for defined groups it is possible to give a tentative outcome. However, if you don't know the outcome, say so. Giving a prognosis helps modify parental expectations.
- Formulate a specific treatment plan that involves the parents. **Rationale**: most parents will be required to actively participate in the care of their child, especially at home (*see* Evidence 2). Active and early parental involvement is essential as is ensuring that the roles of the various team members and their involvement in care provision to the family are explained. This plan may involve screening family members, if the aetiology of the developmental delay is genetic in origin.
- Providing clinical letters to parents. **Rationale**: many parents are their own case managers, consequently providing them with clinic letters is appropriate and essential.
- Care of the acutely ill hospitalised child with developmental delay. **Pitfall**: parents of children with developmental delay are usually used to hospitalisation and are aware how their child responds to illness. They are usually tuned in to soft signs of clinical deterioration (especially if an early warning score is not in use in the paediatric unit); therefore, if they feel that their child is clinically deteriorating, assess the child with care, paying attention to the child's physiological parameters. This helps to avoid the 'I told you so but you did not listen!' scenario.
- The concept of the home hospital. **Rationale**: many children requiring complex care are not looked after at home by their parents, with the support of community resources. This places significant stress on these families and if the child becomes ill direct admission to hospital is required. This should be formalised in a written treatment plan.

- Dealing with the difficult parent encounter. **Pitfall**: *see* Chapter 2: Communication.

Specific issues for families include the following points.
- Adapting to the new reality. **Rationale**: the diagnosis of developmental delay is devastating for parents and time is required to adapt to the diagnosis. Providing accurate information is helpful and putting them in touch with support groups is beneficial.
- Impact of the diagnosis on the parents. **Rationale**: mothers and fathers adapt at different rates to the diagnosis of developmental delay. Appropriate support should be offered to parents and they have the opportunity to accept or reject it.
- Impact of diagnosis on siblings. **Pitfall**: the diagnosis of a major illness or disability will stress parents, and siblings may be negatively impacted as the child with the disability will require more of the parents' time. This issue should be discussed with parents to enhance their awareness. Many families actively involve siblings in the care of the disabled child with positive benefits.
- Burden of medical care at home. **Rationale**: physicians and healthcare teams must be aware of the burden of care provision that is undertaken by parents. Parents will vary in their abilities and the treatment regime must be practical if parents are to achieve success. Prior to discharge assess the time that will be required to provide the child's care: if this time is exceeded by parents, evaluate the reasons.
- Provision of respite care. **Rationale**: parents of a child with a major disability should have access to respite care on a regular basis. This allows parents a 'holiday' from their role as carers. Some may choose not to avail of the service but providing the option is crucial.
- Communication with parents. **Rationale**: clinic visits need to be structured, therefore it is best if the child and parents attend a multidisciplinary meeting on a regular basis where treatment option, progress, and clinical difficulties can be discussed. Determining the role and responsibilities for agreed actions is required.
- Financial impact of a child with developmental delay. **Rationale**: parents need to be informed of resources that are available to them if their child has a major disability. This needs to be done proactively to avoid financial hardship.

Early intervention services
Referral to the early intervention service is indicated if a child has delay in two domains (e.g. if both motor delay and delayed speech). The child developmental team is a multidisciplinary team involved in both the assessment and management of children with developmental delay. The professionals involved include the following.
- *Developmental paediatrician*: diagnostic testing, support and advice on medical issues
- *Paediatric physiotherapist*: assessment and management of gross motor difficulties, provision of special equipment and prevention of deformities
- *Occupational therapist*: advice on toys, play and appliances to aid daily living

- *Speech and language therapist*: advice on feeding and assessment and management of speech problems, strategies for communication
- *Clinical psychologist*: cognitive and neuropsychological assessment
- *Special needs teacher*: advice on special educational needs
- *Social worker*: support to the family and advice regarding benefits and respite care

Autism and autism spectrum disorder

The treatment of autism will require input from a multidisciplinary team but the goals are:

- improved social functioning
- improved communication
- improved cognitive ability
- reduced obsessional and co-morbid behaviours.

To achieve these goals, a clinical psychologist and a speech therapist need to be involved.

Attempting to determine a successful comprehensive intervention to date has not been successful (*see* Evidence 3), although small randomised controlled trials of poor quality have shown effect. Children and adolescents with repetitive behaviours can be prescribed risperidone (*see* Evidence 4) but they need to be under the care of a specialist. Some autistic children with hyperactivity will benefit from methylphenidate, but often a therapeutic trial is required. An N = 1 study should be used to evaluate this intervention.

Children with autism experience sleep disturbances and melatonin is of value (*see* Evidence 5). Parents frequently find that they themselves are sleep deprived due to their child's disturbed sleep and will wish a specific intervention.

Parents of children with autism may wish to discuss the influence of the MMR (measles, mumps and rubella) vaccine on their child's symptoms and the role of diet in treatment. There is no temporal relationship between MMR vaccine administration and autism. There is no evidence that dietary manipulation affects outcome in children with autism.

General principles for management of inborn errors of metabolism

- Supportive care
- Reduce metabolic load
- Remove toxic metabolites
- Stimulate residual enzyme activity
- Enzyme replacement therapy
- Organ transplantation
- Gene therapy

FOLLOW-UP

The follow-up of these children depends on their primary diagnosis.

CLARIFICATION STATEMENTS FOR PARENTAL MISCONCEPTIONS

'Is there an epidemic of autism?'

Certainly autism is being recognised with increased frequency, but the reasons are uncertain. The use of the word 'epidemic' here is incorrect.

'Why is it that some causes of developmental delay are unknown?'

The potential causes of developmental delay is very extensive and the list is getting longer as our knowledge increases; however, knowing the cause does not allow (as yet) a specific treatment to be administered that reverses the developmental delay.

SUMMARY PRACTICE POINTS
- Developmental screening tools should be used rather than global assessments.
- The 'red flags' provided for child development are very useful.
- The 'red flag' list for autism will assist in the diagnosis.
- If worried about autism, refer early for an Autism Diagnostic Observation Schedule or Autism Diagnostic Interview – Revised.
- Global delay affects 1%–3% of 5-year-old children.
- Inborn errors of metabolism are individually rated but as a group they are more common than expected.
- Plot growth parameters inclusive of head circumference.
- Refer hypotonic infants promptly for assessment.

EVALUATING THE EVIDENCE

Evidence 1	
Theme E1	*Can parents identify cognitive delay?*
Question	Can parental reports identify children with cognitive delay?
Design	Cohort study
Level of evidence	
Setting	Paediatric centres in England, Australia and New Zealand
Participants	Infants who participated in the International Neonatal Immunotherapy Study (INIS) were eligible for enrolment. The INIS was a double-blind randomised controlled trial that evaluated immunoglobulin therapy for neonatal sepsis and an end point was cognitive function at 24 months.
Intervention	Participants were evaluated by the Parent Report of Children's Abilities – Revised (PARCA-R) and the Bayley Scale of Infant Development 2 (BSID 2). The PARCA-R consists of 34 items that assess non-verbal cognition (score 0 or 1), a 100-word list to assess vocabulary (score 0 or 1), and an 18-item assessment of sentence complexity (items 1–6, score 0, 1 or 2; items 7–18, score 0 or 1).
Outcomes	The primary outcome was the ability of the PARCA-R to define major cognitive delay, indicated by a BSID 2 Mental Development Index <55. Data from the PARCA-R and the BSID 2 administered within a month of each other achieved the greatest area under the receiver operator curve. With a targeted specificity of 0.9, the cut-off for the PARCA (Parent report composite) subgroup was ≤37, the sensitivity was 0.82, the positive predictive value was 0.37 and the negative predictive value was 0.99.
Main results	Five hundred and thirty-seven children had the BSID 2 completed and PARCA-R was obtained on 476 (88.6%). On the BSID 2 Mental Development Index only 29 (6%) had a score <55% and 71 (15%) had a score <70.
Conclusion	The PARCA-R is a practical tool to assess cognitive function at 2 years of age.
Commentary	Researchers are increasingly faced with the need to follow up infants to determine the outcome several years after the intervention. These assessments are expensive and time-consuming. The development of effective tools to allow parental assessment of cognitive impairment serves a dual function: (a) it allows researchers an alternate strategy for assessment and (b) it also allows the practising physician access to a cognitive assessment tool. If this assessment raises concerns a formal evaluation may then be requested. These evaluations may not be readily available therefore prudence is required when they are requested. The early detection of cognitive disabilities allows an opportunity for remediation prior to the child attending school.
Reference	Martin AJ, Darlow BA, Salt A, et al.; INIS Trial Collaborative Group. Identification of infants with major cognitive delay using parental report. *Dev Med Child Neurol.* 2012; **54**(3): 254–9.

Evidence 2	
Theme E2	*Home-based intervention for developmental delay*
Question	What is the impact of home-based visits for children with developmental delay?
Design	Randomised controlled trial
Level of evidence	Jadad 3
Setting	Department of paediatrics, child development and rehabilitation, academic medical centre, Australia
Participants	Children aged 3–5 years of age, attending a child development centre, with communication disorders, developmental delay, physical disabilities and pervasive developmental delay were eligible for inclusion.
Intervention	Both groups received standard care interventions, which included multidisciplinary team involvement for 5 hours per week over the school terms. Each child had an individualised programme developed with input from the parents. The home-based programme was for 1–1.5 hours per week for 40 weeks, focused on the needs of the child by reinforcing centre-based activities and developing new goals and objectives at home, e.g. enhancing the skills of daily living. Parents were helped to understand the meaning of difficult behaviour and coached in coaxing strategies, e.g. offering a choice with regard to clothes preferences. Cognitive development was assessed using the Bayley Scales of Infant Development for children functioning less than 3.5 years and the Wechsler Preschool and Primary Scale of Intelligence for those who were older. The child's behaviour was assessed using the Preschool Behavior Checklist, which was completed by the teachers at the centre.
Outcomes	The primary outcome was the change in cognitive development and behaviour of the participants.
Main results	Twenty-nine children received the centre-based intervention and 30 received both centre and home interventions. In the intervention group the intelligence quotient (IQ) pre-intervention was 60.2 and improved by 4.7 points post intervention. For the control group the pre-intervention IQ was 60.6 but fell by 3.5 points over the year. In the intervention group the Preschool Behavior Checklist was 19.2 pre-intervention and fell by 7.2 post intervention; for the control group it was 17.4 pre-intervention and it increased by 0.3.
Conclusion	This study suggests that reinforcing the skills learnt by children and families during centre-based programmes through a home visiting programme is beneficial to both child and parent.
Commentary	This study indicated that children with disabilities can have improved functioning with the addition of a home programme. This may influence parents in their choice of schooling for their children. More intensive intervention at home could allow some of these children to attend mainstream schools. An added benefit of the home intervention was the ability to tackle difficult behaviour, which parents found demanding. The reduction in IQ of the control group of 3.5 points was less than 0.5 standard deviations, which the authors defined as no change.
Reference	Rickards AL, Walstab JE, Wright-Rossi RA, *et al*. A randomized, controlled trial of a home-based intervention program for children with autism and developmental delay. *J Dev Behav Pediatr*. 2007; **28**(4): 308–15.

Evidence 3	
Theme E3	*Social communication and autism*
Question	How effective is parent-mediated communication-focused treatment (PACT) in children with autism?
Design	Randomised controlled trial
Level of evidence	Jadad 5
Setting	Primary care centres, three academic medical centres, England
Participants	Families with a child aged between 2 years and 4 years 11 months with autism diagnosed according to the international standard diagnostic test (social and communication domains of the Autism Diagnostic Observation Schedule – Generic and two of the three domains of the Autism Diagnostic Interview Revised Algorithm) were eligible for inclusion. Endpoint assessments were videotaped, and anonymised for assessment.
Intervention	The intervention group received usual care plus the PACT intervention where the control group received the usual intervention only. The PACT intervention targets social interactive and communication impairments in autism.
Outcomes	The primary outcome was the Autism Diagnostic Observation Schedule – Generic social communication algorithm score which is a measure of the severity of the symptoms of autism. Secondary outcomes were (a) parent–child interaction during naturalistic play in a standard non-therapy setting, (b) change in the child's language and social communication and (c) the adaptive functioning in the school beyond the family.
Main results	Of 252 families assessed for eligibility, 90 were excluded (35 declined, 27 did not meet inclusion criteria and the remainder for 10 other reasons) and 152 were randomised. Seventy-seven were allocated to the PACT, with 74 (96%) completing the study, and 75 were allocated to the control group, with 72 (96%) completing the study. At the end of the study most children were still classified as autism (65% in PACT group and 71% in the usual treatment group); however, 30% of the PACT group, compared with 22% of the usual treatment group (absolute risk reduction = 8%; number needed to treat = 13), had changed to autism spectrum disorder and 5% of the PACT group had changed to non-spectrum, compared with 7% of the usual treatment group. There were positive effects for the secondary outcome parent–child social communication.
Conclusion	On the basis of this study the PACT intervention cannot be recommended as an add-on intervention for the reduction of autism symptoms.
Commentary	The PACT interventions aim to increase parental sensitivity and responsiveness to child communication and reduce mistimed parental responses by working with the parents and using video feedback methods to address parent–child interaction. They also aim to improve the child's communication by a range of strategies such as action routines, familiar repetitive language and pauses. This was an intensive intervention with a 2-hour clinic visit every 2 weeks for 6 months, followed by a monthly booster session for 6 months. Between sessions parents were requested to do 30 minutes per day of home practice. Usual treatment resulted in 10 hours of speech and language therapy. Families had access to group based psychoeducation, communication-focused interventions.

(*continued*)

Evidence 3	
Theme E3	*Social communication and autism*
Commentary (*cont.*)	Initial studies of the PACT intervention indicated a significant treatment effect, which was not replicated in this large and well-designed study, outlining the pitfalls of basing treatment strategies on poor evidence.
Reference	Green J, Charman T, McConachie H, *et al.* Parent-mediated communication-focussed treatment in children with autism (PACT): a randomised controlled trial. *Lancet.* 2010; **375**(9732): 2152–60.

Evidence 4	
Theme E4	*Drug therapy in children with autism*
Question	Is risperidone effective in the treatment of autism?
Design	Randomised controlled trial; secondary outcomes being reported, separate from original study)
Level of evidence	
Setting	Five departments of psychiatry, academic medical centres, the United States
Participants	Children aged 5–17 years were eligible for inclusion if they met the Diagnostic and Statistical Manual of Mental Disorders, Fourth Edition, criteria for autism and they experienced impairing behavioural symptoms such as severe tantrums, aggression or self-injurious behaviour.
Intervention	Participants were randomised to 8 weeks of risperidone or placebo, and subsequently entered the open-label phase of the study. The Ritvo-Freeman Real Life Rating Scale (RFRLR scale) was modified to convert it from a self-reporting scale to allow parents to report their observations. The scale assesses sensory motor behaviours, social relatedness, affectual reactions, sensory reactions and language.
Outcomes	The paper reports on the secondary outcomes of the original study as measured on the RFRLR scale, the Children's Yale Brown Obsessive Compulsive Scale and the Maladaptive Behaviour domain of the Vineland Adaptive Behaviour Scale.
Main results	Of the original 270 patients screened, 112 did not meet the inclusion criteria and the parents of 57 declined to participate. One hundred and one patients entered the double-blind component of the study. The mean age of the children was 8.8 years (range 5–17 years). The RFRLR scale scores were significantly reduced in the sensory motor behaviours, affectual reactions and sensory response after treatment with risperidone.
Conclusion	Risperidone led to significant improvement in the restricted, repetitive and stereotypical patterns of behaviour interests and activities of autistic children but did not change the deficits in social interaction and communication.
Commentary	The RFRFL scale used was adapted to allow assessment of a clinical response. The actual items evaluated were sensory motor behaviours included hand flapping, rocking and pacing. Social-relatedness behaviours include appropriate responses to interaction attempts and the initiation of appropriate physical contact. Affectual reactions are abrupt changes in affect, e.g. crying and temper tantrums.

(*continued*)

Evidence 4	
Theme E4	*Drug therapy in children with autism*
Commentary *(cont.)*	Sensory responses include being agitated by noises, rubbing surfaces and sniffing self or objects. Language evaluates communication skills and the appropriateness of language. In dealing with families with autistic children, there may be a multitude of symptoms and classifying them into groups is useful for both parents and clinicians.
	In studies the primary outcomes are the most relevant but in some studies (as in this case) the secondary outcomes have relevance that can be translated into clinical practice.
Reference	McDougle CJ, Scahill L, Aman MG, *et al.* Risperidone for the core symptom domains of autism: results from the study by the Autism Network of the Research Units on Pediatric Psychopharmacology. *Am J Psychiatry.* 2005; **162**(6): 1142–8.

Evidence 5	
Theme E5	*Melatonin in children with autism spectrum disorder and fragile X syndrome*
Question	In children with fragile X or autism with sleep problems, is melatonin treatment effective?
Design	Randomised controlled trial
Level of evidence	Jadad 5
Setting	Paediatric clinic, academic medical centre, the United States
Participants	Children and adolescents with sleep problems who were diagnosed with autism, fragile X syndrome or autism and fragile X were eligible for enrolment.
Intervention	Participants received melatonin or placebo for 2 weeks and then alternated for another 2 weeks after a 1-week baseline assessment period.
Outcomes	The primary outcomes were changes in sleep duration, sleep-onset latency and sleep-onset time, which were measured by an Actiwatch and sleep diaries completed by parents.
Main results	Eighteen patients were enrolled, of whom 12 completed the study, with a mean age of 5.47 years (range 2–15.25 years). Five participants met the diagnostic criteria of autism spectrum disorder, three for fragile X syndrome, three for fragile X syndrome and autism spectrum disorder, and one for fragile X permutation. Melatonin treatment increased sleep by 21 minutes, mean sleep-onset latency was reduced by 28 minutes and mean sleep-onset time was earlier by 42 minutes. No adverse effects from melatonin treatment were reported. There were no differences in the frequency of sleep awakenings between the two groups.
Conclusion	The use of melatonin lessened the sleep difficulties experienced by the participants and can be offered as a therapeutic option.
Commentary	Children with autism and fragile X syndrome have cognitive and behavioural problems; however, the presence of associated sleep disturbances increases the stress levels in families and contributes to sleep deprivation in the parents as well as the child.

(continued)

Evidence 5	
Theme E5	*Melatonin in children with autism spectrum disorder and fragile X syndrome*
Commentary (*cont.*)	The use of melatonin is a therapeutic option available for treatment of the sleep difficulties that these children experience. The dose utilised in this study was 3 mg of melatonin.
Reference	Wirojanan J, Jacquemont S, Diaz R, *et al.* The efficacy of melatonin for sleep problems in children with autism, fragile X, or autism and fragile X. *J Clin Sleep Med.* 2009; **5**(2): 145–50.

DEVELOPMENT DELAY: MULTIPLE-CHOICE QUESTIONS

Q1 Which of the following statements should raise concerns regarding appropriate development?
a) Lack of head control at 3 months
b) Persisting primary reflexes at 6 months
c) Hand preference at 6 months
d) No pincer grasp at 6 months
e) No sitting at 9 months

Q2 Which of the following statements should raise concern regarding appropriate development?
a) Hand preference at 6 months
b) No tuneful babbling at 12 months
c) No pointing at 15 months
d) Absence of symbolic play at 2 years
e) No sentences at 18 months

Q3 Which of the following statements is/are true for a normal child 18 months of age?
a) The child has 6–20 words
b) The child walks carrying a toy
c) The child can build a tower of six bricks
d) The child can walk up and down stairs holding on
e) The child feeds him- or herself independently

Q4 Features of autism include which of the following?
a) Ritualistic play
b) Poor eye contact
c) Failure to thrive
d) Lack of empathy
e) Macrocephaly

Q5 Features of Williams's syndrome include which of the following?
  a) Congenital heart disease
  b) Overfriendly personality
  c) Widely spaced teeth
  d) Sensitivity to noise
  e) Cleft palate

Q6 Inborn errors of metabolism should be considered in children with which of the following symptom complexes?
  a) Developmental regression
  b) Recurrent vomiting and failure to thrive
  c) Unusual body odours
  d) Cataracts, corneal opacities
  e) Recurrence episodes of coma

Q7 Features of Rett's syndrome include which of the following?
  a) Epilepsy
  b) Developmental regression at 4–6 years of age
  c) Macrocephaly
  d) Intermittent hyperventilation
  e) Autism

Q8 Which of the following statements on chromosomal microarray CGH analysis are correct?
  a) It is first-line genetic testing for unexplained developmental delay.
  b) It detects chromosomal imbalances better that karyotyping.
  c) It detects almost all cases of mosacism.
  d) It detects balanced translocations.
  e) It requires a relatively large blood sample (7 mL).

Answers

A1	a, b, c, e		**A2**	a, b, c, d
A3	a, b, e		**A4**	a, b, d
A5	a, b, d		**A6**	a, b, c, d, e
A7	a, d, e		**A8**	a, b

SLIDES

1. Myelomeningocoele 1
2. Myelomeningocoele 2
3. Talipes equinovarus
4. Kyphoscoliosis
5. Partial lipodystrophy
6. Absent red reflex (toxocariasis)

Chapter Twenty-three

THE CHILD WITH DOWN'S SYNDROME

COMMON SCENARIO

An infant, born at term to a 38-year-old mother, is noted by the midwife to have dysmorphic features that include flattening of the skull and upward-slanting palpebral fissures, and he also has low tone.

LEARNING OBJECTIVES

- Recognise Down's syndrome (DS) and be able to describe the three types
- Develop a strategy to explain the diagnosis to the parents
- Be aware of potential complications in the neonatal period
- Anticipate the future care requirements of children with DS
- Devise a strategy for when to order laboratory tests for children with DS

BACKGROUND

Children with DS are easily recognised. Typical features include:

- hypotonia
- microcephaly with brachycephaly
- epicanthic folds
- flat nasal bridge
- upward-slanting palpebral fissures
- Brushfield's spots (in the eyes)
- small mouth
- small ears
- excessive redundant skin at the nape of the neck
- single palmar crease
- a short fifth finger with clinodactyly.

Genetically, three forms of DS are recognised. The most common, in 95%, is a non-familial trisomy 21 (47 chromosomes are present with an extra chromosome 21, hence the name). In 3%–4% of children with DS phenotype there is an unbalanced translocation between chromosome 21 and another chromosome, usually number 14. The majority of these (75%) are de novo but a minority are the result of familial translocations and as a consequence, genetic studies on the parents need to be performed to further counsel and advise them. In the remaining 1%–2% of children with DS, mosacism is present (two cell lines are present: one normal and one with trisomy 21). The risk of having a child with DS increases in a linear fashion up until the age of 30 and increases exponentially thereafter.

Children with DS have variable degrees of cognitive impairment, which may be mild (IQ of 50–70), moderate (IQ of 35–50) or severe (IQ of 20–35).

The approximate risks of associated impairment are:
- hearing loss (75%)
- visual problems (60%)
- cataracts (15%)
- refractive errors (50%)
- obstructive sleep apnoea (OSA) (50%–75%)
- otitis media (50%–70%)
- congenital heart disease (40%–50%)
- hypodontia and delayed dental eruption (23%)
- gastrointestinal atresias (12%)
- thyroid disease (4%–18%)
- seizures (1%–13%)
- haematological problems inclusive of anaemia (3%)
- iron deficiency (10%)
- transient myeloproliferative disorder (10%)
- leukaemia (1%)
- coeliac disease (5%)
- atlantoaxial instability (1%–2%)
- autism (1%)
- Hirschsprung's disease (<1%).

The most widely used antenatal screening test for DS is the triple test: alpha-fetoprotein, unconjugated oestriol and human chorionic gonadotropin. This is usually performed at 15–18 weeks' gestation. The likelihood of trisomy 21 is determined based on the level of each serum marker and the mother's age. The triple test has a false positive rate of 5%. A normal result reduces the likelihood of trisomy 21 but does not exclude it. Definitive prenatal diagnosis requires foetal karyotyping. This can be performed by chorionic villus sampling or amniocentesis.

The diagnosis of DS is usually made after birth, given that the features are readily recognisable to experienced midwifery staff. Communicating the diagnosis to the parents requires sensitivity and should be delivered by an experienced doctor who will be able to address the parents' concerns. It is not appropriate to withhold the diagnosis until the chromosome analysis is available. Parents will remember how the diagnosis is disclosed to them for many years; therefore, due care must be exercised. The meeting should take place in a private setting and the parents should first be congratulated on the birth of their child. The discussion will include certainty that the diagnosis is correct, why it happened, could it happen again, the likely developmental progress and the immediate health concerns, if present. The doctor should employ a balanced approach to the information given, ensuring that it is current, and avoid personal bias. Explaining to parents the available local resources is helpful and many have a preference to meet with a parent who has a child with DS, which should be facilitated if possible. A specific meeting with the parents prior to discharge is helpful and any unasked or unanswered questions can be addressed. All children with DS must have a specific plan at discharge, which includes the timing of the next visit, what to do if problems arise and who to contact. Communicating the diagnosis to the family doctor is important, as is outlining the current clinical issues at discharge.

The healthcare needs of the child with DS are varied and potential complications must be anticipated; therefore, follow-up in a specialty clinic is advised.

HISTORY

KEY POINTS IN THE NEWBORN PERIOD				
Antenatal history	Scans performed during pregnancy Triple test Chorionic villus sampling Amniocentesis Antenatal diagnosis made	**Birth History**	Gestation Birthweight Delivery mode Apgar score	**🔴 Red flags** Poor weight gain Failure to pass meconium at 24 hours Bilious vomiting
Maternal history	Previous pregnancies Age	**Feeding history**	Breast- or bottle-fed Number of wet nappies Weight loss Shortness of breath with feeds	
Family history	Previous children with DS Children with disabilities	**Vomiting**	Frequency Volume Bile Passed meconium	

(continued)

KEY POINTS IN THE NEWBORN PERIOD				
Diagnosis and expectations	How was diagnosis made? Parental understanding of DS Acceptance of diagnosis Written information on condition Awareness of support groups	**Special care baby unit or neonatal intensive care unit admission**	Admitted to special care baby unit or neonatal intensive care unit Breathing difficulties Blue or cyanotic episodes	
		Follow-up	Appointments Local services Who to contact if have concerns	

EXAMINATION

- Plot length, weight and head circumference on DS growth charts
- Evaluate for features of DS (*see* Background) and specifically assess
- Check primitive reflexes, e.g. Moro reflex, assess tone (ventral and vertical suspension, head lag) and observe suck and swallow co-ordination
- Eyes: red reflex
- Cardiovascular exam: heart rate, precordial activity, murmur, pre- and post-ductal saturations, femoral pulses
- Respiratory exam: respiratory rate, stridor, work of breathing
- Abdominal exam: distended abdomen, bowel sounds, hernia orifices
- Check hips for dislocation (Incidence in DS is 6%): Ortolani and Barlow tests

---

Red flags

- Failure to gain weight
- Tachypnoea with a cardiac murmur
- Abdominal distension
- Absent red reflex
- Respiratory distress

SCREENING AND COMPLICATIONS IN DOWN'S SYNDROME

Early months		
	Health issue	*Intervention*
Ensure enrolment in early intervention services	Developmental delay	Children with DS must be involved in an early intervention team that is multidisciplinary in nature to ensure growth and development are enhanced
Cardiac disease	Respiratory syncytial virus infection	Palivizumab prophylaxis
Ear, nose and throat concerns	Serous otitis media OSA Hearing deficit	Formal audiology assessment Ear, nose and throat review Assess need for grommets Consider adenotonsillectomy Sleep studies
Immunisations	Increased risk of infections	Immunisations
Years 1–5		
Visual issues	Refractive errors (50%) Strabismus Ambylopia	Ophthalmology review
Spine abnormalities	Atlantoaxial instability (usually asymptomatic at this age) Symptoms include neck pain, abnormal neck posture, torticollis, reduced neck movement, gait deterioration, increasing fatigability on walking, deterioration in handling skills	X-ray neck in neutral position If abnormal obtain paediatric orthopaedic or neurosurgical opinion
Thyroid function	Hypothyroidism (often asymptomatic)	Thyroid function texts: thyroid hormone T4, thyroid-stimulating hormone, thyroid antibodies (for autoimmune disease)
Gastrointestinal tract	Coeliac disease	Coeliac screen
Central nervous system	Seizure	Obtain electroencephalogram and paediatric neurology consultation
Ear, nose and throat	OSA (restless sleep, snoring and daytime sleepiness)	Refer for sleep study Evaluate for associated obesity Consider adenotonsillectomy
Cardiovascular	Congenital heart disease	Ensure cardiology follow-up and antibiotic prophylaxis (if required)
Gastrointestinal tract	Constipation	Exclude organic aetiology hypothyroidism and coeliac disease Treat with laxatives and diet modification, if appropriate

(*continued*)

	Health issue	*Intervention*
Behaviour	Assess social progress and developmental progress	Ensure follow-up with local support services
Dental	Dentition often delayed and irregular and hypodontia occurs	Dental consultation
Skin	Dry skin, keratosis pilaris	Education regarding regular use of moisturisers, avoidance of soap products
Years 6–13		
Growth	Growth parameters, assess if overweight or obese	Weight reduction strategies
Academic performance (inclusive of speech attainment)	Performance in school	Requirements in school Special needs assistant Access to resource hours Individualised educational programme
Behavioural concerns	Potential attention deficit hyperactivity disorder or autistic symptoms	If considered, likely assessment should be undertaken
Developmental status	Gross motor function	(*See* Evidence 2)
Self-care skills	Self-care skills	Parents of children with DS should encourage self-care skills and foster independence. Parents play an important role in establishing these characteristics

INVESTIGATIONS

Chromosomal analysis

Fluorescent in situ hybridisation can give results in 24–48 hours, but it only detects an extra copy of chromosome 21 and not translocations; therefore, it is prudent to await a complete chromosomal analysis report.

How often should a full blood count be performed?

Polycythaemia occurs frequently in DS (18%–64%), with transient myeloproliferative disorder being recognised in approximately 10%. Children with DS should have a full blood count on a yearly basis, as they are prone to iron-deficiency anaemia.

How often should thyroid function tests (T4, TSH, thyroid antibodies) be performed?

Congenital hypothyroidism occurs in 1% of children with DS.

Echocardiogram

Children with DS have a heart defect in 50% of cases. While clinical examination is useful in detecting murmurs and electrocardiograms are helpful, an echocardiogram is prudent even if the child is asymptomatic.

(*continued*)

INVESTIGATIONS *(cont.)*

When should children be screened for coelic disease?

The risk of coeliac disease in DS is 6% and it should be considered if the child presents with symptoms of coeliac disease.

Neck X-ray for atlantoaxial instability

Children with symptoms should be X-rayed; however, 30% will have radiological evidence of increased movement at the craniovertebral junction but few will have symptoms. Routine X-rays are not recommended, except for those involved in contact sports.

Sleep studies

Children presenting with symptoms of OSA should have a sleep study performed. Despite this being a recommendation, it may not always be possible to have it performed.

Hearing assessments

Children with DS need full audiological review by 10 months of age, which includes hearing test, otoscopy and typanometry, given their high prevalence of deafness and associated ear infections.

MANAGEMENT PLAN: TWO-STEP APPROACH

1. Adaptation to the diagnosis
2. Treatment of specific issues for children with Down's syndrome
   a) development progress
   b) cardiac disease
   c) recurrent infections
   d) behavioural problems
   e) growth
   f) obstructive sleep apnoea

Adaptation to the diagnosis

While healthcare professionals are used to dealing with children who have special needs and their families, for the affected family beginning this journey it is daunting task. Explain the concept of the multidisciplinary team (*see* Evidence 1), and outline the roles of each team member and why they are involved. It is prudent to outline the roles of the primary care provider and the lead paediatrician and to explain the role of each. This will avoid confusion for the parents. The involvement of other consultants will be determined by the clinical needs of the child with DS, and parents will become aware of this with the passage of time. Information transfer between care providers of the child with DS is crucial, and parents should not be the sole conduit of information; therefore, reports and clinical updates should be communicated promptly. Many units have specific booklets that they give to parents of a child with DS and most parents will make contact with their local DS association; however, they often require a specific meeting to clarify specific issues. Often the lead paediatrician is best placed to clarify their concerns.

Treatment of specific issues for children with Down's syndrome
Development progress
While parents are aware that children with DS have developmental delay, they invariably desire data on specific rates of progress and what interventions should be put in place. The involvement of the multidisciplinary team is helpful but physicians should be able to explain the achievement of gross motor skills and why the delay is accentuated in some areas (*see* Evidence 2).

Cardiac disease
While the occurrence of cardiac disease is 40%–50% of all children with DS, even if asymptomatic, all require an echocardiogram (*see* Evidence 3). Occasionally parents may be reluctant to have this done, especially if the infant is thriving; however, the risk of cardiac disease needs to be explained.

Recurrent infections
Children with DS are prone to ear infections, and hearing loss is common (*see* Evidence 4). It is difficult to assess the tympanic membranes because of the narrow auditory canals. When acute otitis is suspected, treatment should be prompt, as the associated hearing loss may have an impact on speech development. They frequently require the placement of ventilation tubes for non-resolving secretory otitis media. The middle secretions are more viscous than in the normal child for uncertain reasons, and this limits the effectiveness of surgery. The active involvement of ear, nose and throat specialists is frequently required. Children with DS also experience rhinosinusitis. The reasons are uncertain but adenoidal hypertrophy, allergy and sinus infections may play a role. They frequently require courses of antibiotics to treat these illnesses. Children with DS who have cardiac disease receive palivizumab as prophylaxis against respiratory syncytial virus; however, deviation from national guidelines is now occurring and clinicians are offering prophylaxis to infants with DS who do not meet the criteria. The impact has been a reduction in hospitalisation for respiratory tract infections.

Behavioural problems
The development of behavioural problems is common in children but increased in those with DS. It is prudent to ask about behaviour at each visit and give parents specific advice. Parents should be educated to use a consistent behavioural approach to these difficulties.

Growth
Short stature is a feature of children with DS. The mean height for males is 157 cm and for females is 145 cm. The aetiology of the short stature is unknown. Children with DS should be plotted on appropriate DS charts and if they experience growth

failure, specific conditions that are more common in DS should be evaluated (coeliac disease, hypothyroidism). Weight should be carefully assessed and attention paid to the child's diet and exercise level, as children with DS have a propensity to obesity. Preventive strategies are best.

Obstructive sleep apnoea

Children with DS are prone to OSA. Parents may report snoring, disturbed sleep, frequent awakenings and apnoeas. During the day the child may have excessive sleepiness, difficulty in concentration and learning. In rare circumstances the child can develop cor pulmonale. Nocturnal pulse oximetry is not helpful in the assessment of OSA and sleep studies are warranted.

FOLLOW-UP

Children with DS need to be seen in a specialty clinic at least on a yearly basis to ensure that their health needs are met. The benefits of such clinics are established. Routine care should be undertaken by the general practitioner.

WHEN TO REFER?

In children with DS the following warrant referral:
- growth failure, either height or weight
- excessive weight gain
- sleep-related symptoms
- impaired communication (missed otitis media)
- behavioural difficulties, new onset
- acute neck pain

CLARIFICATION STATEMENTS FOR PARENTAL MISCONCEPTIONS

'Can Down's syndrome be prevented?'

No, it is not possible to prevent DS. Prenatal diagnosis is available (*see* Background).

'How well do families cope with the unexpected diagnosis of Down's syndrome?'

Families are resilient and, after an initial phase of adaptation, cope very well. The divorce rate for families with a child with DS is lower than the average. Children who have a sibling with DS tend to be more empathic and caring than their peers. Children with DS have a good temperament and are generally happy and content, despite having associated medical co-morbidities. Involvement with the local chapter of the DS association offers parents and families opportunities to share experiences and to network.

> *'Are all children with Down's syndrome the same?'*

No, not all children with DS are the same. The expression of co-morbidities varies, as does academic achievement. Consequently the developmental gains achieved in the first 2 years offer an insight into the child's ability.

SUMMARY PRACTICE POINTS

- The diagnosis of DS is made on clinical grounds, but the exact type requires chromosomal analysis.
- Relaying to parents that their child has DS needs to done with sensitivity and to be undertaken by an experienced physician.
- A normal cardiac examination does not mean the absence of cardiac disease.
- Hearing deficits are common in DS.
- OSA may be subtle in its presentation.
- Routine X-rays for atlantoaxial instability in an asymptomatic child are not required.
- Anticipating potential complications is aided by age-appropriate screening.

EVALUATING THE EVIDENCE

Evidence 1	
Theme E1	**Specialty clinics for Down's syndrome (DS)**
Question	What is the impact of specialty clinics for patients with DS?
Design	Retrospective cohort study
Level of evidence	
Setting	Department of paediatrics, children's hospital, the United States
Participants	New patients with DS older than 3 years of age seen in this specialty clinic were eligible for inclusion.
Intervention	The adherence to healthcare recommendations was evaluated.
Outcomes	The primary outcome was adherence to healthcare recommendations for children with DS proposed by the American Academy of Pediatrics and the Down Syndrome Medical Interest Group.
Main results	One hundred and five children, with an average age of 9.5 years (range, 3–20.9), were included in the analysis. Pertaining to healthcare recommendation and percentage up to date, the results were as follows: thyroid function tests (56.3%), audiograms (47.1%), coeliac screen (45.2%), ophthalmological examination (55.8%), cervical spine X-ray (77.9%) and all of these (9.8%).

(continued)

Evidence 1	
Theme E1	***Specialty clinics for Down's syndrome (DS)***
Main results (*cont.*)	Parental concerns were behavioural problems (54.3%), language concerns (53.3%), eating, weight and diet issues (19%), orthopaedic issues (16.2%), educational issues (15.2%), sleep issues (12.4%) and constipation (9.5%). New clinician diagnoses included xerosis (54.3%), expressive language disorder (53.3%), disruptive behaviour (not otherwise specified) (37.1%), obesity (>95% body mass index) (25.7%), overweight (85%–95% body mass index) 21%, constipation (19%), seasonal allergies (18.1%), obstructive sleep apnoea (14.3%), thyroid conditions (8.6%), coeliac disease (5.7%) and autism spectrum disorder (5.7%).
Conclusion	A specialty DS clinic can identify and address many healthcare needs of children and adolescents with DS not identified in primary care settings.
Commentary	This was a tertiary care DS clinic that was commenced to provide care for children and adolescents with DS. Many of the children would have had significant contact with the healthcare system prior to attending this clinic. This clinic had a physician with a special interest in DS in attendance, supported by a dietitian, audiologist and resource specialists and accessed other specialists as needed. An important finding was the high number of children and adolescents with disruptive behaviours; however, some of these were secondary to expressive language frustrations, which can be mitigated with the assistance of augmented communication devices and additional speech and language services. The findings of this study pertaining to obstructive sleep apnoea have resulted in a recommendation that all children with DS have a sleep study by the age of 4 years. Children who attend DS clinics still need quality primary care and as such, their specialty clinic visits should focus on ensuring healthcare recommendations are adhered to and potential co-morbidities are recognised.
Reference	Skotko BG, Davidson EJ, Weintraub GS. Contributions of a specialty clinic for children and adolescents with Down syndrome. *Am J Med Genet A*. 2013; **161A**(3): 430–7.

Evidence 2	
Theme E2	***Down's syndrome (DS) and gross motor skill acquisition***
Question	What is the difference in motor milestones between children with DS and typical children?
Design Level of evidence	Longitudinal cohort study
Setting	Department of physiotherapy, academic medical centre, Brazil
Participants	Infants with DS were eligible if under 3 months of age and if they had no neurological, sensory or orthopaedic alterations unrelated to DS. The control group were typical infants whom had no risk factors for developmental delay.
Intervention	Infants with DS and normal infants were assessed using the Alberta Infantile Motor Scale (AIMS) on a monthly basis from 3–12 months of age. The DS group received physiotherapy based on the Bobath concept and the sensory integration method.

(*continued*)

Evidence 2	
Theme E2	*Down's syndrome (DS) and gross motor skill acquisition*
Outcomes	Differences in age and percentage of infants who acquired motor skills in prone, supine, sitting and standing positions.
Main results	Eighty-six infants were enrolled, 26 of these with DS, of whom 20 completed the study, and 60 typical infants, of whom 25 completed the study. Infants who missed three consecutive assessments were excluded from the study. Skill acquisition in the prone position was 1–3 months delayed compared with normal infants. There was no difference in skill acquisition in the supine position at 8 months (all infants were rolling prone to supine without rotation). While 100% of typical infants were rolling prone to supine with rotation at 1 year, only 69% of children with DS achieved this skill. Motor skill acquisitions in the sitting position were delayed by 1–4 months in the DS group. Eighty-eight per cent of typical infants were sitting with arm support at 1 year, compared with 29% of infants with DS. Skill acquisition in the standing position was the most difficult for DS infants to acquire, and no child with DS was able to do this at 1 year.
Conclusion	Children with DS acquire motor skills at different ages. The more complex the skill the greater time differences are likely to be present between the typical child and those with DS. Therapeutic interventions should be initiated before 6 months of age.
Commentary	AIMS is a validated observational scale that assesses infants from birth to achieving independent gait and indentifies risks of developmental delay. The domains assess infant motor behaviour in supine (9 skills), prone (21 skills), sitting (12 skills) and standing (16 skills) subscales. Having this scale available allows the progress of the infant with DS to be monitored. Typically, parents wish to know when their child will sit up and when they can expect the child to walk. The AIMS outlines the intermediate skill set that needs to be achieved in order to achieve these goals. It also allows the parents to be aware of the complexity of motor skill acquisition.
Reference	Pereira K, Basso RP, Lindquist AR. Infants with Down syndrome: percentage and age for acquisition of gross motor skills. *Res Dev Disabil.* 2013; **34**(3): 894–901.

Evidence 3	
Theme E3	*Cardiac disease in children with Down's syndrome (DS)*
Question	What is the effectiveness of clinical examination, chest radiography and electrocardiography compared with echocardiography in detecting congenital heart disease early in the life of children with DS?
Design	Prospective 2-year screening survey
Level of evidence	
Setting	Department of paediatric cardiology, academic medical centre, Northern Ireland
Participants	Newborn infants, diagnosed with DS, were eligible for enrolment if born within the 2-year screening period.
Intervention	All infants with DS had a clinical examination, chest X-ray and electrocardiogram performed soon after birth, followed by a 2-D echocardiography examination.

(*continued*)

Evidence 3

Theme E3	Cardiac disease in children with Down's syndrome (DS)
Outcomes	The primary outcome was the diagnostic ability of the clinical examination, chest X-ray and electrocardiogram to diagnose congenital heart disease compared with the 2-D echocardiography examination.
Main results	Over the 2-year period, 81 infants with DS were identified, giving an annual incidence of 1.50/1000 births. Thirty-four (41.9%) infants had congenital heart disease diagnosed (13 atrioventricular septal defects, seven secundum atrial septal defects, six large solitary patent ductus arteriosus and five isolated ventricular septal defects and 3 with a combination of defects). Twenty-one infants had an abnormal clinical examination (18 had heart disease but two had cyanosis related to polycythaemia and had persistent foetal circulation). Of the 60 thought to have no heart disease, 16 (26.5%) were diagnosed with structural heart defects (five atrioventricular septal defects, six secundum atrial septal defects, one patent ductus arteriosus and one had a combination of defects). Of 65 infants with a chest X-ray reported as normal, 19 had an abnormal echocardiography. Seventy-nine babies had electrocardiograms performed, of which 13 (16.5%) were regarded as abnormal (defined as abnormal QRS axis or evidence of ventricular hypertrophy), as were subsequent echocardiograms. Of the 66 normal electrocardiograms, 19 (29%) had abnormal echocardiograms.
Conclusion	Echocardiography performed early (within 6 weeks) in DS infants can identify cardiac disease that might otherwise have been missed.
Commentary	Screening for congenital heart disease through clinical examination, electrocardiograms and chest X-ray only will fail to identify all DS infants with congenital heart disease and therefore echocardiography is warranted. The tests used had low sensitivity; however, the symptoms and signs of congenital heart disease evolve, and evidence of left-to-right shunts may not have developed in the neonatal period because of high pulmonary vascular resistance, which falls over a period of time.
Reference	Tubman TR, Shields MD, Craig BG, et al. Congenital heart disease in Down's syndrome: two year prospective early screening study. BMJ. 1991; 302(6790): 1425–7.

Evidence 4

Theme E4	Hearing loss in Down's syndrome (DS)
Question	In children with DS, what are the causes of hearing loss and how frequently do they occur?
Design Level of evidence	Case series with chart review
Setting	Department of otolaryngology, academic medical centre, the United States
Participants	Children with DS born in Utah between January 2002 and December 2006, identified through the state newborn screening database and birth defects registry, were eligible for inclusion.
Intervention	Newborn hearing screening for DS and follow-up to assess hearing loss (if present)

(continued)

Evidence 4	
Theme E4	**Hearing loss in Down's syndrome (DS)**
Outcomes	The types and frequency of hearing loss in infants with DS
Main results	Of an eligible 344 patients, 332 were included in the analysis. Eighty-seven (26.2%) infants did not pass the newborn screening. Thirty-three (37.9%) had a conductive hearing loss, 16 (18.4%) had normal hearing, 5 (5.7%) had sensorineural hearing loss (SNHL), three (3.4%) had mixed hearing loss, eight (9.2%) had indeterminate hearing loss and 22 (25.3%) were lost to follow-up. Of those who passed their newborn screening, 124 (54.3%) had normal hearing, 101 (43.5%) had conductive hearing loss, one (0.4%) had sensorineural hearing loss, one (0.4%) had indeterminate hearing loss and five (2.5%) had no follow-up. Of the 123 infants who did not have newborn screening, one (7.5%) had normal hearing, four (30.8%) had conductive hearing loss and eight (61.5%) were lost to follow-up. Of 101 infants with conductive hearing loss, 97 (96%) had ventilation tubes inserted to aid resolution of the hearing loss. Most children with SNHL were diagnosed beyond 90 days but associated medical and surgical conditions contributed to the delay.
Conclusion	Patients with DS present with relatively high incidence of conductive hearing loss, mixed hearing loss and SNHL compared with patients without DS. The high loss to follow-up in those who failed newborn screening (25.3%) is worrisome.
Commentary	Infants with DS are prone to hearing loss. The anatomy of the ear canal (excessive narrowing) can make visualisation of the tympanic membrane difficult. If the tympanic membrane cannot be visualised, referral to an ear, nose and throat specialist is warranted. When serous otitis media does occur, the fluid that accumulates is more viscous that in children without DS and it is more difficult to aspirate. In this study, five infants had SNHL but it was unilateral in three, which has major implications for the speech development of a child with developmental delay. The finding of one child who passed the newborn screening but was subsequently diagnosed with SNHL supports the regular assessment of hearing in children with DS.
Reference	Park AH, Wilson MA, Stevens PT, *et al.* Identification of hearing loss in pediatric patients with Down syndrome. *Otolaryngol Head Neck Surg.* 2012; **146**(1): 135–40.

DOWN'S SYNDROME: MULTIPLE-CHOICE QUESTIONS

Q1 Features of DS include which of the following?
 a) Microcephaly with brachycephaly
 b) Hypotonia
 c) Upward-slanting palpebral fissures
 d) Short fifth finger with clinodactly
 e) Brushfield's spots

Q2 In DS which of the following statements is/are true?
 a) The triple test is effective in prenatal diagnosis.
 b) In 95% there is non-familial trisomy 21.

c) In 1%–2% mosacism is present.

d) The risk of DS increases with advancing maternal age.

e) Unbalanced translocations are de novo in 75% of cases.

Q3 Which of the following statements is/are true?

a) DS is associated with a 3% failure in newborn hearing screening.

b) Children with DS have narrow ear canals, which makes visualisation of the tympanic membranes difficult.

c) Children with DS with otitis media have more viscous fluid than normal children.

d) Antibiotic treatment is not effective for otitis media in DS.

e) Congenital deafness occurs in 3.5% of children with DS.

Q4 With regard to heart disease in DS, which of the following statements is/are correct?

a) Sixty-five per cent of patients have congenital heart disease.

b) Seventy per cent of patients have an atrioventricular septal defect.

c) If the clinical examination is normal, 25% will have unrecognised cardiac disease.

d) The electrocardiogram is a good predictor of cardiac disease.

e) An echo should be done on all children with DS before 6 months of age.

Q5 With regard to atlantoaxial instability in DS, which of the following statements is/are true?

a) All DS should be screened before 10 years of age.

b) Neck pain is an indicator for screening.

c) Lower limb involvement presents with intermittent numbness.

d) The presence of impaired hand movement is an indicator of atlantoaxial instability.

e) Non-steroidal anti-inflammatory drugs are helpful in 35%.

Q6 Which of the following statements is/are correct in regard to OSA in children with DS?

a) Snoring is a major symptom.

b) Cor pulmonale is a rare feature.

c) Oxygen saturation monitoring is an effective screening to tool to detect OSA.

d) Formal sleep studies are required in all patients with DS who have symptoms and signs suggestive of OSA.

e) Tonsillectomy is the treatment of choice for OSA.

Q7 Which of the following statements with regard to DS is/are correct?

a) Refractive errors occur in 50% of patients.

b) Keratosis pilaris is frequently present.

c) Delayed dentition is frequent.

d) Coeliac disease occurs in 20% of children.

e) Hypothyroidism occurs in 30% of patients by 15 years of age.

Q8 Which of the following statements with regard to height in DS is/are correct?

a) The short stature is related to growth hormone insensitivity.

b) Growth hormone treatment is effective only in 15% of DS patients.

c) The mean final height for a male with DS is 157 cm.

d) The mean final height for a female with DS is 153 cm.

e) Final height in DS is strongly influenced by the mother's height.

Answers

A1	a, b, c, d, e	**A2**	a, b, c, d, e
A3	b, c	**A4**	c, e
A5	b, d	**A6**	a, b, d, e
A7	a, b, c	**A8**	c

SLIDES

1. Down's syndrome
2. Brushfield's spots
3. Single palmar crease

Chapter Twenty-four

THE CHILD WITH A LIMP

COMMON SCENARIO

'Over the past few days, he's started limping. At first, I thought he was just putting it on to get attention, but he's been persistently limping now for 2 days. He's not complaining of any pain and he definitely didn't injure himself or fall.'

LEARNING OBJECTIVES

- Understand the causes of limp in childhood
- Identify key points in the history or examination that might lead to a diagnosis
- Recognise 'red flags' in the history or diagnosis that require further investigation or specialist referral
- Explain what investigations are indicated
- Understand when and what treatment is required for the management of common causes of limp

BACKGROUND

Limp or refusal to walk in children is a common reason for referral for assessment. Gait reflects the coordinated action of the lower extremities. A limp is an asymmetrical gait caused by pain, weakness or deformity. Normal gait is bipedal, rhythmical and effortless. There are two phases involved: stance and swing. During the stance phase the foot is in contact with the ground; during the swing phase it is in the air. Normally, the stance phase forms 60% of the gait cycle and the swing phase forms 40%. Limb advancement occurs during the swing phase. Abnormal gait can be antalgic or non-antalgic.

An antalgic gait is caused by pain. In order to minimise pain and weight-bearing, less time is spent in stance phase, with a resultant increase in swing phase in the painful limb. Non-antalgic gaits include circumduction gait (knee is hyperextended, locked and affected leg is circumducted during swing stage), equinus gait (toe walking), Trendelenburg gait (pelvis tilts toward unaffected side during swing stage)

Toddler (1–3 years)
Toddler's fracture
Developmental dysplasia of the hip (DDH)
Cerebral palsy
Congenital malformation
Intravertebral discitis
Leg length discrepancy

Child (4–10 years)
Transient synovitis
Perthes disease

Adolescent
Slipped upper femoral epiphysis (SUFE)
Osgood–Schlatter's disease
Osteochondritis dissecans

To be considered in all age groups
Septic arthritis/osteomyelitis
Trauma
Non-accidental injury
Haematological disease
Inflammatory disease: juvenile idiopathic arthritis (JIA)
Referred pain: appendicitis, hernias, testicular torsion
Malignancy (solid bone tumours, space-occupying lesion in brain or spine, neuroblastoma, leukaemia, metastatic tumour)
Meningococcal disease
Neuromuscular disease (cerebral palsy, Duchenne's muscular dystrophy)
Metabolic disease (rickets)

and steppage gait (hip and knee flexed excessively to allow the toes to clear the ground).

Proper evaluation of limp in childhood requires knowledge of the normal developmental stages of gait. At approximately 10–12 months of age, the normal child begins cruising; at 12–14 months of age they can stand unaided and walk for short distances. Toddlers initially walk with a broad-based gait. To improve their balance, they tend to flex their hips, knees and ankles to lower their centre of gravity. By 3 years of age, most children have developed sufficient balance for a normal gait posture.

Limp is never normal and a cause should be established. There is a long list of possible diagnoses and a complete history and thorough examination are very helpful tools in reaching a diagnosis. Serious and life-threatening conditions including malignancy, bone and joint infections, connective tissue disease and non-accidental injury must be considered and excluded. Certain causes of limp can be diagnosed immediately. Some cases require a period of observation and additional investigations. Many resolve spontaneously or require minimal intervention.

It is important to remember that if pain is present, the location of pain does not always reflect the location of pathology, e.g. hip pathology can present with knee pain. The differential diagnosis for limp in childhood is extensive and should take into account the age of the child and the presence of pain. Limp can be the presenting complaint in a variety of haematological, neurological and gastrointestinal conditions.

Toddler (1–3 years)

Trauma

Trauma (including non-accidental injury and toddler's fracture) is the commonest cause of limp in childhood. There is usually a clear history of trauma consistent with the injury. In pre-ambulatory children, where the history is inconsistent or not compatible with the injury, non-accidental injury needs to be considered. A toddler's fracture, also known as CAST (childhood accidental spiral tibial) fracture, is common in children aged 9 months to 3 years. It occurs after low-energy trauma, often with a rotational component, so there may not be a clear history of trauma. A sudden twisting of the tibia causes a fracture in the distal third of the tibia, in a spiral pattern.

Developmental dysplasia of the hip

DDH includes a spectrum of abnormalities of the hip joint that varies from mild to severe. The femoral head has an abnormal relationship to the acetabulum. The hip may be dysplastic, fully or partially dislocated (subluxation). DDH is four times more common in girls and is twice as common on the left. Additional risk factors include firstborn, breech delivery, positive family history, the presence of oligohydramnios antenatally and associated neuromuscular or neural tube defects. All children are clinically screened at birth for DDH, and in many countries universal screening for DDH with ultrasound has been introduced; however, many cases are not diagnosed in the newborn period and present in later childhood with a painless limp. On examination there may be asymmetric gluteal and thigh skin folds and a Trendelenburg gait. In the newborn period, they may have a positive Barlow or Ortolani finding.

Discitis

Although discitis can occur at any age, the incidence is increased in the toddler age group. Discitis is inflammation of the intervertebral disc space or vertebral end plate and occurs most commonly in the lumbar region. It is an uncommon condition with a good prognosis. Presentation is usually non-specific and gradual. Toddlers present with limp or refusal to walk. They are systemically well and may have a low-grade fever. Examination may reveal restricted spinal mobility and loss of lumbar lordosis. There may be tenderness at the site of the lesion. The key is to distinguish discitis from vertebral osteomyelitis. Vertebral osteomyelitis affects older children, who are systemically unwell with high fever and complain of pain in the lumbar, thoracic or cervical spine. The white cell count (WCC) and C-reactive protein (CRP) are usually normal or slightly elevated; the erythrocyte sedimentation rate (ESR) is usually raised and can be used to monitor response to treatment. Blood cultures are usually negative. Spinal X-rays can be normal initially; however, after 2–4 weeks, disc space narrowing and irregular end plates of neighbouring vertebrae can be seen. Magnetic resonance imaging (MRI) of the spine is the investigation of choice to detect early discitis and rule out spinal tumours. The aetiology is unknown. Although an infectious cause has been proposed, organisms are rarely isolated and children recover without antibiotics.

Cerebral palsy

Mild cerebral palsy is the most common neurological disorder that leads to asymptomatic limping in the toddler age group.

Child (4–10 years)

Transient synovitis

Transient synovitis or 'irritable hip' is the most common cause of acute hip pain in childhood. It is a diagnosis of exclusion. It occurs in children aged between 2 and 10 years and affects boys more than girls. It is commonly preceded by a viral infection (7–10 days before). The child is usually comfortable at rest, is systemically well and may have a low-grade fever. There may be a decreased range of movement of the hip, especially internal rotation. The child usually prefers to keep the hip abducted and externally rotated.

Legg–Calvé–Perthes disease

Perthes disease results from idiopathic avascular necrosis of the femoral epiphysis, which in turn impairs the endochondral ossification on the femoral head. Typically, it presents in boys aged 2–10 years. It is bilateral in 10%–15% of cases. The onset is usually insidious. Limp is usually the presenting complaint; however, the child may also complain of pain in the knee, hip, groin or thigh. Examination may be normal initially, apart from the limp, but later there is loss of internal rotation, muscle wasting and a Trendelenburg gait. Limb length discrepancy may be evident because of adduction contracture or a collapsed epiphysis. Anteroposterior (AP) and lateral X-rays should be performed. X-ray changes vary depending on the radiological stage of the disease. During the early stage, joint space widening can be seen. This is followed by stage 2, where sclerosis secondary to necrosis and marrow calcification can then be detected. In stage 3, fragmentation of bone can be observed. Finally, in stage 4, healing occurs as reossification takes place. MRI is useful in the early stages of the disease or when changes are absent on the plain film.

Adolescent

Slipped upper femoral epiphysis

SUFE is the most common hip disorder occurring in adolescents. It is frequently misdiagnosed. Untreated, it can lead to permanent limb shortening, loss of internal rotation and abduction, and increased susceptibility to avascular necrosis and early-onset degenerative hip arthritis requiring hip reconstruction. The mean age at diagnosis is 13.5 years in boys and 12 years in girls, with boys being more commonly affected. Risk factors include obesity, hypothyroidism, pituitary deficiency, growth hormone supplementation and renal osteodystrophy. In 25% of cases it is bilateral. It affects the epiphyseal plate of the proximal femur with displacement of the epiphyses of the femoral head posteroinferiorly.

Adolescents can present with a limp, inability to weight-bear and pain in the hip, thigh, groin or knee. It can be caused by trauma or it can occur gradually. Presentation can be acute (<3 weeks) or chronic (>3 weeks). If children are able to weight-bear (with or without crutches), it is described as stable; an unstable hip cannot weight-bear. Limited internal rotation of the hip is the most consistent finding on examination. AP and frog leg lateral X-rays of the hip should be taken to grade the severity of the slip. The Southwick grading system is used to measure the degree of displacement of the epiphysis, which can be mild (<30°), moderate (30°–60°) and severe (>60°).

Osgood–Schlatter's disease

Osgood–Schlatter's disease is inflammation at the site of insertion of the patellar tendon. It is an overuse injury presenting with pain and swelling localised to the tibial tuberosity, in children aged 10–14 years. It is more common in boys and athletes and it is associated with growth spurts. The pain is exacerbated by strenuous exercise. Examination reveals tenderness at the tibial tuberosity with pain elicited on straight leg raising test.

Osteochondritis dissecans

Osteochondritis dissecans is complete or incomplete separation of a portion of joint cartilage and underlying bone, causing a loose body in the joint space. It usually affects the knee joint in athletic teenagers. Adolescents present with knee pain or discomfort and swelling. Pain is usually worse after exercise. There may be a history of a clicking or popping sensation of the knee joint. Boys are more commonly affected than girls. The aetiology is unknown but may be related to repetitive micro-trauma or stress. AP, lateral and tunnel-view (knee in flexion) X-ray views should be taken. If a lesion is noted, an MRI should be requested to determine the stage of the lesion.

All age groups

Septic arthritis

Although more than one joint can be involved, septic arthritis usually affects a single joint, with the knee, hip and ankle being most commonly involved. Joint sepsis can be caused by pathogenic inoculation of the joint by direct or haematogenous spread. The child is usually systemically unwell, with joint pain, pseudoparesis and high fever. To maximise intracapsular volume, the hip is usually kept flexed, abducted and externally rotated.

- In the newborn period, group B streptococcus and *Escherichia coli* are important pathogens.
- After the newborn period, *Staphylococcus aureus* is the most common causative organism.

The joint is red, hot, swollen and tender (if the hip is involved, limited movement may only be found on examination). Inflammatory markers and peripheral white cell counts are raised. Urgent intervention is required to prevent long-term joint destruction and disability. The diagnosis is confirmed by ultrasound-guided aspiration of the joint fluid and positive identification of the causative organism.

Osteomyelitis

Osteomyelitis most commonly occurs at the metaphysis of the distal femur or proximal tibia but any site can be affected. It generally follows haematogenous spread and is most often due to *S. aureus*. In children with sickle-cell disease, salmonella may be the causative organism.

Children with osteomyelitis present with a high swinging fever and an acutely painful limb, which they are unwilling to move. Examination reveals an unwell, febrile child with exquisite tenderness, erythema and swelling over the site affected. Pseudoparalysis is an early sign in newborns or infants. A raised white cell count with neutrophilia, a high ESR and CRP is found. Blood cultures are commonly positive. Diagnosis is made by technetium bone scan, which shows a 'hot spot' of increased uptake at the site of infection. Intravenous antibiotics are given until the clinical signs have resolved and the acute-phase reactants have returned to normal, and then oral antibiotics are continued for several weeks.

Juvenile idiopathic arthritis

JIA is diagnosed if arthritis is present for more than 6 weeks in a child less than 16 years of age, once other causes have been excluded. The incidence is 1 in 10 000. In oligoarticular arthritis, fewer than four joints are involved. In polyarticular arthritis, more than four joints are involved.

JIA can be classified as:
- systemic onset
- polyarticular (rheumatoid factor negative or positive)
- oligoarticular
- enthesitis-related arthritis
- psoriatic arthritis.

Systemic onset accounts for 15% of cases. Any number of joints can be affected. It affects males and females equally. Rheumatoid factor and antinuclear antibody tests are negative. It is associated with fever, a salmon-pink effervescent rash, hepatosplenomegaly and lymphadenopathy. Oligoarticular JIA accounts for 40%–50% of cases. Females are more commonly affected and present at 1–5 years of age. The large joints are usually affected. A positive antinuclear antibody test is associated with an increased risk of uveitis. Rheumatoid factor is negative. Remission rates of up to 60% can occur in puberty. Polyarticular arthritis can be rheumatoid factor positive (5% of cases) or negative (30% of cases). It affects both small and large joints. Rheumatoid positive arthritis is similar to adult rheumatoid arthritis and carries a poorer prognosis.

Malignancy (solid bone tumours, space-occupying lesion in brain or spine, neuroblastoma, leukaemia, metastatic tumour)

Systemic symptoms such as fever, weight loss, night sweats and bone or back pain, particularly at night, should prompt investigation to exclude neoplastic causes of limp. A history of bleeding or easy bruising suggests a haematological malignancy. Acute lymphoblastic leukaemia is the most common malignancy to present with bone pain in children. Acute lymphoblastic leukaemia can mimic osteomyelitis, septic arthritis and JIA. It may be associated with anaemia, thrombocytopenia, leukopoenia, blast cells on the blood film and raised inflammatory markers.

Malignant bone tumours (osteosarcoma and Ewing's sarcoma) usually present with localised, progressive dull ache that disturbs sleep and is not relieved by rest or analgesia. Osteosarcomas are aggressive.

Osteoid osteomas are uncommon in children younger than 5 years. Pain is the most frequent presenting complaint, although children may present with a limp. Pain secondary to an osteoid osteoma classically responds well to non-steroidal anti-inflammatory drugs (NSAIDs).

Lyme disease

In endemic areas, and if there is a history of recent travel to endemic areas, Lyme disease should be considered. Lyme disease is caused by *Borrelia burgdorferi* and is the most common tick-borne infection in the United States. Three stages of the disease are described. Usually within 14 days of a tick bite, stage 1 is seen. It is characterised by erythema migrans (small erythematous macule or papule that enlarges with central clearing) associated with fever, arthralgia, headache and fatigue. Untreated, patients can go on to develop neurological and cardiovascular complications and arthritis.

HISTORY

KEY POINTS					
Limp	Onset Ability to weight-bear Limitation of activities Time of day when limp is worse	Growth and development	Milestones achieved Delayed walking Pubertal stage	**�︎ Red flags** History of asymptomatic limp in a toddler who is walking Acute-onset pain and limp Chronic limp in an obese patient
Pain	Onset Location Abdominal or back pain Severity Course over the day Exacerbating and relieving factors Response to NSAIDs	Family history	Arthritis DDH Psoriasis Haemoglobinopathy or bleeding disorder Inflammatory diseases	
Associated symptoms	Weakness Fever Decreased appetite Joint swelling, pain or stiffness Weight loss Night sweats Rash Visual disturbance Morning stiffness Voiding or stooling problems Bruising	Birth history	Breech Oligohydramnios Complications at birth Resuscitation required	
Trauma	Recent trauma Mechanism Witnessed fall or injury	Medical and surgical history	Recent infections Psoriasis History of bleeding disorder	
		Social history	Recent travel Sporting activity	

EXAMINATION

All children should have their height and weight plotted on an appropriate centile chart. Document vitals including temperature.

- Observe gait with shoes off; ask child to run, hop, skip, walk heel to toe
- Perform Gowers's test
- Measure limb length

- Full neurological examination
- Full musculoskeletal exam
- Examine spine
- Examine the abdomen for masses or hepatosplenomegaly and check the hernia orifices for tender lymph glands
- Examine skin for bruising or petechiae
- Feel for lymphadenopathy

❗ Red flags

- Abnormal neurological examination
- Pyrexia
- Generalised lymphadenopathy and/or hepatosplenomegaly
- Pallor, excessive bruising or petechiae
- Muscle wasting
- Gowers's test positive
- Joint swelling, tenderness or heat
- Localised bony tenderness
- Limitation of movement

DIFFERENTIAL DIAGNOSIS OF LIMP

The differential diagnosis of a child with limp is presented in the background section. This table includes causes of limp that are not included in that section.

Clinical condition	Typical features	Differentiating features
Foreign body in the foot	Acute onset of limp but pain located in the sole of the foot	Local swelling in the sole of the foot, from a foreign body
Inguinal lymphadenitis	Reluctance to walk as pain occurs and child consequently rests	Tender lymph nodes in the inguinal region. Check for skin abrasion in the affected leg
Acute meningococcal disease	Acute onset of leg pain with reluctance to bear weight and walk	Pain can be severe but other features of sepsis appear within hours
Influenza infection with myositis	Acute onset of leg pain and limp if attempt to walk	Tenderness of muscle with gentle compression

Clinical signs or tests	Description
Gowers's sign	The child climbs to the standing position.
Galeazzi's sign (leg length discrepancy)	The child should lie supine with his or her knees and hips flexed. The test is positive for leg length discrepancy if the knee on the affected side is lower than that on the normal side.

(continued)

Clinical signs or tests	Description
Trendelenburg's test (weakness of hip abductors)	The child should stand on the affected limb and lift the unaffected limb off the floor. The test is positive if the pelvis drops down toward the unaffected side.
FABER test (sacroiliac joint assessment)	Place the ipsilateral ankle on the contralateral knee in the supine patient. Provide gentle downward pressure on the knee. The test is positive if pain is elicited (hip flexion, abduction and external rotation).

INVESTIGATIONS

What laboratory investigations are required?

In children with limp and fever, a full blood count, blood film, ESR and CRP, and blood cultures should be performed. In septic arthritis blood cultures are positive in only 30% of cases.

Four clinical predicators of septic arthritis (*see* Evidence 1):
1. fever
2. non-weight-bearing
3. ESR >40 mm/hour
4. WCC >12 × 10⁹/L.

If none are present, the risk of septic arthritis is <0.2%. If one is present, the risk increases to 3%, 40% with two factors, 93.1% with three factors and 99.6% when all four factors are present.

CRP, ESR and WCC can also be increased with inflammation and malignancy.

When should plain X-rays of the hip be performed?

If an area of pathology such as the hip joint is localised by history or examination, AP and frog leg lateral view X-rays should be obtained. These films should be reviewed for evidence of femoral head fragmentation, trauma, joint space widening or structural abnormalities. Plain X-rays do not differentiate between transient synovitis, septic arthritis and osteomyelitis.

If JIA is suspected, what laboratory investigations should be performed?

JIA is a diagnosis of exclusion and there is no diagnostic test. It is important to note that inflammatory markers and autoantibody screens may be normal. However, in cases where JIA is clinically suspected the diagnosis is not excluded by a negative test.

When should an ultrasound scan be performed?

An ultrasound scan is useful for detecting joint effusions. However, ultrasound is unable to distinguish between an effusion caused by transient synovitis and one caused by septic arthritis.

If the scan is normal, but clinically septic arthritis or osteomyelitis is suspected, a bone scan or MRI should be performed.

When should an isotope bone scan be performed?

Isotope bone scan is a sensitive means of detecting alterations in the metabolic rate of bone, and bone scanning is an important modality in identifying osteomyelitis (see 'hot spots') or Perthes disease (diminished uptake on bone scan), stress fracture or a toddler's fracture. Bone scanning may also detect infiltrative bone disease such as leukaemia or neuroblastoma.

When should a joint be aspirated?

In those presenting with a septic arthritis, joint aspiration should be undertaken under strict aseptic conditions.

MANAGEMENT PLAN: FOUR-STEP APPROACH

1. Clarifying and pitfall avoidance strategies:
   a) parent
   b) doctor
2. Conservative management
3. Medical management
4. Surgical management

Clarifying and pitfall avoidance strategies

Parent

- Limp is a symptom and not a disease. **Rationale**: parents may want specific treatment for their child's limp but a clear aetiology must be discerned prior to any treatment being prescribed.
- Missed DDH. **Pitfall**: parents will expect DDH to be diagnosed at birth but in a percentage of patients, despite screening and examination, a diagnosis is not made. The term 'developmental dysplasia of the hip' is used, rather than congenital dislocation of the hip, as the condition is not always present at birth.

Doctor

- Documentation of musculoskeletal examination. **Pitfall**: musculoskeletal examination is often suboptimal in clinical practice; therefore, exercise due care in the assessment of the child with limp.
- Limp, fracture and potential non-accidental injury. **Rationale**: in the child who presents with limp the possibility of non-accidental injury needs to be entertained and the doctor needs to be guided by the history presented.
- Referred pain in the child with limp. **Rationale**: in children with limp, pain can be referred to another joint region (e.g. hip to knee).
- Limp in the obese child. **Pitfall**: do not assume that the limp is related to his or her weight, as the child or adolescent may have SUFE.
- Joint pain at night and the child with limp. **Pitfall**: children with benign nocturnal limb pains, which can be located in the thigh, shin and calf region, do not have a limp. If the pain is located in a joint region, then investigation is required to exclude a malignancy.
- The limping but well toddler. **Pitfall**: consider cerebral palsy in this child. A careful examination will usually give the diagnosis.
- Limp post transient synovitis. **Pitfall**: the occurrence of limp months after an episode of transient synovitis may reflect the presence of avascular necrosis of the femoral head. It is prudent to follow up children with transient synovitis at least once, to make sure all is well.
- The child with an absent limp. **Rationale**: children with arthritis may have morning stiffness and initially a transient limp. Specifically ask if morning stiffness is present and how long it takes to improve with activity.

Conservative management

- Transient synovitis is managed with reassurance, bed rest and analgesia (*see* Evidence 2). The prognosis is excellent and most cases resolve within a week.
- Management of Osgood–Schlatter's disease is rest and anti-inflammatory medication. Sporting activity and exercise should be gradually lessened until the pain resolves or is tolerated. Once resolved, activity can resume again, with levels of activity titrated to maintain symptom control. Physiotherapy can be helpful.
- The management of discitis is controversial. Bed rest and adequate analgesia is recommended. However, the use of broad-spectrum antibiotics remains controversial, as children recover well without antimicrobial treatment and a causative organism is rarely found.
- Management of Perthes disease depends on the age of the child, the amount of the femoral head involved and the radiographic stage of the disease. The aims of treatment are to improve mobility, reduce mechanical stress and preservation of joint congruence. Milder disease in younger children can be managed conservatively with observation, analgesia and physiotherapy. In some cases, limitation of weight-bearing with best rest and the use of crutches is required. Revascularisation and resossification takes place over 18–36 months.
- In the newborn period, mild hip instability usually resolves spontaneously over time. Infants with dislocated or subluxable hips are treated with a Pavlik harness or abduction splint, usually for a period of 3 months.
- Milder cases of osteochondritis dissecans, in which the physis is still open, can be managed conservatively with rest, avoidance of competitive sports and low-intensity physical rehabilitation.

Medical management

- Septic arthritis and osteomyelitis require prompt treatment with broad-spectrum intravenous antibiotics (*see* Evidence 3). Ideally, articular fluid is sent for Gram stain, culture and sensitivities prior to commencement of antibiotics. Arthrotomy with drainage of the joint and washout should be performed. The addition of steroid therapy is advantageous in the resolution of septic arthritis (*see* Evidence 4).
- JIA will require treatment with NSAIDs as part of the initial strategy pending rheumatology consultation (*see* Evidence 5). If only one joint is affected, intra-articular steroid injections (triamcinolone hexacetonide) are used. When methotrexate is used there is a lag of up to 3 months before a therapeutic effect is evident.

Surgical management

- More severe cases of Perthes disease require surgical intervention; this is more likely in older children and if more than 50% of the femoral head is involved. Surgical options include femoral and pelvic osteotomies.
- The management of SUFE is surgical. The goal of treatment is to prevent slip progression and associated complications. Treatment of stable SUFE is in situ

fixation with a screw. The risk of avascular necrosis is greatly increased in unstable slips and they require urgent fixation. This is usually performed within 24 hours. Prophylactic fixation of the contralateral hip is controversial, although it is performed in some centres and in certain circumstances.

- Children with DDH who present after 6 months of age or fail to respond to conservative management usually require open or closed reduction. The hip is then placed in a cast, which is worn for several months. Children presenting after 18 months of age may require femoral and/or pelvic osteotomy.
- More severe cases of osteochondritis dessicans, when the physis is closed, require arthroscopy or open removal.

FOLLOW-UP

- Follow-up is dependent on the primary condition.
- Children with arthritis will need to see a paediatric rheumatologist and ophthalmologist to ensure potential eye complications are avoided (iritis).
- Many children will require orthopaedic follow-up to ensure that the primary condition does not deteriorate and some will require surgery should this occur.

WHEN TO REFER?

- Abnormal hip examination at any time
- Limp that recurs in any child previously diagnosed with transient synovitis
- Limp with constitutional symptoms
- Limp in the overweight child
- Limp that occurs independent of trauma
- Nocturnal bone pain
- Suspected malignancy

CLARIFICATION STATEMENTS FOR PARENTAL MISCONCEPTIONS

'I thought this hip problem was called congenital dislocation of the hip, so why was it missed?'

In many but not all cases, it is recognised soon after birth by examination of the hips or through screening; however, not all cases are evident at that time. Consequently, the name has been changed to 'developmental dysplasia of the hip' to reflect the current reality.

'There must be a reason for these pains at night, and what do you mean by growing pains?'

The term 'growing pains' is not used that much anymore; as the term benign nocturnal limb pain is preferred. These pains do not reflect any underlying disease, and gentle rubbing of the area often improves the discomfort. They are more likely to occur after periods of significant activity and some parents find paracetamol prior to bedtime helpful.

> *'Yes, I know she is overweight, but how can the weight be causing the limp? We thought that she strained a muscle or something.'*

Overweight children and adolescents are at risk of SUFE and the first sign is often limb pain with the occurrence of a limp.

SUMMARY PRACTICE POINTS

- DDH will not all be recognised in the newborn period (hence the label of congenital dislocation of the hip has been abandoned).
- Knee pain may be referred hip pain.
- Limp always requires a diagnosis.
- Limp must be considered in terms of the child's development.
- Osteomyelitis and septic arthritis are emergencies, so prompt referral is required.
- If NSAIDs do not relieve pain related to limp, assume a sinister aetiology.
- Musculoskeletal examination is often poorly performed; have a system of examination.

EVALUATING THE EVIDENCE

Evidence 1	
Theme E1	*Septic arthritis and transient synovitis of the hip*
Question	Can septic arthritis be differentiated from transient synovitis of the hip?
Design	Development of a clinical prediction rule
Level of evidence	
Setting	Children's hospital, academic medical centre, the United States
Participants	The charts of patients admitted with an acutely irritable hip for whom the differential diagnosis involved transient synovitis and septic arthritis were reviewed.
Intervention	Diagnoses of true septic arthritis, presumed septic arthritis and transient synovitis were explicitly defined on the basis of the white blood cell count in the joint fluid, the result of joint fluid cultures and the clinical course. A probability algorithm was constructed for differentiation between septic arthritis and transient synovitis, based on independent multivariate predictors.

(continued)

Evidence 1

Theme E1	*Septic arthritis and transient synovitis of the hip*
Outcomes	The primary outcome was the development of a clinical prediction rule to differentiate patients with septic arthritis from those with transient synovitis.
Main results	The clinical notes of 282 patients were reviewed; however, 114 were excluded, 82 patients had a septic arthritis and 68 had transient arthritis. The clinical features were collated and analysed. Four features predicted outcome and these were (1) history of fever, (2) non-weight-bearing, (3) an erythrocyte sedimentation rate of >40 mm/hour and a white blood cell count of >12 × 10^9/L. The predictive value of septic arthritis with no predictor is <0.2%, with one predictor it is 3%, with two predictors it is 40%, with three predictors it is 93.1% and with four predictors it is 99.6%.
Conclusion	The use of clinical prediction rules can aid the clinician in diagnosing or excluding septic arthritis.
Commentary	The child who presents with an irritable hip can have several potential aetiologies, including Legg–Perthes disease, juvenile rheumatoid arthritis; however, it is the differentiation between septic arthritis and transient synovitis that is the most important, as the demographics are similar but the prognosis, if an incorrect diagnosis is made, is significantly different. The provided algorithm is a significant aid to the doctor assessing the child.
Reference	Kocher MS, Zurakowski D, Kasser JR. Differentiating between septic arthritis and transient synovitis of the hip: an evidence-based clinical prediction algorithm. *J Bone Joint Surg Am.* 1999; **81**(12): 1662–70.

Evidence 2

Theme E2	*Treatment of transient synovitis of the hip*
Question	Does ibuprofen shorten the duration of pain in children with transient synovitis?
Design	Randomised controlled trial
Level of evidence	Jadad 5
Setting	Emergency department, academic medical centre, Australia
Participants	Children aged 1–12 years were eligible for inclusion based on a clinical diagnosis of transient synovitis, with the presence of a pain, limp or both, and an examination revealing limitation of hip movement or pain localised to the hip joint by the child. All children had an ultrasound at 24 hours and day 7. Tests performed included full blood count, erythrocyte sedimentation rate, C-reactive protein and a hip X-ray (anteroposterior and frog leg lateral). Children who required hospitalisation were ineligible for enrolment.
Intervention	Children diagnosed with transient synovitis received either ibuprofen (10 mg/kg, three times a day) or an identical placebo.
Outcomes	The primary outcome was the mean duration of symptoms in both groups. Parents, twice daily, completed a symptom diary inclusive of a pain scale and the presence of standard symptoms. Resolution was defined as absence of pain, normal gait and normal activity.

(continued)

Evidence 2	
Theme E2	*Treatment of transient synovitis of the hip*
Main results	Of the 121 patients who met the entry criteria, 40 were randomised: 20 to the ibuprofen group, of whom 17 completed the study, and 20 to the placebo group, of whom 19 completed the study. The mean duration of symptoms was 2 days in the ibuprofen group and 4.5 days in the placebo group. In the ibuprofen group, seven (41%) patients reported adverse symptoms, of whom four had mild gastrointestinal symptoms and three disliked the taste.
Conclusion	Ibuprofen shortens the duration of symptoms in children with transient synovitis of the hip.
Commentary	Ibuprofen was effective in the resolution of symptoms of children with transient synovitis through its anti-inflammatory effect. This study had a potential group of 121 eligible children but the requirement to have ultrasonography of the hip performed excluded those presenting out of hours. The importance of small asymptomatic hip effusions in children with transient synovitis remains unclear. Ibuprofen is beneficial in the treatment of children with transient synovitis who are discharged home.
Reference	Kermond S, Fink M, Graham K, *et al.* A randomized clinical trial: should the child with transient synovitis of the hip be treated with nonsteroidal anti-inflammatory drugs? *Ann Emerg Med.* 2002; **40**(3): 294–9.

Evidence 3	
Theme E3	*Dexamethasone and septic arthritis*
Question	What is the impact of dexamethasone treatment in children with septic arthritis?
Design	Randomised controlled trial
Level of evidence	Jadad 5
Setting	Department of paediatrics, rheumatology and orthopaedic, academic medical centre, Israel
Participants	Patients aged 6 months to 18 years diagnosed with septic arthritis were eligible for inclusion. Septic arthritis was defined as: (a) acute onset of swelling, pain, local warmth and severe limitation of motion in any joint except for hip and shoulder, in which case severe pain and limitation of motion were sufficient for diagnosis; (b) turbid fluid from joint aspiration containing ≥50 000 white blood cells/mm³; (c) elevated acute-phase reactants erythrocyte sedimentation rate, C-reactive protein or white blood cell count.
Intervention	At diagnosis all patients received intravenous (IV) cefuroxime 150 mg/kg/day in three divided doses and either IV dexamethasone (0.15 mg/kg/dose every 6 hours for 16 doses) or an identical placebo.
Outcomes	The primary outcomes were (a) time to clinical and laboratory normalisation and (b) the duration of hospitalisation.
Main results	Sixty patients were eligible for inclusion, but 11 refused and 49 were randomised: 24 to the dexamethasone group and 25 to the placebo group. There were no treatment withdrawals.

(*continued*)

Evidence 3	
Theme E3	**Dexamethasone and septic arthritis**
Main results (*cont.*)	The mean age at enrolment was 33 ± 42 months (range 6–161 months). Relating to clinical outcomes normal full range of movement and first day of normal function were achieved on days 7 and 6.6 for dexamethasone and days 12.2 and 8.7 for placebo. Relating to normalisation of C-reactive protein, for dexamethasone it was 3.1 days, compared with 5.5 days for placebo (absolute risk reduction (ARR) = 77%; number needed to treat (NNT) = 2). The difference in duration of IV antibiotic treatment between dexamethasone and placebo was 2.7 days (dexamethasone, 9.9 days; placebo, 12.6 days; ARR = 27%; NNT = 4).
Conclusion	The use of dexamethasone in the treatment of septic arthritis leads to a more rapid improvement in clinical and laboratory markers with a reduction in the duration of IV antibiotic treatment.
Commentary	Septic arthritis is a severe and rapidly progressive erosive disease. Despite the use of antibiotic treatment the inflammatory process can continue with resulting residual joint damage. In this particular study there was no difference in outcome in the long-term follow-up of these patients.
Reference	Harel L, Prais D, Bar-On E, *et al.* Dexamethasone therapy for septic arthritis in children: results of a randomized double-blind placebo-controlled study. *J Pediatr Orthop.* 2011; **31**(2): 211–15.

Evidence 4	
Theme E4	**Antibiotic treatment for osteomyelitis**
Question	What is the optimal duration of antibiotic treatment in acute haematogenous osteomyelitis (AHOM)?
Design	Randomised controlled trial (non-inferiority)
Level of evidence	Jadad 1
Setting	Seven academic medical centres and regional hospitals, Finland
Participants	Infants, children and adolescents, aged 3 months to 15 years, were eligible for inclusion in this study if they had clinical features of AHOM (characterised by fever; painful and swollen limb without trauma; restriction of motion, often with a tender and warm area); and a positive culture (this was included to avoid discussion on the accuracy of diagnosis).
Intervention	Participants were assigned to either a 20- or a 30-day antibiotic treatment regimen, with the initial 2–4 days intravenously administered and the remainder orally administered. Antibiotic choice was clindamycin (40 mg/kg per day every 6 hours) or a first-generation cephalosporin. Due to cephalosporin drug availability, the initial choice of cephradine was switched to cephalothin).
Outcomes	The primary outcome was full recovery (having no symptoms or signs of AHOM at the end of the follow-up period, with no re-administration of antimicrobials for an osteoarticular indication since the primary treatment) at 12 months after the primary treatment.

(*continued*)

Evidence 4	
Theme E4	*Antibiotic treatment for osteomyelitis*
Main results	AHOM was clinically diagnosed in 183 cases but only 131 (72%) were culture positive, and of these, 67 were randomised to the short antibiotic course and 64 to the long course.
Conclusion	Most cases of AHOM can be treated for 20 days including a short 2- to 4-day course of intravenous antibiotics and the remainder as orally administered clindamycin and first-generation cephalosporins at high doses, provided the clinical response is good and the C-reactive protein normalises in 7–10 days.
Commentary	AHOM is a relatively rare condition, with an incidence of 4.5 per 100 000, but is a potentially devastating disease and consequently has been treated with prolonged courses of intravenous and oral antibiotics. A clinical caveat from this study is separating out tests that measure infection and inflammation. The use of C-reactive protein as the guide to improvement, as opposed to the erythrocyte sedimentation rate, allowed antibiotics to be discontinued earlier (a value under 20 mg/L on two successive measurements is correlated with marked clinical improvement at 7–10 days of antibiotic treatment).
Reference	Peltola H, Pääkkönen M, Kallio P, *et al.* Osteomyelitis–Septic Arthritis Group. Short-versus long-term antimicrobial treatment for acute hematogenous osteomyelitis of childhood: prospective, randomized trial on 131 culture-positive cases. *Pediatr Infect Dis J.* 2010; **29**(12): 1123–8.

Evidence 5	
Theme E5	*The treatment of rheumatoid arthritis*
Question	Which is more effective in the treatment of rheumatoid arthritis: ibuprofen or aspirin?
Design	Randomised controlled trial
Level of evidence	Jadad 5
Setting	Multicentre setting, academic medical centres, the United States and Finland
Participants	Children and adolescents 15 years and under were eligible if they met the American College of Rheumatology guidelines for juvenile rheumatoid arthritis. Patients with any of the subtypes (systemic, pauciarticular or polyarticular) were included, provided that they had evidence of a minimum of one joint of active arthritis.
Intervention	Patients received either ibuprofen (30–40 mg/kg/day) or aspirin (60–80 mg/kg/day) for 12 weeks.
Outcomes	The following variables were used as the primary outcomes: (a) duration of the morning stiffness, (b) the number of joints with swelling, (c) the number of joints with pain on motion, (d) the total number of joints with active arthritis and the overall severity score.
Main results	Sixteen centres contributed 92 patients: 45 received Ibuprofen and 47 received aspirin. The juvenile rheumatoid arthritis types were pauciarticular in 48%, polyarticular in 44% and systemic disease in 8%.

(*continued*)

Evidence 5	
Theme E5	**The treatment of rheumatoid arthritis**
Main results (*cont.*)	The global responses to treatment for ibuprofen were 79%, 79% and 85% when assessed by the investigator, parent and child, as compared with aspirin, where response rates were 77%, 83% and 90%. There was no difference clinically. Seventeen patients experienced significant side effects: four (9%) related to ibuprofen and 13 (27.5%) from aspirin (absolute risk reduction (AAR) = 18.5%; number needed to harm (NNH) = 6). Six (13%) patients on aspirin withdrew because of side effect severity, compared with 0 in the ibuprofen group (ARR = 13%; NNH = 8).
Conclusion	Ibuprofen is as effective as aspirin in the treatment of rheumatoid arthritis and has a better safety profile.
Commentary	Rheumatoid arthritis is a chronic disease, which impairs the quality of the child's life. Utilising medications that have a good safety profile is imperative. The study demonstrated the effectiveness of non-steroidal anti-inflammatory drugs, and their safety profile has been further enhanced over the years with the introduction of enteric-coated tablets.
Reference	Giannini EH, Brewer EJ, Miller ML, *et al.* Pediatric Rheumatology Collaborative Study Group. Ibuprofen suspension in the treatment of juvenile rheumatoid arthritis. *Pediatrics.* 1990; **117**(4): 645–52.

LIMP: MULTIPLE-CHOICE QUESTIONS

Q1 In DDH, which of the following is/are true?
a) It is more common in boys.
b) Breech position in utero is a risk factor.
c) Polyhydramnios is a risk factor.
d) Painless limp is a late presentation.
e) The incidence is 1:250 children.

Q2 In transient synovitis, which of the following is/are true?
a) It is often preceded by an upper respiratory tract infection.
b) The child is comfortable at rest.
c) There is reduced internal rotation.
d) Steroids reduced the inflammation in 80% at 24 hours.
e) It is a risk factor for aseptic necrosis of the femoral head.

Q3 In septic arthritis, which of the following is/are true?
a) It is caused by group B streptococcus in the newborn period.
b) It is caused by *S. aureus* in childhood.
c) The hips and knees are most commonly affected joints.
d) The hip, if affected, is often internally rotated.
e) Forty per cent of patients present with associated headache.

Q4 Which of the following is/are true of Osgood–Schlatter's disease?
a) It affects 1:300 children.
b) Steroid treatment is a causative factor.
c) It affects the patellar insertion.
d) Pain is worse with activity.
e) Tenderness of the tibial tuberosity is a key feature on physical examination.

Q5 Which of the following statements is/are true pertaining to toddler's facture?
a) Toddler's fracture occurs in the middle third of the tibia.
b) It often requires a cast.
c) The child often presents with crying.
d) A history of trauma is often absent.
e) It may indicate non-accidental injury.

Q6 Which of the following statements regarding JIA is/are true?
a) Arthritis must be present for more than 6 weeks.
b) A salmon-pink rash occurs in systemic-onset disease.
c) The incidence is 1:1500.
d) Forty to fifty per cent of cases are oligoarticular.
e) NSAIDs are first-line treatment.

Q7 Which of the following is/are true with regard to Lyme disease?
a) It is the most common cause of reactive arthritis.
b) It is associated with erythema migrans.
c) It is associated with erythema multiforme.
d) Ten per cent of patients develop an erosive arthritis in the hands.
e) It is caused by *Borrelia burgdorferi*.

Answers

A1	b, d	**A2**	a, b, c, e
A3	a, b, c	**A4**	b, c, e
A5	c, d, e	**A6**	a, b, d, e
A7	b, e		

SLIDES

1. Anterior uveitis
2. Idiopathic juvenile arthritis
3. Juvenile idiopathic arthritis
4. Neuroblastoma (proptosis)

Chapter Twenty-five

THE PALE CHILD

COMMON SCENARIO

'He looks so pale and yet he has a good appetite and drinks a lot of milk.'

LEARNING OBJECTIVES

- Understand the red blood cell indices
- Develop a strategy to problem solve microcytic, normocyctic and macrocytic anaemias
- Understand what tests should be performed in a child with anaemia
- Have a treatment strategy for iron-deficiency anaemia
- Be able to recognise and treat the presentations of sickle-cell anaemia
- Have a strategy to recognise treatment options in thalassaemia

BACKGROUND

Anaemia is defined as a haemoglobin concentration two standard deviations below the mean allowing for age and sex of the child. Normal haemoglobin varies with age and sex.

- From birth to 3 months of age, the haemoglobin level drops from a mean level of 16.5 g/dL at birth to a nadir of 11.5 g/dL at 3 months.
- At 6 months of age, the mean haemoglobin level is 12.0 g/dL and remains stable until 6 years of age.
- From 6 to 12 years, the mean haemoglobin rises to 13.5 g/dL.
- From 12 to 18 years of age, the mean haemoglobin is higher in boys (14.5 g/dL) than girls (14.0 g/dL).

Most children with mild anaemia are asymptomatic with minimal signs including pallor. Symptoms of moderate to severe anaemia vary depending on the child's age but include exertional dyspnoea, palpitations, easy fatigability, failure to thrive and poor weight gain. Signs of anaemia include pallor, pale conjunctiva and nail beds, a flow murmur, tachycardia and in extreme cases signs of heart failure.

Anaemia can be classified according to interpretation of the mean corpuscular volume (MCV), i.e. are the red blood cells microcytic, macrocytic or normocytic.

Red blood cell indices	Explanation
Reticulocyte count	Bone marrow activity
RDW (red cell distribution width)	Shows if cells are the same or different size or shape
MCV (normocytic, macrocytic, microcytic)	Size or volume of the red blood cell
Mean corpuscular haemoglobin concentration (normochromic, hyperchromic, hypochromic)	Concentration of haemoglobin in the red blood cell
Haematocrit	Fractional volume of whole blood occupied by red blood cells
Haemoglobin	Concentration of the red blood cell pigment haemoglobin in whole blood

MICROCYTIC ANAEMIA

Iron-deficiency anaemia

The commonest cause of microcytic anaemia in Europe is iron deficiency. A 1-year-old requires approximately 8 mg/day of iron. Absorption of iron takes place in the jejunum and duodenum. Iron is mainly stored in haemoglobin (70%), with the rest found in the liver and spleen. Fifty per cent of available iron is absorbed from breast milk, while only 10% is absorbed from cow's milk. Iron absorption is increased by vitamin C, fructose and citrate and inhibited by tannins and high-fibre foods. Although the majority of cases are secondary to nutritional insufficiency, iron deficiency can also be due to underlying medical conditions causing occult gastrointestinal (GI) blood loss, malabsorption or menorrhagia.

A careful history, including a detailed dietary history, should identify those at risk of iron deficiency. Risk factors include prematurity, low birthweight, maternal iron deficiency, delayed weaning onto solids, excessive or early introduction of cow's milk, tea drinking, iron-deplete diet lacking in iron-fortified cereals. The full blood count (FBC) shows a low haemoglobin, with a low MCV, raised red cell distribution width, low reticulocyte count and hypochromia.

In at-risk ethnic groups thalassaemia syndromes should be considered. Thalassaemias are most common in the Indian subcontinent, the Mediterranean and the Middle East. Normal haemoglobin (HbA) has four protein chains, two alpha and two beta globin chains. Four genes (two from each parent) are needed to make the two alpha globin chains. Thalassaemia is a spectrum of disease characterised by decreased or absent production of alpha or beta globin chains.

Alpha thalassaemia

- Children with an absence of one alpha gene or alpha thalassaemia minima are silent carriers and have a normal haemoglobin and MCV.
- Children with two absent alpha genes have alpha thalassaemia trait and a mild microcytic anaemia.
- Loss of three alpha chains or HbH (beta 4 tetramers) results in moderate to severe anaemia.
- Loss of four alpha chains results in hydrops foetalis and haemoglobin Bart's (gamma 4 tetramers). The condition is incompatible with life as alpha globin is essential for the formation of foetal haemoglobin.

Beta thalassaemia

Children with beta thalassaemia minor or beta thalassaemia trait have one normal beta globin allele and one beta globin thalassaemia allele. Most patients are asymptomatic or have a mild hypochromic anaemia.

Children with beta thalassaemia intermediate are compound heterozygote for two different beta globin chain mutations and have mild to moderate anaemia, however they do not require transfusion during early life and so do not become transfusion dependent till the second decade of life.

Beta thalassaemia major is the most severe form, with children homozygous for mutations associated with absent or severely reduced production of beta chains. Children have severe haemolytic anaemia, hepatosplenomegaly with little HbA and HbF and A2 only. It presents during the first year of life with failure to thrive and irritability.

Anaemia of chronic disease

A number of chronic diseases can cause anaemia for different reasons including hypoactivity of the bone marrow, poor response to erythropoetin or shortened red blood cell survival. Causes include infections such as tuberculosis, HIV, endocarditis and osteomyelitis, inflammatory conditions such as inflammatory bowel disease or juvenile idopathic arthritis, neoplasms and chronic renal failure.

Lead poisoning

Although public health interventions have removed many sources of lead from the environment, children can still be exposed to harmful levels usually in the home. Lead can be absorbed by ingestion of lead-containing particles or inhalation of lead dust or fumes. Ingestion of lead-containing paint is the commonest cause of exposure in children. Exposure to lead is associated with cognitive impairment and adverse neurodevelopmental outcomes. In severe cases anaemia may develop as lead inhibits haeme synthesis.

MACROCYTIC ANAEMIA

Macrocytic red blood cells may be a normal variant in newborns and children with Down's syndrome.

Common pathological causes of macrocytic anaemia include:

- vitamin B_{12} and folate deficiency
- hypothyroidism
- liver disease
- anticonvulsant medications.

Rarer causes of macrocytic anaemia include the following.

- **Transient erythroblastopaenia of childhood** is a rare acquired red cell aplasia of unclear aetiology occurring in previously healthy children under 4 years of age. The disease is self-limiting and normally resolves within weeks to 2 months. It is frequently associated with viral illnesses.
- **Diamond–Blackfan's anaemia** is a congenital erythroid aplasia that presents in infancy with severe anaemia, often in association with physical anomalies (in 50% of cases) and short stature. Children often have typical craniofacial features and a classical triphalangeal thumb.
- **Severe aplastic anaemia** is a syndrome of bone marrow failure with peripheral pancytopenia and marrow hypoplasia. It can be congenital or acquired.
- **Fanconi's anaemia** is an autosomal recessive bone marrow failure syndrome with an increased risk of developing acute myeloid leukaemias and certain solid tumours. Most patients are diagnosed before 7 years of age. It is a heterogeneous condition, with chromosomal instability. Hypoplasia of the thumb and radius are common. Abnormalities in skin pigmentation are commonly seen including café au lait macules.
- **Myelodysplastic syndromes** are clonal disorders characterised by ineffective haematopoiesis and subsequent development of acute myeloid leukaemia. It is uncommon in childhood and extremely heterogeneous in terms of its presentation and outcome. The most common genetic abnormality is a mutation on chromosome 7. In over 50% of cases a stem cell transplant is curative.

NORMOCYTIC ANAEMIA

In considering normocytic anaemias, a useful approach is to look at the reticulocyte count. An elevated reticulocyte count indicates effective erthyropoeisis, with a low or normal reticulocyte count indicating ineffective erythropoeisis.

Haemolytic anaemias and anaemia due to acute blood loss are associated with a high reticulocyte count. Serum bilirubin and lactate dehydrogenase are increased and haptoglobin is decreased. A wide variety of conditions can cause haemolysis, however the clinical context, blood film and Coombs' test or direct antiglobulin test results will often provide clues as to the cause of the haemolysis. There may be a history of jaundice, splenomegaly, gallstones or a significant family or neonatal history.

Haemolytic anaemias can be hereditary or acquired. Hereditary casues of haemolytic anaemias include membrane defects such as hereditary spherocytosis or elliptiocytosis, enzyme defects such as G6PD deficiency or pyruvate kinase deficiency and haemoglobinopathies.

Hereditary spherocytosis is the most common cause of haemolytic anaemia in children. It is inherited in an autosomal dominant pattern, but due to phenotypic variations, there may not always be a positive family history. Abnormal membrane proteins result in rigid red blood cells with a spherical shape that are trapped and destroyed in the spleen, resulting in haemolytic anaemia. Children present with jaundice, anaemia and splenomegaly. An elevated mean corpuscular haemoglobin concentration strongly suggests spherocytosis. Peripheral smear shows spherocytes. Patients can present with a 'hyperhaemolytic crisis' where haemolysis is accelerated as a result of infection, commonly, non-specific viral infections. Splenectomy is curative; however, because of the risk of sepsis this is reserved for severe cases. Indications for splenectomy include frequent hyperhaemolytic crises, symptomatic anaemia, gallstones or growth retardation.

G6PD deficiency is an X-linked recessive disorder caused by mutations in the G6PD gene. More than 300 varieties of G6PD deficiency have been identified. Clinical manifestations include:

- asymptomatic
- neonatal jaundice
- haemolysis – episodic or chronic.

Haemolysis can be triggered by certain drugs, infections and foods, such as:

- dapsone
- antimalarials
- antibiotics – sulphonamides, nitrofurantoin, co-trimoxazole, chloramphenicol
- aspirin
- naphthalene
- vitamin K
- chemicals in mothballs
- fava beans.

Sickle-cell disease is an autosomal recessive disease prevalent in children of African or Caribbean descent. Sickle-cell haemoglobin is caused by a mutation in the beta globin gene on chromosome 11, causing a substitution of valine for glutamate. Patients homozygous for the sickle-cell gene have sickle-cell disease. The majority of centres now offer some form of antenatal and newborn screening either universal or selectively. Without screening, children usually present at 6–12 months with a moderate anaemia of 6–8 g/dL.

Four types of crisis can occur:

1. vaso-occlusive: acute chest syndrome, dactylitis, stroke, priapism, painful crisis
2. aplastic: can be triggered by parvovirus B19
3. haemolytic
4. splenic sequestration.

Acquired immune haemolytic anaemias

Auto-immune haemolytic anaemia is characterised by the presence of autoantibodies that bind to the surface membrane of the erythrocyte leading to premature red cell destruction. Autoimmune haemolytic anaemias are classified based on the temperature at which the antibody optimally binds to the erythrocyte. Warm autoimmune haemolytic anaemias are associated with lymphoid malignancies. Cold autoimmune haemolytic anaemias can be seen following infection with mycoplasma pneumonia or Epstein–Barr virus. Alloimmune haemolytic anaemias can occur as a result of haemolytic transfusion reactions or in the newborn due to ABO or Rhesus incompatibility.

Drug-induced haemolysis can be immune mediated or non-immune mediated.

Acquired non-immune haemolytic anaemias

Can be caused by infections, such as malaria, drugs or as a result of mechanical destruction in thrombotic thrombocytopenic purpura, haemolytic-uraemic syndrome, disseminated intravascular coagulation, patients with prosthetic heart valves.

Normocytic anaemia with a low reticulocyte count

Children with a normal or low reticulocyte count require bone marrow evaluation as this may indicate marrow infiltration such as leukaemia or neuroblastoma.

HISTORY

KEY POINTS				
Pallor	Duration Acute or sudden onset Present since birth	Symptoms of bleeding	Malaena Haematemesis Nosebleeds Menorrhagia Mucosal bleeding	**🔴 Red flags** Rapid onset of pallor Jaundice Chest pain Fever in a child with sickle cell disease
Dietary history	Duration of breastfeeding Timing of introduction of solids Iron-rich foods (meat and green vegetables) Cow's milk intake	Symptoms of pica	Eat paper or dirt Chew on ice	

(continued)

KEY POINTS				
Family history	Race and ethnic background Anaemia Jaundice Early onset gallstones Splenectomy Blood transfusions	**Past medical history**	Recurrent upper respiratory tract infections Recurrent episodes of jaundice and pallor	
Symptoms of leukaemia?	Easy bruising Swellings Bone pain Limp	**Birth and maternal history**	Mother vegetarian Prematurity Jaundice Transfusion	
Lead exposure	Housing Paint exposure	**General health**	Lethargy Similar energy levels to siblings and peers? Recurrent infections Fainting or light-headedness	
		Drugs	Regular medication Recent antibiotics	

EXAMINATION

All children presenting with pallor should have a full systemic examination.

- Look for signs of iron deficiency (leuconychia/koilonychia/angular stomatitis, painful glossitis, pale palmar creases/pale conjunctivae/soft systolic murmur)
- Look for evidence of jaundice (suggests haemolysis)
- Check for lymphadenopathy and bruising or petechiae
- Examine for hepatomegaly and splenomegaly
- Fundoscopy for retinal haemorrhages
- Signs of heart failure: tachypnoea, oedema, crepitations, hepatomegaly, murmur
- Signs of hypovolaemia: heart rate, respiratory rate, blood pressure, capillary refill time, temperature

INVESTIGATIONS

What are first-line investigations that should be performed in a child with pallor?

FBC, paying particular attention to the MCV, blood film and reticulocyte count

If the haemoglobin is low, but the WCC and platelets are normal, then the child is anaemic

However, if pancytopenia is present, then bone marrow involvement is likely and urgent specialist referral is required for further investigation and management

In children with microcytic anaemia, what further investigations should be performed?

Serum iron, total iron binding capacity and serum ferritin

In iron-deficiency anaemia, the serum iron and ferritin will be low, with a low percent transferrin saturation and a high total iron binding capacity. Zinc protoporpyrin levels are raised. Reticulocyte haemoglobin and transferrin 1 receptor levels (if available) are useful. They measure iron deficiency at a cellular level

Haemoglobin electrophoresis in at-risk ethnic groups

In children with macrocytic anaemia, what further investigations should be performed?

B_{12}, folate, red cell folate, liver function tests, thyroid function tests

In children with normocyctic anaemia and a high reticulocyte count, what further investigations should be performed?

G6PD screening

Osmotic fragility test for hereditary spherocytosis

Coombs' test for haemolytic anaemia (a direct Coombs' test detects antibodies on red cells; washed red blood cells are mixed with antihuman globulin, which reacts with antibodies on the red blood cell surface, causing them to clump together; a positive direct Coombs' test indicates an immune haemolytic anaemia)

Serum haptoglobin level

In newborns: maternal and foetal blood groups

What further findings might indicate a haemolytic anaemia?

Blood film – showing red cell fragments

Bilirubin – raised unconjugated bilirubin

Haptoglobin – reduced

Haptoglobins are proteins that bind free haemoglobin. In the presence of haemolyis, when haemoglobin is released, it is bound by haptoglobin and so levels are reduced.

MANAGEMENT PLAN: TWO-STEP APPROACH

1. Clarifying and pitfall avoidance strategies
2. Management of specific conditions:
   a) iron-deficiency anaemia
   b) sickle-cell disease
   c) hereditary spherocytosis
   d) thalassaemia

Clarifying and pitfall avoidance strategies

- The presence of pallor is not diagnostic for anaemia. **Rationale**: the presence of marked pallor may be genetic in the Caucasian population. Other causes include nausea, pain and oedema of the skin. The sensitivity and specificity of pallor to identify anaemia is poor.
- Cow's milk ingestion and iron-deficiency anaemia. **Rationale**: the ingestion of cow's milk contributes to iron-deficiency anaemia as it is low in iron. Occult blood loss occurs in 40% of infants who drink cow's milk and the non-haeme iron absorption is inhibited by calcium and casein (which are present in cow's milk).
- Screening for iron-deficiency anaemia. **Rationale**: the best parameters to define the presence of iron-deficiency state are (a) serum ferritin, since this is an acute-phase reactant protein, the result must be interpreted in terms of a normal C-reactive protein level; (b) serum reticulocyte haemoglobin concentration; and (c) red cell membrane transferrin receptor, which currently is not widely available.
- The need to treat iron-deficiency anaemia. **Rationale**: iron-deficiency anaemia is associated with both cognitive and behavioural problems in children and, as a consequence, needs to be treated.
- Looking at the FBC to assess iron-deficiency anaemia. **Rationale**: the FBC report should be assessed for the Mentzer index (MCV/number of red cells in millions). A Mentzer score <13 suggests thalassaemia.
- Non-responding iron-deficiency anaemia. **Rationale**: iron deficiency that does not respond to oral iron should prompt the following response: (a) ensure that the iron is being consumed in therapeutic doses, (b) consider the possibility of an anaemia of chronic disease, e.g. lead poisoning, (c) consider the presence of excessive milk consumption, (d) consider missed coeliac disease and (e) consider the possibility of ongoing iron loss from the gut due to Meckel's diverticulum or inflammatory bowel disease. Iron in such cases can be administered intravenously after an initial test dose of intravenous iron to ensure the absence of an anaphylactic event.
- Sickle-cell disease. **Rationale**: those children with sickle-cell disease present many challenges for the doctor especially when infection or acute painful episodes occur.

Management of specific conditions

Iron-deficiency anaemia

Anaemia secondary to iron deficiency is important to treat, as iron deficiency is shown to decrease cognitive and motor function. Dietary measures alone cannot treat iron-deficiency anaemia and supplemental elemental iron is required. Parents should be given written information on iron-rich foods, which should be an essential part of their child's diet. Iron-rich foods include green leafy vegetables, iron-fortified cereals, lean meats, beans, eggs and raisins.

Oral iron should be prescribed at 6 mg/kg/day for 1 month followed by 3 mg/kg/day for 2–3 months to replete iron stores. It is important to advise parents that iron, like all medicine, should be kept out of reach of children. Accidental overdoses of oral iron can be life-threatening. One week after initiation of treatment, repeat FBC, film and reticulocyte count – rise in HB is 1 g/week. The child should be followed up until the haemoglobin, MCV and serum ferritin normalise. Compliance can be an issue because of poor palatability and adverse GI side effects (*see* Evidence 1). If response to treatment is poor, non-compliance or ongoing undetected GI tract blood loss should be considered.

Parenteral iron therapy is seldom required. It is generally reserved for severe anaemia with poor compliance or intolerance of oral supplements. Red cell transfusion should be reserved for severe, symptomatic anaemia compromising end organ function.

Sickle-cell disease

With the advent of screening the management of sickle-cell disease has been modified. Early diagnosis has allowed for parental education on the disease, recognition of complications and for the commencement of prophylactic antibiotics to prevent pneumococcal disease, which is 600 times more common in children with sickle-cell disease.

- *Infection prevention*. In children with sickle-cell disease there is splenic hypofunction and antibiotic prophylaxis is required. Penicillin is the antibiotic of choice. It should be taken until the child is 5 years of age, as after this age the risk of pneumococcal disease decreases. Adherence rates are 70% and at each clinic visit adherence should be discussed. The use of antibiotics will not impact on viral illnesses. To further reduce the risk of pneumococcal disease, pneumococcal vaccination must be administered. Adherence and completeness of immunisation in a timely fashion is required. For children travelling abroad with sickle-cell disease malaria, prophylaxis is required, as is prophylaxis against meningococcal disease.
- *Sickle-cell in the emergency department*. While the majority of patients with sickle-cell disease receive their care in a tertiary centre, they can present acutely to emergency departments. There are three complications of sickle-cell that need to be treated promptly: (1) acute painful episodes, (2) fever (rule out infection) and (3) acute chest syndrome or pneumonia. The child with sickle-cell attending the emergency department suggests that they are unwell. Many parents of children with chronic diseases attempt to maximise out of hospital treatments prior to attending the emergency department and prolonged waiting times are likely to adversely affect the outcome for the child.

ACUTE PAINFUL EPISODES IN SICKLE-CELL DISEASE

Acute painful episodes are the most frequent complication of sickle-cell disease. Obstruction of blood flow by sickled erythrocytes leads to hypoxia and acidosis and eventually to ischaemic injury. The presenting symptoms and signs are pain in the extremities with swelling, low-grade fever with associated redness and warmth. If it

occurs in the abdomen there may be mild to severe pain. Patients who have experience of these episodes usually have taken paracetamol and codeine prior to presenting
to the emergency department and require adequate analgesia – usually morphine
intravenously with continuous infusion thereafter (for other options, *see* Evidence 2).
Discharge is possible once the pain has abated and the child is adequately hydrated.
If inpatient treatment is required, (a) ensure adequate hydration (fluids, intravenous
and oral) 1–1.5 times maintenance, (b) commence stool softeners while on narcotic
medications, (c) use oxygen if hypoxaemia is present (oxygen saturation ≤94%), (d) use
incentive spirometry for those able to co-operate (usually 5 years of age and older) –
10 breaths every 1–2 hours while awake or five breaths every 15 minutes, (e) monitor
pain (utilising an age-appropriate pain scale) and (f) ambulate as soon as is practical.

FEVER IN PATIENTS WITH SICKLE-CELL DISEASE

Patients with sickle-cell disease, despite prophylactic antibiotic therapy and full immunisations develop fever and are at risk of overwhelming sepsis. When these children
present in a febrile state they should be seen promptly and assessed. A FBC and blood
cultures should be drawn and the child immediately commenced on intravenous antibiotics (often a third-generation cephalosporin) prior to the FBC result being known
and investigations, e.g. a chest X-ray being performed. Fever should be treated with
paracetamol in standard doses. All febrile children with sickle-cell disease should be
admitted for at least 48 hours while awaiting blood culture reports.

Children who look toxic, are non-adherent to penicillin prophylaxis, are under
1 year of age, have respiratory distress or have had previous meningitis warrant consideration of vancomycin treatment. Consultation should occur with the tertiary care
team responsible for the child's care if hospitalisation in another facility has occurred.
The potential aetiologies of the fever are varied (*see* Evidence 3) but the risk of true
bacteraemia is 4%.

ACUTE CHEST SYNDROME

Acute chest syndrome is the second most frequent cause of admission to hospital
of children with sickle-cell disease. The aetiologies include bacteria (pneumococcus,
Gram-negative bacteria, chlamydia and *Mycoplasma pneumoniae*) and viruses (respiratory syncytial virus, influenza and parainfluenza). Non-infectious causes include
pulmonary infarction, pulmonary oedema from fluid overload, hypoventilation from
pain or narcotic administration. Children under 4 years of age present with cough
fever and upper lobe disease. Older children present with dyspnoea, chills, no fever
and multiple lobes involved (inclusive of lower lobe) on chest X-ray. Tenderness over
the ribs is frequently noted.

The initial management consists of monitoring vitals, obtaining FBC, blood
culture, chest X-ray, nasopharyngeal swab, and group and crossmatch. Treatment
consists of intravenous fluids at maintenance rate (excessive fluid administration wors-
ens symptoms and fluid overload can trigger acute chest syndrome), oxygen to keep

oxygen saturation ≥94% and intravenous antibiotic (third-generation cephalosporin). All children require admission to hospital, but if unstable they should be transferred to a tertiary care centre. Patients who are moderately ill and whose haemoglobin is <1.5 g/L below baseline should be transfused with 10 mL/kg. Patients should not be transfused to a haemoglobin >10 g/L or a haematocrit >30%). Morphine for analgesia is required and incentive spirometry should be undertaken.

Hereditary spherocytosis

In the management of hereditary spherocytosis (HS) several issues need to be considered that involve folate treatment, splenectomy and prophylaxis against infection. Folate therapy is recommended in moderate to severe cases of HS. A reasonable daily dose is 2.5 mg for a child younger than 5 years and 5 mg for a child older than 5 years. Splenectomy is very effective in reducing haemolysis and the risk of gallstones in HS but it is associated with an increased risk of sepsis. In moderate HS (characterised by haemoglobin 10–15 g/L, reticulocyte count >6% and serum bilirubin >34 μmol/L) is usually necessary during school age before puberty. In severe HS (characterised by a haemoglobin of 6–8 g/L, reticulocyte count >10% and a serum bilirubin >51 μmol/L) splenectomy is necessary but should be delayed until 6 years if possible. Infection risks are reduced through prophylactic antibiotic use and a pneumococcal vaccination (which must be updated on a regular basis) but not completely eliminated. In children undergoing a splenectomy, a cholecystectomy should also be performed.

Thalassaemia

In beta thalassaemia the cornerstone of management is regular blood transfusions. However, this is associated with iron overload and the need to use iron chelation therapy. The use of desferrioxamine subcutaneously for 8–10 hours a day, 5 days a week is arduous and adherence to treatment can be difficult. The use of oral iron chelation therapy has not been successful (*see* Evidence 4). For children who require very frequent transfusions, hydroxyurea offers an alternative treatment option (*see* Evidence 5). It has also been used in patients with sickle-cell disease.

For those children with thalassaemia intermedia there may not be a requirement for blood transfusion and if there is, it is usually irregular.

FOLLOW-UP

Short-term follow-up of dietary iron deficiency with follow-up FBC after 3 months. Beware that the most common reason for failure to respond is non-compliance. Always also consider occult blood loss or malabsorption if the patient is not responding.

WHEN TO REFER?

- Iron-deficiency anaemia that fails to respond to treatment with oral iron (6 mg/kg/day of elemental iron for 8 weeks)
- All macrocytic anaemias
- Children with sickle-cell disease (should be assessed by paediatric haematologist)
- Children with thalassaemia
- Children with evidence of red cell haemolysis

CLARIFICATION FOR PARENTAL MISCONCEPTIONS

'My child's blood count could not be that low just due to dietary causes.'

Iron deficiency due to dietary lack of iron may cause, if prolonged, marked drops in haemoglobin down to 2–3 g/L and will respond to alteration of the diet and oral elemental iron.

'When should I worry about the possibility of leukaemia?'

In general terms, the great majority of anaemia seen in primary care is related to iron deficiency and is dietary in origin. Pallor is a feature of leukaemia but the blood count and film will show not just anaemia but also alterations in the white cell count or platelet count.

'What do I need to know if my child has a diagnosis of sickle-cell anaemia?'

The most important aspects of management are strict adherence measures to prevent sickle-cell disease-related problems including prophylaxis with oral penicillin once the diagnosis is made, folic acid supplementation and trying to reduce risks of crises by avoiding cold, dehydration and over-exertion with hypoxia, recognising and promptly responding to the signs of splenic sequestration (sudden drop in haemoglobin). If a child with sickle-cell anaemia has a stroke, they should receive monthly exchange transfusions for 3 years to reduce the risk of recurrence.

'Is the anaemia due to blood loss?'

Usually GI blood loss perhaps relating to reflux oesophagitis or gastritis. Meckel's diverticulum bleeds are rare and GI bleeding due to inflammatory bowel disease is usually characterised by blood and mucus in the stools. Coeliac disease is relatively common and may present with anaemia and thus a coeliac screen is warranted, especially if there is a positive family history.

SUMMARY PRACTICE POINTS

- Anaemia is relatively common in childhood, especially in toddlers.
- It is usually due to dietary lack of iron.
- Treatment is with oral elemental iron for 3 months.
- Non-response is usually due to non-compliance with treatment.
- Occult GI blood loss or malabsorption should be suspected if not responsive to oral iron.
- Bone marrow failure is very rare and may be suspected if the neutrophil count or platelet count is also low.
- Haemolytic anaemias have significant racial predilection (hereditary spherocytosis in northern Europeans, sickle-cell anaemia in Afro-Caribbeans and beta thalassaemia in southern Europeans and in the Middle East, G6PD in the Indian subcontinent).

EVALUATING THE EVIDENCE

Evidence 1	
Theme E1	**Treatment of iron-deficiency anaemia**
Question	What is the most effective form of iron therapy to treat iron-deficiency anaemia?
Design	Randomised controlled trial
Level of evidence	Jadad 1
Setting	Rural communities, Mexico
Participants	Anaemia was defined as haemoglobin <11.7 g/dL (based on the children's age and the altitude of 1600 m).
Intervention	Children with iron deficiency were randomised to receive iron supplements (ISs), iron supplements plus folic acid (IFSs), a multiple micronutrients supplement (MMS), a micronutrient-fortified complementary food as a porridge powder (FCF) or water-fortified zinc, iron and ascorbic acid (FW). The IS was ferrous sulphate.
Outcomes	The primary outcome was the resolution of the iron-deficiency anaemia after 4 months of treatment with one of the five treatment regimens. Secondary outcomes included patient acceptability and tolerance of the treatment.
Main results	Of the 577 children screened for iron-deficiency anaemia, 266 were anaemic and were included in the study. Fifty were assigned to the IS group, with full data on 40 (80%); 49 to the IFS group, with full data on 42 (86%); 51 to the MMS group, with full data on 36; 58 to the FW group, with full data on 48; and 59 to the FCF group, with full data on 51. The reduction in the prevalence of anaemia was as follows: IS 58%, IFS 69%, MMS 72%, FW 52%, FCF 45%. Assuming IS to be the standard of care, IFS 69%–IS 58%, absolute risk reduction (ARR) = 11%, number needed to treat (NNT) = 10; MMS 72%–IS 58%, ARR = 14%, NNT = 8. There were no significant differences in adherence rates among treatments; however, FCF and FW were preferred as IF, IFS and MMS were not palatable because of the high content of minerals in the solution.

(continued)

Evidence 1	
Theme E1	**Treatment of iron-deficiency anaemia**
Conclusion	IFS and MMS were more effective that IS in treating anaemia. The study participants accepted the fortified foods more readily than the supplements.
Commentary	Iron deficiency is common in childhood and is associated with developmental delay. Iron deficiency may be related to the low content of iron in the commonly used weaning foods for children. The diagnosis of iron deficiency in the early stages can be difficult. Serum iron is a reflection of the dietary iron consumed and the serum ferritin is an acute phase reactant thus, if the child has recurrent illnesses, cannot be relied on for diagnosis. Serum ferritin should be used in conjunction with C reactive protein levels. The use of zinc protoporphyrin levels are useful. Zinc protoporphyrin is an early product of impaired haem synthesis as is elevated in iron deficiency anaemia. Iron supplements are effective in the treatment of iron deficiency anaemia, however parental adherence to treatment has to be assessed and haemoglobin levels should rise by 1 g/dL per week. Treatment should be continued for 6 weeks to ensure normal iron stores
Reference	Rosado JL, González KE, Caamaño Mdel C, *et al.* Efficacy of different strategies to treat anemia in children: a randomized clinical trial. *Nutr J.* 2010; **9**: 40.

Evidence 2	
Theme E2	**Analgesia and acute sickle-cell pain**
Question	How effective is intranasal diamorphine (IND) for acute sickle pain?
Design	Cohort study
Level of evidence	
Setting	Department of haematology and emergency medicine, academic medical centre, the United Kingdom
Participants	Children with acute painful sickle-cell crises not responding to home analgesia and who were presenting to the emergency department were eligible for inclusion, provided they were over 1 year of age and not in shock or experiencing airway compromise or respiratory depression.
Intervention	Two interventions were utilised. • Intervention 1: IND (0.1 mg/kg) given as a single dose immediately on presentation to the emergency department, followed if required by intravenous morphine bolus (100 µg/kg) and infusion via patient-controlled analgesia once intravenous access was secured. • Intervention 2: IND (0.1 mg/kg) given simultaneously with oral morphine (0.4 mg/kg) immediately on arrival and followed by a further dose (0.4 mg/kg) at 1 hour if required.
Outcomes	The primary outcome was the reduction in pain experienced from time 0 minutes to 2 hours, utilising the British Association of Emergency Medicine paediatric pain assessment tool, and also the effectiveness and acceptability of the nasal administration route.

(*continued*)

Evidence 2	
Theme E2	*Analgesia and acute sickle-cell pain*
Main results	In intervention 1, nine patients were recruited and 13 were recruited in phase 2. The mean age was 10 years (range 2–16). The proportion of children in severe pain, in phase 1, at time 0, 15, 30 and 120 minutes were 78%, 11%, 0% and 11%, respectively, while in phase 2 they were 77%, 30%, 15% and 0%, respectively. There were no episodes of sedation or respiratory depression related to morphine. Two children in phase 1 received oral morphine, as successful cannulation was not achieved. The mean score for medication effectiveness out of 10 was 8.2 and for acceptability it was 8.5.
Conclusion	IND can be recommended for acute control of sickle-cell pain in children presenting to hospital.
Commentary	Children who present to the emergency department with acute sickle-cell crisis experience significant pain. The ability to relieve the pain, without the need to establish intravenous access is desirable especially as intravenous access may be difficult to establish, because of recurrent cannulation, in children who have recurrent crises. Many of these children will have used oral analgesics (paracetamol, ibuprofen, and codeine) at home without effect and the combination of intranasal diamorphine with oral morphine administered at presentation by the nursing staff was noted to be highly valued by both patient and parent. While pain scores appeared to improve more quickly in phase 1, the numbers treated were too small for statistical analysis.
Reference	Telfer P, Criddle J, Sandell J, *et al*. Intranasal diamorphine for acute sickle pain. *Arch Dis Child*. 2009; **94**(12): 979–80.

Evidence 3	
Theme E3	*Pneumococcal disease in sickle-cell disease*
Question	What is the prevalence of pneumococcal bacteraemia in children with sickle-cell disease?
Design	Retrospective chart review
Level of evidence	
Setting	Depart of paediatrics, academic medical centre, the United States
Participants	Children, previously diagnosed with sickle-cell disease, seen in the emergency department with fever >101°F were included.
Intervention	Charts of all children seen with pyrexia (temperature >101°F) were assessed and the following data abstracted: demographics (age, gender and ethnicity), variant of sickle-cell disease, duration of hospitalisation, temperature on admission, laboratory results: initial white blood cell count, C-reactive protein, blood culture report, time to positive blood culture.
Outcomes	The primary outcome was the prevalence of bacteraemia.
Main results	Over a 78-month period, 134 children had 458 episodes of febrile admissions. Two admissions were removed from the analysis, as no blood cultures were drawn.

(*continued*)

Evidence 3	
Theme E3	***Pneumococcal disease in sickle-cell disease***
Main results (*cont.*)	Of the 456 blood cultures, 37 (8%) grew bacterial organisms; however, only 19 (4%) were true pathogens. Three of the 19 infections were port infections. An analysis of infections pre- and post-introduction of the pneumococcal polysaccharide conjugate vaccine (PCV13) in 2010 (replacing the PCV7) indicated two (0.4%) cases of pneumococcal bacteraemia pre 2010 and none post. All febrile children were treated with a third-generation cephalosporin for at least 48 hours. Age, temperature on admission, white blood cell count and C-reactive protein did not differentiate positive cultures with true pathogens from the others. The time to positive blood cultures in true bacteraemia was 22.6 hours and 32.6 in those considered contaminants. The aetiologies of the febrile illnesses were lobar pneumonia, 82 (18%); acute chest, 47 (10%); occult bacteraemia, 19 (4%); viral infection, 13 (3%); urinary tract infections, 12 (3%); and no cause found, 283 (62%). All children were treated with intravenous antibiotics.
Conclusion	The prevalence of bacteraemia was 4% but since 2010 and the introduction of the PCV13 no cases of pneumococcal bacteraemia have been identified (compared with two (0.4%) from 2006–10).
Commentary	Children with sickle-cell disease develop functional asplenia at a very early age and are at high risk of death from infection by encapsulated bacteria. The two major advances have been prophylactic penicillin for children under 5 and primary vaccination. The introduction of the PCV7 reduced the rate of pneumococcal infection, and with the extended coverage offered by PCV13, this is likely to further lessen pneumococcal infection rates. The findings of positive blood cultures at 24 hours, may allow for the modification of the inpatient treatment strategy in selected patients given that 62% have no source identified.
Reference	Patel A, Zuzo A, Imran H, *et al*. Prevalence of pneumococcal bacteremia in children with sickle cell disease. *Pediatr Hematol Oncol*. 2013; **30**(5): 432–6. Epub 2013 Apr 9.

Evidence 4	
Theme E 4	***The treatment of iron overload in children with thalassaemia***
Question	What is the comparative efficacy of desferrioxamine (DFX), deferiprone (L1) and in combination on iron chelation thalassaemic children?
Design	Randomised controlled trial
Level of evidence	Jadad 1
Setting	Department of paediatrics and pathology, academic medical centre, India
Participants	Children were eligible for inclusion if they had received more than 20 blood transfusions and the serum ferritin was greater than 1500 ng/mL.
Intervention	Children were allocated to one of three groups: 1. subcutaneous DFX at a dose 40 mg/kg day over a period of 8–10 hours for 5 days a week 2. oral L1 at a dose of 75 mg/kg/day in two to three doses

(*continued*)

Evidence 4	
Theme E 4	**The treatment of iron overload in children with thalassaemia**
Intervention (*cont.*)	3. combined subcutaneous DFX at a dose of 40 mg/kg/day over an 8- to 10-hour period 2 days a week and oral L1 at a dose of 75 mg/kg day in two to three divided doses.
	Treatment was for a 6-month period.
Outcomes	The primary outcome measure was the change in serum ferritin over the 6-month period.
Main results	Initially 10 patients were in group 1, but two were excluded (reasons not stated) and one transferred to group 2; consequently, seven were analysed in this group. There were 11 patients in group 2 and 10 in group 3. In group 1 the initial mean serum ferritin (mean ± standard deviation (SD)) was 5077.18 ± 1714.99 ng/mL and post treatment was 3718 ± 738.39 (a 26.7% reduction). In group 2 the initial serum ferritin (mean ± SD) was 2672.9 ± 886.44 and post treatment was 3422 ± 886.42 (a 28% increase). In group 3 the initial serum ferritin (mean ± SD) was 3347.78 ± 1526.46) and post treatment was 3376.57 ± 1222.41 (a 0.008% increase). Adverse effects included two (9.5%) patients who experienced arthropathy related to L1, which was transient.
Conclusion	DFX is the most effective chelating drug for iron overload therapy in multi-transfused patients with beta thalassaemia. Oral chelation treatment on its own did result in a therapeutic benefit.
Commentary	There are few studies on chelation therapy in children and treatment is based on expert opinion due to a lack of evidence. The gold standard for measuring and monitoring total body iron is a liver biopsy, which was not done in this study. Currently (if available) magnetic resonance imaging can assess liver iron levels non-invasively. Children who have been transfused with more than 10 units of blood or have serum ferritin levels >100 ng/mL should commence chelation therapy. Subcutaneous DFX is the best strategy; however, adherence is difficult, given the infusion duration. Children undergoing chelation therapy require periodic serum ferritin monitoring and assessment of liver iron content. DFX treatment is expensive, being twice as expensive as the combination treatment and seven times as expensive as the oral therapy. Cost of therapy will influence choice of treatment is some countries and combination therapy may be chosen. Oral therapy (at least in the short term of 6 months) is ineffective.
Reference	Gomber S, Saxena R, Madan N. Comparative efficacy of desferrioxamine, deferiprone and in combination on iron chelation in thalassemic children. *Indian Pediatr.* 2004; **41**(1): 21–7.

Evidence 5	
Theme E5	**The role of hydroxyurea (HU) in the treatment of thalassaemia**
Question	What is the efficacy of HU in treating transfusion-dependent children and adolescents with beta thalassaemia?
Design	Case series
Level of evidence	

(*continued*)

Evidence 5	
Theme E5	***The role of hydroxyurea (HU) in the treatment of thalassaemia***
Setting	Department of paediatric haematology, academic medical centre, Pakistan
Participants	Children older than 1 year of age with a diagnosis of beta thalassaemia major (defined as a haemoglobin <7 g/dL, high HbF, absent or very low HbA, and more than eight transfusions per year) and beta thalassaemia intertmedia characterised by haemolytic disease but with a maintenance haemoglobin between 7 and 10 g/dL without transfusion at least until 2 years of age were eligible to participate. Responders were defined as children who were transfusion independent, with haemoglobin >7 g/dL. They were subclassified into two groups: (1) children who before HU usage were transfusion dependent and became transfusion independent on treatment with HU or (2) children who were never transfused but their haemoglobin increased – this was the beta thalassaemia intermedia group. Partial responders were defined as those who had a 50% reduction in their transfusion requirement compared to the control period. Non-responders were defined as those whose blood transfusion requirements were less than 50% reduced compared with the control period.
Intervention	Participants received HU at an initial dose of 10 mg/kg/day, increased by 1 mg/kg/week until a dose of 20 mg/kg/day was reached or until myelotoxicity occurred (which was defined as white blood cell count <1500/µL, or platelet <80 000 µL, haemoglobin of 6 g/dL, a twofold increase in alanine aminotransferase or aspartate aminotransferase, and a 50% increase in serum creatinine.
Outcomes	The primary outcome was the change in packed red cell transfusions required in the 24 months of follow-up compared with the 6 months prior to study enrolment.
Main results	One hundred and fifty-two patients were enrolled, of whom 146 completed the study (of the six, three were non-compliant, two were under splenectomy and one died from complications related to haemochromatosis). Sixty-six children (41.1%) responded to treatment (33 in group A and 27 in group B). The mean packed red cell (transfused in the control period of 6 months) was 965.6 mL. A decrease in serum ferritin occurred in groups A and B. Fifty-seven (39.0%) patients were partial responders, with a reduction in packed red cells of 60%. While desferoxamine was recommended as iron chelation therapy, families were non-compliant because of cost. Twenty-nine (18.9%) children were non-responders. Response to treatment occurred at 65 days (range 30–180). Only four (2.7%) of children developed myelosuppression and two (1.7%) developed diarrhoea. Symptoms abated after temporarily discontinuing the HU.
Conclusion	HU was found to be safe in patients with beta thalassaemia major, with the majority achieving a reduction in transfusions.
Commentary	HU acts by reversing the switch from gamma to beta globin chain synthesis in red cell precursors; this results in enhanced production of haemoglobin F. The most common side effect is myelosuppression. However, if the white blood cell count falls with intercurrent infections, then the HU should be temporarily stopped. Other features noted in this study were the cessation of facial features related to thalassaemia, improved exercise tolerance, increase in height and better school attendance. An assessment of quality of life measures related to HU should be undertaken. HU can also be used with effect in children with sickle-cell disease.

(continued)

Evidence 5

Theme E5	*The role of hydroxyurea (HU) in the treatment of thalassaemia*
Reference	Ansari SH, Shamsi TS, Ashraf M, *et al.* Efficacy of hydroxyurea in providing trans-fusion independence in β-thalassaemia. *J Pediatr Hematol Oncol.* 2011; **33**(5): 339–43.

PALE CHILD: MULTIPLE-CHOICE QUESTIONS

Q1 Clinical features of anaemia include:
   a) Pale conjunctiva
   b) Flow murmur
   c) Resting tachycardia
   d) Pedal oedema
   e) Fatigability

Q2 Which of the following statements is/are correct with regard to iron?
   a) Absorption occurs in the jejunum and duodenum.
   b) Seventy per cent of the body's iron is found in haemoglobin.
   c) Fifty per cent of iron from breast milk is absorbed.
   d) Ten per cent of iron from cow's milk is absorbed.
   e) Vitamin C increases iron absorption.

Q3 Risk factors for iron-deficiency anaemia include which of the following?
   a) Prematurity
   b) Maternal iron deficiency
   c) Excessive cow's milk intake
   d) Tea drinking
   e) Obesity

Q4 Causes of a macrocytic anaemia include which of the following?
   a) B_{12} deficiency
   b) Liver disease
   c) Meckel's diverticulum
   d) Hypothyroidism
   e) Folate deficiency

Q5 With regard to hereditary spherocytosis, which of the following statements is/are correct?
   a) The inheritance is autosomal recessive.
   b) Jaundice is a presenting feature.
   c) Splenomegaly is frequently present.

d) Increased mean corpuscular haemoglobin concentration suggests the diagnosis.

e) Infections can provoke a haemolytic crisis.

Q6 With regard to G6PD deficiency, which of the following statements is/are correct

a) It is inherited as autosomal recessive.

b) The MCV is increased.

c) Antimalarial drugs should be avoided.

d) Sulphonamides should be avoided.

e) Joint pains occur in 15% of children.

Q7 With regard to sickle-cell disease, which of the following statements is/are correct?

a) Neonatal screening is available.

b) Splenic sequestration is a recognised feature.

c) The primary mutation is a defect of the beta globulin gene on chromosome 12.

d) Aplastic crises can be triggered by parvovirus B19.

e) Patients develop acute chest pain with infection.

Q8 Which of the following statements is/are correct with regard to haemolytic anaemia?

a) Mycoplasma infections are associated with cold agglutinins.

b) Warm agglutinins are associated with Epstein–Barr infections.

c) Cold agglutinins are associated with lymphoid malignancy.

d) Prosthetic heart valves are associated with haemolytic anaemia.

e) Acquired non-immune haemolytic anaemia occurs in haemolytic-uremic syndrome.

Answers

A1	a, b, c, e		**A2**	a, b, c, d, e
A3	a, b, c, d, e		**A4**	a, b, d, e
A5	b, c, d, e		**A6**	c, d
A7	a, b, d, e		**A8**	a, d, e

SLIDES

1. Scleral icterus
2. Jaundice
3. Nephrotic syndrome (oedema of face)

Chapter Twenty-six

SHORT STATURE

COMMON SCENARIO

'James is one of the oldest is his class, but he is also one of the shortest. He has always been short, but we didn't think much of it, as he is otherwise a very well boy. However, since he's gone to secondary school the other children have started teasing him and he is becoming more self-conscious. We are worried that something might be wrong.'

LEARNING OBJECTIVES

- Understand normal growth patterns in childhood
- Identify key points in the history and examination which point to a diagnosis of idiopathic short stature
- Recognise 'red flags' in the history or examination that require further investigation
- Explain what investigations are needed in children with short stature
- Evaluate the available evidence to support your investigation and treatment options

BACKGROUND

Height is a human characteristic that varies greatly within and between different ethnic groups. Short stature is a term applied to a child 2 standard deviations (SDs) or more below the mean height for children of the same sex and chronological age. Short stature is a common problem in paediatrics since any disease process can affect growth. In the assessment of a short child, the key factor is to differentiate short children who are healthy from those who have an underlying illness or disease.

Growth

Growth in children is divided into three stages:
1. growth in infancy
2. growth in childhood
3. growth in puberty.

Growth in infancy

From conception until the end of the first year of life, growth is dependent upon nutrition. Therefore, in order to grow at a normal rate, infants need adequate caloric intake. The growth rate in the first year of life is, on average, 25 cm.

Growth in childhood

During childhood, growth is dependent upon the action of growth hormone.

The average child grows 5–7 cm a year. Around the age of 6–8 years, children have a mid-childhood growth spurt.

Growth in puberty

Pubertal hormones are responsible for the pubertal growth spurt. The average child grows 9–10 cm a year. Girls enter puberty at 8–12 years of age, at which time they develop secondary sexual characteristics and have a pubertal growth spurt. Boys enter puberty, on average, 2 years later at ages 9–14 years. They have a greater pubertal growth spurt concentrated over a shorter period. Once the epiphyses fuse, growth ceases.

Idiopathic short stature

Idiopathic short stature is defined as height >2 SDs below the corresponding mean height for a given age, sex and population group without evidence of systemic, endocrine, nutritional, or chromosomal abnormalities, and normal stimulated growth hormone levels. Children with idiopathic short stature can be classified as having either familial short stature or constitutional delay of growth.

- **Familial short stature**: children with familial short stature have a normal growth velocity, a bone age appropriate for their chronological age and a predicted adult height appropriate to the familial pattern.
- **Constitutional delay of growth**: the diagnosis of constitutional delay of growth is suggested by a similar growth pattern in the family. Children have a normal growth velocity up to the age of 6 to 36 months, at which time their growth velocity reduces and the child grows at a slower but consistent rate. These children will have both a delayed bone age and pubertal development but a normal adult height.

Isolated growth hormone deficiency

Isolated growth hormone deficiency is a clinical diagnosis, supported by auxological, biochemical and radiological findings. Growth hormone deficiency can be divided into three categories; congenital, acquired and idiopathic. Congenital causes can be the result of genetic mutations or structural defects. Known genes include those that code for growth hormone (GH1), growth-hormone-releasing hormone receptor (GHRHR) and transcription factor SOX3. Acquired causes of growth hormone deficiency include space occupying lesions, head trauma, infection, radiation therapy, infiltrative disease such as histiocytocis and autoimmune conditions such as lymphocytic hypophysitis. Idiopathic growth hormone deficiency is where no known cause is found. The phenotype of children with growth hormone deficiency is highly variable. However, they have a characteristically immature facies with a prominent forehead and depressed midline development. When other pituitary hormone deficiencies are present, there may be a history of neonatal jaundice, hypoglycaemia, micropenis with undescended testes and hypothyroidism.

HISTORY

KEY POINTS				
Growth history	When short stature first noticed Any previous height measurements	**Nutritional history**	Meal patterns Calorific intake Appetite Weight loss/gain	**❓ RED FLAG** Different growth pattern from parents Significantly shorter than siblings Poor feeding in infancy
Past history	Previous illness or disease Coeliac disease Renal disease	**Family history**	Ethnicity Height of parents and siblings History of pubertal delay	
Birth history	Prematurity Intrauterine growth restriction Hypoglycaemia Jaundice	**Psychosocial history**	Impact on child Relationship with peers Bullying at school Problems at home	
Medication history	Steroid use	**Systems review**	Energy levels, sleep patterns, overall health	

EXAMINATION

All children presenting with short stature should have a full systemic examination performed. All measurements should be accurately plotted on an appropriate centile chart.

There are three key questions to answer:
1. Is the child dysmorphic?
2. Is the child proportionately or disproportionately small?
3. Is the child overweight or underweight?

Examinations to cover:
- standing height
- upper to lower body segment ratio
- arm span
- weight measurement
- head circumference

- pubertal staging
- visual acuity and visual fields
- parental heights.

---

❶ Red flags
- Dysmorphic child
- Disproportionately small
- Overweight or underweight
- Abnormal visual acuity or restricted visual fields

HEIGHT MEASUREMENTS

Accurate height measurement is important for growth assessment.

Standing height

Standing height is measured using a Harpenden stadiometer however supine length is used for children under 18 months of age. The stadiometer should be regularly calibrated and used by a trained professional. The child must be positioned with their legs straight and feet together and flat on the ground. Their heels should touch the back plate of the stadiometer. Their buttocks and, if possible, scapula should touch the backboard, with their arms loosely at their side. The child's head must be positioned with the lower margins of the orbit in the same horizontal plane as the external auditory meati. Gentle traction should be applied to the mastoid process as the child breathes in and out. The measurement should be recorded from the scale at the end of expiration.

Upper to lower body segment ratios

Calculating upper to lower body segment ratios can help differentiate skeletal dysplasias causing disproportionate limb shortening from other conditions. The upper to lower body segment is determined by first measuring the lower body segment (i.e. from the top of the symphysis pubis to the plantar surface of the foot). To calculate the upper body segment value, the standing height should be subtracted from the lower segment value. The ratio is then determined by dividing the upper segment value by the lower segment value. Alternatively, the sitting height or upper body segment can be measured and subtracted from the standing height to obtain the lower body segment value. Body proportions change during childhood. The average upper to lower body segment ratio at birth is 1.7. By age 5, the ratio decreases to 1.17, and it decreases to 1 by the age of 10 years.

Arm span

Arm span is calculated by measuring the distance between the tips of the left and right middle fingers when a child is standing flat against a wall, with their arms outstretched and at a 90° angle to their torso. The arm span should be less than height before puberty and greater than height after puberty.

Mid-parental height (in cm)

The height of both parents should be measured and plotted on the growth chart at 19 years of age, with the following adjustments made for the sex of the child.

To calculate the mid-parental height for a boy:

Father's height + (Mother's height + 12.5) / 2

To calculate the mid-parental height for a girl:

Mother's height + (Father's height − 12.5) / 2

The child's height centile should fall within 8.5 cm either side of this centile line.

DIFFERENTIAL DIAGNOSIS

Ninety-five per cent of cases are due to familial short stature, constitutional delay of growth or a combination of the two.

Rare causes	Warning signs or symptoms
Endocrine causes: hypothyroidism, growth hormone deficiency or insensitivity, Cushing's	Decreased growth rate and overweight
Chronic illness: chronic renal failure, renal tubular acidosis, coeliac disease, inflammatory bowel disease, cardiac or respiratory disease, other inflammatory condition	Decreased growth rate and underweight
Genetic: Turner's, Russell–Silver's, pseudohypoparathyroidism, Prader–Willi's syndrome, neurofibromatosis, Noonan's syndrome	Dysmorphic features
Acondroplasia, mucopolysaccharidosis	Disproportionate short stature
Psychosocial deprivation	Decreased growth rate

INVESTIGATIONS

What radiological investigations should be performed?

An X-ray of the left wrist and hand should be taken to determine the child's bone age or level of skeletal maturity. The two most widely used systems are the 'Greulich and Pyle atlas' method and the Tanner–Whitehouse 2 individual bones method (or the TW2 method). A delay in bone age indicates that the child's short stature is partially reversible, as linear growth will continue until closure of the epiphyses.

(continued)

INVESTIGATIONS (*cont.*)

Are laboratory investigations required?

If the history or examination findings are suggestive of a particular aetiology for the short stature, appropriate diagnostic tests should be performed. If there are no clues on history or examination, baseline screening tests are advisable. These include:

- full blood count
- inflammatory markers: erythrocyte sedimentation rate and C-reactive protein
- urea and electrolytes
- calcium, phosphate and bicarbonate
- liver function tests
- coeliac screen
- karyotype (in females)
- thyroid function tests.

How is the growth hormone axis investigated?

Growth hormone secretion is mainly nocturnal and occurs in a pulsatile manner. Therefore, accurate assessment of the growth hormone axis can be difficult and 12- to 24-hour growth hormone profiles are labour intensive, impracticable and of limited value.

Measurement of serum IGF-1 and IGFBP-3 can be useful screening tests to determine whether further investigation is warranted.

Growth hormone provocation tests should only be performed under expert supervision and in centres familiar with its use. The insulin tolerance test remains the gold standard in children over 5 years of age.

In order for results to be meaningful, symptomatic hypoglycaemia needs to be achieved.

After 30–60 minutes, growth hormone concentrations in normal children should rise to greater than 15 mU/L.

Growth hormone deficient patients show an inadequate response, less than 7 mU/L, while partial growth hormone deficient patients achieve levels between 7 and 15 mU/L. However, cut-off values vary depending on local assays used and therefore peak growth hormone concentrations less than 20 mU/L have been used to support the diagnosis of growth hormone deficiency.

What tests are required to diagnose growth hormone deficiency?

Growth hormone deficiency is a clinical diagnosis, supported by auxological, biochemical and radiological findings. Current recommendations are the performance of two provocation tests and an evaluation of other aspects of pituitary function. However, if the child has known central nervous system pathology or known multiple pituitary hormone deficiencies, history of cranial irradiation or a genetic defect affecting the growth hormone axis, only one test is required.

MANAGEMENT PLAN: THREE-STEP APPROACH

1. Clarifying and pitfall avoidance strategies:
   a) parents
   b) doctor
2. Education and reassurance
3. Growth hormone treatment indications

Clarifying and pitfall avoidance strategies

Parents

- Explain growth in terms of genetic potential. **Rationale**: explain to parents their child's genetic growth potential, using the formulae provided. This will put the short stature in context and frame the discussion with them.
- When did the parents become concerned about their child's height? **Rationale**: surprisingly parents do not recognise that their child is short until middle childhood (*see* Evidence 2).
- What are the indications for growth hormone? **Rationale**: the parameters for growth hormone therapy are established and adherence is recommended (*see* Growth Hormone Treatment Indications below).
- Is their child concerned about his or her height? **Rationale**: some children will want to know their final height, especially if they are utilising growth hormone treatment.

Doctor

- Recognising short stature. **Pitfall**: for short stature to be recognised, the child's height and weight must be plotted on the appropriate growth chart. If this is not done routinely, the fall-off in growth will not be recognised early.
- Adequacy of growth. **Pitfall**: to determine height velocity, two accurate height measurements A and B, at least 6 months apart, are needed. Height velocity is calculated by the following equation: B – A / interval in years. Results should be plotted on an appropriate centile chart. Growth velocity charting allows the interval growth to be more appropriately assessed in children with faltering growth.
- Clinical assessment of the short patient. **Rationale**: consider (a) the explanation for the height being less than the child's genetic potential, (b) risk of chronic disease and (c) presence of small for gestational age (SGA) or genetic syndromes, when assessing the patient with short stature.

Education and reassurance

Children with idiopathic short stature do not require any treatment. However, for many children, short stature can affect their self-esteem and impact upon their psychosocial adaptation. Children and their parents need detailed explanation and reassurance that there is no underlying medical condition, that treatment is not indicated and that taller stature is not necessarily associated with positive changes in quality of life. Children and their parents must be provided with realistic expectations for adult height gain.

Growth hormone treatment indications

Growth hormone is licensed for the treatment of short stature caused by:
- growth hormone deficiency
- Turner's syndrome

- chronic renal insufficiency
- Prader–Willi's syndrome
- Russell–Silver's syndrome
- SGA children who fail to achieve catch-up growth by 2 years.

In the United States, growth hormone is also licensed for the treatment of idiopathic short stature. Growth hormone is given as a daily subcutaneous injection and treatment is usually prescribed for a number of years until growth is complete. Parents should be given realistic predictions of potential height gains and counselled that outcomes can vary considerably.

Children with growth hormone deficiency have the greatest outcome from treatment, with an average height gain of 9–10 cm.

In girls with Turner's syndrome, height gain following treatment with growth hormone can be variable. On average, following treatment, a gain of approximately 6 cm can be expected in adult height. GH treatment commenced in early childhood achieves improved growth but there is an increased risk of side effects (*see* Evidence 1).

In Prader–Willi's syndrome, growth hormone treatment increases height velocity although the final expected height gain remains unknown. Growth hormone treatment has additional benefits in children with Prader–Willi's syndrome. Treatment decreases body mass index and increases lean body mass.

The majority of small for gestational age children catch up growth within the first 2 years. However, approximately 15% of children fail to reach their potential. Although the final expected height gain remains unknown, studies have found an increase in height of 2–2.7 SDs compared with baseline after treatment (*see* Evidence 3).

CLARIFICATION STATEMENTS FOR PARENTAL MISCONCEPTIONS

> *'What do you mean he has delayed bone age? Will he ever catch up?'*

For some children who are short, they make take 15 months to grow what the average child will grow in 12 months. As a consequence when they are 6 years, their bone age will be 4.5 years. They will enter puberty later but their final height will reach their genetic potential.

> *'I know he is short but GH treatment will improve his self-esteem. Being short can be so hard for older children and adolescents.'*

Children and adolescents, as a consequence of their short stature, suffer no adverse behavioural or no psychosocial problems. Large studies indicate a slight increase in self-perception of peer victimisation. The use of growth hormone in children with idiopathic growth hormone is controversial, as these children have normal growth hormone levels (*see* Evidence 4).

SUMMARY PRACTICE POINTS

- Growth is a sensitive indicator of good health in childhood.
- Growth parameters height, weight and head circumference should be plotted at 6-month intervals on appropriate growth charts.
- Short stature is a common presentation in paediatrics.
- The vast majority of children have idopathic short stature.
- Specialist referral is indicated if the child is dysmorphic or has SGA with no growth spurt at 2 years.
- Growth hormone treatment is not without complications.

EVALUATING THE EVIDENCE

Evidence 1	
Theme E1	*Growth hormone (GH) treatment for children with Turner's syndrome*
Question	What is the height gain in children with GH treatment?
Design	Randomised controlled trial
Level of evidence	Jadad 3
Setting	Endocrine clinics in multiple children's hospitals, Canada
Participants	Well children with Turner's syndrome, aged 7–13 years were eligible for inclusion if their height was less than the 10th percentile for chronological age on the growth charts of the National Center for Health Statistics of the United States and an annualised height velocity less than 6 cm a year during the 6-month pre-randomised period.
Intervention	Eligible subjects, stratified for height relative to chronological age, were randomised to receive recombinant GH (Humatrope) by daily subcutaneous injection six times weekly (0.30 mg/kg/week, maximum weekly dose 15 mg) or no GH treatment. Girls with primary ovarian failure received standardised sex steroid replacement at age 13 years. Protocol completion required annualised height velocity less than 2 cm/year and a bone age of 14 years or greater. Patients were also assessed 1 year post protocol.
Outcomes	The primary outcome was the height difference between the two groups at protocol completion.
Main results	One hundred and fifty-four patients were randomised, 76 to the GH group, with 61 (80%) completing the protocol, and 78 to the control group, with 43 (55%) completing the protocol. The mean duration of treatment was 5.7 years. The gain in height was 7.2 cm (95% confidence interval: 6.0–8.5).
Conclusion	GH treatment, with the induction of puberty at a near physiological age, increases final adult height of girls with Turner's syndrome.

(*continued*)

Evidence 1	
Theme E1	**Growth hormone (GH) treatment for children with Turner's syndrome**
Commentary	This study outlines the value of GH treatment in girls with Turner's syndrome. This study revealed an advantage in starting treatment early at 7 years rather than at 12–13 years. The commencement of treatment in the early years of life is likely to produce a better outcome. While young children with Turner's syndrome do not consider their height to be a problem, maximising growth will lessen the social difficulties that they experience related to their short stature. A height of 152.4 cm (5 feet) is desirable. The use of GH was associated with increased ear disorders especially otitis media and the need for surgical procedures (mostly ears, nose and throat related). Possible explanations for this may be increased size of the tonsils and adenoids from GH therapy. Regular assessment of hearing is required in girls with Turner's syndrome given their predisposition to otitis media and hearing loss.
Reference	Stephure DK; Canadian Growth Hormone Advisory Committee. Impact of growth hormone supplementation on adult height in Turner syndrome: results of the Canadian randomized control trial. *J Clin Endocrinol Metab*. 2005; **90**(6): 3360–6.

Evidence 2	
Theme E2	**Short stature and parent and child perceptions**
Question	When do parents recognise their child is short?
Design	Randomised controlled trial
Level of evidence	Jadad 5
Setting	Department of paediatric endocrinology, academic medical centre, Sweden
Participants	Ninety-nine 3- to 11-year-old short prepubertal children with either isolated growth hormone deficiency (n = 32) or idiopathic short stature (n = 67) participated in a 2-year trial where they received either individualised or fixed-dose growth hormone treatment. The study assessed height perceptions of both child and parent.
Intervention	Parents and child were asked to complete three scales: (1) the Silhouette Apperception Test, (2) sense of tallness scale and (3) a binary (yes/no) appropriate height scale. The Silhouette Apperception Test has five randomly ordered silhouettes representing the 3rd, 25th, 50th, 75th and 97th percentile. The sense of tallness is a 100 mm visual analogue scale between the bipolar adjectives 'short' and 'tall'. When responding to the visual analogue scale item, respondents indicate their level of agreement, making a point on the line between tall and short.
Outcomes	The perception of height by parent and child.
Main results	Children and parents overestimated height at the start of treatment (72%, 54%) and at 24 months (52%, 30%). Short children described themselves as tall until 8.2 years (girls) and 9.0 years (boys).
Conclusion	At the age of 8–9 years children on average change from finding their height appropriate to finding it inappropriate.
Commentary	The recognition of being short has important implications for families.

(*continued*)

Evidence 2

Theme E2	*Short stature and parent and child perceptions*
Commentary *(cont.)*	In children with syndromes such as Turner's and Russell–Silver's, or those who are small for gestational age, the lack of concern voiced by the child may influence the parents' decision; however, parents should be informed that the child's concerns with regard to their size will be evident at 8–9 years. Parents should take this fact into account when making decisions related to growth hormone treatment for short stature.
Reference	Chaplin JE, Kriström B, Jonsson B, *et al*. When do short children realize they are short? Prepubertal short children's perception of height during 24 months of catch-up growth hormone treatment. *Horm Res Paediatr.* 2012; **77**(4): 241–9.

Evidence 3

Theme E3	*The impact of growth hormone (GH) on small for gestational age (SGA) infants*
Question	What is the adult height after GH treatment in children who are SGA?
Design	Randomised controlled trial
Level of evidence	Jadad 5
Setting	Paediatric endocrine clinic, children's hospital, the Netherlands
Participants	Prepubertal short children born SGA were eligible to participate who met the following criteria: • birth length standard deviation score (SDS) below −1.88 • chronological age 3–11 in boys and 3–9 in girls at the start of the study • height SDS for chronological age (height SDS) below −1.88 • height SDS for chronological age zero or less to exclude children presenting spontaneous catch up growth • no evidence of pubertal commencement.
Intervention	Participants received GH at 0.033 mg/kg/day (group A) or 0.067 mg/kg/day (group B) or no treatment (group C).
Outcomes	The impact of GH treatment on final adult height
Main results	Of the 79 enrolled in the GH treatment arms, 54 completed the study and 15 similar SGA children served as controls. In the GH group A, 28 children after a mean (±SD) of 7.9 (1.7) years of treatment had an adult height (AH) SDS of 1.8 (0.7). In group B, 26 children after a mean (±SD) of 7.5 (1.7) years of treatment had an AH SDS of 2.1 (0.8). In group C, for the 15 children the mean (±SD) AH SDS was −2.3 (0.7). There were no differences in outcome between groups A and B. There were no major adverse effects reported in this study.
Conclusion	Long-term continuous GH treatment in children born SGA without catch-up growth leads to a normalisation of adult height.
Commentary	Most children born SGA will achieve catch-up growth by the age of 2 years, but approximately 15% do not. While there is considerable variability in the response to GH, children with the greatest parental height adjusted deficit will have the best responses to treatment. Early GH commencement will enhance the final outcome in terms of adult height.

(continued)

Evidence 3	
Theme E3	**The impact of growth hormone (GH) on small for gestational age (SGA) infants**
Commentary (cont.)	If children commence GH treatment at least 2 years before the onset of puberty the AH SDS is 1.7, which is equivalent to 12 cm compared with pre-treatment predictions. If it is started later the AH SDS is 0.9 corresponding to a 6 cm increase in adult height (Dahlgren, 2005). Final height for males born SGA is on average 7.5 cm shorter and for females born SGA is 9.6 cm shorter than their mid-parental height if they are untreated.
References	Van Pareren Y, Mulder P, Houdijk M, *et al.* Adult height after long-term, continuous growth hormone (GH) treatment in short children born small for gestational age: results of a randomized double-blind, dose-response GH trial. *J Clin Endocrinol Metab.* 2003; **88**(8): 3584–90.
	Dahlgren J, Wikland KA; Swedish Study Group for Growth Hormone Treatment. Final height in short children born small for gestational age treated with growth hormone. *Pediatr Res.* 2005; **57**(2): 216–22.

Evidence 4	
Theme E4	**Growth hormone in children with idiopathic short stature**
Question	How effective is growth hormone in the treatment of idiopathic short stature?
Design	Randomised controlled trial
Level of evidence	Jadad 5
Setting	Department of endocrinology, academic medical centre, the United States
Participants	Children aged 9–16 with non-growth hormone-deficient short stature, were eligible if height or predicted height was ≤2.5 standard deviation score (SDS). Criteria were modified to include six participants with height SDSs between −2.25 and −2.25.
Intervention	Participants were randomised to receive either recombinant human growth hormone 0.22 mg/kg/week subcutaneously three times a week or placebo. The study continued until growth rate decreased to 1.5 cm a year, indicating near-adult height.
Outcomes	The primary outcome was the difference in adult height attributable to growth hormone therapy.
Main results	Sixty-eight patients were randomised, 37 to growth hormone treatment, with final height measurements available in 22 (59%). Of the 31 in the placebo group, only 11 (35%) had a final height measurement. The mean age of the treatment group was 12.5 years at the start of treatment and the mean duration of treatment was 4.6 years. The intention to treat analysis of patients (who had at least 6 months of growth hormone treatment) revealed a 3.7 cm difference in height between treatment and control group. Compliance with growth hormone treatment was estimated at 89% and 81% for placebo. No patient experienced benign intracranial hypertension, diabetes mellitus or slipped capital epiphysis.
Conclusion	Growth hormone treatment increases growth by 3.7 cm in children and adolescents with idiopathic short stature.

(*continued*)

Evidence 4	
Theme E4	*Growth hormone in children with idiopathic short stature*
Commentary	Children and adolescents with idiopathic short stature have normal growth hormone levels. Using the criterion of height −2.25 standard deviation score (SDS) or less as eligibility for growth hormone therapy is equivalent to including 1.2% of all children. The final height gain may not warrant the economic cost. Children with idiopathic short stature are healthy, and subjecting them to a treatment with potential side effects (*see* Main Results) may not be appropriate. Ethical questions relating to the value of height are also raised.
Reference	Leschek EW, Rose SR, Yanovski JA, *et al.* Effect of growth hormone treatment on adult height in peripubertal children with idiopathic short stature: a randomized, double-blind, placebo-controlled trial. *J Clin Endocrinol Metab.* 2004; **89**(7): 3140–8.

SHORT STATURE: MULTIPLE-CHOICE QUESTIONS

Q1 Recognised causes of growth hormone deficiency include which of the following?
  a) Idiopathic short stature
  b) Cranial irradiation
  c) Histiocytosis
  d) Lyme disease
  e) Lymphocytic hypophysitis

Q2 Which of the following features should raise concerns related to growth hormone deficiency?
  a) Intrauterine growth retardation
  b) Hypoglycaemia
  c) Midline facial defects
  d) Conjugated hyperbilirubinaemia
  e) Post maturity

Q3 Causes of short stature include which of the following?
  a) Coeliac disease
  b) Chronic renal failure
  c) Crohn's disease
  d) Irritable bowel disease
  e) Bronchiectasis

Q4 Syndromes associated with short stature include which of the following?
  a) Prader–Willi's syndrome
  b) Russell–Silver's syndrome
  c) Noonan's syndrome
  d) Down's syndrome
  e) Turner's syndrome

Q5 Appropriate tests in a child with short stature include which of the following?
a) Bone age of the right wrist
b) Serum calprotectin
c) Karyotype assessment
d) Anti-endomesial antibodies
e) Thyroid function tests

Q6 Which of the following statements is/are true?
a) Growth hormone secretion occurs mainly at night.
b) Twenty-four-hour growth hormone profiles are useful to assess growth hormone levels.
c) Assay of IGF1 and IGFBP-3 are useful screening test for growth hormone deficiency.
d) The insulin tolerance test is useful in assessing growth hormone deficiency.
e) Growth hormone levels are reduced in children with Down's syndrome.

Q7 Risk associated with growth hormone treatment includes which of the following?
a) Hypoglycaemia
b) Hyponatraemia
c) Intracranial hypertension
d) Dilatation of the aortic root in children with Turner's syndrome
e) Slipped capital femoral epiphysis

Q8 Which of the following statements is/are correct?
a) Growth hormone in Turner's should start at 6 years of age.
b) Overgrowth of the feet is a recognised complication.
c) Growth hormone treatment in Turner's syndrome is associated with increased episodes of otitis media.
d) The mean adult height in Turner's syndrome without growth hormone treatment is 143 cm.
e) Alopecia is a complication of growth hormone treatment in Turner's syndrome.

Answers

A1	b, c, e		A2	a, b, c
A3	a, b, c		A4	a, b, c, d, e
A5	c, d, e		A6	a, c, d
A7	a, c, d, e		A8	b, c, d

Chapter Twenty-seven

THE CHILD WITH A PUBERTAL DEVELOPMENT DISORDER

COMMON SCENARIO

'She's only a year old and I wasn't too sure initially whether to be concerned, but now it's really obvious that she has swollen breasts, at first I thought it was normal or would just go away, but it hasn't and I just don't know what to think.'

LEARNING OBJECTIVES

- Understand normal pubertal development
- Recognise the cause of disordered pubertal development
- Recognise 'red flags' in the history or examination that require further investigation
- Outline appropriate investigation for precocious and delayed puberty

BACKGROUND

Puberty is the physiological sequence of events leading to physical and sexual maturation. It involves the development of secondary sexual characteristics as well as growth, changes in body composition and psychological maturation. Tanner stages are used to evaluate pubertal development.

The start of puberty is heralded by the appearance of a palpable breast bud in girls and a testicular volume over 3.5 mL in boys. These changes occur in response to the secretion of gonadotropin-releasing hormone from the hypothalamus which stimulates the release of gonadotropin follicle-stimulating hormone (FSH) and luteinising hormone (LH) from the anterior pituitary gland. LH increases oestrogen secretion in females and testosterone secretion in males. FSH acts on the gonads to produce ova and sperm. FSH is usually higher than LH in pubertal children, this ratio reverses in puberty.

Oestrogen and testosterone levels rise progressively as puberty progresses. Oestrogen is responsible for breast development and androgens are responsible for pubic and axillary hair, adult body odour, acne and genital enlargement. The pubertal growth spurt lasts for approximately 2 years, after which growth continues at a slower rate until epiphyseal fusion.

In girls, normal puberty is signalled by breast development (known as thelarche) followed within 6–12 months by the appearance of pubic hair. The attainment of fertility is signalled by the onset of menstruation (menarche). Onset of puberty in girls normally occurs between the ages of 9–13 years with menarche occurring 2 years later. Onset of puberty in girls is associated with rapid linear growth. The peak growth rate for girls is 6–11 cm year. After menarche, growth velocity progressively declines until epiphyseal fusion marks the end of growth, typically about 18 months later.

In boys, puberty is signalled by testicular enlargement. Puberty starts when testicular size reaches 3.5 mL and progresses through puberty to 15–25 mL. In boys, puberty normally starts between 10 and 14 years of age. The first visible sign of puberty is the appearance of pubic hair, followed by growth of the penis. The peak growth rate for boys is 7–12 cm. Growth continues until epiphyseal fusion in mid to late teens. The timing of puberty relates to ethnicity (Afro-Caribbean or mixed race early menarche more common), genetic and nutritional factors.

Several abnormalities in the process of sexual maturation can occur in children, the commonest conditions presenting in childhood are precocious and delayed puberty.

Pubertal development in girls			
Stage	Breast development	Pubic hair	Other changes
1	Prepubertal	None	None
2	Breast bud	Minimal hair around labia	Growth spurt
3	Enlargement of breast and areola	Darker and extends across the midline	Peak growth, axillary hair
4	Secondary mound of areola and papilla	Increased but less than adult pattern	Menarche
5	Adult size and shape	Adult distribution including medial thighs	

Pubertal development in boys				
Stage	Genital development	Pubic hair	Testicular size (mL)	Other changes
1	Prepubertal	None	<4	None
2	Early penile and scrotal growth	Minimal hair at base of penis	4–8	None
3	Increase penile length, further scrotal rugosity	Darker, extending across midline	10–15	Light facial hair, growth spurt
4	Increased penile width, scrotal pigmentation	Increased but less than adult pattern	15–20	Sideburns
5	Adult size and shape	Adult distribution, including medial thighs	20–25	Facial hair and change in voice

PRECOCIOUS PUBERTY

Precocious puberty is defined as the appearance of secondary sexual characteristics before the age of 8 years in girls and 9 years in boys. However, a trend toward earlier onset of puberty has been seen in a number of countries. There is an association between early sexual maturation and obesity. Precocious puberty may be central, peripheral or incomplete.

- **Central (complete) precocious puberty**: due to premature activation of the hypothalamic-pituitary-gonadal access (gonadotropin dependent). Central causes account for over 80% of cases of precocious puberty. Pulsatile hypothalamic secretion of gonadotropin-releasing hormone (GnRH) stimulates pituitary secretion of LH and FSH. Secondary sexual characteristics develop in a concordant manner (i.e. breast bud followed by pubic hair and menarche in girls or testicular enlargement followed by penile growth and pubic hair in boys). Progression can be rapidly or slowly progressive. It is 5 to 10 times more common in girls than boys. Most cases in girls are idiopathic (90%) and there is often a positive family history. It is a diagnosis of exclusion. The long-term complication of idiopathic precocious puberty is compromised adult height. An underlying cause is more likely in males (90% of cases). Boys typically have symmetrically enlarged testicular volumes. Causes of central precocious puberty due to central nervous system (CNS) abnormalities including CNS tumours (optic glioma (neurofibromatosis), astrocytoma, hypothalamic hamartomas, craniopharyngioma, ependynoma) cranial irradiation, previous meningitis or encephalitis, abscess, trauma, hydrocephalus, congenital abnormalities, prolonged primary hypothyroidism and longstanding peripheral precocious puberty.
- **Peripheral precocious puberty**: is due to increased production of sex steroids (adrenal or gonadal sex steroids or exposure to exogenous steroids) in the absence of reactivation of the hypothalamic-pituitary gonadal access (gonadotropin independent). FSH and LH levels are low. It may present with some or all of the physical changes of puberty. It can be congenital or acquired. In boys, it is caused by secretion of androgens from the testes or adrenal glands or, rarely, from secretion of human chorionic gonadotropin (hCG) or LH, which stimulates Leydig cell production of testosterone. Testes are usually small in size unless a tumour is present. In girls, it is caused by excessive oestrogens. They may have pubic and axillary hair before breast development, or menses without breast development.
- **Incomplete precocious puberty/normal variant puberty**: incomplete pubertal development in the absence of other stigmata of puberty.
- **Premature thelarche**: premature breast development in the absence of other signs of sexual development. It may be unilateral or bilateral, and breast size may wax and wane although never more than stage 3 breast development. Premature thelarche is usually noted between 6 months and 4 years of age. Growth velocity and bone age are normal for age. Pelvic ultrasound shows prepubertal findings.

Gonadotropin levels are prepubertal and resolve spontaneously or progress to puberty at a normal age. No treatment is required.

- **Premature adrenarche**: increased levels of adrenal DHEA and its sulphate ester DHEAS before the age of 8 years in girls and 9 years in boys and the concurrent presence of signs of androgen action including adult-type body odour, pubic and axillary hair, mood changes and oily skin and hair. There is no associated testicular growth or breast development. Bone age and linear growth are normal for age. There is an association between the premature adrenarche and low birth weight and the later development of polycystic ovarian syndrome. Congenital adrenal hyperplasia or adrenal tumours need to be outruled.

- **Premature menarche**: isolated vaginal bleeding without breast or pubic hair. No history of genital trauma, suspicion of child sexual abuse, foreign body or tumour. Bone age normal and prepubertal uterus ultrasound scan finding. Vaginal bleeding, very occasionally, can be the presenting sign of profound hypothyroidism in girls.

Causes of peripheral precocious puberty	
Congenital causes	
Non-classical congenital adrenal hyperplasia	Pubarche and advanced growth
	In girls amenorrhoea, oligomenorrhoea, acne and hirsutism
	Mineralocorticoid usually unaffected
McCune–Albright's syndrome	Females more commonly affected, but it also occurs in males. In girls, presenting feature is often menses with or without thelarche. Polyostotic fibrous dysplasia of skull and long bones, irregular café au lait spots and precocity due to autonomously functioning ovarian cysts
	Ovarian cysts
	May be associated with hyperthryoidism, Cushing's syndrome, hyperprolactinaemia, pituitary gigantism, hypophosphatemic rickets
	Underlying defect is mutation of G protein
Familial male precocious puberty	Autosomal dominant, mutation in LH receptors, prepubertal levels of LH and FSH, pubertal testosterone levels
Testotoxicosis	Symmetrical testicular enlargement
Hypothyroidism	Growth retardation, delayed skeletal maturation
Acquired causes	
Exogenous exposure to sex steroids	Ingestion of oral contraceptives or anabolic steroids
	Skin to skin transmission: topical preparations (testosterone gel, oestrogen cream) hair products, lavender and tea tree oil
Endogenous exposure to sex steroids	Sex steroid secreting tumours:
	Ovarian: granulosa-theca cell tumours are the most common, ovarian cysts
	Testicular: Leydig cell adenomas
	Adrenal: oestrogen- or androgen-secreting adrenal tumour
	Germ cell tumours: gonadal or extragonadal, increased secretion of hCG and testosterone

DELAYED PUBERTY

In girls, delayed puberty is defined as absence of any breast development by 13 years of age or more than 5 years between initial breast development and the onset of menses. Primary amenorrhoea occurs when girls develop secondary sexual characteristics but fail to achieve menses by 16 years of age. In boys, delayed puberty is defined as absence of testicular enlargement by 14 years of age or more than 5 years between the initial development of secondary sexual characteristics and the final stages of pubertal development. Delayed puberty affects 2.5% of adolescents and is more common

Hypergonadotropic hypogonadism: high FSH and LH, low sex steroids	
Klinefelter's	Tall stature, cryptorchidism or small testes, gynaecosmastia, pubic hair sparse
Triple X syndrome	Tall, amenorrhoea, infertility
Turner's	45XO, webbed neck, widely spaced nipples, coarcation of the aorta
Gonadal failure	Chemotherapy, radiotherapy, infections (mumps), autoimmune, galactosaemia
Androgen insensitivity syndrome	Androgen receptor gene mutations
Gene mutations	FSHR and LHR gene mutations
Hypogonadotropic hypogonadism: low FSH, LH and sex steroids	
Constitutional delay in growth and puberty	Mainly boys, positive family history
Structural brain abnormalities	Tumours, infiltrations, infections Panhypopituitarism, septo-optic dysplasia
Chronic diseases (if end stage or severe)	Inflammatory bowel disease, coeliac, cystic fibrosis, diabetes mellitus, chronic renal failure, systemic lupus erythematosus, juvenile idiopathic arthritis
Endocrine	GH deficiency, hypothyroidism
Excessive exercise	Thin, competitive sports, athletics, ballet
Eating disorders	Food restriction, purging, poor self image
Kallmann's syndrome	Anosmia or hyposmia
Bardet–Biedl's and Laurence–Moon's syndrome	Obesity, polydactyl
Prader–Willi's	Obesity, hypotonia, mental retardation
Gene defects	DAX-1, LHR, FSHR, leptin and leptin receptor, FSH and LH gene mutations
Eugonadotropic hypogonadism: normal FSH and LH	
Congenital anatomic abnormalities	Imperforate hymen, vaginal atresia, vaginal aplasia
Polycystic ovarian disease	Overweight, hirsutism
Hyperprolactinaemia	Pituitary adenoma

in boys. In most cases, no pathological cause is found and adolescents will go on to have normal progression of puberty once it starts.

Delayed puberty is most commonly due to constitutional delay of growth and puberty (90%–95%). It is due to persistence of the prepubertal hypogonadotropic state. In 60% of cases there is a family history in parents or siblings of delayed puberty. It is a diagnosis of exclusion. Bone age is delayed and consistent with the degree of pubertal maturation. Therefore it is associated with short stature. Sexual maturity and final height are not adversely affected.

A useful approach in the child with delayed puberty is to look at the baseline biochemistry results. There may also be clues in the history and examination. A micropenis will be seen in congenital hypopituitarism.

HISTORY

KEY POINTS				
Pubertal signs	What features of puberty are present? Duration Rate of progression Sequence of events	**Development**	Delayed milestones Learning difficulties	**🔍 Red flags** Dysmorphic features Headache Early-morning vomiting
Growth	Size of clothes bought Recent growth Any previous height measurements	**Medical and surgical history**	CNS trauma, infection, radiation Congenital adrenal hyperplasia	
Associated symptoms	Visual problems Headaches Early-morning vomiting Abdominal pain Seizures Sense of smell	**Medications**	Oral contraceptive pill Testosterone gel Steroids	
Family history	Onset of puberty in parents Maternal history of early menarche Age at which father started shaving Parents' height	**Social history**	Intense or excessive exercise	
Diet	Concerns about weight Calorie intake	**Systems review for chronic disease**	Chronic cough Recurrent infections Joint swelling Fatigue Bowel habit	

(continued)

KEY POINTS				
Impact on child	Impact on self-esteem and self-image			
	Relationship to peers			
	Bullying or teasing			

EXAMINATION

- Height, weight and head circumference should be recorded and plotted on an appropriate centile chart
- Plot mid-parental height
- Tanner staging
- Phallic length and width
- Testicular volume (use Prader orchidometer)
- Cliteromegaly
- Labial fusion
- Pubic hair
- Skin exam: acne, oily skin or hair, axillary hair, hirsutism, odour, café au lait macules
- Neurological exam: visual fields and fundi, sense of smell
- Examination of thyroid gland
- Gastrointestinal exam: abdominal masses

Red flags

- Contrasexual development
- Dysmorphic features
- Macrocephaly
- Restricted visual fields
- Papilloedema
- Hypertension
- Café au lait macules

INVESTIGATIONS

When is a pelvic ultrasound indicated in girls?

A pelvic ultrasound is indicated to determine whether pubertal changes have occurred in the uterus and ovaries, to evaluate for ovarian tumours and enlarged cysts.

- Ovary volume: prepubertal, <1.5 mL; postpubertal, >3–4 mL
- Follicle size: prepubertal, <6 mm; postpubertal, >6 mm
- Uterus to cervix ratio: prepubertal, <1; postpubertal, >1
- Endometrial thickening: prepubertal, none; postpubertal, present

(continued)

INVESTIGATIONS (*cont.*)

If the ovaries have a multicystic appearance and the uterus is enlarging (>2 mL) it is likely that puberty is imminent.

What information does a bone age provide?

Children with suspected precocious puberty should have a bone age checked by taking an X-ray of the left wrist. In precocious puberty the bone age is usually more than 2 standard deviations above the chronological age. Exceptions are GnRH dependent precocious puberty with growth hormone deficiency, slowly progressive precocious puberty in which the bone age may be normal and hypothyroidism in which the bone age is delayed.

What investigations should be performed in the investigations of precocious puberty?

X-ray of left wrist to determine bone age

Thyroid function tests

Low in hypothryoidism

LH and FSH and GnRH testing

GnRH testing distinguishes between central and peripheral precocious puberty – basal LH and FSH are measured before and after stimulation with GnRH or GnRh agonist.

In central precocious puberty, LH and FSH are pubertal and will increase.

In peripheral precocious puberty, LH and FSH will remain low or unchanged.

Determining whether precocious puberty is central or peripheral will help guide further investigations.

hCG and alfa fetoprotein

Elevated levels are seen with germ cell tumours.

Testosterone and oestradiol

Oestradiol: elevated levels indicate increased production or exposure. In girls, very high oestrogen levels can indicate an ovarian cyst or tumour.

Testosterone: in boys, elevated levels indicate testicular activation; in girls, elevated levels indicate adrenal disorder.

DHEA, DHEAS, 17-OHP, androstenedione, urinary steroid profile

Elevated with adrenal tumours or adrenal enzyme defects

MRI brain in central precocious puberty

May show pathological cause of central precocious puberty

Abdominal/pelvic ultrasound scan

May show tumours

Pelvic ultrasound scan in girls

Looking for tumours, cysts, pubertal changes

What investigations should be performed in hypergonadotropic hypogonadism?

Bone age

Karyotype: chromosomal disorders

Pelvic ultrasound scan: uterine volume and ovaries, presence of intra-abdominal testes

Abdominal MRI: further intra-abdominal imaging

hCG test: causes an increase in testosterone and oestrogen if the gonads are present and functioning

(continued)

In males:

Inhibin B detects presence of Sertoli cells or secretory follicles (measure of testicular function)

Inhibin A detects presence of corpus luteum

Anti-Müllerian hormone detects presence of testicular tissue

Urine steroid profile: steroid synthesis disorder

What investigations should be performed if chronic disease is suspected?

Targeted investigations should be performed if chronic disease is suspected. Useful routine baseline investigations include:

- full blood count, C-reactive protein and erythrocyte sedimentation rate to exclude anaemia, inflammatory disease
- urea and electrolytes and liver function tests to exclude liver disease
- bone profile – may show inappropriate alkaline phosphatase
- coeliac screen
- thyroid function tests.

What investigations should be performed in hypogonadotropic hypogonadism?

Bone age

GnRH or LH-releasing hormone test to stimulate release of LH and FSH

If short stature or signs of other endocrine deficiency, full pituitary workup should be done

If CNS abnormality suspected: MRI brain

MANAGEMENT PLAN: THREE-STEP APPROACH

1. Clarifying and pitfall avoidance strategies
2. Treatment of precocious puberty
3. Treatment of delayed puberty

Clarifying and pitfall avoidance strategies

- Parental response to disordered puberty. **Rationale**: parents may be more distressed than the child when disordered puberty occurs. To address this effectively parental education needs to be undertaken with an explanation of how the process has deviated from the norm and ensuring that the normal process is known to them.
- The benign nature of premature adrenarche and thelarche need to be explained to the parents and child (premature adrenarche). Explain clearly the maximal progression of symptoms to the parent at the initial consultation to inform and reassure them.
- Precocious puberty and special circumstances. **Rationale**: some children will be predisposed to the development of precocious puberty, e.g. post meningitis and if there are early signs parents should be informed.
- Delayed puberty and the adolescent. Explain to the adolescent that puberty will occur but that it will be delayed. Indicate that when puberty is complete, growth

is also almost completed; therefore, they will continue to grow while awaiting pubertal onset. The occurrence of sweating that requires the use of a deodorant heralds the onset of puberty.

- Puberty and chronic disease. **Rationale**: some children with chronic diseases, e.g. Crohn's disease, or those treated with oral steroids may experience delayed puberty and or short stature. The potential impact of such treatments needs to be explained to parents prior to their commencement.

Treatment of precocious puberty

Principles of treatment in precocious puberty:

- stop progression of secondary sexual characteristics
- increase final adult height
- promote psychological well-being
- treat underlying cause if known.

Adolescents with precocious puberty and significantly advanced bone age, decreased predicted adult height and a pubertal response to gonadotropin testing should be treated with GnRH agonists to supress pubertal regression and improve final adult height. GnRH provides constant serum levels of GnRH activity and overrides the pulsatility of endogenous GnRH, which is required to trigger pubertal progression. The most widely used GnRH agonists are triptorelin and leuprorelin (*see* Evidence 1). It takes 1–2 years for the growth rate to decrease and reach a normal rate for chronological age. After an initial surge of LH, LH and sex steroid levels decrease to suppressed levels in approximately 15 days. GnRH agnonists are generally well tolerated, common side effects include headaches. Favourable outcome in adult height (based on predicted final height), reproductive function, bone mineral density and body composition have been demonstrated. Treatment is expected to result in cessation of pubertal development but may not cause regression of all features.

- Congenital adrenal hyperplasia is treated with hydrocortisone replacement therapy and may also require fludrocortisone.
- Tumours of the testes, adrenal glands and ovaries should be resected if possible.
- Conservative management of ovarian cysts is usually appropriate, with follow-up to ensure spontaneous regression occurs.
- hCG secreting tumours may require chemotherapy and radiotherapy in addition to surgery.
- Treatment of testotoxicosis and McCune–Albright's syndrome is required to prevent the synthesis or action of gonadal steroids. Treatment options include ketoconazole, cyproterone, androgen receptor blockage (spironolactone) and aromatse inhibition (testolactone, letroxole, anastozole).

Treatment of delayed puberty

Principles of treatment in delayed puberty include:

- ensuring attainment of secondary sexual characteristics
- induction of the growth spurt
- promote psychosocial well-being
- treat underlying cause if known.

If an underlying cause is identified, specific treatment should be initiated. In children with an underlying illness, management should focus on maximising their nutritional status and the use of additional supplements where appropriate.

The management of children with constitutional delay is controversial, as many recommend conservative management with observation alone, while others advocate for induction of puberty with sex steroids (*see* Evidence 2). Most cases can be managed with a full explanation of the processes of normal puberty, the variations of normal, and reassurance that full secondary sexual development will occur with time.

If treatment is required, puberty can be induced. In males, increasing doses of intramuscular testosterone can be given. Testosterone:

- does not increase testicular size
- causes virilisation (increased phallic size and scrotal rugae)
- accelerates development of secondary sexual characteristics
- stimulates growth spurt
- is usually continued until there is evidence of spontaneous puberty, i.e. testicular growth.

hCG in males helps to maintain spermatogenesis.

In females, increasing doses of oestrogen (transdermal and oral preparations) can be given. Oestrogen helps to:

- develop secondary sexual characteristics
- attain menses
- stimulate pubertal growth
- attain bone mineral mass
- promote uterine development.

For females, pulses of GnRH may be required to promote fertility.

FOLLOW-UP

- Children with precocious puberty require follow-up with a paediatric endocrinologist to ensure regression of symptoms.
- Adolescents with delayed puberty, should have their growth and pubertal status assessed yearly, if they are anxious.

WHEN TO REFER?

- All girls younger than 8 years and boys younger than 9 years with signs of secondary sexual development require evaluation
- Children with premature thelarche
- Children with premature adrenarche
- Adolescents with delayed onset puberty

CLARIFICATION STATEMENTS FOR PARENTAL MISCONCEPTIONS

'How can she have breast development? She's only 2 years of age!'

Premature thelarche is a benign entity. The breast size may fluctuate but will never exceed stage 3 development. Children will be unaware of this development and parents can be reassured that the child will progress to puberty at a normal age. Blood tests will be unhelpful to explain the breast enlargement and suggestions that premature thelarche is related to increased sensitivity to oestrogens is speculative.

'Is puberty starting earlier in girls now?'

The age of onset of puberty is reducing and this is noted especially in the United States in the Hispanic population. The age is reducing in Europe but to a lesser degree. Improved nutrition is probably a major contributing factor to the age reduction of puberty.

'Are mood changes in adolescents related to hormone changes?'

Mood changes are evident in adolescents and adolescents have marked changes in various hormones; however, this temporal relationship has not been proved to be cause and effect.

SUMMARY PRACTICE POINTS

- Tanner staging is used to assess pubertal status.
- Precocious puberty occurs in girls under 8 and boys under 9 years.
- Baseline tests for precocious puberty include FSH, LH, serum testosterone and hCG level.
- Central causes account for 80% of cases.
- Thelarche occurs from 6 months to 4 years.
- Adrenarche occurs at <8 years in girls and <9 years in boys.
- For children with precocious puberty, check visual fields and assess for papilloedema and café au lait macules.

- Parents are frequently stressed by disordered puberty; therefore, clarify the significance and implications of the findings.
- Delayed puberty rarely requires treatment.

EVALUATING THE EVIDENCE

Evidence 1	
Theme E1	***The treatment of precocious puberty.***
Question	In the treatment of precocious puberty, which is more effective: monthly depot injection or tri-monthly deposition therapy of leuprolide?
Design	Randomised controlled trial
Level of evidence	Jadad 2
Setting	Department of paediatric endocrinology, academic medical centre, the United States
Participants	Children diagnosed with central precocious puberty (CPP) were invited to participate. CPP was defined clinically as the onset of breast development before 8 years of age in girls and in boys was defined as Tanner 2 genital stage and testicular volume >4 cc before 9 years of age. Minimal laboratory inclusion criterion was a random LH level >0.3 IU/L or aqueous leuprolide-stimulated LH >15 IU/L performed with immunochemiluminometric assay.
Intervention	Participants were randomised to either monthly depot leuprolide acetate 7.5 mg every 4 weeks or depot leuprolide acetate (DL) 11.25 mg 3-month preparation every 12 weeks. Subsequently, a third arm was added, which was 22.5 mg of DL. At 48 weeks, subjects in the 7.5 mg 1-month dose were converted to the 11.25 mg 3-month dose and in the final year of randomisation the 7.5 mg 1-month DL arm was terminated. Participants were followed for 96 weeks, with assessment every 12 weeks.
Outcomes	The primary outcome was the suppression of puberty.
Main results	Fifty-four patients were randomised (5 males, 49 females) with a mean age of 8.1 ± 1.9 years. Forty-one children had idiopathic CPP, four had central nervous system tumours, and nine had other causes, which included seizure disorders, congenital infection, meningitis, holoprosencephaly and primary hypothyroidism. Mean stimulated levels of LH, FSH and E2 decreased significantly in all dose groups between baseline and all subsequent treatment visits. Height velocity was similar in all groups and regressed to normal prepubertal rate during treatment.
Conclusion	All doses of DL were effective in prompt and effective treatment of precocious puberty, but higher LH and FSH levels were seen with the 11.5 mg 3-month DL dose.
Commentary	Central precocious puberty is defined as the activation of the hypothalamic–pituitary–gonadal axis leading to the development of early sexual maturation. The GnRH analogues are the mainstay of treatment, as they are potent inhibitors of gonadotropin secretion, leading to a decrease in sex steroid production and cessation of pubertal progression. In the treatment of CPP, suppression of stimulated LH is regarded as the best short-term evidence of treatment adequacy.

(*continued*)

Evidence 1	
Theme E1	*The treatment of precocious puberty.*
Commentary (*cont.*)	This study introduces a new option in the treatment of CPP with a 3-month depot injection as compared with the approved monthly and annual histrelin implant.
Reference	Fuld K, Chi C, Neely EK. A randomized trial of 1- and 3-month depot leuprolide doses in the treatment of central precocious puberty. *J Pediatr.* 2011; **159**(6): 982–7.

Evidence 2	
Theme E2	*Therapy for delayed puberty and short stature*
Question	What is the impact of androgen therapy in constitutionally delayed growth and puberty?
Design	Randomised controlled trial
Level of evidence	Jadad 5
Setting	Fourteen paediatric endocrine clinics, the United States
Participants	Boys who met the following criteria were eligible: • age between 11 and 14 • height more than 2 standard deviations below the mean height for age • a bone age greater or equal to 9 years of age • a bone age delay of more than 1 year • pubertal stage development of Tanner 2 or less • normal intellectual skills • normal thyroid function.
Intervention	Oxandrolone at a dose of 0.1 mg/kg/day or an identical placebo were used. All participants had self-image measured using the Piers-Harris Children's Self-Concept Scale and social competence measured using the Child Behaviour Profile.
Outcomes	The primary outcome was growth velocity after 1 year of treatment.
Main results	Forty-four boys were enrolled 23 to the oxandrolone group and 21 to the placebo group. Two in each group did not complete the study. The mean change in height was 9.5 ± 1.7 cm in the oxandrolone group and 6.8 ± 2.8 cm in the placebo group. Mean predicted heights did not change in each group. The Piers-Harris Children's Self-Concept Scale and the Child Behaviour Profile did not differ at baseline or at the end of the study. There were no complications detected during the study.
Conclusion	Oxandrolone increased height velocity but did not result in improvement in psychosocial status.
Commentary	While oxandrolone increased height, these changes may be too small for the individual boy to notice over the short term. Curently, most adolescent males are counselled not to seek treatment for delayed puberty. There is no convincing evidence that treatment will produce a measurable gain from a psychological perspective. Concerned adolescents should be followed to ensure that growth is occurring and reassured accordingly.
Reference	Wilson DM, McCauley E, Brown DR, *et al.* Oxandrolone therapy in constitutionally delayed growth and puberty. *Pediatrics.* 1995; **96**(6): 1095–100.

PUBERTY: MULTIPLE-CHOICE QUESTIONS

Q1 Tests for precocious puberty include which of the following?
   a) X-ray of the right wrist
   b) FSH and LH levels
   c) Testosterone levels
   d) hCG levels
   e) Computed tomography of the brain

Q2 Which of the following statements relating to Prader–Willi's syndrome is/are correct?
   a) Hypotonia is a feature.
   b) Obesity is a recognised feature.
   c) Short stature is a feature.
   d) Obstructive sleep apnoea occurs.
   e) Developmental delay is a feature.

Q3 Which of the following statements on precocious puberty is/are true?
   a) It begins before the age of 8 in girls.
   b) It begins before the age of 9 in boys.
   c) Central causes account for 75% of cases.
   d) It is 20 times more common in girls.
   e) Compromised adult height is a long-term complication.

Q4 Causes of precocious puberty include which of the following?
   a) Previous meningitis
   b) Irradiation
   c) Retinoblastoma
   d) Chronic active hepatitis
   e) Craniopharyngioma

Q5 Which of the following statements on premature thelarche is/are true?
   a) Bone age is normal.
   b) Gonadotropin levels are prepubertal.
   c) Breast development occurs only.
   d) Pelvic ultrasound is normal.
   e) Breast stage 4 occurs in 25%.

Q6 In premature adrenarche, which of the following statements is/are true?
   a) Pubic and axillary hair develop.
   b) Children have an adult body odour.
   c) Testicular enlargement occurs.
   d) Levels of DHEA are increased.
   e) There is an association with polycystic ovarian syndrome.

Q7   Which of the following statements is/are true with regard to McCune–Albright's syndrome?
   a) The male to female ratio is 6:1.
   b) Menses occur without thelarche.
   c) Polyostic fibrous dysplasia occurs in the long bones.
   d) Polyostic fibrous dysplasia occurs in the skull.
   e) Functioning ovarian cysts lead to precocious puberty.

Q8   Which of the following statements relating to delayed puberty is/are true?
   a) No breast development by 13 years.
   b) More than 3 years from breast development to menses.
   c) There is a positive family history in 85%.
   d) Equally as common in males and females.
   e) The child reaches normal final height.

Q9   Which of the following is/are features of Klinefelter's syndrome?
   a) Increased adult height
   b) Small testes
   c) Gynaecosmastia
   d) Ventricular septal defect in 25%
   e) Sparse pubic hair

Q10   Which of the following statements is/are true of Turner's syndrome?
   a) Short stature occurs in 80%.
   b) Webbing of the neck is a characteristic feature.
   c) Coarctation of the aorta occurs.
   d) Growth hormone treatment is indicated in 65%.
   e) Lymphoedema is noted at birth in 80%.

Answers

A1	b, c, d		A2	a, b, c, d, e
A3	a, b, e		A4	a, b, e
A5	a, b, c, d		A6	a, b, d, e
A7	b, c, d, e		A8	a, e
A9	a, b, c, e		A10	b, c, e

SLIDES

1. Bilateral undescended testis
2. Precocious puberty
3. Precocious puberty

Chapter Twenty-eight

THE CHILD WITH DIABETES MELLITUS

COMMON SCENARIO

'She just hasn't been right over the past few weeks. She's exhausted, she started wetting the bed and she's constantly thirsty, and even though her appetite has increased enormously, I think she's losing weight.'

LEARNING OUTCOMES

- Understand how children with diabetes present in clinical practice
- Conduct a treatment plan for the effective management of children with newly diagnosed diabetes
- Understand the treatment options for diabetic control
- Explain the complications associated with poor glycaemic control

BACKGROUND

Diabetes mellitus is defined as either a blood glucose >11.1 mmol/L or a fasting glucose >7.0 mmol/L with glycosuria plus or minus ketonuria and symptoms of hyperglycaemia. Type 1 diabetes is the commonest type of diabetes in childhood. The age at presentation of type 1 diabetes has a bimodal distribution, with a peak at 4–6 years and a second peak at 10–14 years.

Type 1 diabetes is caused by an absolute deficiency of insulin due to destruction of insulin-producing pancreatic beta cells. Genetic and environmental factors are implicated in the pathogenesis of the disease.

In 5% of cases there is a positive family history. HLA genes of DR3-DQ2 and DR4-DQ8 are present in 90% of children with type 1 diabetes. Exposure to one or more environmental agents may trigger the immune system response to beta cells. Several environmental factors, including viruses (Coxsackie B, enteroviruses, cytomegalovirus, mumps and rubella), immunisations, dietary factors and perinatal factors, have been implicated.

The incidence of type 1 diabetes varies between northern and southern hemispheres.

In Europe, the incidence of type 1 diabetes in children aged 0–14 years is highest in Finland, at 57/100 000; in the United Kingdom, Canada and the United States the incidence is similar, at 22/100 000; in Ireland it is 16/100 000 and in Venezuela it is 0.1/100 000.

Type 1 diabetes is associated with other autoimmune disorders such as Hashimoto's and Graves's disease (3%–5%), coeliac disease (2%–5%) and Addison's disease (<1%). Autoantibodies identified in newly diagnosed diabetics include islet cell antibodies, anti-insulin and glutamic acid decarboxylase autoantibodies (85%–98% of cases).

In children with type 1 diabetes, insulin deficiency results in hyperglycaemia. Once the renal threshold for glucose is exceeded, osmotic diuresis occurs, resulting in polyuria and polydipsia. The classic presentation of diabetes is with polyuria, polydipsia and weight loss. Insulin deficiency also causes lipolysis and the production of excess fatty acids and ketone bodies. The accumulation of ketoacids in the blood leads to the development of a metabolic acidosis, which results in compensatory rapid deep breathing or Kussmaul's respiration. Diabetic ketoacidosis (DKA) is the leading cause of morbidity and mortality in children with type 1 diabetes. Progressive dehydration, acidosis and hyperosmolality cause decreased consciousness leading to coma and, if untreated, death.

DKA is frequently the initial presentation in children of new-onset diabetes mellitus. Younger children and children whose families do not have access to medical care for social or economic reasons are more likely to present with DKA. Protective factors that decrease the risk of DKA include a first-degree relative with type 1 diabetes and higher parental education. In children presenting with and without ketoacidosis, the mean duration of symptoms is similar (16.5 and 17.1 days, respectively), with 40% of children having been seen by a doctor at least once before diagnosis. The risk of DKA in children with known diabetes is 1–10 per 100 person years and is usually due to either inadvertent or deliberate insulin omission. The risk is higher in teenagers, those with a history of poor control, difficult family circumstances, psychological or psychiatric disorders and those on insulin pump therapy.

The incidence of type 2 diabetes has increased in recent years, especially in certain ethnic groups such as African and Asian-American children, although it remains rare in the general paediatric population.

Diagnosis of diabetes

Type 1 diabetes may present with symptoms ranging from incidental glycosuria to life-threatening DKA.

- When symptoms of hyperglycaemia are present, a random plasma glucose of >11.1 mmol/L is diagnostic.
- An oral glucose tolerance test is rarely needed, except in atypical cases or very early disease in which plasma glucose levels are normal. A 75 g glucose load should be given and blood glucose measured 2 hours post administration.
- A fasting blood glucose (at least 8 hours) of >7 mmol/L is an indicator of diabetes.

- HbA1c of >6.5% is an indicator of diabetes.

HISTORY

KEY POINTS				
Urinary symptoms	Night-time awakening Frequency of urination Episodes of incontinence Secondary nocturnal enuresis	**Family history**	Diabetes Hypothyroidism Coeliac disease Addison's disease	**❶ Red flags** Polyuria Polydipsia Weight loss
Fluid intake	Thirst Fluid intake Type of fluid – water, fizzy drinks	**Symptoms of DKA**	Vomiting Abdominal pain Respiratory distress	
Weight loss	Loose-fitting clothes Previous recorded weights Appetite	**Symptoms of intercurrent infection**	Fever, rash, upper respiratory tract infection symptoms, vomiting, diarrhoea	
Current or recent use of medication that may affect blood glucose	Steroids Atypical antipsychotics Chemotherapeutic agents	**Social history** (factors that might influence management of diabetes)	Family structure Difficulties at school Hobbies and activities – sports and so forth	

EXAMINATION

All children presenting with suspected diabetes should have a full systemic examination.

- Height, weight and body mass index should be obtained and plotted on an appropriate centile chart
- Blood pressure
- Fundoscopy
- Signs of dehydration (decreased skin turgor, sunken eyes, absence of tears, sunken fontanelle, dry mucous membranes, lethargy)
- Kussmaul's respiration (tachypnoea and hyperventilation)
- Level of consciousness

---

❶ Red flags

- Decreased level of consciousness
- Signs of dehydration
- Kussmaul's respiration
- Epigastric pain (indicator of hypovolaemic shock)

DIFFERENTIAL DIAGNOSIS

Organic causes	Symptoms seen
Pneumonia	May also have symptoms of tachypnoea and hyperventilation – however, in diabetes no cough is evident
Acute appendicitis	May have abdominal pain and tenderness in DKA – appropriate fluid, insulin and electrolyte therapy will ameliorate the abdominal symptoms within hours
Nocturnal enuresis	May be confused but urinalysis will distinguish from diabetes
Severe sepsis	If severe acute sepsis, hyperglycaemia, glycosuria and ketonuria may occur
Psychogenic or compulsive polydipsia	Classically a toddler who drinks lots of fluids both day and night but remains well, has normal urinalysis and never loses weight
Diabetes insipidus	Large volumes of dilute urine passed with associated poor weight gain Will see very significant hypernatraemia Diagnosed by formal fluid fast for 4 hours If central will respond to DDAVP

INVESTIGATIONS

What biochemical criteria are required for the diagnosis of DKA?

- Hyperglycaemia, with a blood glucose >11 mmol/L
- Metabolic acidosis with a venous pH <7.3 and/or plasma bicarbonate <15 mmol/L

In children presenting with suspected diabetes, what investigations should be performed?

- Plasma glucose
- Venous blood gas
- Serum electrolytes
- Urea and creatinine
- Full blood count
- Urinalysis and urine microscopy (if evidence of infection)
- Blood cultures (if signs of sepsis)
- Islet cell antibodies, glutamic acid decarboxylase and insulin autoantibodies
- Thyroid function tests
- Coeliac antibodies

How often should glucose and ketone levels be monitored?

Frequent testing is the only way to manage blood glucose levels safely. Most children need to test a minimum of four times a day, prior to each meal and before bed. If they are unwell, on pump therapy or their blood glucose levels are difficult to control, more frequent monitoring is required. Ketones should be monitored during illness and if glucose levels are high. HbA1c reflects average blood glucose values over the preceding 6–8 weeks. HbA1c should be monitored every 3 months.

MANAGEMENT PLAN FOR TYPE 1 DIABETES: FIVE-STEP APPROACH

1. Clarifying and pitfall avoidance strategies
2. Education and multidisciplinary support:
   a) intensive education of parent and child

3. Blood glucose monitoring:
   a) standard monitoring of glucose
   b) continuous glucose monitoring
4. Insulin therapy:
   a) standard insulin therapy
   b) insulin pump therapy
5. Follow-up and management of acute and chronic complications

Clarifying and pitfall avoidance strategies

- Explain to the parents that diabetes can be insidious in its presentation, especially if the child presents in coma, as they may be feeling guilty that the diagnosis was not make earlier.
- Diabetes needs to be actively managed to ensure optimal outcome for the child; therefore, all units caring for children and adolescents with diabetes should have multidisciplinary teams with a paediatrician, a dietitian and a clinical nurse specialist in diabetes, at a minimum.
- Traditional hospital care of children with diabetes is lessening; therefore, if they attend the emergency department because of illness or are admitted for surgery, appropriate standards of care must be met (*see* Evidence 1). This is not always achieved.
- Parents and child must be empowered to manage their child's diabetes. **Rationale**: the level of diabetes control determines prognosis, in terms of occurrence of complications.

Education and multidisciplinary support

Optimal management of diabetes requires a dedicated multidisciplinary team consisting of:

- consultant paediatric endocrinologist or paediatrician with special interest in paediatric diabetes
- paediatric dietitian
- diabetes nurse specialist
- psychosocial support.

Intensive education of parent and child

Self-management of diabetes is the ultimate goal for all patients with diabetes. To achieve this goal, the carers of a young child need to be able to balance insulin replacement with dietary intake and exercise levels, in order to maintain blood glucose control and to prevent and recognise the occurrence of complications. Blood glucose testing and the incidence of acute and chronic complications measure the success of self-management.

Education is essential at diagnosis. The family must be given basic survival education, including:

- what is diabetes? The consequences of having diabetes and the lifelong complications
- the role of insulin and delivery methods, administration, injection sites and storage/disposal, adjustments
- recognising glucose homeostasis patterns through review of food intake, blood glucose levels, insulin dosage and activity
- blood glucose monitoring and HbA1c – targets, technique and actions based on results (including relationship to food and exercise)
- the diabetes support team, importance of regular review, when and how to access help
- causes, symptoms, treatment, prevention of hypo- and hyperglycaemia – DKA and sick day management
- importance of carrying identity bracelet, support and entitlements for daily living with diabetes
- management of diabetes in crèche, at school or on holidays.

Dietitian education can help people to balance and adjust their food choices according to their activity and insulin levels, to avoid and treat high blood glucoses and low blood glucoses and to adjust meal patterns when feeling unwell. Initially the education given should focus on recognising food types and how they influence blood glucose levels. Topics should include:

- healthy eating and food groups
- effects of different food groups on blood glucose levels
- carbohydrate sources and tools to calculate carbohydrate content per serving
- options for meals, snacks and drinks
- estimating carbohydrates in recipes and complex meals
- insulin to carbohydrate ratio and correction doses
- carbohydrate adjustment when exercising or eating out.

Blood glucose monitoring

Standard monitoring of glucose

Daily blood glucose levels are used to monitor control and adjust insulin dosages. In general, we aim for glucose levels between 4.5 and 9 mmol/L. Frequent testing is the only way to manage blood glucose levels safely. Most children need to test a minimum of four times a day. There is good correlation between frequency of monitoring and glycaemic control. Glucose levels should be used to determine immediate adjustments to short- or rapid-acting insulin and after observing patterns of blood glucose over several days, make adjustments to long-acting insulin.

HbA1c levels are used to evaluate long-term glycaemic control over the preceding 2–3 months and are currently considered the best index of metabolic control for diabetic patients in the clinical setting, as well as a measure of the risk for the development of micro- and macrovascular complications. In children, higher HbA1c targets are used to minimise the risk of hypoglycaemia, as children may be too young to recognise symptoms of hypoglycaemia and/or to independently seek attention for prompt treatment. For children <6 years of age: target HbA1c levels of 7.5%–8.5% are used. Progressively lower targets are used as children get older; for children 5–13 years of age, <8% is the target; for children 13–18 years of age, <7.5% is the target.

Continuous glucose monitoring

Continuous blood glucose monitoring (*see* Evidence 2) is potentially useful in children, but as yet it has not been incorporated into standard practice.

Insulin therapy

Standard insulin therapy

Standard insulin regimens include:

- twice-daily injections with a mixture of short- and intermediate-acting insulin (usually younger children)
- multiple daily injections of a long-acting insulin at night and a rapid-acting insulin at mealtimes.

Twice-daily injections:

- children are usually started on a total daily dose (TDD) of 1 unit/kg/day
- two-thirds of the TDD is given in the morning, with one-third given at night
- one-third of each dose if short-acting and two-thirds if long-acting.

Multiple daily injections:

- children are usually started on a TDD of 1 unit/kg/day
- 0.4 units/kg is given as a long-acting injection at night
- 0.2 units/kg is given as a rapid-acting insulin at mealtimes.

Insulins are categorised by:

- onset (speed of onset)
- peak (how long it takes to achieve maximum impact)
- duration (how long effect lasts for)
- concentration (units per millilitre)
- route of delivery (subcutaneous or intravenous).

Rapid-acting insulin such as NovoRapid starts to work within 10 minutes, peaks at 1–2 hours and lasts for 4–6 hours.

Short-acting insulins such as Actrapid start to work in 30 minutes to 1 hour, peak at 2–4 hours and last 6–8 hours.

Intermediate-acting insulins such as Insulatard start to work within 1–2 hours, peak at 6–10 hours and last over 12 hours.

Long-acting insulins such as Levemir start to work in 1 hour, have a relatively flat action profile and last for 24 hours.

Insulin pump therapy

Continuous subcutaneous insulin infusion (CSII) therapy has a number of theoretical advantages over multiple daily injections in the care of young children with type 1 diabetes, particularly in children less than 5 years of age, and it is favoured by parents (*see* Evidence 3).

Insulin pumps deliver continuous (basal) insulin; pumps can be programmed to deliver different basal rates of insulin at different times of the day or night. Pumps must be activated to deliver preprandial boluses. Children and their families need to be competent in carbohydrate counting and the use of insulin to carbohydrate ratios. Subcutaneously placed cannulae need to be re-sited every 2–3 days.

Follow-up and management of acute and chronic complications

At 3-monthly reviews, the following should be addressed:
- HbA1c measurement and review of home monitoring records
- frequency and awareness of hypoglycaemic episodes should be determined
- injection sites and technique
- diet
- exercise
- school and family issues.

Hyperglycaemia management

Parents of children with diabetes often phone healthcare professionals for advice regarding hyperglycaemia. It is important to try to determine the cause of hyperglycaemia by reviewing previous blood glucose readings, determining if (a) insulin therapy had been omitted, (b) dietary intake had been modified, (c) problems with glucometer or injection methods had been noted or (d) intercurrent illness was present. First, it is important to determine if the child is well, i.e. not vomiting and with a normal conscious level. If there is concern, the child should be referred immediately to his or her local emergency department. If the blood glucose is >15 mmol/L, blood ketones should be checked. If ketones are negative, no additional insulin is required and the blood glucose should be rechecked in 2 hours. If blood ketone levels are >0.6 mmol/L, 10% of the TDD of insulin should be given as fast-acting insulin (in addition to normal insulin). The blood glucose and ketone levels should be rechecked in 2 hours. If they remain elevated, with ketones and/or vomiting, a further 10% of the child's total daily insulin should be given and he or she should be referred to the emergency department. If the blood glucose remains above 15 mmol/L but the ketones have cleared, both should be reassessed in 2 hours. If the blood glucose has decreased below 15 mmol/L, no further action is required; however, the parents should be advised to contact their diabetes team.

Hypoglycaemia management

Parents of children with diabetes often phone healthcare professionals for advice regarding the management of hypoglycaemia, which is an anxiety-provoking event for parents (*see* Evidence 4). It is important to determine the cause of hypoglycaemia by reviewing previous blood glucose readings, determining if insulin intake has been sufficient, the amount of exercise the child has had, assessing potential alcohol taken or whether the child has an intercurrent illness. Hypoglycaemia is more common in children with lower HbA1c levels, a previous history of hypoglycaemic episodes, higher insulin doses and younger age. There are concerns over the impact of hypoglycaemia on the developing brain and on cognitive function; severe hypoglycaemia can cause convulsions, coma and even death, and the risk is higher in children under 5 years of age.

If the child has a decreased level of consciousness or is confused, intramuscular glucagon should be given and an ambulance called.

If the child is well and able to eat and drink, provide a high glycaemic index food or fluid, such as 50 mL of Lucozade or 100 mL of 7 Up, followed by one to two servings of low glycaemic index foods, such as two to three digestive biscuits. Blood sugar levels should be rechecked 30 minutes later. If unable to eat or drink, or glucose fails to increase, a whole tube of Glucogel should be given. If unconscious, intramuscular glucagon should be administered and an ambulance called.

Sick day management

Management of sick days requires more frequent monitoring of blood glucose and ketones to avoid hyperglycaemia or hypoglycaemia and prevention of DKA. During sick days, insulin should never be stopped but may need to be adjusted in response to blood glucose and ketone levels.

Illness can cause hyperglycaemia or hypoglycaemia. During times of acute illness, children's calorific intake may be decreased due to nausea or vomiting or decreased appetite. As a result their insulin requirements decrease. However, the stress of illness may cause an increase in counter-regulatory hormones, resulting in increased insulin needs. In younger children, counter-regulatory responses are not well developed and therefore hypoglycaemia is more common. In older children, hyperglycaemia is more common.

One strategy that parents can follow with intercurrent illness is outlined as follows. Stress the importance of adjusting insulin in terms of blood sugars and urine ketone levels:

a) for blood glucose <6 mmol/L and urine ketones positive or negative, decrease the daily insulin by 20% until blood glucose 6–11 mmol/L

b) for blood glucose 6–13 mmol/L and urine ketone positive or negative, continue to monitor blood glucose levels, while giving usual insulin dose

c) for blood glucose 13–17 mmol/L and urine ketone negative, give the usual insulin and at the same time add 10% of the total insulin dose as a rapid-acting insulin

d) for blood glucose >11 mmol/L and urine ketones 2+ or 3+, give the usual insulin dose and add 20% more (of TDD) as a rapid-acting insulin every 4 hours until the ketones are negative and blood glucose <11 mmol/L

e) for blood glucose >17 mmol/L and urine ketones positive or negative, use the strategy outlined for option d.

Diabetic ketoacidosis

DKA should be managed according to locally agreed protocols that reflect the current evidence for most appropriate management. Complications of hypoglycaemia, hypokalaemia and idiopathic cerebral oedema may occur during treatment of DKA. Children with DKA require close cardiac monitoring, including observation of their heart rate, respiratory rate, blood pressure, neurological status, fluid status, glucose, ketones, electrolytes and blood gasses. Following initial resuscitation, intravenous fluids should be replaced over a 48-hour period with close monitoring of potassium levels and potassium replacement initiated once urine output has been established. Insulin should be given by continuous intravenous infusion.

FOLLOW-UP

Long-term complications may be:
- microvascular – retinopathy, nephropathy, neuropathy
- macrovascular – ischaemic heart disease or peripheral vascular disease.

Microvascular complications may develop in puberty or early adulthood (*see* Evidence 5). Nephropathy is preceded by the development of persistent microalbuminuria, affecting about 10% of children and adolescents with type 1 diabetes. It is detected by measuring the albumin to creatinine ratio in the first voided morning urine sample (the upper limit of normal being 1.5 mg/mmol). Persistent microalbuminuria predicts progression to gross proteinuria within 6–14 years. Microalbuminuria is reversible with good glycaemic control and blood pressure control. Patients with persistent microalbuminuria should have blood pressure checked, serum urea, electrolytes and creatinine measured and a renal ultrasound performed. If microalbuminuria persists, treatment with angiotensin-converting enzyme inhibitors (e.g. captopril) should be considered, even in the absence of hypertension.

Retinopathy is usually not recognised until diabetes has been present for 5–10 years. Risk factors include poor glycaemic control, increased duration of diabetes, hypertension, hyperlipidaemia and cigarette smoking. Children should have annual ophthalmology examinations performed once the child is 10 years of age and has had diabetes for 3–5 years. The earliest sign of diabetic eye disease is the development of background retinopathy (microaneurysms and haemorrhages with exudates not involving the macula). This stage is asymptomatic and does not damage vision. Improvements in glycaemic control reduce the risk of the development of retinopathy and limit progression of established retinopathy. Background diabetic retinopathy may progress to proliferative retinopathy, which can be successfully treated in its early stages with laser photocoagulation therapy.

The earliest symptoms of neuropathy are numbness and paraesthesia of the hands and feet, with evidence of decreased vibration sense, loss of ankle jerks and diminished pinprick sensation. Children with type 1 diabetes should have annual foot exams from puberty, looking at sensation, pulses, skin integrity and nail problems. Clinically significant neuropathy is very rare in adolescence.

WHEN TO REFER?

- Any child with suspected diabetes mellitus should be referred immediately for specialist assessment.
- Children with risk factors for type 2 diabetes mellitus should be referred for screening.

CLARIFICATION STATEMENTS FOR PARENTAL MISCONCEPTIONS

'Why are the blood glucose recordings so good and yet the HbA1c is high?'

This is not uncommon and the most likely explanation is the blood sugars are not being performed and fictitious results are being offered. The HbA1c result is very reliable as an index of glycaemic control over the previous 6–8 weeks.

'What about inhaled insulin?'

There have been some trials but in general terms, inhaled insulin has not proved successful.

'What about pump therapy?'

Insulin pump therapy is very effective and is especially useful in those children under 5 years old with type 1 diabetes. A very intensive educational effort is required prior to commencing pump therapy. Overall glycaemic control is improved and the risk of hypoglycaemia is lessened.

'Does every child with diabetes have to be admitted to hospital for treatment, even when they do not have diabetic ketoacidosis?'

No, some units utilise an outpatient or day ward management process to educate, stabilise and treat the child who develops diabetes. This process normalises the condition for parents more quickly than does management on an inpatient ward.

SUMMARY PRACTICE POINTS

- Diabetes mellitus type 1 is increasing in incidence.
- Children presenting for the first time may present in DKA or with the classical symptoms of polyuria, polydipsia and weight loss.
- Children with suspected diabetes mellitus require immediate referral for specialist assessment.
- Multidisciplinary team treatment involves a dedicated paediatrician or endocrinologist, dietitian, psychologist and clinical nurse specialist in diabetes.
- Improved glycaemic control lessens the risks of microvascular complications.
- Insulin pump therapy is recommended for children under 5 years of age.

EVALUATING THE EVIDENCE

Evidence 1	
Theme E1	*The care of patients with diabetes mellitus in hospital*
Question	How does the care offered to children with diabetes mellitus compare with the care standards that have been developed?
Design	Audit (evaluation of standards of care against actual practice)
Level of evidence	
Setting	Twenty-seven diabetes services in three regions, England
Participants	Children and adolescents with diabetes mellitus who were hospitalised (for a period >4 hours) for either aspects of their diabetes (including diabetic ketoacidosis (DKA) or hypoglycaemia) or reasons unrelated to their diabetes (including elective and emergency surgery) were eligible for inclusion.
Intervention	Standards for inpatient care of children with diabetes, developed by the Children and Young People's Diabetes Implementation Support Group of the Department of Health were assessed against actual practice in the selected hospitals.
Outcomes	The primary outcome was adherence rates to the standards of care.
Main results	All 27 centres provided responses. Of the 29 locations for the 27 services, 21 (73%) always send and four (14%) generally send copies of letters to family.
	For emergency department standards, nine (33%) had a trained paediatric nurse on each shift, 25 (93%) had DKA protocol, 19 (70%) had a newly diagnosed protocol, 19 (70%) had a hypoglycaemias protocol, 18 (67%) had a surgery protocol and 14 (52%) had all four protocols. Twenty-four (89%) had ensured ED staff and had educational modules on diabetes management, and 24 (89%) had a paediatric consultant responsible for emergency department liaison on diabetes care.
	For ward management, 26 (96%) had a DKA protocol, 24 (89%) had a newly diagnosed protocol, 22 (82%) had a hypoglycaemic protocol, 23 (85%) had a surgery protocol and 19 (70%) had all four protocols.

(continued)

Evidence 1	
Theme E1	*The care of patients with diabetes mellitus in hospital*
Main results (*cont.*)	Only four (15%) services always enabled parents to manage their child's diabetes, 20 (70%) had a diabetes link nurse, 25 (93%) had an inpatient paediatric nurse specialist, 10 (37%) had adequate dietetic support for ward staff and 29 (100%) had paediatric nurses looking after the child with diabetes. Twenty-five (93%) services provide regular diabetes education to ward staff, and eight (30%) provide 24 hour access to ward staff; however, only seven (26%) services discuss promptly (within 2 hours) the reason a child with diabetes is admitted. Sixteen insulin errors were noted among the 115 patients admitted to the 27 services.
Conclusion	The audit (the first of diabetes inpatient services in England) demonstrates that some standards can be met but others that are resource related will be more challenging to meet.
Commentary	Diabetes care in children and adolescents is increasingly becoming an outpatient-based process; however, hospitalisation is required periodically. Consequently familiarity with management strategies (insulin pump therapy, carbohydrate counting) will decrease as exposure lessens. Unforeseen consequences could include parents being responsible for calculating insulin doses, which may not be appropriate in all situations. The development of e-learning modules could help address the knowledge deficit. Themes that emanate from this study are the importance of cohorting children with diabetes on the same ward, early involvement of the diabetes link nurse and having available a specialist paediatrician in diabetes for consultation and advice – these all add to enhanced appropriate patient care.
Reference	Edge J, Ackland FM, Payne S, *et al.* Inpatient care for children with diabetes: are standards being met? *Arch Dis Child.* 2012; **97**(7): 599–603.

Evidence 2	
Theme E2	*Continuous glucose monitoring (CGM) in diabetes mellitus*
Question	How effective is real-time CGM in children with diabetes mellitus?
Design	Randomised controlled trial
Level of evidence	Jadad 3
Setting	Diabetes Research in Children Network (DirecNet), the United States
Participants	Children with diabetes for at least 1 year, aged between 4 and 10 years, with a HbA1c ≥7%, treated with basal bolus therapy either using an insulin pump or at least three multiple daily injections of insulin for the prior 3 months and with no plans to switch the insulin modality for the next 6 months were eligible for inclusion. Prior to randomisation, eligible participants had to wear a CGM device for a minimum of 7–14 days, have no severe skin reactions at the insertion site, have at least 96 hours of CGM readings, and to have performed at least three blood glucose meter readings per day.
Intervention	Participants in the intervention group were given a CGM device and a new blood glucose monitoring device with test strips, whereas the control group were given a new blood glucose measuring device and test strips.

(*continued*)

Evidence 2	
Theme E2	*Continuous glucose monitoring (CGM) in diabetes mellitus*
Outcomes	The primary outcome was a binary variable, defined as a reduction in the HbA1c of ≥0.5% from baseline to 26 weeks and no severe hypoglycaemic events.
Main results	Of the 146 children randomised, 74 were in the CGM group and 72 in the control group, with 69 (93%) and 68 (94%), respectively, completing the study. The primary outcome was achieved in 13 (19%) of the CGM group and 19 (28%) of the control group (absolute risk reduction = 9%; number needed to treat = 12). Severe hypoglycaemic events occurred in three (4%) of the CGM group and in five (7%, six total events) of the control group. While 65 (91%) were wearing the CGM sensor at least 1 day per week at the end of the study, only 41% averaged 6 days/week during the study.
Conclusion	The use of CGM did not improve glycaemic control in the population studied, despite a high degree of parental satisfaction.
Commentary	CGM has made it possible to assess the patterns and trends of blood glucose and the substantial variability that occurs throughout the day in patients with diabetes mellitus. The benefits of this technology are most apparent with near-continuous wear of the sensors, as glycaemic patterns related to exercise and meals can be incorporated into the daily management of an individual's diabetes. In this study the data, obtained from the monitoring, were not incorporated into the day-to-day management and as a consequence, the primary outcome favoured the non-use of CGM. Parents were favourably disposed to CGM but there appears to be an unremitting fear of hypoglycaemia (unchanged with enhanced data compared with the control group) on the part of parents of these young children and consequently they may have used the data to decrease the risk of this event. Aiding parents to overcome their fear and integrate the use of this data remains a significant challenge.
Reference	Mauras N, Beck R, Xing D, *et al.* Diabetes Research in Children Network Study Group. A randomized clinical trial to assess the efficacy and safety of real-time continuous glucose monitoring in the management of type 1 diabetes in young children aged 4 to <10 years. *Diabetes Care.* 2012; **35**(2): 204–10.

Evidence 3	
Theme E3	*Insulin pump therapy in children with diabetes mellitus*
Question	Is insulin pump therapy more effective than intensive insulin injection therapy?
Design	Randomised controlled trial
Level of evidence	Jadad 3
Setting	Endocrinology clinic, academic medical centre, the United States
Participants	Children <5 years of age with type 1 diabetes for at least 1 year and who received two or more insulin injections per year were eligible to participate.
Intervention	Participants were randomised to receive continuous subcutaneous insulin infusion (CSII) or intensive insulin injection therapy.
Outcomes	The primary outcome was change in HbA1c, with secondary outcomes being severe hypoglycaemic events, meter-detected hypoglycaemia, blood sugar variability, body mass index and satisfaction with therapy at 6 months.

(*continued*)

Evidence 3	
Theme E3	*Insulin pump therapy in children with diabetes mellitus*
Main results	Of 50 eligible patients, 42 were randomised: 21 to the pump group and 21 to insulin injections. In the pump group, 20 children completed the study and one developed a tape allergy and quit. Seventeen of the insulin injection group completed the study (one failed to commence the study, two dropped out because of family difficulties and one was non-compliant). Mean HbA1c at the start of the study was 9.0% (±0.6%) for both groups; at 6 months mean HbA1c for the pump group was 8.5% ± 0.6 and for the injection group it was 8.7% ± 0.7% (no difference). Except for an increase in meter-detected hypoglycaemic episodes in pump treatment versus injection (18.5% versus 14.5%), all secondary outcomes were similar. Nineteen (95%) of parents opted to continue with pump therapy beyond the study period.
Conclusion	Pump therapy in preschool children was not associated with clinically significant differences in glycaemic control compared with intensive insulin injection therapy; however, parents reported satisfaction with CSII.
Commentary	CSII is able to closely simulate the normal pattern of insulin secretion through the delivery of basal insulin doses with the addition of prandial boluses. Such a system offers the possibility of more flexibility and more precise insulin delivery than multiple daily injections. CSII is increasing in popularity with families despite the intensive training necessary, and once using it, few switch back to multiple injections of insulin. CSII should be considered for children with recurrent severe hypoglycaemia, wide fluctuations in blood glucose, suboptimal glucose control (HbA1c exceeding age-related targets), microvascular complications and/or risk factors for macrovascular complications. Children with good metabolic control but insulin regimen that compromises lifestyle can also be considered for CSII (Phillip *et al.*, 2007).
References	DiMeglio LA, Pottorff TM, Boyd SR, *et al.* A randomized, controlled study of insulin pump therapy in diabetic preschoolers. *J Pediatr.* 2004; **145**(3): 380–4.
	Phillip M, Battelino T, Rodriguez H, *et al.* Use of insulin pump therapy in the paediatric age-group: consensus statement from the European Society for Paediatric Endocrinology, the Lawson Wilkins Pediatric Endocrine Society, and the International Society for Pediatric and Adolescent Diabetes, endorsed by the American Diabetes Association and the European Association for the Study of Diabetes. *Diabetes Care.* 2007: **30**(6): 1653–62.

Evidence 4	
Theme E4	*Hypoglycaemia in children and adolescents with diabetes mellitus*
Question	How frequent are episodes of hypoglycaemia in children and adolescents?
Design	Prospective observational study
Level of evidence	
Setting	Two paediatric diabetes centres, the United States
Participants	Persons aged 9–15 years with type 1 diabetes for over 1 year, with a most recent HbA1c <13% and no major chronic medical or psychiatric disease were eligible.

(continued)

Evidence 4	
Theme E4	*Hypoglycaemia in children and adolescents with diabetes mellitus*
Intervention	None
Outcomes	The primary outcome was the frequency of severe hypoglycaemia, which was defined as episodes requiring help from another person for oral treatment or episodes resulting in seizures and/or coma. Outcome rates were calculated and compared with those of insulin regimens.
Main results	Overall, 255 were followed for a median of 1.2 years. The distribution of participants across the regimen, which were NPH, basal bolus injections and pump therapy, was 44%, 20% and 36%, respectively, at study commencement and 31%, 25% and 44%, respectively, at its completion. There were 145 episodes of severe hypoglycaemia among 64 participants (31 had one episode, 14 had two, 8 had three and 11 had four or more). The overall incidence was 37.6/100 patient years (pump therapy, 31.8/100 patient years; basal bolus injections, 34.4/100 patient years; NPH, 46.1/100 patient years). There were 37 episodes of seizure or coma in 22 participants (pump therapy, 4.5/100 patient years; basal bolus, 11.1/100 patient years; NPH, 14.4/100 patient years).
Conclusion	The rate of severe hypoglycaemia in children and adolescents remains high but it was lowest with pump therapy. Patients transition between treatment options, in their pursuit of suitable therapy options.
Commentary	Balancing the risks of hypoglycaemia with the goal of optimal glycaemic control is a major challenge for those with diabetes, and for those who provide their care. Anxiety related to hypoglycaemia may increase patient's fear and discourage tight glycaemic control. It is recognised that severe hypoglycaemia in children and adolescents (if repeated) may lead to subtle problems in learning and in their ability to remember. The advent of continuous glucose monitoring may prove a valuable tool in the reduction of severe hypoglycaemic rates.
Reference	Katz ML, Volkening LK, Anderson BJ, *et al.* Contemporary rates of severe hypoglycaemia in youth with type 1 diabetes: variability by insulin regimen. *Diabet Med.* 2012; **29**(7): 926–32.

Evidence 5	
Theme E 5	*Complications in diabetes in children and adolescents*
Question	How can the risk of complications be assessed in diabetes in children and adolescents?
Design	Prospective observational study
Level of evidence	
Setting	Department of paediatrics, academic medical centre, the United Kingdom
Participants	A total of 527 children with diabetes were included in this study, which commenced in 1986 and reported results to 2005.

(continued)

Evidence 5

Theme E 5	*Complications in diabetes in children and adolescents*
Intervention	All participants had annual assessments. Data collected included height, weight, and blood pressure, with first voided urines collected on 3 consecutive mornings for an albumin to creatinine ratio and blood drawn for HbA1c. Microalbuminuria was defined as albumin to creatinine ratio of 3.5–35 mg/mmol in males and 4.0–47 mg/mmol in females. Persistent microalbuminuria was defined as the presence of microalbuminuria at every subsequent annual visit. Intermittent microalbuminuria was defined as a positive result during an annual assessment followed by regression to normal albuminuria, and then recurrence of microalbuminuria at a later date.
Outcomes	The primary outcome measures were annual glycated haemoglobin (HbA1c) and an assessment of urinary albumin to creatinine ratio.
Main results	Of the 527 participants, 135 (26%) met the study definition of microalbuminuria and the cumulative follow-up period was 5182 years. The cumulative presence of microalbuminuria was 25.7% (95% confidence interval (CI): 21.3–30.1) after 10 years and 50.7% (95% CI: 40.5–60.9) after 20 years with diabetes. The mean age of onset of microalbuminuria was 16.1 ($\pm$4.3) years. The major predictor of microalbuminuria was poor glycaemic control (35% risk increase for each 1% increase in HbA1c). Of the 135 with microalbuminuria, 65 (48%) developed persistent microalbuminuria, 17 (13%) had intermittent microalbuminuria and 53 (39%) had transient microalbuminuria, giving a cumulative prevalence of regression to the normal albuminuric range of 51.9% (95% CI: 42.3–61.5) after 4.9 years after the onset of microalbuminuria. Eighteen (13%) of those with microalbuminuria developed macroalbuminuria (3% of the inception cohort) at a mean age of 18.5 years with a 10.0 year duration of diabetes.
Conclusion	The only modifiable predictor to prevent the development of microalbuminuria and preventing progression to macroalbuminuria is poor glycaemic control.
Commentary	In adults with type 1 diabetes, microalbuminuria is an early marker of structural renal disease and a risk factor for the development of microalbuminuria. The presence of microalbuminuria is associated with the subsequent development of end-stage disease. Glycaemic control is unequivocally linked to the development of microalbuminuria and the progression to macroalbuminuria; however, less than 50% of adolescents achieve HbA1c levels of <9%, which is a worrying trend. Enhanced glycaemic control at diagnosis needs to be the goal to prevent complications and this may well influences choices in insulin therapy.
Reference	Amin R, Widmer B, Prevost AT, *et al.* Risk of microalbuminuria and progression to macroalbuminuria in a cohort with childhood onset type 1 diabetes: prospective observational study. *BMJ.* 2008; **336**(7646): 697–701.

DIABETES MELLITUS: MULTIPLE-CHOICE QUESTIONS

Q1 Which of the following statements is/are correct with regard to diabetes mellitus in children and adolescents?
a) The peak incidence is 7–10 years of age.
b) Five per cent have a positive family history.
c) Type 1 diabetes accounts for 4% of all new cases in adolescents.
d) HLA typing is routinely performed in children with new-onset diabetes mellitus.
e) Glutamic acid decarboxylase autoantibodies are associated with the development of diabetes mellitus.

Q2 Which of the following conditions is/are associated with diabetes mellitus in children?
a) Thyroid disease
b) Addison's disease
c) Ankylosing spondylitis
d) Coeliac disease
e) Cystic fibrosis

Q3 Which of the following statements is/are true with regard to the incidence of diabetes mellitus?
a) In Europe the incidence is highest in Finland.
b) The incidence in the United States is twice that of the United Kingdom.
c) The incidence is lowest in South America.
d) Diabetes mellitus in children and adolescents has a bimodal distribution at the ages of 4–6 years and 10–14 years.
e) The incidence in the United Kingdom is 24/100 000 from 0 to 14 years.

Q4 Clinical features of DKA include which of the following?
a) Polydipsia
b) Weight loss
c) Epigastric pain
d) Kussmaul's breathing
e) Coma

Q5 The differential diagnosis of DKA includes which of the following?
a) Acute appendicitis
b) Sepsis
c) Diabetes insipidus
d) Pneumonia
e) Conversion reaction

Q6 Which of the following statements is/are correct with regard to diabetes management?
a) All children must be admitted to hospital for education and stabilisation.
b) In the initial months (while adapting to the diagnosis) blood glucose control can be lax.
c) Insulin pump therapy is only for the older child with diabetes (>8 years).
d) Parents are fearful of hypoglycaemic episodes.
e) Intramuscular injections twice a day is acceptable treatment.

Q7 Which of the following statements is/are true with regard to diabetes mellitus in children and adolescents?
a) HbA1c levels must be performed every 3 months.
b) During intercurrent illnesses, insulin requirements increase.
c) Microalbuminuria is a complication of diabetes mellitus.
d) Microalbuminuria is reversible with improved blood glucose control.
e) Microalbuminuria ideally should be assessed through assessment of the first voided urine in the morning.

Answers

A1	b, e	**A2**	a, b, d, e
A3	a, c, d, e	**A4**	a, b, c, d, e
A5	a, b, c, d	**A6**	d
A7	a, b, c, d, e		

Chapter Twenty-nine

CHILDHOOD AND ADOLESCENT OBESITY

COMMON SCENARIO

'What do you mean that my child is overweight? I am worried that his shortness of breath is related to asthma – if that were fixed, he would be able to keep up with his friends playing soccer.'

LEARNING OBJECTIVES

- Understand the aetiology of obesity
- Learn to classify obesity
- Recognise the clinical presentation and evaluation of obesity
- Establish the differential diagnosis
- Establish a treatment plan for the obese child
- Develop awareness of the psychosocial impact of obesity on children and adolescents

BACKGROUND

The prevalence of obesity is increasing over the last 3 decades. Currently one-third of the paediatric population is considered to be overweight, with 20% classified as obese.

The aetiology of obesity is multifactorial, with the main factors being genetic, environmental (inclusive of sedentary lifestyle), reduction in exercise and modified dietary habits.

Genetic factors

Parents who are obese are likely to have children who are obese.

Environmental factors

- *Sedentary behaviour.* In the last 2 decades there has been a significant change in the activity levels of children and adolescents. With advances in technology, children's leisure activities now revolve around watching television and playing video games; as a consequence, the time devoted to outdoor activities has lessened. This has also coincided with societal changes where children less readily play adjacent to their homes with their friends but, rather, undertake structured, organised activities. These factors all have combined to a more pervasive sedentary lifestyle.
- *Dietary habits.* With the development of industrialised societies has come a change in the eating habits of populations, which has been associated with the development of obesity. Currently children and adolescents eat large amounts of calorie-dense foods and also have preferences for soft drinks and juices. Calorie-dense foods are palatable, readily available and enjoyable to eat; consequently, children and adolescents are less likely to refrain from eating when advised to do so.

Strategies to problem-solve obesity

When dealing with the obese paediatric patient, determining the aetiology (primary or secondary) and the presence of associated co-morbidity is important.

Obesity in the paediatric population differs from adults, as children and adolescents need to grow. In adolescent years weight doubles and height increases by 20%. The use of body mass index (BMI) alone is not adequate to assess the severity of the obese state. Instead, BMI percentiles for age and sex are more appropriate – these are derived from the UK 1990 reference chart.

Definition of obesity

There is a difference between the epidemiological assessment of obesity and how the issue is defined in a clinical context. Epidemiological studies have used the following parameters to define excessive weight:
- overweight for a child and adolescent is a BMI of >85th centile but <95th centile
- obesity for a child and adolescent is a BMI of >95th centile.

In clinical practice the following parameters are used:
- overweight child or adolescent is a BMI of >91st centile
- obese child or adolescent is a BMI of >98th centile
- severe obese child or adolescent is a BMI of >99.6th centile
- very severe obese child or adolescent is a BMI of >3 standard deviations above the reference mean
- extreme obesity for child or adolescent is a BMI of >4 standard deviations above the reference mean for the standard population.

HISTORY

KEY POINTS			
Weight	When did they start to be concerned about weight? Always been overweight? Previous measurements How concerned are the parents and child?	**Birth history**	Maternal gestational diabetes Intrauterine growth restriction
Dietary history	Meal patterns Snacks Quantity and portion size Typical meal Fast-food intake Intake of fruit and vegetables Types of fluids drunk: fizzy drinks, juice	**Social history**	Meals eaten together as a family What activities do the family enjoy together?
Activity levels	Exercise during day Exercise tolerance Participate in sports Walk to school Amount of time spent watching TV or playing video games	**Impact on child**	Bothered by weight Bullying or teasing at school Poor self-confidence
Family history	Obesity in parents or siblings Diabetes Cardiovascular disease Ethnicity	**Systems review**	Snoring at night Daytime sleepiness Difficulty concentrating at school Limp Knee or ankle pain Abdominal pain Visual disturbance Excessive hair growth Acne Mood disturbance
Medications	Steroids Sodium valproate Risperidone	**Interventions tried**	What have they tried?
Growth and development	Age at onset of puberty Learning difficulties Developmental delay Menorrhagia Are periods regular?	**Past medical history**	Headaches Cranial surgery or irradiation Head trauma Cold intolerance Constipation

EXAMINATION

- Height, weight
- BMI centile
- Dysmorphic features
- Pubertal staging
- Waist circumference (useful in serial follow-up only)
- Pulse rate, blood pressure (use age-appropriate cuff and check age-specific norms)
- Abdominal examination check for liver enlargement
- Skin check for:
  - striae
  - acanthosis nigricans (located in flexures and dorsum of hand)
  - hirsutism
  - intertrigo
- Gait assessment
- Fundoscopy

Red flags

- Short stature
- Intellectual disability
- Dysmorphic features
- Abnormal fundoscopy
- Snoring
- Hepatomegaly

DIFFERENTIAL DIAGNOSIS

Aetiology	Differentiating features
Hypothyroidism	Faltering growth (assess centiles), constipation, reduction in activity, learning difficulties, cold intolerance
Growth hormone deficiency	Short stature
Hypercortisolism	Short stature, purple striae
Hypothalamic damage	Medical history
Prader–Willi's syndrome	Hypotonia
	Developmental delay
	Narrow bifrontal diameter
	Almond shaped palpebral fissures
	Narrow nasal bridge
	Small narrow hands and feet

(continued)

Aetiology	Differentiating features
Cohen's syndrome	Developmental delay, thin arms and legs, high-arched palate, short philtrum
Laurence–Moon–Biedl's syndrome	Developmental delay, poor vision, anosmia, polydactyly, syndactyly, urogenital anomalies
Down's syndrome	Dysmorphic features, short stature
Pseudohypoparathyroidism	Short stature, carpopedal spasm (hypocalcaemia), seizures, developmental delay

INVESTIGATIONS

For children with a BMI above the 97th centile, blood glucose, serum cholesterol (high-density lipoprotein) and triglycerides, and liver function tests should be undertaken.

Full blood count

In children with obesity, iron deficiency is relatively common. While children with obesity have caloric intake, the quality of the foods ingested are variable.

Blood glucose

The information gained from blood glucose is limited. If it is elevated, a glucose tolerance test should be undertaken.

Glucose tolerance test

Altered glucose metabolism occurs in patients with severe obesity, often with a family history of diabetes mellitus, and consequently a glucose tolerance test is warranted.

Lipid profile (cholesterol and triglyceride levels) after an overnight fast

Many obese children and adolescents will have abnormal lipid profiles but appropriate management of their weight will result in normalisation of these abnormalities.

Thyroid function test inclusive of thyroid antibodies

In children with short stature, thyroid function test should be undertaken to exclude hypothyroidism. Thyroid antibodies, if present, suggest an autoimmune aetiology.

Liver function tests

The presence of hepatomegaly in the obese child and adolescent is associated with liver dysfunction with elevation of liver enzymes – in particular, alanine transaminase.

MANAGEMENT PLAN: THREE-STEP APPROACH

1. Clarifying and pitfall avoidance strategies
2. Non-pharmacological approach:
   a) nutritional advice
   b) physical activity
   c) weight management goals
   d) psychosocial advice

3. Pharmacological approach:
   a) drug treatment for obesity
   b) bariatric surgery

Clarifying and pitfall avoidance strategies

- Clarify obesity status. **Rationale**: parents of children and adolescents may not realise that their child is overweight and they may be unaware that the complications of obesity are asymptomatic in the paediatric age range.
- Encouraging change. **Rationale**: dealing with obesity is a family issue, and simply telling a parent that their child is overweight will not result in change. Other strategies, such as motivational interviewing techniques, can be useful in this situation (*see* Chapter 2: Communication).
- Goal setting. **Rationale**: the management goals in paediatric obesity differ from those for adults, and physicians need to have adequate knowledge to address their concerns (*see* Evidence 3) in this area. In the young obese patient, dramatic weight loss is discouraged and weight maintenance is the preferred outcome, while ensuring that growth is preserved. To address the needs of the obese paediatric patient, involvement of a team including physician, dietitian and exercise specialist improves the outcomes (*see* Evidence 2).

Non-pharmacological approach

Nutritional advice

The nutritional advice that is given to families with an obese child or adolescent reflects the changes that must be made by the family as a unit and is not designed for the obese child or adolescent alone. Before offering advice, clarify the eating habits of the family – especially the length of time devoted to meals, the portion sizes offered at mealtimes and the social interaction that occurs. Parents need to support and act as role models for their children.

A meal schedule must be established with minimal snacking between meals. Family meals should not take place in front of the television. (Often it is best to have the television turned off for a specific length of time). At mealtimes water should be drunk rather than sweetened beverages or milk. Fruit and vegetables should be incorporated into the diet. Foods containing complex carbohydrates should be used, rather than those with simple carbohydrates. Low-fat consumption should be encouraged. Portion sizes offered by parents are often too large and need to be reduced. Having a dietitian review this concept with parents is important in reducing caloric intake. Parental role modelling for children is important in modifying family eating habits (*see* Evidence 1).

Physical activity

Prior to instituting any changes, parents should assess the length of time spent watching television and time dedicated to organised sports and to family activities, which should include the child's travel to school, whether they are brought by car, are brought by bus, use a bicycle or walk. It is appropriate to advise parents to restrict television viewing to a maximum of 2 hours per day and to increase the family activity levels. Promoting walking at a moderate to vigorous pace is useful and this should be undertaken by both parents and children as far as is practicable. Evaluate other options to increase activity by promoting walking to school (if practicable) and involvement in sporting activities on a regular basis. Promote the concept of at least 1 hour of activity per day every day and emphasise the concept that all activity counts. To sustain increased activity levels for children, a fun element must be incorporated into the activities. Physicians may want to assess the child's physical activity level and the 6-minute walk test can serve as a useful tool to monitor progress (*see* Evidence 4).

Weight management goals

In children, weight maintenance rather than weight loss is the goal, as normal growth must be preserved. The parents and child need to understand this concept. When reviewing the overweight paediatric patient, all progress, no matter how small, should be acknowledged and patients should not be reprimanded for non-adherence but be encouraged to continue trying.

Psychosocial advice

The impact of obesity on the child and adolescent must be assessed in terms of its social impact. Specific inquiry must address teasing and bullying. Adolescents who are losing weight may be subject to bullying (*see* Evidence 5) and strategies to address this must be discussed with them.

Pharmacological approach

Drug treatment for obesity

Drug therapy (orlistat) in for paediatric obesity is limited to those with morbid obesity and is moderately successful (*see* Evidence 6). A paediatrician with a special interest in obesity should undertake the treatment and follow-up.

Bariatric surgery

Surgery for the obese adolescent is now being considered for some patients. Selection criteria include (a) BMI >35 with co-morbidities of type 2 diabetes, moderate or severe obstructive sleep apnoea, pseudotumour cerebri, severe non-alcoholic steatohepatitis and (b) BMI >40 with co-morbidities of mild obstructive sleep apnoea, hypertension, insulin resistance, glucose intolerance, abnormal lipid profile and impaired quality of life. The procedure of choice is the sleeve gastrectomy and adjustable gastric banding. While the initial results are encouraging, only a few studies have been performed in adolescents; however, it is likely to become an option for those obese patients who have failed medical treatment.

FOLLOW-UP

Follow up should be on a 3-monthly basis, with a focus on weight maintenance, evaluation of parental modelled behaviour and assessment of exercise undertaken.

WHEN TO REFER?

- The majority of patients with obesity can be managed in primary care.
- Only about 2% of obese patients have an underlying pathology (hypothyroidism, growth hormone deficiency, hypercortisolism, hypothalamic damage and the outlined syndromes) and require referral.
- Obese patients with complications should also be referred (hepatomegaly with liver dysfunction, evidence of diabetes mellitus, raised intracranial pressure, orthopaedic problems, snoring that may be related to sleep apnoea).

CLARIFICATION STATEMENTS FOR PARENTAL MISCONCEPTIONS

'What is wrong with giving him juice? After all, it is natural.'

The issue is not whether it is natural but, rather, it is related to the caloric intake. In the treatment of the obese child the aim is to reduce the amount of simple carbohydrate that the child ingests. Substituting water for juice is an appropriate strategy.

'I know my child is overweight. What diet should I use?'

In children and adolescents with obesity, dieting is only part of the solution, in conjunction with exercise and a reduction in sedentary behaviour. Severe food restriction to achieve weight loss is not good clinical practice, as the weight loss is rarely maintained and the weight problem is addressed utilising only one strategy.

'I know he is overweight, but he looks healthy. Why make a big deal about it?'

Many of the complications of obesity are subclinical in children and adolescents but will become manifest over time. We try to prevent the development of problems rather than attempt corrective action once they have occurred. Before you decide about doing anything about obesity, ask yourself, is this how your child wants things to be?

SUMMARY PRACTICE POINTS

- Obesity in the paediatric patient is defined in terms of BMI centiles, not BMI alone.
- Waist circumference should not be used as a primary indicator of obesity assessment in the paediatric patient.

- Secondary causes, while uncommon, are recognised if attention is focused on height, developmental assessment and presence of dysmorphic features.
- Use motivational interviewing to induce change even if the parents and patient are not ready.
- Weight maintenance rather than weight loss should be the goal.
- Recognise the psychosocial impact of obesity and ask specifically about teasing and bullying.
- Be realistic in the goal setting with the family.

EVALUATING THE EVIDENCE

Evidence 1	
Theme E1	*The impact of dietary modification and exercise in obese children*
Question	What is the impact of parent diet modification and exercise in children with obesity?
Design	Randomised controlled trial
Level of evidence	Jadad 3
Setting	Department of paediatrics in two academic medical centres, Australia
Participants	Prepubertal children, aged 5.5–9.9 years, who were overweight, as defined by the International Obesity Task Force cut-off points, were eligible for enrolment.
Intervention	This study had three intervention arms: a parent-centred dietary modification programme (the diet group), a child-centred physical activity skill development programme (the activity group) and a combination of both (the diet and activity group). The programmes were of 6 months' duration.
Outcomes	The primary outcome measure was change in the body mass index z-score at 2 years.
Main results	Five hundred and five were assessed for eligibility, of whom 319 were eligible, with 206 consenting to enrolment and being randomised (73 to physical activity, 63 to diet and 70 to physical activity and diet). Sixty-three (86%) of the activity group, 42 (66.6%) of the diet group and 60 (85.6%) of activity and diet group completed the study. The body mass index z-score change from baseline to 2 years for activity was −0.19 (−0.30 to −0.07), for diet was −0.35 (−0.48 to −0.22) and for diet and activity was −0.24 (−0.35 to −0.13).
Conclusion	The greatest effects were achieved from the parent-centred diet programme. The primary hypothesis was that the combination of diet and activity would produce the most effect.
Commentary	This study was designed to avoid the pitfalls of previous studies of the overweight and their families, in that the numbers enrolled were large, the follow-up period was 2 years (studies suggest that weight loss is not maintained after 1 year) and dropouts were accounted for. All three groups achieved clinically important gains and it would have been unethical to use a control group, especially for a 2-year period where overweight children and their families would have been denied care. This study underscores the important role that parents play in facilitating behavioural change in their prepubertal children and reducing their caloric intake.
Reference	Collins CE, Okely AD, Morgan PJ, *et al.* Parent diet modification, child activity, or both in obese children: an RCT. *Pediatrics.* 2011; **127**(4): 619–27.

Evidence 2

Theme E2	Modifying models of obesity care
Question	Can a hospital-based childhood obesity clinic be transferred to primary care?
Design	Randomised controlled trial
Level of evidence	Jadad 1
Setting	Hospital-based paediatric department and primary care centre, England
Participants	Children and adolescents aged 5–16 years, with a body mass index (BMI) ≥98th centile and referred by their family doctors were eligible for inclusion.
Intervention	Participants were randomised to receive five visits over a 1-year period, either at a hospital-based childhood obesity clinic with a multidisciplinary team (doctor, specialist obesity nurse, dietitian and exercise specialist) or a nurse-led clinic in primary care (supported by an exercise specialist and dietitian). The nurses in the primary care centres were mentored initially by the hospital-based multidisciplinary team.
Outcomes	The primary outcome was the measured change in BMI standard deviation scores at 12 months.
Main results	One hundred and fifty-two patients were eligible, having been referred by their family doctors, but 31 (20%) were screened out and 45 (30%) declined to participate. Seventy-six patients were randomised, and baseline data were available on 68: 42 in primary care, with 26 (69%) completing the study, and 26 in the hospital clinic, with 23 (88.4%) completing the study. The mean change in BMI standard deviation scores was −0.17 (95% confidence interval (CI): −0.27 to −0.07) for those in primary care and −0.15 (95% CI: −0.26 to −0.05) for the hospital group.
Conclusion	Primary care settings have the potential to be effective in the management of child obesity and are acceptable to parents.
Commentary	This study addresses the transfer of hospital-based obesity clinics for children to the community. The nurse-led approach was successful when compared with the hospital setting and represents a potential strategy to address the childhood obesity. An important aspect of this study was the high rate of withdrawal (29; 43%), with many parents highlighting poor motivation where parents struggled to motivate and positively influence their children between visits and the development of parent–child conflict as a consequence. Associated with this (for some families) was the belief the attendance was optional and that obesity has few medical consequences.
Reference	Banks J, Sharp DJ, Hunt LP, *et al.* Evaluating the transferability of a hospital-based childhood obesity clinic to primary care: a randomised controlled trial. *Br J Gen Pract.* 2012; **62**(594): e6–12.

Evidence 3	
Theme E3	**Paediatricians and obesity**
Question	Are paediatricians competent to address the needs of the overweight or obese child?
Design	Online survey of Australian paediatricians' self-perceived competence and training in management of obesity, with a prospective patient level practice audit.
Level of evidence	
Setting	Secondary care centres, Australia
Participants	Paediatricians providing secondary care
Intervention	National audit of paediatric practice in outpatient settings for 2 weeks or evaluating 100 consecutive patients' visits, whichever was reached first
Outcomes	The primary outcomes were 1) a survey: self-reported competencies, training in and use of clinical skills in obesity and its co-morbidities, and 2) an audit that assessed paediatricians' reported assessment of each child's height, weight, age, sex and diagnoses including overweight/obesity.
Main results	Of 166 (44.7%) paediatricians, most felt very or quite competent in assessing (89%) and managing (68%) obesity, but few (20) felt that they would make a difference. Perceived competency management of co-morbidities were obstructive sleep apnoea (37.9%), depression (34.3%), bullying and social difficulties (33%), insulin resistance (19.2%), hypertension (27.1%), fatty liver (13.2%), dyslipidaemia (<12%). The audit of 200 paediatricians resulted in 8345 patient encounters being assessed – height and weight were recorded in 66%. Based on the audit data, of 296 children who would have been assessed as being overweight or obese, only 118 (39.9%) were similarly classified by the paediatrician.
	Many paediatricians (71%) were interested in participating in obesity research, with two-thirds expressing a specific interest in obesity-related co-morbidities.
Conclusion	There is a clear need for improved paediatrician training in obesity management, but this alone will not improve outcomes for the overweight or obese child.
Commentary	Despite the recognition of long-term complications of obesity in children, less than 2% of overweight or obese Australian children receive help with weight management when they attend primary care services, despite national guidelines existing for over a decade. While most agree the issue must be addressed, there is no effective programme that can address all aspects of this issue, further increasing the challenge for the paediatrician. For the practising clinician, dealing with the individual family with an overweight or obese child, knowledge is important but addressing the issue in a holistic fashion is required, and the involvement of dietitians and exercise specialists. Motivating the child and family to persevere is often required and the skills of motivational interviewing are needed (*see* Chapter 2: Communication).
Reference	Wake M, Campbell MW, Turner M, *et al*. How training affects Australian paediatricians' management of obesity. *Arch Dis Child*. 2013; **98**(1): 3–8.

Evidence 4	
Theme E4	*Exercise capacity in the obese child*
Question	Does exercise capacity improve in obese children with weight reduction?
Design	Cohort study
Level of evidence	
Setting	Department of paediatrics, academic medical centre, Germany
Participants	Overweight children and adolescents with a body mass index above the 85th centile were eligible for enrolment to participate in a 3-week residential program.
Intervention	The primary intervention was a residential weight loss programme consisting of regular physical exercise, moderate dietary restriction (1400–1600 kcal/day), and comprehensive dietary and behavioural support.
Outcomes	The primary outcome in this study was the change in distance walked in the 6MWT (6-minute walk test). This was compared with the results of age- and sex-matched normal-weight children and adolescents (n = 353).
Main results	One hundred and thirty-two overweight children and adolescents were eligible, of whom 113 completed the study and their mean age was 12.9 years (range 8–17 years). The pre-intervention 6MWT for the overweight group was 631 ± 88 m versus 675 ± 70 m for control group. The post-intervention 6MWT was 667 ± 90 m ($P < 0.001$). Participants reduced their body weight from 80.9 ± 19.8 kg to 75.6 ± 19 kg, and body mass index centiles from $98.2\% \pm 2.1\%$ to $96\% \pm 3.8\%$.
Conclusion	The 6MWT improved during the weight reduction process and represents a useful and practical tool to assess exercise performance in overweight children.
Commentary	With the publication of a reference range, the 6MWT is a valuable and practical tool to measure exercise performance in overweight children to a sub-maximal level. It can be used by the individual child to monitor progress and to serve as a marker of exercise tolerance.
Reference	Geiger R, Willeit J, Rummel M, *et al*. Six-minute walk distance in overweight children and adolesents: effects of a weight-reducing program. *J Pediatr.* 2011; **158**(3): 447–51.

Evidence 5	
Theme E5	**The social impact of being overweight and obese in adolescents**
Question	What are the social impacts of being overweight or obese?
Design	Web-based questionnaire
Level of evidence	
Setting	Adolescents who had attended two weight loss camps, the United States
Participants	Adolescents aged 14–18 years who had attended one of two weight loss camps were invited to participate in an online survey to assess their experiences with weight-based victimisation.
Intervention	The survey explored provided a definition of bullying, and then explored the participants' experiences in terms of frequency, perpetrators, location and methods employed. Perceived parental weight status was also assessed as research, suggesting a negative relationship between maternal BMI and child self-esteem and adaptive skills.
Outcomes	The reported reasons for being bullied or teased, the perpetrators of weight-based victimisation and the different forms of weight-based bullying or teasing.
Main results	Three hundred and sixty-one adolescents responded: 44% male, 40% female and 16% not reported. Most participants self-reported as white (71%), with the remaining 18% black/African/American, 6% Latin/Hispanic, 2% Asian/Pacific Islander and 3% others. While most participants reported being teased or bullied in relation to their weight, for 21% it was very often. For those who experienced bullying or teasing very often, it was perpetrated by a peer (30%), friend (8%), unknown (15%), physical education teacher (6%), parent (11%) and a teacher (3%) and consisted of verbal teasing (28%), relational victimisation (30%), cyberbullying (17%) and physical aggression (17%).
Conclusion	Weight loss victimisation is a prevalent experience for weight loss treatment seeking youth, even when they are no longer overweight.
Commentary	The response rate to this survey seems low but the authors indicate that it is acceptable for Internet-based surveys. The participants for this study had attended camps specifically designed to achieve weight loss, and while data are provided in relation to ethnicity, no socio-economic data are provided. The self-reported format may introduce a bias in the reporting of victimisation, but the message is clear: the overweight adolescent experiences weight-based torment and the authors provide data related to frequency, perpetrators and methods, which can be useful in discussions with an adolescent or which can be introduced when assessing the psychosocial impact of being overweight or obese. Having these data at hand can allow for potential strategies for this bullying or teasing to be developed.
Reference	Puhl RM, Peterson JL, Luedicke J. Weight-based victimization: bullying experiences of weight loss treatment-seeking youth. *Pediatrics*. 2013; **131**(1): e1–9.

Evidence 6	
Theme E6	***Drug therapy for adolescent obesity***
Question	How effective is orlistat in the treatment of the obese adolescent?
Design	Randomised controlled trial
Level of evidence	Jadad 5
Setting	Thirty-two academic medical centres, Canada and the United States
Participants	Adolescents aged 12–16 years who had a body mass index (BMI) 2 units above the 95th percentile were eligible for inclusion. Those with a BMI of >44% were excluded.
Intervention	Participants received a 120 mg dose of orlistat three times a day or placebo in conjunction with a mildly hypocaloric diet (with the aim to secure weight loss of 0.5–1 kg/week), exercise and behavioural therapy for a 1-year period.
Outcomes	The primary outcome was a reduction in body mass index (BMI) at 1 year.
Main results	Five hundred and eighty-eight adolescents were screened, with 539 meeting the inclusion criteria: 182 were assigned to the placebo group, with 117 (65) completing the study, compared with 357 assigned to the orlistat group, with 232 (66%) completing the study. The primary outcome in the placebo group was a gain in BMI of 0.31 compared with a BMI loss of 0.55 in the orlistat group. A loss of BMI of ≥5% was achieved in 15.7% of the placebo group, compared with 26.5% in the orlistat group (absolute risk reduction (ARR) = 10.5%; number needed to treat (NNT) = 11). A BMI reduction of ≥10% occurred in 4.5% of the placebo group, compared with 13.3% of the orlistat group (ARR = 8.8%; NNT = 13). Gastrointestinal side effects included fat (oily) stool, 50.3%; oily spotting, 29%; oily evacuation, 23.3%; abdominal pain, 21.9%; faecal urgency, 20.7%. There were no clinically relevant non-gastrointestinal side effects recorded.
Conclusion	Orlistat was effective in reducing BMI in obese adolescents when combined with a hypocaloric diet and a behavioural programme.
Commentary	Orlistat is a gastrointestinal tract lipase inhibitor that decreases fat absorption by 30%.
Reference	Chanoione JP, Hampl S, Jensen C, *et al.* Effects of orlistat on weight and body composition in obese adolescents: a randomized controlled trial. *JAMA.* 2005; **293**(23): 2873–83.

OBESITY: MULTIPLE-CHOICE QUESTIONS

Q1 Which of the following statements is/are true?
   a) Seven per cent of 7-year-olds are obese.
   b) Obese parents are likely to have obese children.
   c) Sedentary behaviour is an important risk factor for obesity.
   d) Four per cent of obese children have an organic aetiology for their obesity.
   e) Eating non-processed foods contributes to obesity.

Q2 Which of the following statements is/are true?
   a) Iron deficiency is common in obese children.
   b) Liver function test abnormalities are found in obese adolescents.
   c) Lipid profiles are abnormal in obese adolescents.
   d) Calprotectin levels are elevated in 5% of obese adolescents.
   e) Creatine phosphokinase levels are elevated in 14% of adolescents.

Q3 Which of the following medications induce weight gain?
   a) Risperidone
   b) Sodium valproate
   c) Oral steroids
   d) Methotrexate
   e) Megace

Q4 In treating the obese child, which of the following strategies is/are helpful?
   a) Reduce portion size
   b) Reduce complex carbohydrate intake
   c) Ask parents to role model for the child
   d) Reduce television viewing
   e) Commence multivitamins

Q5 Complications of obesity include which of the following?
   a) Depression
   b) Obstructive sleep apnoea
   c) Insulin resistance
   d) Hepatomegaly
   e) Raised intracranial pressure

Q6 Clinical findings in the obese adolescent include which of the following?
   a) Gait abnormalities
   b) Acanthosis nigricans
   c) Psoriasis
   d) Fundoscopic abnormalities
   e) Hirsutism

Q7 Recognised causes of obesity include which of the following?
   a) Hypothyroidism
   b) Pseudohypoparathyroidism
   c) Cohen's syndrome
   d) Prader–Willi's syndrome
   e) Adrenal insufficiency

Q8 Features of Prader–Willi's syndrome include which of the following?
  a) Hypotonia
  b) Developmental delay
  c) Early failure to thrive
  d) Small, narrow hands
  e) Macroglossia

Q9 Features of hypothyroidism include which of the following?
  a) Faltering growth
  b) Learning difficulties
  c) Deafness
  d) Constipation
  e) Vaginal bleeding (in girls)

Q10 Which of the following statements is/are correct?
  a) Paediatricians feel competent to address childhood obesity.
  b) Hospital-based clinics are more effective than community clinics.
  c) Adolescents who achieve weight loss are subjected to bullying.
  d) Orlistat use is an effective long-term treatment in the obese adolescent.
  e) Obese patients who achieve rapid weight loss initially, have a better outcome than those who reduce weight consistently.

Answers

A1	b, c	**A2**	a, b, c
A3	a, b, c, e	**A4**	a, c, d
A5	a, b, c, d, e	**A6**	a, b, d, e
A7	a, b, c, d	**A8**	a, b, c, d
A9	a, b, d, e	**A10**	a, c

Chapter Thirty

THE CHILD WITH AN ACUTE RASH

COMMON SCENARIO

'She's had a fever for the past few days, but I've been managing to control it with paracetamol. This evening she just broke out all over in a rash.'

LEARNING OBJECTIVES

- Identify common exanthems presenting in childhood
- Recognise serious and potentially life-threatening acute rashes
- Explain what investigations are required

BACKGROUND

Acute rashes are extremely common in childhood and a common reason for presentation to primary care physicians and emergency departments. The differential for acute rashes in children is extensive. Most acute rashes are benign and self-limiting. This chapter provides an overview of common rashes and highlights the important and potentially serious and life-threatening diseases that should not be missed.

VIRAL EXANTHEMS

An exanthem is any eruptive skin rash that may be associated with fever or other systemic symptoms. Exanthem comes from the Greek word *exanthema*, meaning 'a breaking out'. They are usually caused by viruses but may also occur secondary to bacteria and drugs. Many of the common exanthems have distinct patterns of rashes or symptoms. Viral exanthems are more common in children, with drug eruptions occurring more frequently in adults. A careful history and examination can help establish the diagnosis in most cases.

Parvovirus B19 (slapped cheek syndrome)

Parvovirus B19 is transmitted by the respiratory route; however, vertical and parenteral transmission can also occur. It commonly occurs in children 4–10 years of age. In 20% of cases the virus is asymptomatic. It is a biphasic illness; in week 1 patients may experience fever, malaise, headache and myalgia, and they then develop an erythematous rash, which resembles the appearance of a 'slapped cheek' on the face, with sparing of the nasal bridge and the periorbital region. As the facial rash fades, an erythematous, reticular-like rash spreads to involve the trunk and limb. The disease is self-resolving. In rare cases, complications such as arthralgia and arthritis may occur. In patients with chronic haemolytic anaemias the virus can cause an aplastic crisis, as it replicates in erythroid precursors. In pregnancy it can lead to foetal demise or hydrops foetalis.

Human herpesvirus 6 (roseola infantum)

The incubation period is 9 days. The mode of transmission is unknown, but it is likely due to nasopharyngeal secretions. Children may be asymptomatic, developing an acute febrile illness without a rash. With roseola infantum (also known as exanthema subitum or sixth disease), children develop a high fever lasting 3–4 days. They generally appear well and may have mild upper respiratory tract symptoms. Once the fever subsides, they develop a generalised macular rash. By the age of 2, almost 100% of children have developed antibodies to the virus. It is a common cause of febrile convulsions. It has been associated with aseptic meningitis, encephalopathy hepatitis, an infectious mononucleosis-like syndrome and haemotological malignancies.

Varicella zoster (chickenpox)

Varicella is transmitted by respiratory droplets, and the incubation period is 14 days. Children develop fever and a rash. The rash initially starts on the scalp and trunk and spreads centrifugally. The rash evolves from maculopapular lesions into vesicles, which then crust over. Complications include secondary bacterial infection with streptococcus and staphylococcus. Rarer complications include cerebellar ataxia encephalitis, purpura fulminans and stroke. Immunocompromised children are at risk of developing haemorrhagic lesions, pneumonitis, pancreatitis, hepatitis, progressive and disseminated disease and disseminated intravascular coagulation.

Mumps

The incubation period is 14–21 days. With routine vaccination, the incidence has dropped dramatically. Children develop fever, malaise and parotitis, which may initially be unilateral. They may complain of an earache or pain on eating or drinking. Children are infectious for 7 days after the onset of parotid swelling. Complications include orchitis, meningoencephalitis and unilateral hearing loss, which is usually mild and transient.

Rubella

The incubation period is 14–21 days. It is spread through direct or droplet contact from nasopharyngeal secretions. With routine vaccination, the incidence has dropped dramatically. Children are infectious a week before the onset of the rash until 3–5 days after the rash. Fifty per cent of cases are asymptomatic. After a prodromal low-grade fever, headache and upper respiratory tract symptoms, a maculopapular rash develops, initially on the face and then spreading centrifugally. The rash spreads quickly covering the body within 24 hours. It fades in 3–5 days, clearing from the head and neck first. Suboccipital and post-auricular lymphadenopathy can be found. Petechiae can be found on the soft palate and uvula (Forchheimer's sign). Complications are rare and include arthritis, encephalitis, myocarditis and thrombocytopenia. Infection in the first trimester can cause foetal demise or congenital rubella syndrome (sensorineural hearing loss, mental retardation, eye abnormalities and congenital heart disease).

Measles

The incubation period is 10–14 days. Children are infectious 1–2 days before the prodrome to 4 days after the onset of the rash. With routine vaccination, the incidence has dropped dramatically. Children are generally miserable with a fever, conjunctivitis coryza, and cough; 7–11 days after the prodrome, the rash begins behind the ears and then spreads cephalocaudally and centrifugally. It is initially maculopapular and then becomes blotchy and confluent. After 3–4 days it begins to spread and may desquamate. Koplik's spots (grey-white papules on the buccal mucosa) can be found in the mouth and precede the onset of the rash. Generalised lymphadenopathy can be found on examination. Respiratory complications include pneumonia, tracheitis, otitis media and a bronchiolitic-type illness. Rarer complications include encephalitis and subacute sclerosing panencephalitis. Immunocompromised patients are at increased risk of developing giant cell pneumonitis and encephalitis. Diarrhoea is a common feature in third-world countries, where the mortality rate is high.

Scarlet fever

Scarlet fever is caused by group A beta-haemolytic streptococcus. The incubation period is 2–4 days. There is a sudden onset of fever associated with marked pharyngitis with exudate, malaise and headache. A finely punctate sandpaper-like rash develops 12–48 hours after the onset of fever. Pastia lines (red streaks) can develop in skin creases. Children have a characteristic strawberry-like tongue associated with circumoral pallor. Purulent complications include otitis media, sinusitis, peritonsillar or retropharyngeal abscess and cervical adenitis. Non-suppurative complications include acute glomerulonephritis and rheumatic fever.

Herpes simplex virus

Manifestations depend on the portal of entry and host factors, including age, immunity and presence of eczema. Herpes simplex virus (HSV) type 1 usually occurs in children, with type 2 infection occurring after puberty. Type 2 infection is usually sexually transmitted and causes genital lesions. HSV type 1 infection in children is usually asymptomatic or non-specific. Herpetic gingivostomatitis is the commonest type of symptomatic herpetic infection occurring in children aged 1–5 years. It presents with painful oral blisters that ulcerate. It is associated with a high fever. Eating and drinking is painful and excessive drooling is commonly seen. The fever generally lasts 3–5 days, with complete resolution of symptoms within 2 weeks. Recurrent HSV infection can cause 'cold sores', which present with grouped vesicles on an erythematous base around the mouth and nose. Vesicles may appear pustular (white or yellow) or erosions may only be seen.

Hand, foot and mouth disease

Hand, foot and mouth disease is caused by Coxsackie A virus. It is highly contagious and commonly occurs during the summer months. Children develop painful vesicular lesions on the hands, feet, mouth and tongue. Systemic features are mild and include a low-grade fever and malaise. Oral lesions resolve spontaneously in 5–7 days.

Gianotti–Crosti's syndrome (papular acrodermatitis of childhood)

Gianotti–Crosti's syndrome most commonly affects children aged 1–6 years. Several viruses have been implicated, including hepatatis B, Epstein–Barr, enteroviruses, echovirus and respiratory syncytial virus. A prodrome of fever and upper respiratory tract symptoms is followed by the development of an erythematous papular rash primarily affecting the face, extremities and buttocks, with sparing of the trunk. It typically resolves in 2–3 weeks but may persist for up to 8 weeks.

Epstein–Barr Virus

Epstein–Barr virus, also know as 'glandular fever' typically affects adolescents. Typically, they develop a fever associated with lymphadenopathy and pharyngitis. Palatal petechia can be found. In approximately 10% of cases, a generalised maculopapular rash develops, initially on the trunk and upper arms, but then spreads to involve the face and forearms. If treated with beta-lactamase antibiotics, an intense, itchy morbilliform rash breaks out on the extensor surfaces.

Papular purpuric gloves and socks syndrome

Papular purpuric gloves and socks syndrome presents as painful, pruritic, symmetrical purpuric erythema and petechiae of the hands and feet in a 'glove and stocking' distribution. There may be associated localised oedema, low-grade fever and oral lesions. The aetiology is unclear and many viruses have been implicated. It is self-limiting, with resolution of symptoms in 1–2 weeks.

NON-PETECHIAL RASH IN THE UNWELL CHILD

Kawasaki's disease

Kawasaki's disease is a diagnosis of exclusion. The criteria for diagnosis are fever lasting for 5 or more days plus four of the following features:

- pleomorphic rash that is of truncal distribution
- involvement of the extremities: erythema, oedema, pain and later desquamation
- mucous membrane injection: strawberry tongue, cracked dry lips, inflammation of the urinary meatus
- cervical lymphadenopathy
- non-purulent conjunctivitis.

One of the most serious complications of Kawasaki's disease is the development of coronary artery aneurysms, leading to coronary thrombosis and acute myocardial infarctions. Aneurysms occur in 30% of untreated cases. Aseptic meningitis, sterile pyuria, hydrops of the gallbladder and hepatitis can also occur.

Staphylococcal toxic shock syndrome

Features of toxic shock syndrome include a high fever, vomiting, abdominal pain, severe muscle ache and headache, profuse watery diarrhoea and rash with rapid progression to severe shock and end organ dysfunction. It is due to the toxic shock syndrome toxin-1 produced by *Staphylococcus aureus*.

The criteria for diagnosis are:

- fever >38°C
- diffuse macular erythroderma
- desquamation 1–2 weeks after onset of illness
- hypotension
- involvement of three or more organs.

Staphylococcal scalded skin syndrome

Staphylococcal scalded skin syndrome is caused by exotoxin-producing *S. aureus*. The toxin causes an erythematous rash and separation of the dermis beneath the granular cell layer, with bullae formation and sheet-like desquamation. Areas of epidermis separate on gentle pressure (Nikolsky's sign), leaving denuded areas of skin that subsequently heal without scarring. There is associated general malaise, irritability, skin tenderness and a fever may or may not be present. It usually presents in children under 5 years of age. In neonates, the lesions are commonly found on the perineum and periumbilically. In toddlers, the extremities are more likely to be affected.

Stevens–Johnson syndrome and toxic epidermal necrolysis

Erythema multiforme, Stevens–Johnson syndrome (SJS) and toxic epidermal necrolysis (TEN) are considered a spectrum of the same condition, with varying degrees of skin and mucosal involvement. TEN is at the extreme end and associated with high morbidity and mortality. In SJS and TEN there is often a prodromal illness with fever, flu-like symptoms or skin tenderness. Drugs are the most common aetiological agents. Erythematous macules evolve into flaccid blister and extensive areas of epidermal detachment, with a positive Nikolsky's sign. Involvement of the oral, genital or ocular mucosa occurs in over 90% of cases. In SJS less than 10% of the body surface area is involved and in TEN more than 30% is involved.

Meningococcal disease

(*See* Chapter 3 regarding the full presentation and management of meningococcal disease.)

In a child presenting with fever, the presence of purpura is highly predictive of meningococcal disease and should be treated as an emergency. Petechiae alone are less predictive but must be taken seriously, especially if there are other features of septicaemia. Onset of a rash in meningococcal disease occurs at a median of 8 hours after the start of the illness in babies. Meningococcal rashes can look different on different skin types and can be difficult to see on dark skin. Purpura fulminans is a severe complication of meningococcal disease occurring in approximately 15%–25% of those with meningococcemia. It is characterised by the acute onset of cutaneous haemorrhage and necrosis due to vascular thrombosis and disseminated intravascular coagulopathy.

SKIN INFECTIONS
Cellulitis

Cellulitis is an infection of the dermis. It presents as a spreading erythematous tender hot plaque. Group A streptococcus and staphylococcus are the commonest causative organisms. Predisposing factors include skin abrasions or lacerations, burns and eczematous skin. However, a portal of entry for infection is often not found.

Erysipelas

Erysipelas is a superficial cellulitis with marked dermal lymphatic involvement. Group A streptococcus is the main causative organism. It presents as erythematous raised plaques with sharply defined borders.

Impetigo

Impetigo is a common skin infection in children. It is highly contagious and spread by close contact. The majority of cases are secondary to *S. aureus*. It presents as papules and plaques with overlying honey-coloured crusts, most commonly around the nose and angles of the mouth. Bullous forms of impetigo can also occur. Systemic symptoms are not seen.

DISEASE CAUSING ACUTE PETECHIAL RASHES

Idiopathic thrombocytopenic purpura

Idiopathic thrombocytopenic purpura (ITP) is a benign self-limiting illness often preceded by a viral upper respiratory tract infection. It presents with cutaneous and mucosal bleeding in an otherwise healthy, afebrile child with no systemic features. Life-threatening bleeding and intracranial haemorrhage are rare. The peak incidence is between 1 and 5 years of age. Chronic ITP occurs in 5%–10% of cases.

Henoch–Schönlein purpura

Henoch–Schönlein purpura (HSP) is diffuse, self-limiting IgA-mediated vasculitis affecting small vessels and capillaries. It is the commonest vasculitis in children. The hallmark of the disease is non-thrombocytopenic purpura. It is commonly preceded by a viral infection. There is multisystem involvement of the skin, joints, kidneys and gastrointestinal tract. Children present with a symmetrical purpuric rash on the extensor surface of the limbs and buttocks, and these are the first signs in 50% of cases. The trunk is usually spared.

Other differentials to be considered	
Acute leukaemia	More insidious onset, associated lymphadenopathy, hepatosplenomegaly, pallor
Petechiae due to viral infections	Well child, well perfused, no signs of shock
Petechiae due to mechanical causes	Well child, history of vomiting or coughing
	Petechiae in superior vena cava distribution (head and neck)
Haemolytic-uraemic syndrome	Bloody diarrhoea, abdominal pain, lethargy, dehydration, pallor, hypertension

URTICARIAL RASHES

Urticarial rashes are common in children. Urticaria is caused by degranulation of mast cells with releases of histamine, causing vasodilation and increased capillary permeability. Angioedema may also occur. Anaphylaxis is the sudden onset of urticaria, angioedema, dyspnoea and hypotension and is a medical emergency. Lesions can vary in size from small papules to larger raised plaques that coalesce. Lesions typically appear within minutes and fade over a few hours. They are intensely pruritic. Urticaria can be acute (<6 weeks) or chronic (>6 weeks). There are two main classifications of urticaria: ordinary (which can be acute or chronic) and physical. Most cases of ordinary urticaria are idiopathic. Acute urticaria is more likely to have an identifiable cause than chronic urticaria. Urticaria can occur due to drugs, infections, foods, bites and bee stings. Physical urticaria occurs in localised areas after contact with a stimulus. Dermatographism is the most common form, triggered by firm scratching of the skin. Physical urticaria may also be triggered by pressure, heat, cold, vibrations, sunlight and friction.

HISTORY

KEY POINTS				
Rash	Time of onset Description Pattern Distribution Progression Pruritus Previous similar rash	**Drugs and allergies**	Recent antibiotics Prescribed drugs Over-the-counter medication Herbal remedies Food allergies Contact allergies Bites or bee stings	**❢ Red flags** History of infectious disease outbreak in the community, for example measles, chickenpox, parvoviral infections High fever, maculopapapular rash Progressive bruising Irritability with a rash Immunodeficiency state in a child
Fever	Onset in relation to rash Pattern Use of antipyretics Response to antipyretics	**Family history**	Family members with similar symptoms or rash Bleeding or thrombotic disorders	
Feeding and fluid intake	Vomiting Diarrhoea Anorexia Fluid intake Lethargy Decreased urine output	**Vaccination**	Up to date	
Associated symptoms	Pain Headache Neck stiffness Photophobia Upper respiratory tract symptoms Joint swelling or stiffness Myalgia	**Social history**	Sick contacts School or crèche outbreaks Contact with pregnant women Recent travel	
General health and development	Recent weight loss Lethargy Recurrent infection Night sweats	**Past medical history**	Immunodeficiency Bleeding or thrombotic disorder	
Treatments tried	Antihistamine use Topical treatments			

EXAMINATION

Glasgow Coma Scale score and vital signs including temperature should be assessed.

- Skin examination: rash morphology, colour, configuration of lesion, distribution
- Look for meningism (neck stiffness, photophobia, nuchal rigidity, positive Kernig's sign and Brudzinski's sign)
- Examine oral cavity for blisters or erosions
- Examine for lymphadenopathy, hepatosplenomegaly or anaemia
- Signs of dehydration or poor perfusion
- Signs of viral upper respiratory tract infection
- Respiratory exam: dyspnoea, wheeze, stridor

Red flags

- Meningism
- Respiratory distress
- Signs of shock or septicaemia
- Moderate to severe dehydration
- Desquamation
- Features of Kawasaki's disease
- Hepatosplenomegaly and lymphadenopathy

INVESTIGATIONS

If Kawasaki's disease is suspected, what investigations should be performed?

There is no diagnostic test for Kawasaki's disease. The diagnosis is made clinically if the criteria are fulfilled and other illnesses are ruled out. Full blood count (FBC), C-reactive protein (CRP), erythrocyte sedimentation rate, throat swab and blood cultures should be taken. Inflammatory markers are raised in the first 2 weeks of the illness; there may be a leukocytosis with a left shift and after the tenth day of the illness thrombocytosis may be found. Values return to normal within 6–8 weeks. A cardiac echo should be performed during the acute phase of the illness and after 6 weeks.

If ITP is suspected, what investigations should be performed?

An FBC and blood film should be taken. Thrombocytopenia is usually the only abnormality detected. The blood film should show no morphological abnormalities in the red or white blood cells. Platelets are often large. A bone marrow biopsy is required if there is doubt about the diagnosis (i.e. if there is a palpable spleen) or leukaemic infiltration is suspected.

If HSP is suspected, what investigations should be performed?

HSP is a clinical diagnosis; the purpose of laboratory investigations is to exclude other causes and assess the degree of renal involvement. An FBC, coagulation profile, renal, liver and bone profile should be performed. Urinalysis should be performed to check for haematuria and proteinuria. If present, an early-morning protein to creatinine ratio should be checked.

MANAGEMENT PLAN: TWO-STEP APPROACH

1. Clarifying and pitfall avoidance strategies:
   a) parents
   b) doctor
2. Management of specific clinical illnesses:
   a) exanthems
   b) Kawasaki's disease
   c) skin infections
   d) urticaria
   e) Henoch–Schönlein purpura
   f) idiopathic thrombocytopenic purpura

Clarifying and pitfall avoidance strategies

Parents

- Explain the concept of a close contact. **Rationale**: A close contact is someone who has been in proximity to the index case for a period of time that results in a high risk of contacting the diseae. Always ask about household contact less than 2 years, childcare or school contacts within the incubation period of an illness and those exposed to direct exposure to secretions.
- Complications of immunisation. **Rationale**: Complications of vaccination are less frequent than those related to the infection that they aim to prevent. Encephalitis occurs in 1 in 1 000 000 vaccinated children. One in 2000 children who develop measles will develop encephalitis, of whom 1 in 10 will die and 4 in 10 will have permanent brain damage.

Doctor

- The immunisation strategy:
  - in infants, encourage breastfeeding or give a sweet-tasting drink to reduce pain
  - give the least painful injection first if a series of injections are being given
  - for intramuscular injections, do not aspirate prior to injection
  - if the child is over 4 years, rub or stroke the injection site prior to injection
  - suggest to the parent the use of distraction techniques
  - *do not say*, 'it won't hurt' – the child or parent may not view this as correct
  - paracetamol has no proven benefit in pain reduction.
- Strategies for dealing with the immunisation-hesitant parent are as follows.
  - **Pitfall**: do not assume that you know why the parent is hesitant (*see* Evidence 1).
  - Determine if the parents have been vaccinated. **Rationale**: if the parents have been immunised and enjoyed good health, it is likely they will want the same for their child.
  - Clarify what they are most worried about. **Rationale**: parents may have some misinformation that can be easily clarified.

- ○ Use motivational interviewing techniques. **Rationale**: change in behaviour is being sought, and motivational interviewing use is suitable.
- ○ Give compelling evidence for immunisation. **Rationale**: the evidence is compelling for the benefit of immunisation; however, it must be structured with specific examples.
- ○ Explain side effects of vaccine. **Rationale**: giving parents specific incidences is helpful, as is the avoidance of non-specific words such as 'rare' (*see* Evidence 2 and Child with a murmur chapter 18).
- Risk of transmission of infections. **Rationale**: if a child presents with an infectious disease, other siblings may already be affected. Inform parents of incubation periods to enhance their awareness.
- Infections and high-risk groups. **Rationale**: children with immunodeficiency states and those on immunosuppression treatment will require assessment and treatment, especially if exposed to varicella.
- The child with persisting pyrexia and a rash. **Pitfall**: in children with persisting pyrexia and a rash consideration needs to be given to Kawasaki's disease. While the criteria for Kawasaki's disease are explicit, early recognition is desirable. Many of these children are irritable, which can serve as an early clinical prompt to consider the diagnosis.
- Non-blanching rash and meningococcal disease. **Rationale**: *see* Evidence 3.
- ITP and leukaemia. **Rationale**: the risk of leukaemia in ITP is 1%. Failure of the child to respond to therapy will warrant further investigation.

Management of specific clinical illnesses

Exanthems

Most exanthems are short-lived and self-resolving. Management is supportive, ensuring adequate analgesia and prevention of dehydration. Antihistamines or calamine lotion can be helpful in pruritic rashes. Topical analgesia and chlorhexidine mouthwashes may help ease painful mouth ulcers. Parental education is important and should address the infectious period, measure to limit spread to other household members, the likely course and the potential complications.

Special considerations are as follows.
- Scarlet fever is treated with a 10-day course of penicillin.
- Recurrent HSV infection may be treated with prophylactic acyclovir.
- Prevention of measles spread is dependent on prompt (within 72 hours) immunisation of unimmunised people at risk for exposure. Intramuscular administration of normal human immunoglobulin can provide short-term protection against infection if given within 7 days of exposure.
- Varicella zoster immune globulin should be given to children who are at increased risk of severe varicella infection, who do not have pre-existing immunity and who have a history of significant exposure to chickenpox.

Kawasaki's disease

Intravenous immunoglobulin infusion has been shown to reduce the incidence of coronary artery aneurysm if given within 10 days of disease onset. It switches off the inflammatory process. Approximately 5% of cases will require a second dose. High-dose aspirin is given for 14 days and then reduced to low dose. If there are no aneurysms detected by 6 weeks, aspirin can be discontinued. The child should remain on low-dose aspirin for as long as aneurysms are present. A cardiac echo should be performed at presentation and 2 weeks later. If there is evidence of coronary dilatation, long-term follow-up is needed. The clinical severity of Kawasaki's disease is variable and some children will benefit from steroid therapy (*see* Evidence 4).

Skin infections

Impetigo is highly infectious, therefore the child should not attend crèche or school until he or she has been started on antibiotics and the lesions are fully covered. Effective treatments are oral flucloxacillin and the application of paraffin gel to soften the crusts. Cellulitis and erysipelas require hospital admission for intravenous antibiotics.

Children with staphylococcal scalded skin syndrome require hospital admission for intravenous antibiotics, fluid management and analgesia control. To prevent pain and further trauma to the skin, handling should be kept to a minimum and bland emollients should be liberally applied.

In children with SJS or TEN, if a causative drug is identified it should be discontinued immediately. SJS and TEN are life-threatening conditions and therefore supportive care should be started immediately. This includes aggressive management of fluid balance and electrolytes, analgesia, and wound and ocular care.

Urticaria

For some patients with urticaria it is a manifestation of anaphylaxis, which is a medical emergency (*see* Chapter 3: First Response). Children with urticaria alone and no signs of respiratory distress can be managed symptomatically. If a trigger is identified, avoidance should be advised. Antihistamines can be prescribed to alleviate itch.

Henoch–Schönlein purpura

Management is symptomatic treatment with bed rest and analgesia. Steroids can be used for severe or prolonged abdominal pain but evidence of benefit from clinical retrospective trials is poor.

Idiopathic thrombocytopenic purpura

Management is supportive for the vast majority of cases with no bleeding or mild bleeding (petechiae and bruising), irrespective of the platelet count. Contact sports should be avoided and activity should be restricted. Non-steroidal anti-inflammatory drugs and drugs with anticoagulant properties should be avoided. Most cases resolve spontaneously within 8–12 weeks. There is no uniform agreement regarding the indications for pharmacological intervention; however, patients with a platelet count <20 000/mm³ should be treated. Intravenous immunoglobulin is superior to steroid therapy (*see* Evidence 5). Intracranial haemorrhage is a rare complication that requires treatment with platelet transfusions, intravenous immunoglobulin and steroids.

FOLLOW-UP

- Most infectious diseases are self-limited and routine follow-up is not required.
- In Kawasaki's disease, if there is evidence of coronary artery aneurysm, then follow-up by a paediatric cardiologist is required.
- In HSP, the skin lesions may remit and relapse over a period of months in a small number of children. The major concerns relate to those with renal involvement. Haematuria may persist but it is the presence of proteinuria that gives rise to clinical concern and this should be quantified. There is no effective treatment for HSP.
- ITP is often self-limited, but 20% of those offered treatment will develop chronic ITP.
- Urticaria is in most cases self-limited and does not require follow-up.

WHEN TO REFER?

Emergency referral of children with suspected:
- meningococcal disease
- staphylococcal scalded skin syndrome
- SJS or TEN
- staphylococcal toxic shock syndrome
- Kawasaki's disease.

CLARIFICATION STATEMENTS FOR PARENTAL MISCONCEPTIONS

> *'But the shots are painful, and he is so young. Therefore, I am reluctant to get him immunised.'*

Yes, all injections can cause pain; however, if you breastfeed your baby during the vaccination or give a sweet-tasting drink, this will significantly reduce the pain.

> *'Infectious diseases are so rare now, so why all the fuss about immunisation?'*

Immunisation policies have greatly reduced the frequency of these illnesses in the community, but they have not disappeared. To ensure that epidemic or clusters do not occur, high levels of immunisation are required in the community.

I have seen on the Internet that the MMR [measles, mumps, rubella] *vaccine is linked to autism.*

The relation between autism and the MMR vaccine has been disproved.

SUMMARY PRACTICE POINTS

- Parvovirus B19 infections are asymptomatic in 20% of infections but can cause foetal hydrops in pregnancy.
- Varicella complications include pneumonia, encephalitis, ataxia, necrotising fasciitis and purpura fulminans.
- Avoid antibiotic use in Epstein–Barr virus infections.
- Children with Kawasaki's disease have high fevers and are irritable.
- In early SJS the skin is tender on palpation.
- Impetigo has usually honey-coloured crusting, but this is absent if the lesions are in moist areas, e.g. the groin of an infant.
- In ITP, intracranial haemorrhage is rare.
- HSP lesions are initially present on the buttocks but 2% will have initial urticaria.
- Elicit the clinical sign of dermatographism in children with physical urticaria.

EVALUATING THE EVIDENCE

Evidence 1	
Theme E1	*Vaccine refusal by parents*
Question	What are the factors associated with vaccine refusal by parents?
Design	Case control study
Level of evidence	
Setting	Community-based study in three states in the United States
Participants	Surveys were mailed to parents of 815 children with vaccine exemptions (cases) and 1630 children who were fully vaccinated (controls).
Intervention	Parents were asked to complete a survey to explore the study aims.
Outcomes	The primary outcomes were (a) the reasons for non-medical exemption and (b) exploration of parental perception relating to vaccines and vaccine information.
Main results	In the inception cohort, there were 20 siblings and when these were removed, 391 of 805 (48.6%) parents of exempted children responded, as did 976 (59.9%) of the parents of fully vaccinated children. Of the 391 parents with reported exemptions, 86 reported their children to be vaccinated and 28 provided medically valid reasons. Of the remaining 277, 68 (24.5%) children received no vaccinations and the remainder had specific exemptions. The most common vaccine not administered was varicella (n = 147; 53.1%) and the least was polio (n = 45; 16.2%).

(*continued*)

Evidence 1	
Theme E1	*Vaccine refusal by parents*
Main results (*cont.*)	The most common reasons for not vaccinating related to (1) perceived safety [potential harm, n = 190 (68.6%) and immune system overload, n = 136 (49.1%)], (2) low disease risk [n = 103 (37.2%)], (3) disease not dangerous [n = 58 (20.9%)], (4) vaccine failure [n = 36 (13.0%)] and (5) ethical or moral beliefs [n = 25 (9.0%)]. The majority of parents (95.5%) of vaccinated children indicated that vaccination was a benefit to the community, compared with 47.0% of the parents of exempted children. Parents of exempted children reported less confidence in medical, public health and government sources of vaccine information.
Conclusion	Continued efforts are required to educate parents regarding the utility and safety of vaccinations.
Commentary	Children in the United States are required to be vaccinated to attend school. Specific exemptions can be applied for and granted in a discretionary fashion. Immunisation success is dependent on the concept of herd immunity, and falling immunisation rates suggest that epidemics are likely to occur with increasing frequency. Healthcare professionals should counsel and advise parents on the benefits of immunisation. The absence of epidemics of disease may produce a false sense of security and these infectious diseases are not without serious complications.
Reference	Salmon DA, Moulton LH, Omer SB, *et al.* Factors associated with refusal of childhood vaccines among parents of school-aged children: a case-control study. *Arch Pediatr Adolesc Med.* 2005; **159**(5): 470–6.

Evidence 2	
Theme E2	*Immunisation-related side effects*
Question	What are the vaccine-attributable events in children immunised with the MMR (measles, mumps, rubella) vaccine?
Design	RCT
Level of evidence	Jadad 5
Setting	Community-based clinics, Finland
Participants	Parents of twins were invited to enrol their infants in this study.
Intervention	Each twin pair was vaccinated at the same time, with one receiving the MMR and the other a placebo. The process was reversed 3 weeks later. Nurse, parent and investigators were all blind to the order of the injections.
Outcomes	The following outcomes were monitored: local reactions (redness with a diameter exceeding 2.5 cm, soreness and swelling), temperature (mild, <38.6°C; moderate, 38.6°C–39.5°C; and high fever, >39.5°C), rhinorrhoea or cough, nausea or vomiting, diarrhoea, rash, arthralgia, conjunctivitis, staying in bed, drowsiness, irritability and other potential symptoms.
Main results	The study enrolled 1162 monozygous and heterozygous twins, whose ages ranged from 14 to 83 months. Most of the eldest had been vaccinated against measles and 50% of the remainder had had the measles.

(*continued*)

Evidence 2	
Theme E2	**Immunisation-related side effects**
Main results (*cont.*)	Overall, 6% had MMR-attributed events. Fever was the most common, occurring in 12% of the vaccinated group and 8% in the placebo group (absolute risk reduction = 4%; number needed to treat = 25). Respiratory symptoms behaved differently, occurring with increased frequency in both vaccinated and unvaccinated groups to levels of 15%–20%. At 6 years of age systemic reactions occurred 5–15 times less frequently than at 14–18 months of age, with only arthralgia being associated with immunisation. Local reactions occurred in the first 2 post-injection days in 4% of participants, regardless of whether placebo or vaccine was administered.
Conclusion	The MMR vaccine was safe. The occurrence of fever attributable to the MMR was 4%. Older children experience little in the way of side effects apart from arthralgia.
Commentary	The study outlines the side effect profile of the MMR. Immunisation in young children occurs at a time when they are prone to viral illnesses; therefore, they are more likely to manifest systems because of their age rather than because of the MMR vaccine. Parents may assume this temporal relationship is cause and effect.
Reference	Virtanen M, Petola H, Paunio M, *et al.* Day-to-day reactogenicity and the healthy vaccine effect of measles-mumps-rubella vaccination. *Pediatrics.* 2000; **106**(5): e62.

Evidence 3	
Theme E3	**Non-blanching rashes and meningococcal disease**
Question	In a child with a non-blanching rash, how likely is meningococcal disease?
Design	Prospective cohort observational study
Level of evidence	
Setting	Department of paediatrics and microbiology, academic medical centre, the United Kingdom
Participants	All children and adolescents, <15 years of age, with a non-blanching rash were eligible for inclusion.
Intervention	This was an observational study; therefore, care was at the discretion of the attending doctor. Data recorded included presenting symptoms and signs, such as axillary temperature, blood pressure (hypotension was defined as two standard deviations or more below the mean for age), capillary refill time (defined as normal if less than 2 seconds), and details of the rash (size and distribution). Children were characterised as being well (smiling or crying but consolable) or ill (toxic, irritable and crying inconsolably, or lethargic). All children had a full blood count, coagulation profile, C-reactive protein (CRP), blood cultures, and polymerase chain reaction for meningococcal DNA. Cerebrospinal fluid analysis was also performed.
Outcomes	The primary outcome was the presence of proven meningococcal infection.
Main results	Over a 1-year period, 233 (2.5% of all medical attendances) had a petechial or purpuric rash.

(*continued*)

Evidence 3	
Theme E3	*Non-blanching rashes and meningococcal disease*
Main results (*cont.*)	Fifteen were excluded because of alternate diagnosis (11 Henoch–Schönlein purpura, one idiopathic thrombocytopenic purpura, one haemolytic-uraemic syndrome, one leukaemia, and one previously diagnosed clotting disorder). Twenty-four (11%) had proven meningococcal disease. In 34% of children who presented with a petechial rash, the lesions were confined to the distribution of the superior vena cava (SVC). None of these children had meningococcal disease and most were well. Thirty-six per cent of patients had purpura, ill appearance, increased capillary refill time, or hypotension and required prompt treatment. Ninety-six per cent of patients with meningococcal disease will lie within this group; however, the remaining 4% will appear among the 30% who appear well, who have no fever and in whom the petechial rash extended beyond the SVC. A normal CRP was a useful predictor of children who did not have meningococcal disease.
Conclusion	Most children with meningococcal disease are clinically ill. A rash confined to the distribution of the SVC suggests meningococcal disease is unlikely, as does a normal CRP.
Commentary	This study was undertaken prior to the introduction of a national immunisation campaign, and consequently the incidence of meningococcal disease will reduce further; however, the occurrence of meningococcal disease in 11% of patients is high. In this study the admission rate for children presenting with a petechial rash was 84%; this may have been influenced by parental anxiety, given the increased awareness of petechial rashes, an indicator of meningococcal disease and the inability of clinical examination alone to confirm the diagnosis. Petechial rashes in the distribution of the SVC reflect raised venous and capillary pressure from coughing, vomiting or crying. An important factor not assessed in this study was the progression of the petechial rash over a period of hours. Progressive rashes most likely indicate invasive disease and require a prompt clinical response.
Reference	Wells LC, Smith JC, Weston VC, *et al.* The child with a non-blanching rash: how likely is meningococcal disease? *Arch Dis Child.* 2001; **85**(3): 218–22.

Evidence 4	
Theme E4	*Steroid therapy in Kawasaki's disease*
Question	Is steroid therapy effective in Kawasaki's disease?
Design	Randomised controlled trial
Level of evidence	Jadad 3
Setting	Department of paediatrics, multiple academic medical centres, Japan
Participants	Children diagnosed with Kawasaki's disease but at high risk of developing coronary artery aneurysms (Kobayashi score >5) were eligible for enrolment. This score predicts resistance to immunoglobulin therapy and scores as follows: 2 points each for serum sodium <133 mmol/L, 4 days or fewer of illness at diagnosis, aspartate aminotransferase concentration of 100 U/L or more, white cell count with >80% neutrophils; 1 point each for platelet count ≤300 000, C-reactive protein concentration ≥100 mg/L and age <1 year.

(continued)

Evidence 4	
Theme E4	*Steroid therapy in Kawasaki's disease*
Intervention	Participants were randomised to receive standard therapy – intravenous immunoglobulin (IVIG) plus aspirin – or IVIG plus prednisolone (dose 2 mg/kg/day) for 5 days. The prednisolone was given intravenously and was tapered over 15 days in a three-step reduction.
Outcomes	The primary outcome was the development of coronary artery aneurysms.
Main results	Of the 2014 assessed for eligibility, 1436 (71%) did not meet the inclusion criteria, as their Kobayashi score was too low). Of the 467 children who were eligible, 248 (53%) consented for enrolment, of whom 125 were assigned to standard therapy and 123 to IVIG therapy plus prednisolone. Six patients were identified as ineligible. Full data were available on 242 patients, 121 in each group. Twenty-eight (23%) in the standard therapy group and four (3%) in the IVIG plus prednisolone group had coronary artery aneurysm detected during the study period [absolute risk reduction =20%; number needed to treat (NNT) = 5]. Six (5%) of the IVIG plus prednisolone group and 36 (30%) of the standard therapy group did not respond to their primary treatment and additional rescue treatment was provided, usually with IVIG.
Conclusion	The addition of prednisolone to the treatment of severe Kawasaki's disease improves outcomes.
Commentary	Kawasaki's disease is a childhood vasculitis of unknown aetiology that leads to the development of coronary artery aneurysms in 20% of untreated children. The use of immunoglobulin therapy and aspirin is accepted as standard therapy and reduces the occurrence of coronary artery aneurysm. The use of prednisolone further reduces the occurrence of aneurysms in high-risk populations (NNT = 5). The Kobayashi score identifies those high-risk populations who display resistance to IVIG treatment; unfortunately, the score does not identify high-risk populations in other racial and ethnic groups accurately. This study does need to be replicated, as it was carried out in a Japanese population and needs to be assessed in mixed ethnic populations.
Reference	Kobayashi T, Saji T, Otani T, et al.; RAISE study group investigators. Efficacy of immunoglobulin plus prednisolone for the prevention of coronary artery abnormalities in severe Kawasaki disease (RAISE study): a randomised, open-label, blinded-endpoints trial. *Lancet.* 2012; **379**(9826): 1613–20.

Evidence 5	
Theme E5	*Treatment of idiopathic thrombocytopenic purpura (ITP) in children*
Question	Which is more effective in ITP treatment: corticosteroids or intravenous immunoglobulin (IVIG)?
Design	Systematic review
Level of evidence	Jadad 2 (range 1–3)
Setting	Paediatric outcomes research team, academic medical centre, Canada

(*continued*)

Evidence 5	
Theme E5	*Treatment of idiopathic thrombocytopenic purpura (ITP) in children*
Participants	Patients with ITP were included in the analysis if they received either IVIG or corticosteroids.
Intervention	The treatments evaluated the clinical impact of corticosteroids and IVIG in producing a clinical improvement in patients with ITP (platelet count >20 000/mm^3).
Outcomes	The primary outcome was the number of patients with a platelet count >20 000/mm^3 at 48 hours after the initiation of treatment.
Main results	Of 10 randomised controlled trials identified, six provided data on the primary outcome being assessed. The studies included 401 patients. One hundred and fifty-seven of 294 (80.9%) achieved the primary outcome in the IVIG group and 123 of 207 (59.4%) in the corticosteroid group (absolute risk reduction = 21.5%; number need to treat = 5). Treatment side effects of IVIG included nausea, vomiting, headache and macular rash. In the corticosteroid group, side effects included weight gain, hyperglycaemia, hypertension and increased appetite. The dose of corticosteroid used did not influence the platelet response in those treated. In the systematic review, 21% of patients developed chronic ITP (25% in the steroid group and 18% in the IVIG group).
Conclusion	In the treatment of ITP, IVIG is superior to corticosteroid therapy.
Commentary	In children presenting with acute ITP and low platelets, the primary concern in the acute phase is the prevention of an acute intracranial haemorrhage. Data from nine studies with 586 patients report three cases of intracranial haemorrhage: two of these children received steroids, both of whom improved, and one who received IVIG, who died. This patient was described as having a 'florid viral illness and ITP'. It is prudent to acknowledge that the use of corticosteroids may potentially mask the presence of leukaemia, although the risk is low (<1%). The risk of chronic ITP is approximately 21% following acute ITP.
Reference	Beck CE, Nathan PC, Parkin PC, *et al*. Corticosteroids versus intravenous immune globulin for the treatment of acute immune thrombocytopenic purpura in children: a systematic review and meta-analysis of randomized controlled trials. *J Pediatr.* 2005; **147**(4): 521–7.

ACUTE RASH: MULTIPLE-CHOICE QUESTIONS

Q1   Which of the following statements with regard to parvovirus B19 is/are correct?
   a) Forty per cent of infections are asymptomatic.
   b) The rash precedes fever, malaise and myalgia.
   c) A reticular-like rash is found on the trunk and limbs.
   d) Children with haemolytic anaemia can develop aplastic crises if infected with parvovirus B19.
   e) Infection in pregnancy can lead to hydrops foetalis.

Q2 With regard to human herpes virus 6, which of the following statements is/are correct?
a) Encephalitis occurs in 30% of children under 10 years of age.
b) It is a frequent cause of febrile convulsions.
c) The rash occurs once the fever subsides.
d) Differentiation from herpes simplex infection is difficult.
e) Vesicles occur in 90% of patients.

Q3 Which of the following statements relating to varicella is/are correct?
a) The incubation period is 7–10 days.
b) Cerebellar ataxia is a complication.
c) Haemorrhagic varicella occurs in immunocompromised patients.
d) Pancreatitis is a recognised complication.
e) A maculopapular rash occurs before vesicular component of the rash.

Q4 With regard to mumps, which of the following is/are correct?
a) The incubation period is 14–21 days.
b) The incidence is increasing.
c) The child is infectious for 7 days post parotid gland swelling.
d) Transient hearing loss is a recognised complication.
e) Orchitis is a complication.

Q5 Which of the following statements with regard to rubella is/are correct?
a) The incubation period is 7–10 days.
b) It is spread by droplets.
c) Fifty per cent of children are asymptomatic.
d) Anterior auricular lymphadenopathy is typically present.
e) Petechiae are typically present on the soft palate and uvula.

Q6 Features of congenital rubella include which of the following?
a) Sensorineural hearing loss
b) Encephalocoele
c) Jejunal atresia
d) Pulmonary atresia
e) Cataracts

Q7 Which of the following statements related to measles is/are correct?
a) The child is infectious 1–2 days before prodromal symptoms and for 7 days after the onset of the rash.
b) The rash typically starts behind the ears.
c) Purulent conjunctivitis is common.
d) Koplik's spots are seen on the buccal mucosa.
e) Acute disseminated encephalomyelitis is a complication of measles.

Q8 Features of Kawasaki's disease include which of the following?
a) Strawberry tongue and cracked lips
b) Cervical lymphadenopathy
c) Non-purulent conjunctivitis
d) Hydrops of the gallbladder
e) Sterile pyuria

Q9 Staphylococcal toxic shock syndrome includes which of the following features?
a) Pyrexia
b) Severe muscle cramps
c) Abdominal pain
d) Erythroderma
e) Abscess formation in the inguinal and axillary regions

Q10 Staphylococcal scalded skin syndrome includes which of the following features?
a) Desquamation of the skin
b) Skin healing without scarring
c) Lesion occurring around the umbilicus and perineum in neonates
d) Lesions produced by a staphylococcal exotoxin
e) Abscess formation in 15% of children under 5 years

Answers

A1	c, d, e	**A2**	b, c
A3	b, c, d, e	**A4**	a, c, d, e
A5	b, c, e	**A6**	a, e
A7	b, d	**A8**	a, b, c, d, e
A9	a, b, c, d	**A10**	a, b, c, d

SLIDES
1. Erysipelas
2. Hand foot and mouth
3. Herpetic gingivostomatitis
4. Herpes simplex (periorbital)
5. Herpes simplex (perioral)
6. Herpes simplex (herpetic whitlow)
7. Herpes simplex (eyes severe)
8. Impetigo
9. Impetigo (back)
10. ITP (idiopathic thrombocytopenic purpura)
11. ITP
12. ITP (subconjunctival haemorrhage)
13. ITP (bruising)
14. Kawasaki's disease (lips)

15. Kawasaki's disease (day 10)
16. Measles (maculopapular rash)
17. Mumps
18. Scarlet fever (circumoral pallor)
19. Shingles
20. Staphylococcal scalded skin (back)
21. Staphylococcal scalded skin (Nikolsky)
22. Varicella (foot)
23. Varicella (neonatal)

Chapter Thirty-one

THE CHILD WITH A CHRONIC RASH

COMMON SCENARIO

'He just can't stop scratching; he's up all night. I've been putting the hydrocortisone cream on but it's doing nothing for the rash. I've had to start giving him antihistamines at night to help him sleep.'

LEARNING OBJECTIVES

- Understand the terminology used to describe skin rashes
- Identify common chronic skin rashes presenting in childhood
- Explain what investigations are needed
- Conduct a treatment plan for the management of eczema, psoriasis, acne and tinea infections

BACKGROUND

Skin rashes are a common presentation in paediatrics. Although the differential is vast, many common skin rashes are easily recognisable, self-limiting and require nothing more than reassurance and observation. Others may be part of a systemic illness requiring further investigation and treatment. Drugs, infections and allergies can cause skin rashes, while others can be genetic. Acute and chronic rashes vary considerably in their aetiology, presentation and management; therefore, skin rashes will be addressed in two separate chapters dealing with acute and chronic common rashes of childhood.

The first key skill in the management of childhood skin rashes is the ability to describe a rash:

- the morphology (i.e. the shape of the lesion)
- the colour (red, orange, yellow, violet, blue, black)
- the configuration (i.e. the arrangement of lesions)
- the distribution (i.e. area of the body affected)
- whether the skin is itchy, non-itchy, painful or asymptomatic.

Morphology: primary lesion	Description
Macule	Smooth, flat circumscribed areas of skin colour change <1.5 cm in diameter
Patch	Large smooth area of colour change
Papule	Small palpable elevation of the skin <1 cm in diameter (domed, flat-topped, umbilicated)
Nodule	Palpable elevation >1 cm in diameter
Plaque	Palpable elevation >2 cm in diameter
Cyst	Fluctuant fluid-filled papule or nodule
Vesicle	Collection of clear fluid <5 mm in diameter
Bulla	Collection of clear fluid >5 mm in diameter
Pustule	Purulent vesicle
Abscess	Localised collection of pus
Wheal	Oedematous papule or plaque caused by dermal swelling
Petechiae	Small, <5 mm, punctate bleeding into the dermis
Purpura	Visible collection of blood under the skin
Burrow	Thin, red or brown linear papule with scales
Telangiectasia	Dilated capillaries visible on the skin surface

Morphology: secondary lesion	Description
Crust	Dried serum (or exudate)
Scale	Thickened, loose, readily detachable fragment of cornified layer
Excoriation	Shallow linear abrasion caused by scratching
Erosion	Loss of epidermis
Ulcer	Loss of epidermis and dermis
Fissure	Linear crack in the skin
Scar	Permanent lesion due to abnormal formation of connective tissue following injury
Keloid	Exaggerated tissue response to injury extending beyond the margins of the original wound
Eschar	Hard, usually darkened plaque covering an ulcer
Atrophy	Superficial or deep thinning of the skin
Lichenification	Thickened skin with accentuated skin markings
Sclerosis	Induration of the skin
Granulation tissue	Mass of new capillaries and fibrous tissue in healing wound

Configuration of lesion	Description
Nummular	Round or coin shaped
Linear	In a straight line
Target	Concentric rings
Reticulated	Lacy or networked pattern
Annular	Grouped lesions in a circle
Clustered	Lesions grouped together
Confluent	Runs together
Dermatomal	Follows a dermatome
Multiform	Variety of shapes
Serpiginous	Wanders as though following the track of a snake
Scarlatiniform	Pattern of scarlet fever, i.e. widely and diffusely distributed
Satellite	A cluster of lesions around a larger central lesion

ECZEMA

Atopic eczema affects up to 15% of children and accounts for approximately 30% of dermatology consultations in general practice. Ninety per cent of cases present under the age of 5, with 60% presenting under the age of 1. Genetic factors, abnormal skin barrier function and immune dysregulation are implicated in the pathogenesis.

Eczema is diagnosed when a child has an itchy skin condition plus three or more of the following:

- visible flexural dermatitis involving the skin creases (or visible dermatitis on the cheeks or extensor areas in children under 18 months of age)
- personal history of flexural dermatitis (or dermatitis on the cheeks or extensor areas in children under 18 months of age)
- personal history of dry skin in the last 12 months
- personal history of asthma or allergic rhinitis (or history of atopic disease in a first-degree relative of children aged under 4 years)
- onset of signs and symptoms under the age of 2 years.

In infants and toddlers, eczematous plaques affect the cheeks, forehead, scalp and extensor surface. In older children and adolescents the flexor surfaces are primarily affected. Up to one-third of children with eczema have food allergies. Infants with early-onset moderate to severe eczema should be treated with a high level of suspicion for food allergy.

Skin can become lichenified (rough and thickened) as a result of scratching. Secondary infection with staphylococcus and group A streptococcus are a common cause of exacerbations. Infection presents as weeping or crusting, failure to respond to treatment, rapidly worsening eczema or systemic signs and symptoms. Eczema herpeticum is important to recognise and is often missed. Signs of eczema herpeticum are areas of rapidly worsening eczema, failure to respond to topical steroids and multiple punched-out crusted superficial erosions. The child may be unwell with a fever. Known eczema triggers include heat, harsh soaps, chlorine, house dust mite, grass pollen and animal hair, cigarette smoke, stress and irritant foods such as tomatoes and citrus fruits. In many cases, eczema improves during childhood, with periods of remission and exacerbation. However, in other cases eczema may persist, with up to 50%–80% of children developing another atopic disease (allergic rhinitis or asthma).

Differential diagnosis of eczematous itchy rash	
Seborrhoeic dermatitis	Involves scalp, face and flexures and gluteal region
	Erythematous patches and plaques with greasy, yellow scale
Psoriasis	Well-demarcated, raised, inflamed, red lesions covered by a silvery white scale affecting the extensor surface of the elbow and knees and scalp
Immunodeficiency syndromes: • Wiskott–Aldrich's syndrome • hyper IgE syndrome • severe combined immunodeficiency • Omenn's syndrome	Failure to thrive Lymphadenopathy, hepatosplenomegaly Recurrent infections
Scabies	Infestation with the female mite *Sarcoptes scabiei*, transmitted by direct person-to-person contact
	Severe pruritus is a prominent feature that is worse at night
	Burrows are pathognomonic
	Papules, vesicles and pustules can also be seen, most commonly on the finger webs, wrist, elbows, ankles and buttocks
Zinc and biotin deficiency	Nutritional zinc deficiency in exclusively breastfed, presents after 3 months of age or can be inherited autosomal recessive zinc deficiency
	Horseshoe appearance of rash on cheeks, no zerosis, no pruritis
	Associated diarrhoea, recurrent skin infections, alopecia and irritability
	Biotin deficiency – autosomal recessive
	Affects face, perianal, hands and feet
	Associated developmental delay, epilepsy, ataxia and vomiting
Contact dermatitis	Localised dermatitis at site of exposure
Ichthyosis	Absence of pruritus
Molluscum dermatitis	Presence of pearly white papules with central umbilication
Mycosis fungoides	Chronic T-cell lymphoma
	Chronic dermatitis, hypopigmented patches
Tinea corporis	Scaly, itchy annular lesions with active, clearly defined borders with central clearing.

PSORIASIS

Psoriasis is a chronic autoimmune skin disease with a variable clinical spectrum. In 30% of cases there is a positive family history of psoriasis. Although it can occur at any age, it is uncommon in children. Chronicity, inflammation and hyperproliferation are distinct characteristics. Classification of psoriasis is based on the morphology of the rash. Plaque psoriasis and guttate psoriasis are the commonest types affecting children. In children the disease is more pruritic and the lesions tend to be less scaly and softer.

Plaque psoriasis is the commonest form (65% of cases) and presents as well-demarcated, raised, inflamed, red lesions covered by a silvery white scale affecting the extensor surface of the elbows, knees and scalp. Nails may show evidence of pitting, thickening or onycholysis, although these features are rare in childhood. Auspitz's sign, bleeding after removal of a scale or Koebner's phenomenon, lesions induced by trauma, may be seen. Scalp involvement occurs in 80% of children, who develop severe thick white adherent scales with associated hair loss. Other areas commonly involved include the extensor surfaces, umbilicus and gluteal cleft. Trauma, infection, drugs, stress, smoking and alcohol may trigger psoriasis.

Guttate psoriasis usually affects the trunk and limbs, with small scaly patches up to 1 cm in diameter. It is usually preceded by an upper respiratory tract infection or streptococcal throat infection. Depending on the percentage of the body surface involved, psoriasis can be graded as mild (up to 3%), moderate (3%–10%) or severe (>10%).

Differential diagnosis of psoriasis scaly rash	
Pityriasis rosea	Begins as scaling herald patch on chest, abdomen or back, followed by appearance of further scaly lesions on the trunk that follows cleavage lines in a 'Christmas tree' pattern
	It is self-limiting, usually resolving within 6 weeks
Tinea corporis	Scaly, itchy annular lesions with active, clearly defined borders with central clearing
	Usually caused by *Microsporum canis* or *Trichophyton tonsurans*
Lichen planus	Uncommon, pathogenesis unknown
	Delicate white lines in a reticulated pattern (Wickham's striae)
	Classic 6Ps: purple, planar, pruritic, plaques and papules, polygonal.
	Mainly affecting flexor surfaces, can spread
	Oral lesions can occur
Nummular (discoid) eczema	Distinct coin-shaped lesions occur anywhere on the body
Pityriasis rubra pilaris	Erythroderma, palmoplantar keratoderma and follicular hyperkeratosis
	Three types occur in children: (1) classic juvenile onset, (2) circumscribed juvenile onset and (3) atypical juvenile onset

(continued)

Differential diagnosis of psoriasis scaly rash	
Seborrhoeic dermatitis	Involves scalp, face and flexures and gluteal region
	Erythematous patches and plaques with greasy, yellow scale
Pityriasis (tinea) versicolor	Hypo- or hyperpigmented, scaly, oval-shaped patches
	Scale may not be visible until skin is rubbed with a finger
	Mainly chest and back, facial involvement is rare
	Caused by malassezia yeast

ACNE

Acne vulgaris is a disease of the pilosebaceous follicles. It commonly affects teenagers. Males and females are equally affected; however, in males it tends to be more severe and in females it tends to be more persistent. In 50% of cases there is a positive family history. It can have a significant psychological impact and may result in scarring. Four pathogenic factors have been implicated:

1. high levels of dehyroepiandrosterone sulphate associated with puberty
2. proliferation of *Propionibacterium acnes*
3. plugging of the hair follicle due to abnormal keratinisation
4. increased sebaceous gland activity.

Lesions vary in their distribution, extent and degree of inflammation, but they commonly affect the face, chest and upper back. Acne begins with non-inflammatory lesions – open (blackheads) and closed (whiteheads) comedones. As debris and bacteria collect in these pores inflammatory lesions develop with papules, pustules, cysts and nodules. Acne is graded as mild, moderate or severe. Classification of acne is based on the morphology of the skin lesions.

It can be:

- comedonal with open and closed comedones
- inflammatory with papules and pustules
- nodulocystic with nodules and cysts.

Differential diagnosis of acneiform lesions	
Acneiform eruptions	Abrupt onset
	History of exposure – improvement on cessation of exposure
Folliculitis	Commonly affects trunk and extremities
Perioral dermatitis	Localised around mouth
Adenoma sebaceum	Other features of tuberous sclerosis

TINEA INFECTIONS

Fungal infections occur in both healthy and immunocompromised children. Superficial infections are limited to the epidermis. Tinea refers to dermatophyte infections and is classified according to anatomic location.

- Tinea capitis: scalp and hair
- Tinea corporis: body
- Tinea cruris: groin
- Tinea pedis: feet
- Tinea manuum: hands
- Tinea unguium: nails

Tinea capitis primarily affects school-age children. It may be inflammatory (kerion), non-inflammatory or a combination of both. Patchy alopecia is frequently found. In inflammatory tinea there may be erythema, pustules and a kerion. A kerion is a painful, inflammatory, boggy mass with broken hair follicles. Non-inflammatory tinea capitis presents with 'black dots' on the scalp. When the hair shaft breaks at the scalp surface, the debris left in the hair follicle appears as black dots. There may be associated lymphadenopathy. *T. tonsurans* and *M. canis* are the commonest causing dermatophytes. Microsporum is spread by animal contact; trichophyton is spread by human contact. Microsporum infections fluoresce green under Wood's light.

Tinea corporis presents with scaly, itchy annular lesions with active, clearly defined borders with central clearing. It is most commonly caused by the *Trichophyton* species.

Tinea pedis or 'athlete's foot' can be acute or chronic. It is rare in prepubertal children. Exposure to a moist environment and maceration are risk factors for tinea pedis. Infection often occurs in swimming pools, public showers and changing rooms. It is most commonly caused by *Trichophyton rubrum*. It presents with macerated skin between the toes with scaling, which may be intensely itchy. Blistering and hyperkeratotic types can also occur.

Tinea unguium is a fungal infection of the toes or fingernails, although toenails are more commonly affected. It is rare in prepubertal children. Risk factors include ill-fitting shoes, sporting activities, diabetes and poor venous or lymphatic circulation. Nails are thickened, discoloured, brittle and dystrophic. There may be associated tinea pedis.

Differential diagnosis of tinea infections	
Alopecia areata	Well-demarcated circular patches of hair loss
	Exclamation mark hairs
Nummular (discoid) eczema	Distinct coin-shaped lesions occur anywhere on the body
Granuloma annulare	Non-scaly, skin-coloured annular plaques and papules
	Usually affects extremities
Seborrhoeic dermatitis, 'cradle cap'	Usually no hair loss
	Involves scalp, face and flexures and gluteal region
	Erythematous patches and plaques with greasy, yellow scale
Plaque psoriasis	Usually no hair loss
Pityriasis versicolor	Hypo- or hyperpigmented, scaly, oval-shaped patches
	Scale may not be visible until skin is rubbed with a finger
	Mainly chest and back, facial involvement is rare
	Caused by malassezia yeast
Dermatitis	Spares the intertriginous areas
Congenital and acquired nail dystrophy	Microscopic exam and culture of nail scrapings or clippings will confirm if fungal infection present
Pityriasis rosea	Begins as scaling herald patch on chest, abdomen or back, followed by appearance of further scaly lesions on the trunk that follow cleavage lines in a 'Christmas tree' pattern
	It is self-limiting, usually resolving within 6 weeks

VASCULAR MALFORMATIONS

Congenital vascular malformations are called capillary haemangiomas and are common in childhood. Haemangiomas result from overgrowth of endothelial cells, and while they may be present at birth, most become obvious at 4 weeks to 3 months. Most are cutaneous and the initial macule, noted by the parent, grows disproportionately in the first year of life. These lesions resolve with time and watchful waiting is advised in most cases. By 3 years of age 30% have resolved; by 5 years, 50% have resolved; and by 9 years, 90% have resolved. While generally benign, the occurrence of a periorbital haemangioma requires magnetic resonance imaging. Occasionally, children develop stridor in the haemangioma located in the lanynx. The presence of hepatic haemangioma occasionally leads to associated hypothyroidism secondary to a high level of triiodothyronine deiodinase activity within the haemangioma. On very rare occasions a large haemangioma, with an associated arteriovenous shunting in the haemangioma, leads to a high-output state of cardiac failure. Ten per cent of children with a haemangioma develop a complication, with infection and bleeding being most common. Frequently parents are concerned that the haemangioma will produce a cosmetic disability.

Port wine stains, named for their purplish colour, are present at birth. They grow with the child. Unlike capilliary haemangiomas, they are not raised. If present in the distribution of the ophthalmic branch of the fifth cranial nerve, there is a 10% risk of Sturge–Weber's syndrome. These children will require magnetic resonance imaging to establish the diagnosis.

Salmon patch (or stork bite) is another vascular malformation seen in 40% of newborns and is usually located at the nape of the neck, the forehead or the upper eyelid. They may become more intense with crying, thereby attracting attention of the parents.

HISTORY: CHRONIC RASH

KEY POINTS				
Rash characteristics	Time of onset Description Pattern Distribution Progression Severity Presence of itch Scale	**Impact on quality of life**	Sleep disturbance Number of school days missed Deterioration in school performance	**Ɋ Red flags** Failure to thrive Recurrent infections Excessive school loss Negative self-perception Overusage of potent steroids
Treatments tried	Over-the-counter preparations Steroid usage and strengths Antihistamine use Herbal remedies Systemic treatments	**Psychosocial impact**	Self-esteem, teasing or bullying Withdrawal from normal activities	
Skin care regimen	Use of emollients Frequency of application Bathing regimen Use of soaps	**Identified trigger factors**	Irritants Skin infections Medications Contact allergens Food allergens Inhaled allergens Stress Alcohol Smoking	

(continued)

KEY POINTS				
Family history	Eczema Asthma Food allergies Allergic rhinitis Psoriasis Acne Family members with similar rash	**Associated symptoms**	Joint pain or swelling Fever Hair loss Nail changes	
Medical history	Asthma Allergic rhinitis Allergies Recurrent infections	**Drugs**	Prescription drugs Steroids Phenytoin Oral contraceptive pill	
Growth and development	Onset of menses Weight gain or loss	**Social history**	Contact with animals or a farm Pets in the house Children with similar rash at school or crèche	

EXAMINATION

All children should have their height and weight plotted on an appropriate centile chart.

- Rash examination: morphology, colour, configuration of lesions, distribution
- Presence of secondary lesions (crust, lichenification, excoriations)
- Evidence of skin thinning
- Scarring
- Nail changes
- Examine scalp and hair
- Lymphadenopathy or hepatosplenomegaly

🛇 Red flags

- Acne with scarring
- Nodulocystic acne
- Erythroderma
- Infected or extensive severe eczema
- Hepatosplenomegaly

INVESTIGATIONS

If a bacterial superinfection is likely, what investigations should be performed?
Skin swabs should be taken and sent for culture.

In pubertal teenagers with acne, are endocrinology investigations needed?
Endocrinology testing is not indicated unless there are signs of androgen excess, i.e. infrequent menses, hirsutism, male or female pattern alopecia, infertility, polycystic ovaries, cliteromegaly, acanthosis nigricans or truncal obesity. Baseline endocrinology tests would include free testosterone, dehydroepiandrosterone sulphate, luteinising hormone and follicle-stimulating hormone.

If a fungal infection is suspected, what investigations should be performed?
- A potassium hydroxide exam and fungal culture should be performed.
- Septate hyphae and arthrospores may be seen.
- Previous treatment with topical antifungals may produce false negative potassium hydroxide examinations.
- In suspected tinea capitis, scalp scale, hair and hair fragments should be sent for microscopy and culture. If it is not possible to take scalp scrapings, brush samples should be sent.
- In suspected tinea corporis, skin scraping from the active edge of the lesion should be taken.
- If tinea unguium is suspected nail clippings and scrapings should be taken.

MANAGEMENT PLAN: SEVEN-STEP APPROACH

1. Clarifying and pitfall avoidance strategies:
   a) parents
   b) doctor
2. Eczema treatment
3. Psoriasis treatment:
   a) scalp treatment
4. Acne treatment
5. Treatment of tinea infections:
   a) tinea capitis
   b) tinea corporis and tinea pedis
   c) tinea unguium
6. Haemangioma treatment
7. Scabies treatment

Clarifying and pitfall avoidance strategies

Parents

- Diet and eczema. **Rationale:** parents who have a child with eczema will enquire about preventive strategies. Current recommendations suggest breastfeeding is beneficial; solids should be delayed until at least 4 months and cow's milk delayed until 1 year. Structured teaching on eczema treatment in a workshop setting is beneficial for both parents and children (*see* Evidence 1).

- Eczema and psoriasis tips for both parents and children:
  - develop a treatment centre in the home
  - make the application of emollients a game (place small amounts on the skin and join the dots)
  - if someone asks about the condition, be able to give a clear, concise explanation of what it is and how it is treated; this indicates that you are informed and the child will be able to role model this approach.
- Dealing with child and adolescent frustration. **Rationale**: chronic rashes inclusive of eczema, psoriasis and acne remit and relapse. Their chronicity, with the associated flare-up, are challenging for both parents and the affected family member. If the child indicates they are frustrated with the treatment, acknowledge that fact, but also indicate that there are other treatment options.
- If the adolescent feels that the rash is the cause of 'all their problems', test the thought by asking the adolescent is he or she making the rash a scapegoat? The informed child and adolescent will be able to explain his or her disease to others. The uninformed child and adolescent are likely to be embarrassed.

Doctor

- Treatment regimens. **Rationale**: outline standard care, intensification for flare-ups and be aware of the time commitments required. Adherence is improved if the treatment plan is practicable.
- Parent education. **Rationale**: appropriate education results in improved outcomes (*see* Evidence 1).
- Non-improving eczema. **Pitfall**: if eczema remains despite appropriate treatment, consider (1) infection, (2) food allergy and evaluate accordingly, (3) reassess your diagnosis and (4) check with parents for changes in detergent that may be relevant.
- The steroid-averse parent. **Rationale**: some parents will be reluctant to use steroids. Clarify their reasons and explain the treatment plan. Explain steroid potency and the differences between preparations. Suggest the use of topical calcineurin inhibitors if appropriate.
- Models of eczema care. **Rationale**: nurse practitioners and dermatologists are both as effective in the treatment of children with eczema (*see* Evidence 2).
- Psoriasis triggers. **Pitfall**: be aware that streptococcal infections can trigger guttate psoriasis. Occasionally trauma or injury to the skin can induce psoriasis (Koebner's phenomenon).

Eczema treatment

The aims of eczema treatment are to replace lost moisture, provide a waterproof barrier, reduce inflammation, break the itch-scratch cycle and improve the child and family's quality of life. Parents and children should be educated on how to care for their skin, apply steroid ointments, recognise when to step up or step down treatments and how to prevent, recognise and treat infection and avoid known triggers.

Written instructions should be given to parents about prescribed treatments and the management of flare-ups. Parents and children should receive a demonstration on how to apply emollients and steroids.

Treatment options include:
- baths
- emollients
- topical steroids
- calcineurin inhibitors
- occlusive therapy
- ultraviolet light
- systemic treatment (for severe cases).

Children with eczema should ideally bath daily in lukewarm water. However, for many families, this may not be practical and therefore family circumstances need to be taken into consideration. Emollients should be added to the bathwater. Children should bath for a maximum of 5–10 minutes, as prolonged periods dry out the skin. The skin should be pat-dried. Bathing cleanses, hydrates and prepares the skin for topical treatments.

Emollients should be applied three to four times a day. To avoid blocking the hair follicles, emollients should be applied in downward strokes in the direction of hair growth.

For short periods of time, sedating antihistamines can be used to provide short-term relief if sleep is disturbed and while trying to gain control of eczema with topical treatments.

Calcineurin inhibitors (tacrolimus) are used as second-line treatment as a steroid-sparing agent or when topical steroids are ineffective in children over 2 years of age (*see* Evidence 3). It is particularly useful for facial eczema, as it has no skin-thinning effects. A burning sensation is common after applying tacrolimus; however, this tends to settle within a few days of usage. It should not be applied to infected skin. Children should exercise strict photoprotection while using tacrolimus.

Topical steroids vary in potency from mild to very potent. Use of steroids should be tailored according to the severity of the eczema, stepping up to more potent agents when it is poorly controlled and stepping down to the lowest-potency steroid to maintain control. Long-term potent steroids should not be used without specialist advice.

Only mild-potency steroids should be used on the face, axilla and groin. Steroids should be applied immediately after a bath or 30 minutes after a topical emollient has been applied. One fingertip unit is equivalent to 0.5 g of steroid cream or ointment.

Wet wraps (whole-body occlusive dressings) are useful in moderate to severe atopic dermatitis. An emollient is applied to the skin, which is then covered by an inner wet and outer dry tubular bandage. Bandages impregnated with ichthopaste can also be used.

Children with eczema are prone to infection with *Staphylococcus aureus* and group

B beta-haemolytic streptococcus. In general, infection is best treated with a combined topical antibiotic and steroid. If the child is systemically unwell, oral or intravenous antibiotics may be required. However, for localised infection in a systemically well child, topical treatment for 7–10 days is the first-line treatment option. In children with recurrent infections, prevention of infection is important. Weekly antiseptic baths with, for example, Milton Sterilising Fluid can help decrease bacterial skin colonisation and prevent infection.

Psoriasis treatment

Most children are managed with topical treatments alone, but more severe cases may respond to phototherapy or systemic treatments. Parental and child education should focus on the nature of the disease, trigger avoidance and the effects of treatment. It is important not to underestimate the significant social and emotional consequences that psoriasis can have on children.

Regular, daily use of emollients is important as they help to remove scale and, in doing so, they allow other topical agents to work more effectively.

A vitamin D derivative (calcipotreine or calcipotriol) is often the first-line treatment in children with plaque psoriasis and is effective in about 65% of cases. It affects cell division and differentiation. It is often used in rotation with steroid-based formulations. As it does not stain or smell it is often preferred over coal tar or dithranol.

Steroids can be used as monotherapy on the face and flexures. They are clean, easy to apply and effective. Ointments work better than creams on thick plaques, as their absorption is better. However, steroids should not be used as monotherapy on the body as, once discontinued, the psoriasis can recur. Therefore they are usually used intermittently.

Coal tar preparations have both anti-inflammatory and anti-scaling properties. However, they are messy and malodourous, and therefore compliance tends to be problematic.

Dithranol is an effective topical treatment that slows down production of new skin cells. It can be used in two ways: (1) short-contact dithranol (applied directly to lesions and washed off after 15 minutes) and Ingram's regimen (a thicker dithranol preparation is applied directly to the lesions, powder is then applied and the skin is covered with a dressing, which is left on for 6–24 hours). This regimen is used primarily in an inpatient setting. It is messy and stains the skin temporarily.

Scalp treatment

To help remove thick, scaly plaques on the scalp, salicylic acid can be applied, left overnight and washed off in the morning, gently combing the hair to remove the scale. Tar-based preparations can then be applied and left overnight. If the scalp is very itchy or sore, short-term treatment with topical steroid scalp applications can be used.

There are two types of phototherapy: UVA and PUVA. PUVA is rarely used in children, as it is more carcinogenic. UVA is safer and is the most common type of phototherapy used in children. It is generally given as a 6- to 8-week course, three times a week. Short-term complications include erythema, itching, tenderness and, rarely, blistering.

If psoriasis becomes very disabling and resistant to treatment, systemic therapy may be indicated. Oral acitretin is effective and one of the safest systemic treatments that is prescribed commonly. It is a vitamin A derivative and teratogenic. Female patients must avoid pregnancy during treatment and for 2 years after drug withdrawal. Side effects include dry lips, hair thinning, photosensitivity and hyperlipidaemia. Alternative treatment options include methotrexate and cyclosporin.

Acne treatment

Acne should be treated aggressively to avoid permanent scarring and cysts

Mild comedonal acne can be treated with topical retinoids and/or topical benzoyl peroxide. Topical retinoids are vitamin A derivatives that reduce obstruction in the follicles. Benzoyl peroxide has both antibacterial and comedolytic properties.

Mild inflammatory acne can be treated with topical retinoids, topical benzoyl peroxide and topical antibiotics (clindamycin and erythromycin). To prevent the development of antibiotic resistance, topical antibiotics should be prescribed with benzoyl peroxidase. Common side effects of topical treatments include dry skin and irritation. Patients should be advised to moisturise their skin and may need to decrease usage to alternate days if poorly tolerated. It takes several months for the effect of treatment to be seen, so patient education is essential to ensure compliance with treatment.

Patients with moderate inflammatory acne should be prescribed oral antibiotics (minocycline, doxycycline and tetracycline) in addition to topical treatments. Tetracyclines are contraindicated in pregnancy and in children less than 8 years of age. Antibiotics are usually prescribed for 6-month courses. If there has been no response after 3 months, ensure compliance and consider increasing the dose or using an alternative treatment.

In patients with severe inflammatory or nodulocystic acne, resistant acne or acne resulting in physical or psychological scarring, isotretinoin should be considered. Isotretinoin is a vitamin A derivative and is usually prescribed for a 20-week course under specialist supervision. Patients should be counselled about potential side effects, which include dry skin, lips and eyes; mood disturbance; muscle aches and photosensitivity. Isotretinoin is teratogenic and therefore all female patients must be advised of the risks of foetal malformation. Female patients must abstain from sexual activity during the course of treatment and for 1 month after. If sexually active, two forms of contraception must be used.

Treatment of tinea infections

Tinea capitis

The goals of treatment are to treat the infection and prevent the spread of infection to other children. Tinea capitis is treated with systemic antifungals and the application of antifungal shampoos. Tinia capitis secondary to trichophyton should be treated with terbinafine for 4 weeks. Terbinafine is not as effective against microsporum infections. Tinea capitis secondary to microsporum should be treated with griseofulvin for 8 weeks. Alternative treatment options include itraconazole and fluconazole. If a kerion is present, longer treatment is required. Selenium sulphide or ketoconazole shampoo or other topical antifungals should be used at least twice weekly during the first 2 weeks of treatment.

To avoid spreading to other members of the household, children should use their own hairbrushes and towels. Family members in contact with tinea capitis should be examined for evidence of infection; if this is confirmed on mycological exam they should be started on oral treatment. Family members without clinical or laboratory evidence of hair shaft invasion, but from whose scalps dermatophytes are grown, from brush sampling, are called carriers. Children with heavy fungal results from brush sampling should be treated. To reduce carriage of organisms, carriers should be treated with topical miconazole, in addition to topical ketoconazole and selenium sulphide shampoos.

Tinea corporis and tinea pedis

Tinea corporis and tinea pedis usually respond to topical antifungal treatment. To prevent recurrence, topical treatments should be continued for 1–2 weeks after the lesion has cleared. When tinea pedis is present, patients should be advised to change socks daily, dry feet fully after showering or bathing, wear open-toe shoes as much as feasible and use foot powder.

Tinea unguium

Asymptomatic children with tinea unguium may not require treatment. The decision to treat should be discussed with parents and children. It is difficult to treat and responds poorly to topical treatment; therefore, systemic treatment is often required. Topical treatments are applied two to three times weekly for 3–6 months for fingernails and 6–12 months for toenails. Poor compliance is common. Nails should be cut as much as possible prior to applying treatment. Systemic treatment is prolonged, expensive and exposes the child to potential drug side effects. First-line treatment is systemic terbinafine or itraconazole.

Haemangioma treatment

Currently propranolol is emerging as the treatment of choice for haemangiomas where treatment is indicated (*see* Evidence 4). Previously, systemic corticosteroids were used with success rates of 80% but with significant side effects.

Scabies treatment

Permethrin is the treatment of choice in children with scabies (*see* Evidence 5). For infants under 2 months of age, a 7% sulphur is recommended. A small percentage of children, having been treated for eczema, may still experience itch and the doctor may be tempted to re-treat them. These children often respond to treatment with 1% hydrocortisone and sedating antihistamine for 2–3 days, as their symptoms are related to their scratching rather than to the scabies infection, which is effectively treated by the permethrin.

WHEN TO REFER?

- The diagnosis is unclear
- Difficult to control acne or acne with scarring
- Children with eczema that is severe, poorly controlled with topical steroids or associated with recurrent infections
- Difficult-to-control psoriasis

CLARIFICATION STATEMENTS FOR PARENTAL MISCONCEPTIONS

> *'I know he has eczema but steroids thin the skin and are harmful.'*

Steroid treatment in conjunction with other treatments forms an important part of the eczema treatment programme. Steroids have different strengths and the focus of treatment is the use of the lowest-potency steroid possible. Low-potency steroids, in general, do not produce thinning of the skin.

> *'The eczema must be related to a food allergy. I think that removing milk and eggs could be a good idea.'*

Children with eczema often have allergies; however, elimination diets are not an effective strategy for treating eczema. There are a small number of children in whom a food allergy results in a flare-up of their condition, but the temporal relationship is often evident from the history.

> *'How can I give him his shots with this eczema?'*

The presence of eczema is not a contraindication to immunisation. All children should be immunised in accordance with national guidelines.

SUMMARY PRACTICE POINTS

- Sixty per cent of eczema commences in <1 year.
- Eczema favours the flexures.

- Failure of eczema to respond to topical steroids suggests there is co-existing infection of the skin.
- Tacrolimus is second-line treatment for eczema and strict photoprotection is required.
- Plaque psoriasis is the most common type of psoriasis in children.
- Psoriasis in moist areas is non-scaly
- Guttate psoriasis is associated with upper respiratory tract infection.
- Vitamin D derivatives are first-line treatment in children.
- Vascular lesions can be treated with propranolol.
- Permethrin is the treatment of choice for scabies.
- After scabies treatment the residual itch can cause post-scabetic eczema.

EVALUATING THE EVIDENCE

Evidence 1	
Theme E1	**Parent education and eczema**
Question	What is the impact of nurse-led eczema workshops for parents of children with eczema?
Design	Randomised controlled trial
Level of evidence	Jadad 2
Setting	Department of dermatology, academic medical centre, Australia
Participants	Infants, children and adolescents with eczema <16 years of age who were new referrals to a department of dermatology were eligible for inclusion.
Intervention	Patients were randomised to receive care in the dermatologist-led clinic, with 40 minutes of patient contact time, or in the nurse-led eczema workshop, with 90 minutes of patient contact time.
Outcomes	The primary outcome was the severity of eczema, determined by using the Scoring of Atopic Dermatitis (SCORAD), from initial assessment to the end of 4 weeks of treatment.
Main results	Of the 182 assessed for eligibility, 165 were randomised (17 were excluded, 16 did not meet criteria and one refused to participate). Eighty were allocated to the nurse-led workshop; however, 26 did not attend, and of the 54 who did attend, full data were available on 49 (91%) at the 4-week follow-up. On the 85 in the dermatologist-led clinic, 27 did not attend, and of the 58 who attended, full data were available on 50 (86%) at the 4-week follow-up. The improvement in SCORAD was −9.93% in favour of the workshop group. On adherence to guidelines, 90% of workshop patients and 78% of clinic patients had a daily bath (absolute risk reduction (ARR) = 12%; number needed to treat (NNT) = 9), 80% of workshop patients and 62% of clinic patients used emollients twice a day (ARR = 18%; NNT = 6), 94% of workshop patients avoided antibiotics, as compared with 80% of clinic patients (ARR = 14%; NNT = 8).
Conclusion	Patients in the nurse-led workshop group had a greater improvement in their eczema than those in the dermatologist-led clinic.

(continued)

Evidence 1

Theme E1	*Parent education and eczema*
Commentary	The factors that influence successful treatment outcome in eczema are parent education, adequate time for explanation and discussion inclusive of demonstration of treatments. In the workshop the applications of creams, cool compresses and wet dressings were demonstrated. The parent or caregiver was an active participant in this process and thus enhanced his or her skills. While both groups watched videos of these processes, those who actually had practised these techniques, under supervision, were likely to be more competent. The current model of Western medicine may be inadequate to address the healthcare needs of children, and more collaborative models (as described in this study) should be developed.
Reference	Moore EJ, Williams A, Manias E, *et al.* Eczema workshops reduce severity of childhood atopic eczema. *Australas J Dermatol.* 2009; **50**(2): 100–6.

Evidence 2

Theme E2	*Treating eczema utilising a nurse practitioner (NP) or dermatologist*
Question	In the treatment of childhood eczema, are there differences between NPs and dermatologists?
Design	Randomised controlled trial
Level of evidence	Jadad 1
Setting	Department of dermatology and epidemiology, academic medical centre, the Netherlands
Participants	Children and adolescents (<16 years) with a diagnosis of eczema (atopic dermatitis) were eligible for inclusion. Parents of children younger than 4 years of age completed the Infants' Dermatitis Quality of Life Index and those aged 4–16 completed the Children's Dermatology Life Quality Index.
Intervention	Eczema care provision to children and adolescents was randomised to a nurse practitioner (NP) or dermatologist.
Outcomes	The primary outcomes were between group (dermatologists and NP) differences in terms of cost-effectiveness and quality-of-life measures of the participants at 12 months.
Main results	One hundred and sixty children and adolescents participated in this study. The mean (± standard deviation (SD)) SCORAD (SCORing Atopic Dermatitis) score were 33.4 (19.3) for the dermatologist and 33.4 (15.6) for the NP in children under 4 years of age. For those older than 4 years the mean SCORAD (±SD) was 35.4 (15.6) for the dermatologist and 29.9 (16.0) for the NP. In terms of clinical effectiveness, the dermatologists offered 4.5 outpatient visits per patient, compared with 3.5 for the NP. In terms of patient contact time, it was 52 minutes per year for the dermatologist compared with 100 minutes for the NP – this included telephone contact time. Cost per patient for the dermatologist was €1409 and per patient for the NP was €981. No differences in Infants' Dermatitis Quality of Life Index and Children's Dermatology Life Quality Index between groups were noted.

(continued)

Evidence 2	
Theme E2	*Treating eczema utilising a nurse practitioner (NP) or dermatologist*
Conclusion	Substituting NPs for dermatologists was effective and care was provided at a lower cost.
Commentary	The severity of eczema was assessed using the SCORAD. This tool calculates: a) the *area* affected using the rule of 9s (head and neck, 9%; upper limbs, each 9%; lower limbs, 18%; anterior trunk, 18%; back, 18%; and 1% for genitals and palm and back of each hand) b) intensity of a representative area of eczema scoring it as none (0), mild (1), moderate (2) or severe (3), (parameters of intensity are redness, swelling, oozing/crusting, scratch marks, skin thickening (lichenification) and dryness, each of which is scored) c) subjective symptoms of itch and sleeplessness (each scored 0–10). The total SCORAD for an individual is a/5 + 7b/2 + c. Eczema is a chronic disease and different models of care provision need to be explored. NPs were cost-effective. Their use of telephone communication to parents reduces direct costs to the parents, in terms of time off work and school loss for the child. It also allows for potential flare-up to be addressed earlier. Such models of care delivery are applicable to other conditions and randomised controlled trials can test their effectiveness.
Reference	Schuttelaar MLA, Vermeulen KM, Coenraads PJ. Costs and cost-effectiveness analysis of treatment in children with eczema by nurse practitioner vs. dermatologist: results of a randomized, controlled trial and review of international costs. *Br J Dermatol.* 2011; **165**(3): 600–11.

Evidence 3	
Theme E3	*Tacrolimus in the treatment of atopic dermatitis (AD)*
Question	How effective is tacrolimus in the treatment of AD compared with 1% hydrocortisone?
Design	Randomised controlled trial
Level of evidence	Jadad 5
Setting	Departments of dermatology, 42 medical centres in 11 European countries
Participants	Children aged 2–15 years of age with moderate to severe AD were eligible for participation. The AD severity was rated on the Rajka and Langeland scoring system. This technique assesses extent, course and intensity of the disease on a scale of 1–3 (maximum 9). A score of 3–4 is mild, 4.5–7.5 is moderate and 8–9 is severe. The extent of the AD had to be >5% on the body surface area.
Intervention	Participants were randomised to 0.03% tacrolimus twice daily or daily, and to 1% hydrocortisone twice daily for 3 weeks. Those on the once-a-day treatment used a placebo ointment once a day also.
Outcomes	The primary outcome was the percentage change in the modified Eczema Area and Severity Index (mEASI) between baseline and at the end of the 3 weeks of treatment.

(continued)

Evidence 3	
Theme E3	*Tacrolimus in the treatment of atopic dermatitis (AD)*
Outcomes (*cont.*)	The mEASI is a composite score comprising severity rating of eczema, scoring 0–3 for (a) erythema, (b) oedema, induration, papulation, (c) excoriations and (d) lichenification. This score was weighted according to the estimated percentage of the affected body surface area. The presence of itch, a key feature of AD, was also assessed on a visual scale, which was converted to an ordinal scale 0–3.
Main results	A total of 624 patients were enrolled, with 210 randomised to tacrolimus twice a day (group 1), 207 to tacrolimus per day (group 2) and 207 to hydrocortisone acetate twice daily (group 3). Withdrawals for group 1 were 21 (10%), group 2 were 26 (12.6%) and group 3 were 41 (19.8%). After 3 weeks of treatment the mean improvement in the mEASI score for group 3 was 47.2%, for group 1 it was 78.7% (absolute risk reduction (ARR) = 31.5%; number needed to treat (NNT) = 4) and for group 2 it was 70.0% (ARR = 222.8%; NNT = 5). The three most common side effects in groups 3, 1 and 2 were (a) skin burning (14.5%, 23.8% and 23.2%, respectively) (number needed to harm (NNH) = 12) for groups 1 and 2; (b) pruritus (15.9%, 21.4% and 18.4%, respectively) (NNH = 18 and 40) for groups 1 and 2; and (c) folliculitis (3.9%, 5.2% and 3.9%, respectively) (NNH = 43 and 0) for groups 1 and 2.
Conclusion	The study found 0.03% tacrolimus ointment is more effective in the treatment of moderate to severe AD than hydrocortisone acetate. Side effects such as skin burning prompted eight (3.8%) patients in group 1 to withdraw from the study.
Commentary	AD in moderate to severe cases will require the usage of more potent topical steroids than hydrocortisone. Tacrolimus offers the physician an alternative strategy for the steroid-averse parent, who is often worried about thinning of the skin from steroid use. The use of once-a-day treatment with tacrolimus would appear to be sufficient in most patients with moderate eczema.
Reference	Reitamo S, Harper J, Bos JD, *et al.* European Tacrolimus Ointment Group. 0.03% Tacrolimus ointment applied once or twice daily is more efficacious than 1% hydrocortisone acetate in children with moderate to severe atopic dermatitis: results of a randomized double-blind controlled trial. *Br J Dermatol.* 2004; **150**(3): 554–62.

Evidence 4	
Theme E4	*Treatment options for infantile haemangiomas*
Question	Which is more effective in the treatment of infantile haemangiomas: propranolol or corticosteroids?
Design	Multicentre retrospective analysis
Level of evidence	
Setting	Departments of dermatology and surgery, academic medical centre, the United States
Participants	Children attending two academic medical centres with infantile haemangiomas were eligible for inclusion.

(*continued*)

Evidence 4	
Theme E4	*Treatment options for infantile haemangiomas*
Intervention	Charts were reviewed to assess for primary treatment with oral steroids or propranolol.
Outcomes	The primary outcome was clearance rates of infantile haemangiomas, which were classified as >75% (in this group there was a proportional decrease in volume, a cosmetically acceptable result determined by physician and/or patient and further treatment was not required) or as <75%.
Main results	One hundred and thirty-nine patient charts were assessed. Of these 139, 22 were excluded because they received alternate treatments, and seven patients were lost to follow-up. Of the 110 patients, 68 received propranolol and 42, oral corticosteroids. In the propranolol group, 59 received only propranolol for an average duration of 7.9 (3.5–14.0) months, and of these, 48 (81%) had >75% clearance and 11 (19%) had <75% clearance. Nine received propranolol but had previously been treated with oral steroids: eight (89%) had >75% clearance and one (11%) had <75%. In those 42 patients treated with oral steroids, only 12 (29%) had >75% clearance and 30 (71%) had <75% clearance. The difference in primary outcome between oral propranolol and oral steroids was absolute risk reduction = 52%, number needed to treat = 2. On discontinuation of propranolol, two patients had relapse. Side effects related to propranolol included one (1.5%) hypoglycaemia and a skin eruption in two (3%). In the oral steroid group, 42 (100%) patients experienced side effects. All had cushingoid features, two had hypertension and one had a life-threatening arterial bleed as a result of an ulceration that eroded through the external carotid artery.
Conclusion	Propranolol is more effective in the treatment of infantile haemangiomas than oral corticosteroids.
Commentary	The majority of infantile haemangiomas regress with time and require intervention. However, in approximately 10% intervention is required. The initial finding of regression with propranolol was noted in a child who was being treated for obstructive cardiomyopathy and high-output cardiac disease with extensive haemangiomas. While propranolol is effective therapy, the mechanism of action is unclear. The evidence from this study, which needs to be confirmed prospectively, indicates the effectiveness and safety of propranolol as first-line treatment in children with haemangiomas. Infants with haemangiomas can develop complications that include ulceration, with resultant bleeding, and infection. Haemangiomas, dependent on their location, can cause airway obstruction. Large haemangiomas can lead to high-output heart failure as a result of arteriovenous shunting.
Reference	Price CJ, Lattouf C, Baum B, *et al.* Propranolol vs corticosteroids for infantile hemangiomas: a multicenter retrospective analysis. *Arch Dermatol.* 2011; **147**(12): 1371–6.

Evidence 5	
Theme E5	**Treatment of scabies**
Question	Which is more effective in treatment of scabies: crotamiton or permethrin?
Design	Randomised controlled trial
Level of evidence	Jadad 5
Setting	Rural community, Panama
Participants	Children with a clinical diagnosis of scabies inclusive of the recovery of one live *Sarcoptes scabiei* mite were eligible for inclusion in the study.
Intervention	Children were randomised to treatment with 10% crotamiton cream or 5% permethrin cream, supplied in identical tubes. Creams were applied in the evening and were washed off the following morning. Clinical photographs were taken to allow independent assessment of disease severity. Also, all lesions were counted, described and recorded on a body chart. To avoid re-infestation from untreated individuals, all household members were treated with open-labelled 5% permethrin.
Outcomes	The primary outcome was cure at 28 days. Participants were assessed at 1 hour and 24 hours post application for evidence of skin irritation and at 14 and 28 days for cure.
Main results	Ninety-six children were enrolled, of whom 94 completed the study. Scabies was classified as mild (fewer than 50 lesions), moderate (50–100 lesions) and severe (>100 lesions). In the permethrin group, 29 were mild, 17 were moderate and two were severe. In the crotamiton group there were 29 mild, 15 moderate and four severely affected children. The age of the children precludes their description of pruritus, but this was inferred from scratching, from visible excoriation and from the opinion of the mother. The active scabetic lesions were 2 mm erythematous papules. In addition, 1–2 mm non-inflammatory papules were also noted, which reflected the host's response to the dead mites. At 28 days, 42 (89%) of the permethrin group and 28 (60%) of the crotamiton group were cured (absolute reduced risk = 28%; number needed to treat = 4). Twelve (17%) of those cured had non-inflammatory papules present at 28 days.
Conclusion	Permethrin is effective and superior to crotamiton in the treatment of scabies.
Commentary	Scabies is a common condition causing intense itching. Permethrin is effective in the treatment of scabies and is not absorbed systemically. It acts by disrupting the sodium channel current, resulting in delayed repolarisation, causing paralysis and death of the parasite in all stages. The non-inflammatory papules post treatments do not reflect treatment failure. A small number of infants, if there is persisting erythema and itch, benefit from 1% hydrocortisone and a sedating antihistamine for 2–3 days, while the skin is healing. Some children will require a second treatment 1–2 weeks later. Permethrin is recommended for infants older than 2 months. For those younger than 2 months, a 7% sulphur is advised.
Reference	Taplin D, Meinking TL, Chen JA, *et al.* Comparison of crotamiton 10% cream (Eurax) and permethrin 5% cream (Elimite) for the treatment of scabies in children. *Pediatr Dermatol.* 1990; **7**(1): 67–73.

CHRONIC RASH: MULTIPLE-CHOICE QUESTIONS

Q1 Which of the following definitions is/are correct?
a) A bulla is greater than 1 cm in diameter.
b) A plaque is a palpable elevation of the skin greater than 2 cm.
c) Petechiae are less than 5 mm in size.
d) Lichenification is thickened skin with accentuation of skin markings.
e) An ulcer of the skin indicates loss of epidermis and dermis.

Q2 Which of the following statements regarding eczema is/are correct?
a) Eczema affects 1% of children and adolescents.
b) Twenty per cent of affected children are under 1 year of age.
c) Itch is a prominent symptom.
d) The flexures of the arms and legs are frequently affected.
e) Eczematous plaques occur in 15% of affected children.

Q3 Which of the following statements is/are correct?
a) Thirty per cent of children with eczema have food allergies.
b) Scratching of eczematous lesions leads to skin lichenification.
c) Triggers of eczema exacerbations include infections.
d) Sedating antihistamines are useful in eczema if used for short periods of time.
e) Blood tests for allergy are preferred to skin prick testing in children with eczema.

Q4 Which of the following statements is/are true with regard to infected eczema?
a) Crusting and weeping of the skin occurs.
b) There is failure of eczema to respond to standard steroid treatment.
c) Fever occurs in 30% of patients.
d) Topical antibiotics are contraindicated.
e) Intravenous antibiotics are required in 15% of children.

Q5 Recognised triggers that aggravate eczema include which of the following?
a) Heat
b) Cold
c) Harsh soaps
d) Chlorine
e) House dust mite

Q6 The differential diagnosis of eczematous lesions includes which of the following?
a) Wiskott–Aldrich's syndrome
b) Scabies
c) Psoriasis
d) Hyperimmune-IgE syndrome
e) Varicella

Q7   Which of the following is/are correct with regard to childhood psoriasis?
   a) Fifty per cent have a positive family history of psoriasis.
   b) Plaque and guttate psoriasis are the most common forms in children.
   c) Koebner's phenomenon is present.
   d) The scalp is involved in 80% of children.
   e) Nail pitting is found in 10% of children.

Q8   The differential of a scaly rash includes which of the following?
   a) Tinea corporis
   b) Lichen planus
   c) Discoid (nummular) eczema
   d) Pityriasis rosea
   e) Urticaria

Q9   Which of the following statements is/are correct regarding acne?
   a) Males and females are equally affected.
   b) It is a disorder of pilosebaceous glands.
   c) It is associated with low levels of dehydroepiandrosterone sulphate.
   d) Plugging of the hair follicles due to abnormal keratin occurs.
   e) The disorder is more severe in males.

Q10 Which of the following statements with regard to tinea infections is/are correct?
   a) Tinea infections are classified by location.
   b) Tinea capitis predominantly affects school-age children.
   c) Tinea capitis is associated with patchy alopecia.
   d) Tinea corporis is characterised by itchy annular lesions.
   e) A kerion is an inflammatory boggy mass on the scalp.

Answers

A1	c, d, e	A2	c, d
A3	a, b, c, d	A4	a, b
A5	a, c, e	A6	a, b, d
A7	b, c, d	A8	a, b, c, d
A9	a, b, d, e	A10	a, b, c, d, e

SLIDES
   1. Acne (facial)
   2. Ammoniacal dermatitis
   3. Eczema (atopic dermatitis)
   4. Eczema trunk
   5. Eczema infected
   6. Eczema herpetic
   7. Eczema infected

8. Eczema hand mittens
9. Pompholyx (dyshidrotic eczema)
10. Pompholyx (dyshidrotic eczema)
11. Granuloma annulare
12. Incontinentia pigmenti (vesicular)
13. Incontinentia pigmenti (papules)
14. Incontinentia pigmenti (linear)
15. Localised scleroderma
16. Morphea
17. Psoriasis legs
18. Psoriasis trunk
19. Psoriasis scalp
20. Psoriasis plaques
21. Psoriasis nails
22. Keloid
23. Kerion
25. Alopecia (early)
26. Alopecia
27. Alopecia (eyebrows)
28. Capillary haemangioma (neck)
29. Capillary haemangioma (eyelid)
30. Kasabach Merritt syndrome
31. Scabies foot (burrow)
32. Scabies sole of foot
33. Scabies interdigital cleft
34. Dermatitis enterohepatica feet (zinc deficiency)
35. Dermatitis enteropathica groin
36. Ichthyosis (neonatal)
37. Raynaud's syndrome
38. Tinea corporis (hand)
39. Mongolian blue spot

Chapter Thirty-two

ATTENTION DEFICIT HYPERACTIVITY DISORDER IN CHILDREN

COMMON SCENARIO

'The teacher says my 7-year-old son has a short attention span and has difficulty keeping up with his classmates academically. On the playground he is very active and is supervised closely, as he has no sense of danger. Recently he ran across the road without looking and was almost hit by a car. Why is he like this?'

LEARNING OBJECTIVES

- Identify the various attention deficit subtypes
- Recognise the conditions that can simulate attention deficit hyperactivity disorder (ADHD)
- Develop awareness of the need treat co-morbid conditions that exist with ADHD
- Understand the treatment options and their effectiveness

BACKGROUND

ADHD is a neurodevelopment disorder characterised by an inability to marshal and sustain attention, modulate activity levels and moderate impulsive actions. It is a common disorder. In the United Kingdom a survey of 10438 children aged 5–15 years found the incidence in boys to be 3.6% and in girls to be 0.85%. This survey used strict criteria. Comparing the epidemiology of ADHD is difficult, as the criteria are symptoms that are continuously distributed across the population. Central to the diagnosis of ADHD is the pervasive nature of the symptoms, which means they must be evident both at school and at home.

ADHD is classified into three subtypes, depending on the distribution of symptoms of specific behaviours: predominantly inattentive, predominantly hyperactive/impulsive and combined types. These three subtypes are not mutually exclusive. The aetiology of ADHD is not understood, but 70% can be attributed to genetic causes and 30% to environmental factors.

The criteria that are required when assessing a child for attention deficit disorder are outlined here.

DIAGNOSIS REQUIRES EVIDENCE OF INATTENTION OR HYPERACTIVITY AND IMPULSIVITY OR BOTH

Inattention

Six or more of the following symptoms of inattention have persisted for at least 6 months to a degree that is maladaptive and inconsistent with developmental level:

- often fails to give close attention to details and makes careless mistakes
- often has difficulty sustaining attention
- often does not seem to listen
- often does not seem to follow through tasks
- often avoids tasks that require sustained attention
- often loses things necessary for activities
- often is easily distracted
- often is forgetful

Hyperactivity and impulsivity

Six or more of the following symptoms of hyperactivity and impulsivity have persisted for at least 6 months to a degree that is maladaptive and inconsistent with developmental level:

- often fidgets
- often leaves seat
- often runs about or climbs excessively
- often has difficulty with quiet leisure activities
- often is on the go or acts if driven by a motor
- often talks excessively
- often blurts out answers
- often has difficulty awaiting turn
- often interrupts or intrudes on others

Symptoms that cause impairment are present before 7 years of age and are present in two or more settings (e.g. home and school).

There are no diagnostic tests for ADHD. The diagnosis is aided by the aforementioned criteria in conjunction with the history, school assessments and psychometric testing. The finding of symptoms at school and at home is paramount in the diagnosis of ADHD therefore parental and school assessments are central to the establishment of the diagnosis. The differential diagnosis section outlines conditions that may resemble ADHD.

HISTORY

KEY POINTS				
Inattention	Six or more of the following: • often fails to give close attention to details • has difficulty sustaining attention • does not listen • does not follow through • has difficulty organising tasks • avoids tasks that require sustained attention • often loses things • easily distracted • forgetful	**Symptom severity**	Ejection from school or play group Injury to others, direct trauma Impact on parent relationship, degree of disharmony Parental respite (if any)	**Q Red Flags** Undertakes dangerous activities e.g running across the road without looking for oncoming traffic Early morning wakening Easily provoked to anger
Hyperactivity/ impulsivity	Six or more of the following: • often fidgets • leaves seat • runs or climbs excessively • has difficulty with quiet leisure • on the go • blurts out answers • difficulty taking turns • interrupts and intrudes	**Academic achievement**	Progress through preschool and school environment Ask about teachers' perceptions compared with others in class	
Age of onset	Present before 7 years	**Peer relationships**	Number of friends, inclusion or exclusion from group and why	
Settings	Present in two or more settings: school, home	**Developmental**	Developmental milestones, activity levels, attention difficulties, impulsivity examples of each Speech delay	

(continued)

KEY POINTS			
Past medical history	Three areas: 1. syndromes inclusive of foetal alcohol syndrome, fragile X, neurofibromatosis, Williams's syndrome 2. medical hypothyroidism, hyperthyroidism 3. deafness	**Systems review**	Focus on: • sleep pattern, when goes to bed, duration of sleep and early awakening • safety issues; ask about dangerous activities undertaken • time taken to complete homework
Family history	Presence of ADHD in parents, especially the father Parent strategies to manage behaviour and success Family history of mental retardation Academic performance of parents Impact of behaviours on parental relationship	**Interventions utilised by parents**	What strategies have they used, for how long, how consistent
Obstetrical history	Three areas: 1. drug consumption – alcohol, cigarettes and heroin 2. prematurity 3. neonatal hypoxia All can be associated with ADHD and learning disabilities	**Styles of parenting**	Do the parents react all the time? Do they lecture the child?

EXAMINATION

- A general physical examination is required in children with suspected ADHD to exclude co-morbid conditions
- Height, weight, head circumference
- Dysmorphic features
- Skin: café au lait lesions in the axilla
- Cardiovascular: pulse rate, blood pressure, murmurs (aortic stenosis)
- Neurological examination

- A developmental examination is essential
- Review of their homework book is important, as well as comments made by their teachers and any reports that are supplied

Red flags

- Macrocephaly fragile X
- Growth failure (foetal alcohol syndrome)
- Dysmorphic features (may be subtle)
- Height/weight discrepancy (hypothyroidism)
- Café au lait spots (neurofibromatosis)
- Murmur of aortic stenosis (Williams's syndrome)
- Developmental delay (on examination)

DIFFERENTIAL DIAGNOSIS

In addressing ADHD, it is best to consider it in the following format.

- Does the child have ADHD alone?
- Does the child have a condition where ADHD symptoms are recognised as occurring with increased frequency?
- Does the child have ADHD and one of its known co-morbidities?

Differential	***Symptoms similar to ADHD***	***Symptoms dissimilar to ADHD***
Hyperthyroidism	Active, usually of recent onset	Sweating, tachycardia, weight loss May have goitre
Fragile X syndrome	Hyperactive and impulsive behaviour	Developmental delay Speech and language delay Physical features: • large forehead, prominent jaw and long face • large head circumference at birth • large testicles after the start of puberty
Neurofibromatosis	Standard features of ADHD	Abnormal physical examination features, e.g. café au lait in the axillary region
Foetal alcohol syndrome	Standard features of ADHD	Growth failure Craniofacial features, smooth philtrum, thin vermilion, small palpebral features Microcephaly This is a spectrum disorder dependent on the amount of alcohol exposure

(continued)

Differential	Symptoms similar to ADHD	Symptoms dissimilar to ADHD
Social immaturity	Many of the features of ADHD are noted but they are not as severe as in ADHD	Parents note has always been behind peers in social skill acquisition, but the skills are acquired albeit at a later date; teachers note slow but steady progress
Learning disorder	See next section in this table This can occur with ADHD or as an isolated condition	

Co-morbid conditions	Symptoms similar to ADHD	Symptoms dissimilar to ADHD
Learning disorder	Poor academic achievement Disruptive in classroom Poor engagement at school and at home	Non-disruptive during non-academic activity
Oppositional conduct disorder	Disruptive behaviour, and frequently breaks rules Refuses to follow directions	Defiant and unreasonable rather than being unsuccessful in engaging the child Ask if argues readily and if uses aggressive tone when responding to requests from parents
Conduct disorder	Disruptive behaviour (extreme)	Lack of remorse Antisocial actions Intent on doing harm to people or animals Aggressive and hostile
Anxiety state, obsessive–compulsive disorder	Poor attention Fidgetiness Difficulty with transition to new activity or environment	Excessive worry and fearful May have difficulty separating from parents
Tic disorder	Poor attention, disruptive actions	Repetitive motor or vocal movements
Adjustment disorder	Poor attention Increased activity Disruptive behaviour Poor academic performance	Precipitating event often of recent origin is evident

INVESTIGATIONS

What is the value of questionnaires?

Rating scales that are specific to ADHD symptomatology are useful in assessing children with ADHD in conjunction to the history, physical examination and other reports. The Conners Rating Scales for parent and teacher are useful, especially when trying to assess the initial severity of symptoms and in follow-up, if on medication, to determine the response. The Home Situation Questionnaire is also useful, as parents are able to reflect the child's behaviour at home.

Is formal psychometric assessment required?

Formal psychometric assessment is required if there is evidence of a learning disability. Data from resource teachers are often valuable in these situations.

What is the value of blood tests?

Few blood tests are required. However, if suspect a full blood count for anaemia (in some areas, lead levels may be performed), T4, thyroid-stimulating hormone, thyroid antibodies for hypothyroidism, genetic assessment for fragile X syndrome. If considering medication, an electrocardiogram may be of some value (evidence lacking).

Is brain imaging required?

Computed tomography of the brain is not required to diagnose ADHD. It may be required if associated conditions, e.g. neurofibromatosis, are suspected.

Is chromosomal analysis of benefit?

Routine chromosomal analysis is of no benefit in the diagnosis of ADHD. If fragile X syndrome is suspected, it must be specifically requested to make the diagnosis.

MANAGEMENT PLAN: THREE-STEP APPROACH

1. Clarifying and pitfall avoidance strategies
2. Non-pharmacological options:
   ○ role of diet
   ○ behavioural strategies
   ○ homework strategies
3. Pharmacological options
   ○ drug treatment for the preschool child
   ○ drug treatment for the school-age child

Clarifying and pitfall avoidance strategies

- Many children have features of ADHD but do not meet the diagnostic criteria.
- To make a diagnosis of ADHD the child must have symptoms both at home and at school.
- Explore with parents what their earliest concerns are with regard to their child's symptoms. **Rationale**: ADHD features evolve and change. Pay attention to anything dangerous the child manifested in his or her early years, and also focus on the child's ability to be safe at home and outside the home.
- Explore with the parents why they think their child's behaviours are a concern. **Rationale**: addressing ADHD requires a change in the family dynamic, especially how parents respond and react to the condition. Their expectations must be realistic.
- Determine the parenting style. **Rationale**: behavioural programmes for ADHD require a modification of parenting behaviours (*see* Evidence 1).

- Explain the absence of a blood test to diagnose ADHD.
- Stress the importance of rating scores in coming to a diagnosis and the role of psychometric testing in assessing for associated disabilities. **Rationale**: the assessment of ADHD and associated conditions can be frustrating for parents, given the absence of a specific test, but it is imperative to a make a correct diagnosis and assess for associated and co-morbid conditions.
- Define what specific changes they would view as positive. **Rationale**: these should form the basis of goal setting. The behaviours of years will not be undone in a few weeks or months.
- Remember parents have been dealing with these challenges for several years and have tried various strategies – therefore, be specific in your recommendations.
- Mention non-verbal communication. **Rationale**: many parents will experience frustration with their child's *behaviour* and they must avoid non-verbal expression of negativity with the child but verbally express their views related to the behaviour.
- Discuss the impact of ADHD symptoms on other children and on the parents' relationship.
- Determine how the family reduces stress. **Rationale**: if stress levels are not reduced then parental effectiveness will lessen. If parents recognise this then they will cope better.

In dealing with an ADHD family, remember the following points.
- The parents are probably tired and frustrated and want a solution.
- The school wants a solution.
- The child is frustrated and may not understand why he or she is experiencing difficulties both at school and school. Have sympathy for the family's challenges and difficulties.

Non-pharmacological options
Role of diet
(*See* Evidence 2)

Behavioural strategies
Behavioural management is the first strategy to aid the family with a child who has ADHD. Knowledge of one behavioural strategy, e.g. 1-2-3 Magic is required to counsel and advise parents. This programme uses a commercial video that has three aims: (1) controlling negative behaviour of the child, (2) encouraging positive behaviour and (3) strengthening the parent–child relationship. Parents when disciplining children show too much emotion and talk too much. In controlling negative behaviour the parents identify these behaviours, the so-called stop behaviours and when they notice them say, 'That's one'. If it continues for 5 more seconds the parents says 'That's two'. If another 5 seconds pass without the behaviour ceasing, they say, 'That's three'. Then the child is placed in time out. There are some 'red card' offences, i.e. an automatic

three, such as hitting a parent, where the child is sent to time out. Positive behaviours are encouraged through (a) positive reinforcement, (b) simple requests, (c) using time frames for task completion, (d) natural consequences and (e) a reward system. The parent–child relationship is strengthened through sympathetic listening, one-on-one fun time. This system is effective when used correctly (*see* Evidence 1). There are other behavioural interventions that are successful (*see* Evidence 3).

Homework strategies

To effectively study, a child must be able to (a) concentrate, (b) have an ability to switch from topic to topic, (c) have specific organisational skills and (d) have a good memory. These four elements provide specific challenges for the child with ADHD. Therefore, to facilitate homework a specific place and time needs to be established, distraction must be minimised, blocks of time for specific tasks should be allocated with appropriately spaced breaks. The use of a 'study buddy' (a child who is reliable in the performance of homework) is useful; to check what work is required to be completed, as the child with ADHD is likely to forget homework requirements. Parents who are involved with their child's homework need to be encouraging and supportive, focusing on what the child is good at first and building on this process.

Pharmacological options

Drug treatment for the preschool child with attention deficit hyperactivity disorder

In the preschooler behavioural management should be the first line of treatment and the parents, preschool and others involved with the child should be supported to ensure it success. If these measures fail then medication can be considered, but the parents need to be counselled on the risk–benefit ratio. In preschool children 30% of children experience significant side effects that include weight loss, emotional lability in the form of outbursts, anxiety and insomnia. One in nine children (number needed to harm = 9) discontinue medication because of the severe side effects. Caution needs to be exercised if medication is prescribed for preschool children and close follow to assess for potential side effects.

Drug treatment for the school-age child with attention deficit hyperactivity disorder

Methylphenidate is a central nervous stimulant that increases the amount of dopamine in the brain. It is generally recommended for children older than 6 years (*see* Evidence 4). Preparations include slow-release dosage forms such as Equasym XL and Concerta XL. Side effects include decreased appetite, insomnia headache and abdominal pain. Recently, short-term reduction in growth has been cited as a side effect. The value of obtaining electrocardiograms in children prior to the institution of medication is uncertain. At follow-up all children need to have their heights and weights measured and side effect profile assessed, and reports from teachers and parents are essential. If a child experiences weight loss due to medication the following strategies should be tried: (a) encourage breakfast with calorie-dense foods, (b) give medication post breakfast, (c) consider shifting dinner to later in the evening, when the effect of the medication is wearing off.

Atomoxetine is a selective noradrenaline reuptake inhibitor. It is useful in children beyond 6 years who have failed to respond to methylphenidate or have developed side effects (*see* Evidence 5). It also causes abdominal pain, reduced appetite, nausea, vomiting and early-morning awakening. Small changes in blood pressure and heart rate have been noted. There is a small risk of hepatic disorders and suicidal ideation, of which parents must be informed.

FOLLOW-UP
- ADHD is a chronic condition and regular follow-up is required.
- If the child is on medication, obtain height and weight at 3-month visits.
- Use rating scale for home, e.g. Barkley's Home Situation Questionnaire; at school the Conners short form rating is useful.
- Titrate dose of medication according to results on rating scales and teacher and parent global assessments.
- Awareness of development of co-morbid conditions.
- Awareness of medication side effects especially in the younger child (<6 years of age). Parental fatigue assessment – how strong is parental relationship ?; assess the need for respite, especially if there are other stressors in the family or if co-morbid conditions are developing.
- Assess impact of condition on family members.
- Doctor will need other to organise family support.

WHEN TO REFER?
Refer to a paediatrician with special interest or to child and adolescent mental health services when the parents or the preschool raise concerns.

CLARIFICATION STATEMENTS FOR PARENTAL MISCONCEPTIONS

'What about colouring agents and excessive sugar intake as a cause of hyperactivity?'

Diet and the amplification of symptoms of ADHD, when assessed in research studies are frequently highlighted by the media. The impact of diet is often overstated and the implication is of a cause-and-effect phenomenon; however, this is untrue. Randomised controlled trials have shown a modest effect on hyperactivity levels in children in the general population and, at most, colouring agents would explain 10% of hyperactivity levels in ADHD. Focusing on diet alone does not address the issues raised by ADHD for families and schools.

'Is ADHD really a diagnosis? Or is it just a way of labelling children who are very active?'

ADHD is a real condition but there is not a blood test to perform to make the diagnosis. Central to the diagnostic criteria is the pervasive nature of the symptoms at home and at school, but their impact on the child's quality of life rather than displaying intermittent symptoms in one location. Parents searching the Internet will find many websites that attempt to discredit the existence of the condition.

'If he would just pay attention, everything would be better.'

The central problem is the ability to pay attention and trying harder often will not correct the problem. If told this repeatedly, some children stop trying, as there seems to be little point.

SUMMARY PRACTICE POINTS
- Remember the diagnostic criteria.
- Be reluctant to use vague terms like 'he is hyper'.
- Think of medical differentials.
- Recognise co-morbid conditions early.
- Know one behavioural strategy to explain to parents – be specific.
- When using medication, titrate for the effective dose but evaluate with objective criteria.

EVALUATING THE EVIDENCE

Evidence 1	
Theme E1	**Brief psycho-educational parent programmes for attention deficit hyperactivity disorder (ADHD)**
Question	What is the impact of brief psycho-educational interventions in children with features of ADHD?
Design	Randomised controlled trial
Level of evidence	Jadad 1
Setting	Community location, metropolitan area, Canada
Participants	Parents of 3- to 4-year-old children who were experiencing behavioural problems were invited to participate and randomised to intervention or wait-list control.
Intervention	The intervention was a video programme called 1-2-3 Magic, which provides simple, clear strategies such as time-out and rewards strategy to reduce both coercive and conflicted patterns of interaction between parent and child.

(continued)

Evidence 1	
Theme E1	***Brief psycho-educational parent programmes for attention deficit hyperactivity disorder (ADHD)***
Intervention (*cont.*)	The programme stresses the importance of eliminating negative parenting strategies such as nagging, hitting the child and voicing critical or hostile comments relating to the child. A major strength of the programme is the provision of both negative and positive parenting examples, to which parents can relate.
Outcomes	The primary outcome was the change in cut-off levels in the Arnold Parenting Scale at 3.1, which indicated the presence of clinically significant behavioural problems. This scale has 30 items and characterises how parents handle their child's behaviour from calm to yelling.
Main results	Of the 220 families who were eligible, 198 were randomised: 89 to the intervention and 109 served as controls. In the intervention group 61% were above the cut-off prior to commencement and this reduced to 26%, a 35% reduction, but in the wait-list control group the percentage above the cut-off was 61% and this reduced to 56% at 3 months (absolute risk reduction = 28%; number needed to treat = 4). Gains were maintained at 1-year follow-up.
Conclusion	The 1-2-3 Magic programme is effective in modifying parent–child interaction when there are behavioural difficulties.
Commentary	Parents found this programme both effective and reasonable to address their children with behavioural problems. Many of the children had features that are common in children with ADHD, in that they were overactive, verbose, were categorised as being difficult in school and easily distractible. This programme is therefore a useful adjunct for parents who are experiencing difficulties addressing their child's behaviour. The video format also is an added advantage especially if access to psychological services is limited. Prior to recommending its use the practitioner needs to asses a copy of the programme, as parents may well have specific questions relating to the strategies used.
Reference	Bradley SJ, Jadaa DJ, Brody J, *et al.* Brief psychoeducational parenting program: an evaluation and 1-year follow-up. *J Am Acad Child Adolesc Psychiatry.* 2003; **42**(10): 1171–8.

Evidence 2	
Theme E2	***Food additives and hyperactivity in children***
Question	Does the ingestion of food additives lead to changes in childhood behaviour?
Design	Randomised controlled trial
Level of evidence	Jadad 5
Setting	Community setting, England
Participants	Two groups of children were eligible: 3-year-olds and 8- to 9-year-olds. Children from a full range of socio-economic backgrounds were included.
Intervention	Children from a general population received a challenge drink with sodium benzoate and one of two artificial food colour and additives mixes (A or B) or a placebo mix.

(*continued*)

Evidence 2	
Theme E2	*Food additives and hyperactivity in children*
Intervention (*cont.*)	Food colouring was removed from the children's diet and they received mix A, mix B or placebo for 1 week, with a 1-week intervening washout period. Mix A contained 20 mg of artificial food colouring (5 mg sunset yellow (E110), 2.5 mg carmoisine (E122), 7.5 mg tartazine (E102), 5 mg ponceau 4R (E124) and 45 mg sodium benzoate). Mix B contained 30 mg of artificial food colouring (7.5 mg sunset yellow, 7.5 mg carmoisine, 7.5 mg quinolone yellow (E110), 7.5 mg allura red AC (E129) and 45 mg of sodium benzoate. For those children aged 8–9 years, the dose was increased by 25%. For 3-year-old children, dose A and dose B were equivalent to the colouring found in two 56 g bags of sweets and for 8- to 9-year-olds, dose A was equivalent to two bags of sweets and dose B equivalent to four bags of sweets.
Outcomes	The main outcome measure was a global hyperactivity aggregate (GHA) based on observed behaviours and rating by teachers and parents, plus for 8- to 9-year-olds a computerised test of attention span.
Main results	In the 3-year-old population, 898 were invited to participate – 209 gave a positive response but only 153 consented and 137 completed the study. In the 8- to 9-year-old group, 633 were invited to participate, 160 gave a positive response and 144 consented, with 130 completing the study. For all 3-year-olds the effect size on GHA was 0.2 (95% confidence interval (CI): 0.01–0.03) for mix A but not for mix B; however, it increased to 0.32 (95% CI: 0.05–0.6) when restricted to those who took more than 85% of the juice. For 8- to 9-year-olds who took more than 85% of the juice, the effect size on GHA was 0.12 (95% CI: 0.02–0.23) for mix A and 0.17 (95% CI: 0.07–0.28) for mix B.
Conclusion	Artificial colours or a sodium benzoate preservative in the diet resulted in a modest increase in activity levels in 3-year-olds and 8- to 9-year-olds in the general population.
Commentary	The impact of food additives in exacerbating activity in children with ADHD has been the subject of debate for a long period of time. Parents of children with ADHD frequently make an observation of a temporal relationship between food additives and activity levels. Temporal relationship does not automatically imply a cause-and-effect relationship. The children in this study did not have ADHD; however, ADHD children have activity levels 2 standard deviations above the norm. An effect size of 0.2 from food additives (as this study found), if found in children with ADHD, would explain 10% of the increased activity. Focusing on diet alone is not a prudent strategy for parents if their child has ADHD.
Reference	McCann D, Barrett A, Cooper A, *et al.* Food additives and hyperactive behaviour in 3-year-old and 8/9-year-old children in the community: a randomised, double-blinded, placebo-controlled trial. *Lancet.* 2007; **370**(9598): 1560–7.

Evidence 3	
Theme E3	*Behavioural programmes for attention deficit hyperactivity disorder (ADHD)*
Question	What is the impact of parenting programmes on children who display features of ADHD in the preschool years?
Design	Randomised controlled trial
Level of evidence	Jadad 1
Setting	Community Setting, Wales
Participants	Families of children aged 3–5 years who presented with symptoms of co-occurring ADHD and conduct disorder were eligible for inclusion. Children were assessed using the Eyberg Child Behaviour Inventory and/or on the hyperactivity subscale of the Strengths and Difficulties Questionnaire.
Intervention	The Incredible Years programme was utilised and consequently parents received individualised (one-to-one) 2-hour coaching/training sessions for 12 weeks to aid their parenting skills.
Outcomes	The primary outcomes were the reduction in parent-reported symptoms on the Conners scale for ADHD at baseline and 6, 12 and 18 months and on the Reliable Change Index for Conduct Disorder.
Main results	Health visitors approached 133 families and 79 fulfilled the eligibility criteria. Fifty received the intervention and 29 served as wait-list controls. Forty-four families (88%) of the intervention group completed the 18-month assessment, as did 27 (93%) of the control group. In the ADHD very large improvements (≥1.5 standard deviation) from baseline were noted in 42% at 6 months, 35% at 12 months and 30% at 18 months (absolute risk reduction (ARR) = 30%; number needed to treat (NNT) = 4). Large improvement (≥0.8 standard deviation) occurred in 58% (ARR = 58%; NNT = 2) at 18 months.
Conclusion	The Incredible Years programme is effective in preschool children with features of hyperactivity, which is a strong marker of ADHD.
Commentary	This study has limitations in that parents rated the children's behaviour and they may have accommodated to it, and also the children may have matured over the study period. The children displayed features of ADHD as measured by the Strengths and Difficulties Questionnaire hyperactivity scale, but this does not automatically imply that the children will develop ADHD. However, as no improvement was noted in the control group, it is reasonable to attribute the gains achieved to the intervention. Given the sustained improvement noted over the 18-month period of the Incredible Years programme, it is of value as first-line treatment in children with ADHD (if available).
Reference	Jones K, Daley D, Hutchings J, *et al.* Efficacy of the Incredible Years programme as an early intervention for children with conduct problems and ADHD: long-term follow-up. *Child Care Health Dev.* 2008; **34**(3): 380–90.

Evidence 4	
Theme E4	*Behavioural and medication treatment of attention deficit hyperactivity disorder (ADHD)*
Question	Which is more effective: medication or behavioural programmes in the treatment of ADHD?
Design	Randomised controlled trial
Level of evidence	Jadad 1
Setting	Community setting, the United States
Participants	Children aged between 7 and 9.9 years were eligible if they met the Diagnostic and Statistical Manual of Mental Disorders, Fourth Edition, criteria for ADHD combined type.
Intervention	Participants were randomly assigned to one of four interventions: (1) medication management, (2) behavioural management, (3) combined medication and behavioural management or (4) community care for 14 months. The behavioural programme included parent training, child-focused training inclusive of a school-based programme integrated within the academic year. The child-focused treatment was a summer camp over 8 weeks, 5 days per week and 9 hours per day, with a focus on social skills training, sports skills, group problem-solving, a positive rewards system and time out. The school-based programme entailed biweekly teacher consultation on classroom behaviour management strategies and 60 school days (on a part-time basis) of direct assistance to the child. Medication was titrated in a double-blind fashion (utilising teacher and parent ratings) until an optional dose was defined. Then the blind was broken and that dose became the subject's initial maintenance dose. If it was a placebo, then alternate medications were used. Doses could be adjusted based on carefully evaluated teacher and parent input. The community care group was provided with a report of their initial assessment and a list of community mental health resources, most community care subjects would receive medication.
Outcomes	This study by the MTA Cooperative Group attempted to answer three questions: (1) How do long-term behavioural and medication treatments compare with each other? (2) Are there additional benefits when they are used together? (3) What is the effectiveness of systematic, carefully delivered treatments versus routine care?
Main results	Of the total group of 579, 145 were assigned to the combined group, 144 to the medication group, 144 to the behaviour group and 146 to the community group. The main domains assessed to evaluate the three questions that were posed were (a) ADHD symptoms, (b) aggression/oppositional defiant disorder, (c) internalising symptoms, (d) social skills, (e) parent–child relations and (f) academic achievement. Medication was superior to behavioural treatments for ADHD symptoms; there were no major differences in other outcomes. Compared with behavioural treatment, the combined treatment was superior in benefiting ADHD symptoms and in reducing oppositional defiant disorder symptoms. Medication management and the combined programme were superior to the community programme for ADHD symptoms where the behavioural programme was not. The combined programme was superior to the community programme for the other five assessment domains.

(continued)

Evidence 4	
Theme E4	*Behavioural and medication treatment of attention deficit hyperactivity disorder (ADHD)*
Main results *(cont.)*	At the end of the study, 212 (73.4%) given medication management and combined treatment were successfully maintained on methylphenidate and 30 (10.4%) on dextroamphetamine. Two hundred and forty-five families provided side effect ratings: 88 (35.9%) none, 122 (49.8%) mild, 28 (11.4%) moderate and 7 (2.9%) severe.
Conclusion	For ADHD symptoms the medication management programme was superior to the behavioural treatment and the routine community programme, which included medication. The combined programme did not yield increased effectiveness over the medication programme.
Commentary	Medication is the first-line treatment in children with ADHD, as this large study indicates, with initial success rates of over 80%; however, the impact of the medication must be assessed and the dose titrated for optimal effect. Up to 10% of children may experience moderate side effects, so regular monthly assessment is prudent in the initial treatment phase.
Reference	MTA Cooperative Group. A 14-month randomized clinical trial of treatment strategies for attention-deficit/hyperactivity disorder. *Arch Gen Psychiatry.* 1999; **56**(12): 1073–86.

Evidence 5	
Theme E5	*The effectiveness of Ritalin and atomoxetine in attention deficit hyperactivity disorder (ADHD)*
Question	Which is more effective in ADHD: Ritalin or atomoxetine?
Design	Randomised controlled trial
Level of evidence	Jadad 5
Setting	20 medical centres, the United States
Participants	Children and adolescents aged 6–16 years who met the Diagnostic and Statistical Manual of Mental Disorders, Fourth Edition, criteria for ADHD, any subtype, were eligible for inclusion.
Intervention	Participants were assigned to receive atomoxetine (dose 0.8–1.8 mg/kg/day), a long-acting methylphenidate preparation (dose 18–54 mg/day) or placebo for 6 weeks. Those assigned to the methylphenidate group were subsequently switched to receive atomoxetine for a 6-week period.
Outcomes	The primary outcome measure was the investigator-administered and investigator-scored version of the ADHD rating scale. A response was defined as a 40% reduction in score or more at 6 weeks compared with baseline.
Main results	Of 635 eligible patients, 516 met the eligibility criteria for study entry, with 222 in the atomoxetine group, 220 in the osmotically released methylphenidate group and 74 in the placebo group.

(*continued*)

Evidence 5	
Theme E5	***The effectiveness of Ritalin and atomoxetine in attention deficit hyperactivity disorder (ADHD)***
Main results (*cont.*)	The response rate for placebo was 24%, for atomoxetine it was 45% (absolute risk reduction (ARR) = 21%; number needed to treat (NNT) = 5), for methylphenidate it was 56% (ARR = 32%; NNT = 3). One hundred and seventy-eight patients in the methylphenidate group were switched to atomoxetine as part of the cross-over design. Of the patients who did not respond to methylphenidate, 30 (43%) responded to atomoxetine.
Conclusion	Methylphenidate outperformed atomoxetine in terms of clinical response.
Commentary	In children and adolescents diagnosed with ADHD, medication is the first-line intervention. Parents will want to balance effectiveness and convenience against potential side effects. This study indicates the effectiveness of treatment, but the crossover component indicates that there is a differential response between ato-moxetine and methylphenidate, which has therapeutic implications, as patients who do not respond to one medication may respond to another. This needs to be explained to parents when discussing treatments.
Reference	Newcorn JH, Kratochvil CJ, Allen AJ, *et al.* Atomoxetine and osmotically released methylphenidate for the treatment of attention deficit hyperactivity disorder: acute comparison and differential response. *Am J Psychiatry.* 2008; **165**(6): 721–30.

ATTENTION DEFICIT HYPERACTIVITY DISORDER: MULTIPLE-CHOICE QUESTIONS

Q1 Which of the following statements is/are correct?
  a) ADHD is more common in boys.
  b) The frequency of ADHD is 4% in children aged 5–15 years.
  c) ADHD is rare in girls.
  d) The aetiology of ADHD is 70% genetic.
  e) The aetiology of ADHD is 30% environmental.

Q2 Which of the following statements is/are correct?
  a) Symptoms of ADHD must be present before 5 years of age.
  b) Symptoms may only be present at school in 15%.
  c) Children with ADHD have above-normal intelligence.
  d) Children with ADHD frequently fail to complete tasks.
  e) Children with ADHD are impulsive.

Q3 Which of the following statements is/are true?
  a) Children with ADHD make friends easily.
  b) Children with ADHD progress normally in school.
  c) Children with ADHD experience sleep disruption.
  d) Children with ADHD have impaired motor skills in 25% of cases.
  e) Children with ADHD suffer from anorexia in 10% of cases.

Q4 There is an increased incidence of ADHD in which of the following conditions?
a) Neurofibromatosis
b) Williams's syndrome
c) Foetal alcohol syndrome
d) Tuberous sclerosis
e) West's syndrome

Q5 Features of foetal alcohol syndrome include which of the following?
a) Growth failure
b) Microcephaly
c) Hyperacusis
d) Short thumbs
e) Brushfield's spots

Q6 Features of fragile X in a 7-year-old boy include which of the following?
a) Macrocephaly
b) Speech delay
c) Large testicles
d) Delayed dentition
e) Short stature

Q7 Which of the following treatments are effective in ADHD?
a) Dietary restriction of food additives
b) Methylphenidate
c) Behavioural programmes
a) Atomoxetine
d) Lithium

Q8 Conditions seen with increased frequency in patients with ADHD include which of the following?
a) Conduct disorder
b) Tic disorder
c) Learning disability
d) Seizures
e) Autism

Q9 Which of the following statements is/are correct?
a) Methylphenidate is effective in 80% of older children with ADHD.
b) Atomoxetine is effective in 40% of older children with ADHD.
c) Placebo is effective in 10% of older children with ADHD.
d) Behavioural therapy is effective in 15% of young children with ADHD.
e) Combined treatment with methylphenidate and behavioural therapy is effective in 75% of older children.

Q10 Methylphenidate side effects include which of the following?
   a) Arrhythmias
   b) Impaired sleep
   c) Weight loss
   d) Diarrhoea
   e) Elevated blood glucose

Answers

A1	a, b, d, e	**A2**	d, e
A3	c	**A4**	a, b, c
A5	a, b	**A6**	a, b
A7	b, c, d	**A8**	a, b, c
A9	a	**A10**	b, c

SLIDES

1. Foetal alcohol syndrome
2. Hyperthyroidism (Graves's disease)
3. Neurofibromatosis (Type 1)
4. Neurofibromatosis (Type 2)

INDEX

5-aminosalicylic acid 188
6-mercaptopurine 188

ABC assessment 28
ABCD mnemonic 56
abdominal distension
 and constipation 223
 and diarrhoea 203, 206
 and DS 453
 and FTT 243
 and intussusception
  99, 176
 and lactose intolerance
  119
abdominal pain
 and anaphylaxis 26–7
 causes of 176–9
 and diabetes 539
 and diarrhoea 209
 differential diagnosis
  for 181–3
 examination for 181
 and failure to thrive
  242
 and food allergy 136–7
 history taking for 180
 investigations for
  183–4
 management of 184–9
 MCQs on 198–200
 parents influencing
  perception of 194–5
 and pharyngitis 45
 and pneumonia 47
 and septicaemia 49
 treatment of 192–3
 types of 175–6
 and vomiting 154–5,
  163, 190
Abdominal Pain Index
 198
abdominal X-ray, and
 constipation 224
absence seizures 383–4,
 391, 394, 396–7, 400
acanthosis nigricans 559,
 570, 604
aCGH (microarray CGH
 analysis) 435–7, 449
achalasia 154, 241, 298,
 317

acitretin 608
acne
 and chronic rash 599
 investigations in 604
 management of 610
 MCQs on 618
 nodulocystic 603, 608
 and puberty 524, 527
 treatment of 608
acute abdominal pain
 175–7, 181–4, 188, 192
acute asthma 21–2, 36–9,
 319
acute chest syndrome
 491, 495–7
acute cough 294, 296, 300,
 304–5, 312
acute diarrhoea 202–3,
 207, 209, 212–14
acute gastroenteritis 166–
 7, 169, 203–4, 209
acute migraine 358–9,
 368, 376–7
acute persistent cough
 294
acute rash
 examination for 580
 forms of 572–9
 history taking for 579
 management of 581–2
 MCQs on 590–2
acute wheeze 20
 and age 314
 differential diagnosis
  of 317
 MCQs on 331
 and saline 324–5
 and steroids 319,
  323–4
Addison's disease 159,
 203, 538–9
adenoidectomy 57, 66
adenotonsillectomy 261,
 411, 454
ADHD (attention deficit
 hyperactivity disorder)
  behavioural
   programmes for 633
  and daytime wetting
   283
  diagnosis of 621–2, 630

differential diagnosis
 for 624–5
 and enuresis 265
 examination for 623–4
 history taking for
  622–3
 investigations for
  625–6
 management of 626–9
 MCQs on 636–7
 medication for 634–6
 parent education for
  630–1
 and seizures 390
 and sleep disorders
  404, 406
 subtypes of 620–1
adolescents, interviewing
 239
adrenaline
 and croup 33, 35–6
 intramuscular 25–7
 nebulised 16, 18–19, 27
 and stridor 34
adrenaline pens 141, 143,
 147–8
adrenarche 524, 529, 532,
 535
AEDs (anti-epileptic
 drugs)
 commencing 391
 and epilepsy
  syndromes 383
 monitoring 389
 in pregnancy 158, 335
 satisfaction with 394–5
 and status epilepticus
  39
 withdrawing 391–2
AHOM, see osteomyelitis,
 acute haematogenous
Aicardi–Goutières
 syndrome 432
albuterol 323–5
Alexander's disease 431
allergen avoidance
 139–41
allergenic food,
 introduction of 144
allergic diseases 122, 128,
 140, 142

allergies, and
 immunodeficiency 87
allergy prevention 122,
 128–9
allergy testing
 and cough 299
 and wheeze 318
alopecia 242, 597, 604
alpha thalassaemia 488
Alport's syndrome 425
amenorrhoea 116, 238,
 241, 252, 525
aminoglycosides 58,
 425–6
amoxicillin 57, 63–4, 67,
 301, 310
anaemia
 and abdominal pain
  179, 181
 and diarrhoea 206
 examination for 492
 and failure to thrive
  244
 history taking for 491–2
 management of 493–4
 MCQs on 505–6
 signs of 486–7
 use of term 486
anal fissures 98, 221–2,
 226
analgesia
 and abdominal pain
  185–6
 and colic 103
 and headache 368, 379
 and migraine 369
 and sickle-cell pain 501
anaphylaxis
 and adrenaline 147–8
 first response to 25–7
 and food allergy 135,
  138, 140–2
 and urticaria 578
Angelman's syndrome
 427–8
angioedema
 and acute rash 578
 and anaphylaxis 26
 and food allergy 136,
  204
 and PIDs 80–1

anorectal malformations 223

anorexia nervosa 159, 238, 249, 252–6

antacids 162

antalgic gait 466

antibiotic-associated diarrhoea 203, 212

antibiotic prophylaxis
  and DS 454
  and recurrent infections 80, 84–5
  and sickle-cell disease 495–6
  and UTIs 70
  and VUR 58

antibiotics
  and acute rash 579
  and AHOM 482–3
  and anaemia 492
  and AOM 63–4
  and CHD 344
  and cough 301, 310
  and fever 59
  and gastroenteritis 161, 164
  and haemolysis 490
  and immune system 85–6
  and PIDs 81
  and pneumonia 67
  and pyelonephritis 69–70
  side effects of 140
  and skin infections 583
  topical 608
  and UTIs 71–2

anticholinergics
  and constipation 223
  and daytime wetting 284–5, 287
  and desmopressin 266, 273

anticonvulsants 31, 39, 162

antidiarrhoeal medications 209–10, 212–13

antihistamines
  and acute rash 579, 582–3
  and anaphylaxis 26–7, 139, 141
  and chronic rash 602
  and eczema 606
  and upper airway cough syndrome 301

antinausea medications 161

antipsychotics 539

antipyretics 55, 63, 395–6, 579

AOM (acute otitis media) 46
  overdiagnosis of 59

recurrent 66
  treatment of 57, 63–4

aorta, coarctation of 337–8, 342, 346

aortic arch, interrupted 335, 338

aortic stenosis 338
  frequency of 335
  MCQs on 356
  murmur of 624
  and syncope 24
  treatment of 346

API (Asthma Predictive Index) 314, 323, 326–8, 332

aplastic anaemia 489

apnoea-hypopnoea index (AHI) 408

appendicitis
  and abdominal pain 177, 182–3
  acute 186, 199
  and diabetes mellitus 540
  and diarrhoea 207
  prediction rules for 190–2
  presentations of 185
  and vomiting 158

appendix, perforated 185, 189, 191

AR, see relaxation, applied

ARR (absolute risk reduction), use of term 5

ASDs (atrial septal defects) 335–7, 345

aspiration pneumonia 317, 332

aspirin
  and haemolysis 490
  and Kawasaki's disease 583
  and rheumatoid arthritis 483–4
  and thrombosis 347

asthma
  and anaphylaxis 25
  and cough 293–5, 297, 301, 303
  and eczema 596–7
  and food allergy 134–5, 138, 140, 142
  management of 321–3
  MCQs on 332
  medication use in 320–1
  in primary care 325–6
  severity of 20–1, 36–7
  step-up therapy for 329–30
  uncontrolled 10, 140, 329–30
  and wheeze 20, 314–15, 318–19

Asthma Action Plans 321

Asthma Control Questionnaire 323

Asthma Control Test 323, 330

ataxia telangiectasia 78, 80, 82, 91

atlantoaxial instability 454, 456, 459, 464

atomoxetine 629, 635–6

atopic dermatitis; see also eczema
  diagnosis of 596
  and food allergy 119, 134–5, 138–40, 142
  treatment of 613–14

audiometry assessment 436

aura, children explaining 364, 366

Auspitz's sign 598

Autism Diagnostic Interview 437, 442, 445

Autism Diagnostic Observation Schedule 437, 442, 445

autism spectrum disorder
  diagnosis of 426, 437
  drug therapy for 446–7
  and insomnia 406
  management of 441–2
  and MMR vaccine 585
  sleep problems in 447–8
  and social communication 445–6
  and speech delay 425

AVPU scale 29

AVSD (atrioventricular septal defect) 335, 343, 345

bacteraemia 61–2, 496, 501–2

bad news, breaking 9–10, 350–1

bariatric surgery 561–2

basilar migraine 360

BEARS instrument 403

behavioural management 254, 414, 627–8, 634

behavioural problems
  and DS 457
  in Lennox–Gastaut's syndrome 385
  sleep-related 404

benign childhood epilepsy 383, 400

benign neonatal sleep myoclonus 387

benign nocturnal limp pain 479

benzodiazepines, and status epilepticus 39–40

benzylpenicillin 67

beta thalassaemia 488, 497, 499, 503–4

BHR (bronchial hyper-reactivity) 314

bilingualism 425

bilious vomiting
  and abdominal pain 176–7, 190
  in neonates 156, 158, 162–4

biofeedback 283–4, 289, 302

bladder
  functioning of 277
  overactive 260, 273, 280, 288
  underactive 280

bladder capacity
  formula for 281
  increasing 265, 268–9
  reduced 260, 284

bladder diaries 263, 283

bladder training exercises 265, 279

bladder ultrasound 279, 281

Blalock–Taussig shunt 342, 346–7

blood loss, occult 494, 497, 499

blood tests, and ADHD 626

bloody diarrhoea 52, 179, 209, 211–12, 217, 578

BMI (body mass index)
  and anorexia nervosa 254–5
  and obesity 557, 563

bone age
  checking 528–9
  delayed 508, 514, 526, 534

bone marrow failure 499

bone pain 50, 472, 478

bone scans 101, 471, 475

bone tumours 472

bowel bladder dysfunction 277

bowel fitness training 226

bowel motility, altered 202

bowel movement frequency 225, 231

bowel obstruction 156, 193

boys, pubertal development in 522

bradycardia
  and anaphlyaxis 26
  and failure to thrive 243, 248
  and food allergy 137

brain damage, and fever 59

brain injury, acquired 427

brain tumours 359, 361, 366, 378
breakthrough seizures 390–1
breast milk
 expressed (EBM) 117
 fortified 247
 insufficient supply of 122–3
breastfeeding
 and acute rash 581
 and anaemia 491
 benefits of 114–16, 131
 and bowel movements 228
 education for 121–2
 and excessive crying 103
 and food allergy 142
 and history taking 120
 problems with 118–20, 123–5
 and rehydration 209–10
 supplementation of 122, 125–8
breath-holding 388
Bristol Stool Chart 222, 225, 277
bronchiectasis
 and cough 294, 299, 301
 and CVID 79, 85
bronchiolitis
 first response to 22
 management of 322, 330–1
 MCQs on 331
 and wheeze 20, 313–15, 317
bronchitis 298, 301, 310
bronchodilators 315, 318, 320, 322, 329, 332
Brudzinski's sign 158, 580
bruising
 abdominal 181
 and acute rash 579
 and NAI 96, 102, 104–6, 112
 tests for 101
budesonide 18, 33, 187, 328
bulimia nervosa 159, 238, 249
bullying
 and chronic rash 602
 and daytime wetting 279
 and FTT 239
 and obesity 562, 568
 and symptoms of stress 370
Burkholderia cepacia 78
burns, accidental and non-accidental 97

C-reactive protein (CRP)
 and abdominal pain 183
 and fever 54
 and Kawasaki's disease 580
 and sepsis 30
café au lait lesions
 and ADHD 623–4
 and anaemia 489
 and pubertal disorders 524, 527, 532
caffeine 262, 278, 359–60, 409
calcineurin inhibitors 606
caloric intake
 and breast milk 118
 and diabetes mellitus 545
 in hospitalisation 248
 inadequate 238–9
 increasing 246–7, 251–2
 MCQs on 256
 and obesity 557, 560–1, 563
CAMHS (Child and Adolescent Mental Health Services) 253, 629
Canavan's disease 431, 434
candidiasis 77–9, 81, 85–6, 92
capillary haemangiomas 601–2
carbamazepine 384, 388, 391
cardiac catheterisation 343
cardiac disease; *see also* CHD; heart failure
 and DS 457, 459, 461–2
 and FTT 119
 and hyperoxia testing 342
cardiac silhouettes 342, 356
cardiomyopathy, obstructive 23–4, 352, 615
carotid bruit 336
CAST fracture 468, 478, 485
cataplexy 404, 407–9, 411, 417–18
CBT (cognitive behavioural therapy)
 and headache 368, 372–3
 and RAP 187, 197–8
 and sleep disorders 410–11
CDS (clinical dehydration scale) 166–7
cefotaxime 19, 30–1
ceftibuten 69

ceftriaxone 69
cellulitis
 and acute rash 577
 signs of 52
centile growth charts
 and FTT 237–8, 249–50
 and short stature 509
central precocious puberty (CPP) 523, 528, 533–4
cephalosporins 482–3
cerebral palsy 430
 and developmental delay 425, 427
 and FTT 240
 and limping 469
 and recurrent infection 76, 82
 and wheeze 316
CGH (comparative genomic hybridisation) 435
CGM (continuous glucose monitoring) 541, 543, 549–50, 552
CH50 83
CHD (congenital heart disease) 334–5; *see also* left-to-right shunts
 cyanotic 339–40, 342, 344
 detection of 349
 and DiGeorge's syndrome 78
 examination for 341–2
 explaining to parents 348, 350–1
 history taking for 341
 investigations for 342
 management of 343–5, 347
 MCQs for 355–7
 and palivizumab 353–4
 and syncope 24
 types of 335
Chédiak–Higashi's syndrome 82
cherry-red spot 431, 435
chest deformity 296, 302, 316, 322
chest infections, recurrent 341
chest pain (CP)
 and CHD 335, 338, 344
 and fever 73
 outcomes for 351–2
 and pneumonia 47
 and syncope 23–4
chest X-ray
 and abdominal pain 183
 and CHD 342, 461
 and cough 299
 and foreign bodies 18

and recurrent infections 82
chickenpox 573, 579, 582
child abuse 105–6, 239
childhood absence epilepsy 383–4, 396–7
Childhood Asthma Control Test 321, 330
chlorhexidine mouth-washes 582
cholecystitis 176
chromosome analysis 83, 435, 452, 455, 459, 626
chronic abdominal pain 183–5; *see also* FAP; RAP
chronic constipation 220–1, 229–32, 235, 279
chronic cough
 and antibiotics 310
 differential diagnosis of 294, 297–8
 and GERD 154
 investigations for 299
 MCQs on 312
 predicting aetiology of 305–6
chronic dermatitis 597
chronic diarrhoea 77, 92, 201–4, 211
chronic disease, anaemia of 244, 488, 494
chronic rash
 examination for 603
 history taking for 602–3
 investigations for 604
 management of 604–5
 MCQs on 617–18
chronic rhinitis 297, 308–9, 314–16
chronic vomiting, *see* recurrent vomiting
ciclesonide 326–7
circumduction gait 466
CIs (confidence intervals) 5, 107
cisplatin 426
clavulanate 301
clindamycin 31, 482–3, 608
clinical letters 439
clinical prediction rule (CPR) 190–2, 286, 479–80
close contact 31, 577, 581
clubbing
 and abdominal pain 181
 and CHD 342
 and cough 296, 298
 and diarrhoea 206
 and failure to thrive 243
cluster headaches 359

coal tar preparations 607
cocaine 31, 359
codeine 300, 496
coeliac disease
    and anaemia 498
    and diabetes 539
    diagnosis of 207, 211
    and diarrhoea 203
    and DS 456
    and FTT 242
    and hypothyroidism
        225
    investigations for 244
    MCQs on 217–18
    pattern of 212
    and short stature 509,
        511
    treatment of 210
    and type 1 diabetes 538
cognitive delay,
    identifying 443
cold intolerance 223, 242,
    558–9
colic
    behavioural
        interventions for 109
    and breastfed infants
        110–11
    diagnosis of 95, 102–4,
        108, 181
    features of 113
    follow-up for 103, 188
    and food allergy 142
    and infant formula 108
    treatment for 102–3
Collaborative
    Management in
    Paediatrics programme
    15
coma
    aetiology of 41–2
    first response to 27–9
combined T- and B-cell
    deficiency 76–7, 82
comedones 599
communication, non-
    verbal 627
conditioning 410
conduct disorder 625, 633
congenital adrenal
    hyperplasia 207, 524,
    526, 530
congenital heart defects
    334–5, 349
conjunctivitis 46, 61, 297,
    574
Conners Rating Scales 625
constipation
    and coeliac disease 203
    and daytime wetting
        277, 282, 284–5
    and dietary fibre 230–1
    differential diagnoses
        of 223–5
    and enuresis 262

examination for 222–3
and failure to thrive
    242
and formula feeding
    229–30
history taking for 222
investigations for 224
management of 224–9
MCQs on 234–6
and overflow diarrhoea
    208–9, 212, 225,
    228–9
and PPIs 162
terminology of 221
treatment of 231–4
and UTIs 57
contact dermatitis 100,
    135, 597
continence, physiological
    development of 260
convulsions, use of term
    380
convulsive seizures 381,
    388–9
Coombs' test 493
corneal abrasion 98,
    100–1, 105, 112
coronary artery
    aneurysms 576, 583–4,
    588–9
corrosive ingestion 315
corticosteroids
    and anaphylaxis 26–7
    and asthma 323
    and cough 301
    and ITP 589–90
    and wheeze 326–7
cough
    and daytime wetting
        278
    differential diagnosis of
        296–8
    duration of 304–5
    examination for 296
    and fever 51
    and GERD 171
    history taking for 295
    investigations for 299
    management of
        299–302
    MCQs on 311–12
    mechanism of 293–4
    normal frequency of
        303–4
    and pneumonia 47
    and stridor 16
    terminology of 294
    and tracheitis 19
cow's milk
    in formula 110, 114,
        116–17, 128–9
    and iron deficiency
        494
cow's milk allergy
    and diarrhoea 204

and feeding problems
    119, 124–5, 132
MCQs on 149
prevalence of 133–4
and sleep disorders
    410, 413
treatment of 210
Coxsackie viruses 537,
    575
cranberry juice 58, 70–1
craniofacial abnormalities
    72, 407–8
Crohn's disease
    and abdominal pain
        179, 183
    and eating disorders
        241
    features of 217
    investigations for 184
    management of 187–8
crotamiton 616
croup
    and adrenaline 35–6
    assessment for 17–18
    and cough 296
    steroid therapy for 33
croup scores 17, 33–6
CSE (convulsive status
    epilepticus) 39–40
CSF (cerebrospinal fluid)
    53
CSII (continuous
    subcutaneous insulin
    infusion) 544, 550–1
Cullen's sign 181–2
CVID (common variable
    immunodeficiency) 77,
    79–80, 85, 90–1
cyclical vomiting
    syndrome 155, 159–60,
    162–3, 173, 195
cyclosporin 608
cystic fibrosis
    and constipation 223
    and cough 295, 298–9,
        311
    and diarrhoea 207
    and failure to thrive
        240, 242
    and fever 55
    and gallstones 177, 183
    and GERD 154
    and recurrent
        infections 76, 84
    and wheeze 317
cystinosis 245

daytime sleepiness 406–7,
    411, 413, 418, 454, 558
daytime wetting 276
    and biofeedback 289
    differential diagnosis
        of 280
    drug therapy for 290
    examination for 279

history taking for
    278–9
investigations for 281
management of 281–5
MCQs on 290–2, 297
terminology of 277–8
and timed voiding
    287–8
DBPCFC (double-blind
    placebo-controlled food
    challenge) 4, 6, 139, 144
DDAVP, see desmopressin
DDH (developmental
    dysplasia of the hip)
    467–8, 473, 476, 478–9,
    484
deafness 426, 456, 623; see
    also hearing loss
deferiprone 502
dehydration
    and acute rash 580
    assessment of 166–7
    and diarrhoea 201
    and failure to thrive
        248
    and fever 54
    hypernatraemic 118–
        19, 125
    investigations in 159
    management of 161
    MCQs on 173–4
    and pneumonia 48
    and syncope 24
    treatment of 167–9,
        209–10, 212
    and vomiting 153–5,
        157, 162–3
dehydroepiandrosterone
    sulphate 599, 604, 618
delayed puberty 525–6
    and brain tumours 361
    and coeliac disease 203
    and Crohn's disease 179
    MCQs on 536
    and short stature 509
    treatment of 531–4
delayed-type
    hypersensitivity skin
    test 83
Dennie–Morgan's folds
    296–7, 316
dermatitis; see also atopic
    dermatitis; eczema
    flexural 596
    perioral 599
    seborrhoeic 597, 599,
        601
dermatographism 138,
    578, 585
dermatologists 605,
    611–13
desferrioxamine 497,
    502–4
desmopressin 261, 264,
    266–8, 271–3, 540

desquamation 576, 580
developmental delay
  and ADHD 624
  degree of 427
  differential diagnosis
    for 425–6, 434–5
  and DS 454
  and enuresis 265
  examination for 433–4
  and FTT 243
  history taking for
    432–3
  home-based
    intervention for 444
  investigations for
    435–8
  management of 439–41
  MCQs on 448–9
  and obesity 559–60
  patterns of 422
  and sleep disorder 410
  syndromes causing 428
  use of term 421–2
  and wheeze 316
developmental milestones,
  normal 421–4
developmental regression
  421, 430–2
developmental screening
  422
dexamethasone 18, 33, 35,
  481–2
dextroamphetamine 411,
  635
diabetes insipidus
  and constipation 223
  and daytime wetting
    278, 280
  and enuresis 261, 263
diabetes mellitus
  complications of
    546–7, 552–3
  and constipation 223
  diagnosis of 538
  and diarrhoea 207
  differential diagnosis
    for 540
  and enuresis 261, 263
  examination for 539
  and failure to thrive
    240
  glucose monitoring in
    549–50
  history taking for 539
  hospital care for 548–9
  hypoglycaemic
    episodes in 551–2
  investigations for 540
  MCQs on 554–5
  and obesity 563
  types of 537–8
diabetes mellitus type 1
  540–2, 547–8
diabetic ketoacidosis
  (DKA)

and abdominal pain
  182–3
and coma 42
diagnosis of 540
first response to 32
and type 1 diabetes 538
and vomiting 158
Diamond–Blackfan's
  anaemia 489
diarrhoea
  and acute rash 579
  and AOM 46
  and cough 295, 298
  and dehydration 201–2
  drug treatment for
    212–13
  examination for 205–7
  and failure to thrive
    240
  and food allergy 119,
    137
  forms of 202–4
  and gastroenteritis
    154, 164
  history taking for 205
  hospitalisation for 211,
    216–17
  and immunodeficiency
    77, 79
  management of 208–9
  MCQs on 217–18
  and measles 574
  and pharyngitis 45
  as side effect 162
diazepam 32, 40–1, 382
diclofenac 395–6
diencephalic syndrome
  241
diet
  and ADHD 629, 631–2
  and diabetes 542
  and eczema 604
  and obesity 557, 564
DiGeorge's syndrome
  and CHD 335
  and developmental
    delay 427–8, 438
  and recurrent
    infections 78, 80, 82–3
digital rectal examinations
  224
dimenhydrinate 161,
  164–5, 174
discitis 468–9, 477
disimpaction 224, 227,
  233
disseminated
  intravascular coagulation
    491, 573
dithranol 607
diuretics 241, 345, 361
doctors
  difficulties with parents
    12
  hostility to 14

dopamine 30, 345, 628
double-blinding, use of
  term 4
double voiding 283
dry skin 455
DS (Down's syndrome)
  and anaemia 489
  and CHD 335, 355,
    461–2
  and constipation 223
  and developmental
    delay 427
  examination for 453
  features of 450–1
  gross motor skills in
    460–1
  investigations in 455–6
  management of 456–9
  MCQs on 463–5
  newborn period of
    452–3
  and obesity 560
  and OSA 406
  screening for 451–2,
    454–5
  specialty clinics for
    459–60
duodenal atresia 158
dysmenorrhoea 182
dysmorphic features
  and ADHD 624
  and CHD 341–2
  and developmental
    delay 428–9, 434
  and DS 450
  and FTT 243
  and obesity 559
  and pubertal
    development 527
  and recurrent
    infections 81
  and seizures 387
  and short stature 511
  and sleep problems
    408
dyspepsia, functional 178,
  195, 200
dyspnoea
  and anaphylaxis 25–6
  and asthma scoring
    21, 37
  and bronchiolitis 317
  exertional 337, 486
  and heart failure 335
  and wheeze 20
dyssomnias 402–4
dysuria 48, 155, 262, 278,
  280

eating behaviours, healthy
  247
eating disorders
  and delayed puberty
    525
  differential diagnosis
    of 241
  features of 238, 242–3
  management of 245–6,
    248–9
  tests for 244
EBM (evidence-based
  medicine) 1–8
Ebstein's anomaly 340,
  342–3, 356
ECG (electrocardiogram)
  and cardiac disease 100
  and CHD 343
  and DS 461–2
  and FTT 244
  pre-medication 628
  and seizures 389
  and status epilepticus
    31
  and syncope 23–4, 388
echocardiogram
  and CHD 343, 461–2
  and DS 455
eczema
  and allergenic food
    144–5
  atopic, see atopic
    dermatitis
  and chronic rash
    596–7
  differential diagnosis
    of 597
  management of 604–7,
    610–11
  MCQs on 617
  nummular 598, 601
  and parental education
    611–12
  and PIDs 78, 81
  professionals treating
    612–13
  and wheeze 314
eczema herpeticum
  596–7
eczematous lesions 617
Edward's syndrome 335
egg allergy 134, 142–3,
  148–9
Ehlers–Danlos's syndrome
  223
electroencephalogram
  (EEG)
  and epilepsy syndromes
    383–5
  and GDD 437
  and headache 370
  MCQs on 401
  and medication
    withdrawal 392
  and seizures 389, 394

electroencephalogram
(EEG) (*continued*)
and status epilepticus
31
and syncope 24
electrolyte disturbances
39, 153, 160–1, 201
electrolyte transport,
alterations in 207
emollients 583, 602,
605–7, 611
encephalitis
and measles 574
and seizures 386
signs of 52
and varicella zoster 585
and vomiting 158
encopresis, *see* faecal
incontinence
endoscopy, and abdominal
pain 184
enemas, and constipation
231–4
enteral feeding 187
enterocolitis
food protein-induced
150
necrotising 61, 90, 240
enuresis alarms 266,
268–70, 272, 274, 284
epigastric pain
and diabetes mellitus
539
and DKA 32
and gallstones 177
epiglottitis 19, 34
epilepsy
co-morbidities of 390
diagnosis of 387, 390
and diet 393–4,
398–9
MCQs on 399
and melatonin 419
and meningitis 49
and migraine 364
pathology of 381
prevalence of 380
refractory 389, 392
epilepsy surgery 392–3
epilepsy syndromes
383–5, 390, 393
epileptic seizures 380–1,
383, 390
Epstein–Barr virus
and acute rash 575
and anaemia 491
and antibiotics 585
and FTT 79
and pharyngitis 45
equinus gait 466
equipoise 6
erysipelas 577, 583
erythema multiforme 56,
179, 576
erythroblastopaenia 489

erythromycin 57, 67, 301,
608
Escherichia coli 48, 79,
471
ESF (energy-
supplemented formula)
251–2
Esomeprazole 171–2
ethosuximide 384, 391,
396–7
eugonadotropic
hypogonadism 525
exanthems, viral 52, 382,
572, 582
excessive crying
causes of 94–5, 104–5
examination for
98–100
history taking for 97
investigations for 101
management of
101–3
MCQs on 112–13
exercise, and obesity
561–2, 564
exercise-induced asthma
321
exercise-induced migraine
360
exercise tolerance 335,
504, 558, 567
eye contact 9, 425–6

faecal impaction 221, 227,
231–2
faecal incontinence
220–1, 225, 232–4, 236
failure to thrive (FTT)
237–8
and abdominal pain
181
and anaemia 486
causes of 238–9, 249
and CHDs 341
differential diagnosis of
240–1
early intervention
programmes in 250–1
examination for 243–4
and feeding problems
119, 123, 247
history taking for
241–2
hospital admission for
247–8
investigations for 244
management of 245,
249
MCQs on 256–8
nutritional intervention
for 246–7
and recurrent
infections 79, 81, 86
and wheeze 315
Fanconi's anaemia 489

FAP (functional
abdominal pain) 175,
178–9, 182, 185–8,
194–7, 200
fat malabsorption 202,
207, 240, 257
FBC (full blood count)
and abdominal pain
183
and anaemia 493–4
and jaundice 121
and Kawasaki's disease
580
and meningococcal
disease 53
and obesity 560
and recurrent
infections 79, 82
and vomiting 159
and wheeze 318
FBT (family-based
treatment) 253–4
FC (faecal calprotectin)
184, 209, 215–16
febrile convulsions 382
age of 394
and EEGs 389
prevention of 390
recurrence of 395–6
and UTIs 48
femoral fractures 96
fever
and acute rash 582
assessment of 44–5, 72
background of 43
differential diagnosis
of 52–3
examination for 51
follow-up for 58–9
history taking in 50–1
investigations of 53–4
management of 54–6
medication for 60
parental
misconceptions about
59
and sickle-cell disease
496, 501–2
treatment of 56–7
fever of unknown origin
43–4
FGIDs (functional gastro-
intestinal disorders)
195–6
fibre, dietary 204–5, 222,
226, 229–31, 277
FIs (febrile infants) 56,
61–3
floppy infant, *see*
hypotonic infant
flow diagrams 4, 7
flucloxacillin 19, 123, 583
fluid intake, optimisation
of 283
fluid resuscitation 161–2

fluorescein 101
fluticosone 329
focal seizures 382
and absence seizures
383
and CSF 53
and neuroimaging 370
origins of 381
foetal alcohol syndrome
355, 623–4, 637
folic acid 499–500
fontanelle
bulging 28, 49, 52, 99,
157
sunken 201, 539
food, as migraine trigger
360; *see also* diet
food allergy
and abdominal pain
189
differential diagnosis of
137–8
and eczema 602, 610
examination for 136
history taking for
135–6
investigations for
138–9
management of
139–42, 145–6
MCQs on 149–50
and oral
immunotherapy
148–9
parental over-
estimation of 142, 144
presentations of 135
prevalence of 133
use of term 134
and wheeze 315, 317
food challenge 138–9,
143–4, 150, 189
food hypersensitivity
(FHS) 143–4
food intolerance 134, 137
food refusal 164, 171, 239,
246, 248
foreign body, in the foot
474
foreign body aspiration
and cough 294, 297–9
first response to 18
MCQs on 332
and wheeze 20, 313–14,
316–17
formula feeding 116–17
and allergies 128–9
and constipation
229–30
and vomiting 160
formula supplementation,
see breastfeeding,
supplementation of
formula thickeners 123,
130–1

fractures
  and head trauma 107
  non-accidental 95–6
  radiological
    investigations for 101
  skull 96
fragile X syndrome 427–8,
  434, 437, 447–8, 623–4,
  637
frontal lobe epilepsy (FLE)
  382, 388
functional constipation
  220–1, 224, 233–4
functional diarrhoea 204,
  208, 210
functional polydipsia 280
fungal infections 76, 79,
  81, 88, 600–1, 604

G6PD deficiency 490, 493,
  499, 506
gait
  unsteady 279
  use of term 466
galactosaemia 428–9, 435,
  438, 525
Galeazzi's sign 474
gallstones 177, 189, 199,
  490, 492
gastro-oesophageal reflux
  and cough 293, 298,
    301
  and failure to thrive
    240
  and feeding problems
    119, 123–4, 132
  and food allergy 142
  and formula thickeners
    130–1
  investigations for 121
  management of 161–2
  and PIDs 76
  prevalence of 164
  and seizures 388
  treatment of 170–1
  and vomiting 154
  and wheeze 315
gastro-oesophageal reflux
  disease (GERD) 154,
  161–2, 164, 171–4
gastroenteritis
  and abdominal pain
    183
  and antidiarrhoeals 210
  bacterial 61, 210
  and dehydration
    166–70
  and fever 52
  and intussusception
    176
  investigations for 183
  juice intake after 212
  and shock 30
  and stool cultures 208
  treatment for 164–5

viral 52, 154, 207
  and vomiting 160–1,
    163–6
gastroschisis 90, 223, 240
Gaucher's disease 429, 431
Gaviscon 170–1
GDD (global
  developmental delay)
  421, 426–7, 435–7, 442
Gianotti–Crosti's
  syndrome 575
Giardia lamblia 77, 79
giggle incontinence 280,
  284
girls, pubertal
  development in 522
Glasgow Coma Scale
  28–9, 41, 50, 580
Glasgow Meningococcal
  Septicaemia Prognostic
  Score 30, 49–50
glomerulonephritis 46,
  574
glucagon 545
glucose
  monitoring levels of
    538, 540, 542–3, 545;
    see also CGM
  and obesity 560
glucose tolerance test
  538, 560
glutaric aciduria 434–5
glycaemic index 545
glycosuria 537–8, 540
goitre 624
gonadal failure 525
Gowers's sign 433, 473–4
graduated extinction 411
granulomatous disease,
  chronic 78
Graves's disease 538
grey matter disease
  430–1, 434
Grey Turner's sign 181–2
gross motor skills 440,
  455, 460–1
group A beta-haemolytic
  streptococcal pharyngitis
  45–6
growing pains 478–9
growth
  faltering 211, 251–2,
    513
  stages of 507–8
growth hormone (GH)
  axis 512
growth hormone (GH)
  deficiency
  diagnosis of 512
  isolated 508–9
  MCQs on 519
  and obesity 559, 563
  and short stature 511
growth hormone (GH)
  treatment 470, 512–20

guttate psoriasis 598, 605,
  618

H2RA (histamine 2
  receptor antagonists)
  162
habit cough 294, 302, 305
haemangiomas 601, 609,
  614–15
haematemesis 130, 196,
  242, 298, 491
haematocrit 159, 487, 497
haematuria 99, 155, 162,
  278, 580, 584
haemoglobin, normal
  486–8
haemolysis 489–92, 497
haemolytic anaemias
  489–91
  and gallstone 177
  MCQs on 506
  and nephrolithiasis 183
  and parvovirus B19 573
  racial predilections
    of 499
  signs of 493
  and thalassaemia 488
Haemophilus influenzae
  19, 46, 67, 79, 310
haemoptysis 295
hair, tuft on spinal
  examination 223, 263
hair loss 598, 601, 603
hair tourniquet syndrome
  100, 105
hallucinations 382, 404
hand foot and mouth
  disease 575
hand washing 84, 209,
  212, 214–15
HbA1c levels 540, 542–3,
  545, 547, 553
hCG 523–4, 528, 531–2
head trauma
  abusive 102, 107
  and phenytoin 31
  and vomiting 157–8
headache diaries 363,
  365–6, 368–9
headaches; *see also*
  recurrent headaches
  and abdominal pain
    178–9
  and acute rash 579
  and fever 52
  and hypertension 156,
    379
  MCQs on 378
  and meningitis 49
  non-pharmacological
    treatment for 371–3
  and pneumonia 47
  and PPIs 162
  and sleep disorders 407
HEADS framework 239

hearing loss; *see also*
  deafness
  causes of 425–6
  and DS 459, 462–3
  and otitis media 46, 65
  and speech delay 425
heart failure
  and anaemia 492
  congestive 337, 340,
    344; *see also* CHD
  and failure to thrive
    243
  and FTT 240, 243
  symptoms of 335
height measurement
  509–11, 513, 526
HELLP syndrome 432
hemiplegic migraine 360
hepatitis 77, 179, 573, 576
hepatomegaly 342, 434,
  563
hepatosplenomegaly 121,
  603
hernias, incarcerated 112
herpes simplex virus
  (HSV) 574–5, 582
hesitancy, use of term 278
hip X-rays 475, 480
Hirschsprung's disease
  223–5, 235
Hirschsprung's
  enterocolitis 181, 207
hirsutism 524–5, 527,
  570, 604
HIV 52, 76, 79, 82–3,
  240, 488
HLA (human leukocyte
  antigen), and coeliac
  disease 207
holding manoeuvres 278,
  285, 291
homework, and ADHD
  623–4, 628
homocystinuria 429, 435
honey
  in infant feeding 118,
    130
  and URTIs 300, 307
Horner's syndrome 360
hospitalisation
  and eating disorders
    248–9, 252–3
  and failure to thrive
    246
  and vomiting 162
HS (hypertonic saline)
  and bronchiolitis 22,
    322, 330–1
  and cystic fibrosis 301
  and wheeze 324–5
HS, *see also* spherocytosis,
  hereditary
HSP (Henoch–Schönlein
  purpura) 182, 578, 580,
  583–5

Hurler's syndrome 435
hydrocephalus 99, 104,
158, 362, 523
hydrops foetalis 488, 573,
585
hydroxyurea (HU) 503–5
hyper-IgE syndrome
78–80, 91–2
hyperactivity; *see also*
ADHD
and autism 441
and food additives
631–2
and sleep problems 407
symptoms of 621–2
hypercalciuria 280
hyperglycaemia 537–8,
540, 542, 544–5, 590
hypergonadotropic
hypogonadism 525,
528–9
hyperlipidaemia 546, 608
hypernatraemia 540
hyperoxia tests 342
hypersomnias 402, 404
hypertension
and CHD 342
and enuresis 263
and IBD 187
and puberty 527
and recurrent headache
365
and retinopathy 546
hyperthyroidism
and ADHD 623–4
and eating disorders
241
hyperventilation 383, 431,
539–40
hypocretin 404, 408
hypoglycaemia
and developmental
delay 432, 438
and DKA 546
frequency of episodes
551–2
and GH deficiency 509
and GH investigations
512
management of 545
monitoring risk of
542–3
and short stature 509
and status epilepticus
39
hypogonadotropic
hypogonadism 525, 529
hypokalaemia
and constipation 223
and DKA 546
and vomiting 159
hypoplastic left heart
syndrome 338, 347, 350
hypotension
and anaphylaxis 25–6

and failure to thrive
243, 248
and hypovolaemia 202
and sepsis 30
hypothermia
and eating disorders
243
and infection 43
hypothyroidism
and ADHD 623
and coeliac disease 203
and delayed puberty
525
and DS 454, 458
and obesity 559, 563,
571
and precocious puberty
524
and short stature 509,
511
hypotonia
and DS 427
and excessive crying
98–9
and fever 52
and obesity 559
and Prader–Willi's
syndrome 525
hypotonic (floppy) infant
429–30, 442
hypovolaemia
and anaemia 492
and DKA 32
and seizures 32
and septicaemia 49
signs of 202
and vomiting 157, 161,
163
hypoxia, neonatal 623
hypsarrhythmia 385

IBD (inflammatory bowel
disease)
and abdominal pain
179
and delayed puberty
525
and diarrhoea 209
and failure to thrive
240, 242
follow-up for 211
investigations for 184,
215–16
management of 187–8
referral for 189
and short stature 511
ibuprofen
and fever 60
and migraine 368, 376
and PDA 345
and rheumatoid
arthritis 484
and transient synovitis
480–1
and vomiting 160

ichthyosis 597
ICSs (low-dose inhaled
steroids) 329–30
idiopathic hypersomnia
404
idiopathic intracranial
hypertension 156, 159,
164, 359, 361, 378–9
idiopathic short stature
508, 513–15, 518
IgA deficiency 76–7, 80,
92, 207, 212
IgE, and food allergies 88,
119, 133, 139, 143
ileal resection 240
ileus 30, 212–13
immotile cilia syndrome
317, 333
immunisation
and acute rash 581–2
and eczema 610
parental refusal of
584–6
side effects of 586–7
immunodeficiency
and chronic rash 597
and diarrhoea 207
immunodeficiency states
55, 76, 84, 582
immunoglobulin levels
82–3, 305
immunoglobulin therapy
83, 85, 90–1, 93, 588–9
immunotherapy, and
chronic rhinitis 309
impetigo 577, 583, 585
inattention 621–2, 625
incontinence, use of term
277
infant feeding
basic principles of
114–15
common problems
with 118–19
examination for
problems 120–1
managing problems in
121–2
MCQs on 131–2
infant formula
cow's milk-based
(CMF) 128–9
hydrolysed 108, 122,
124, 127–8
Infant Gastroesophageal
Reflux Questionnaire
171
infant regurgitation 119,
130–1
infantile spasms 384, 391,
394, 397–8
infants, clinically unwell
74
infections; *see also*
recurrent infections

and acute crying 112
congenital 425, 533
frequency of 75, 86–7
and hand washing
214–15
and sleep disorder 410,
413
transmission of 582
inflammatory diarrhoea
202
infliximab 187–8
inguinal hernia,
incarcerated 183
inhaler technique 301,
316, 320–1, 323
inhalers, dependency on
322–3
insomnia, chronic 406,
409, 412–13, 418–19
insulin
and coma 28
deficiency of 537–8
and DKA 32, 540
and glucose levels
544–6
inhaled 547
insulin therapy 542–4,
548, 550–1
insulin tolerance test 512,
520
intellectual disability
426–7, 439, 559
intermittency, use of term
277
International Headache
Society criteria 3, 362–3,
375–7
intracranial haemorrhage
101, 578, 584–5, 590
intranasal diamorphine
(IND) 500–1
intubation, and epiglottitis
19
intussusception
and abdominal pain
176
and coma 28
and diarrhoea 207
ileocolic 178
investigations for 184
management of 186
MCQs on 198–9
vaccine-related 217
X-rays in 190–1
ipratropium, and asthma
37–8
ipratropium bromide 22
iron chelation therapy
497, 503–4
iron deficiency
and diet 498
follow-up of 497
MCQs on 505
and obesity 560
signs of 492

iron-deficiency anaemia 487
  and coeliac disease 203
  and DS 455
  examinations in 493
  follow-up for 498
  management of 494–5
  treatment of 499–500
iron overload 497, 502–3
iron supplements (ISs) 499–500
iron therapy, parenteral 495
irritability, causes of 112
irritable bowel syndrome (IBS)
  and abdominal pain 178, 185
  and diarrhoea 202, 206, 215
  and food allergy 137
  and probiotics 187, 196–7
  and vomiting 155
isotretinoin 608
ITP (idiopathic thrombocytopenic purpura) 578, 580, 582–5, 589–90
IVIG (intravenous immunoglobulin) 90–1, 589–90

Jadad score 6–7
Janz's syndrome 384, 400
jaundice
  and anaemia 490–2
  and developmental delay 433
  follow-up on 124
  in infants 118, 123, 125, 131
  investigations for 121
  and short stature 509
JIA (juvenile idiopathic arthritis) 471–2
  and anaemia 488
  and delayed puberty 525
  investigations for 475
  and limp 467
  management of 477
  MCQs on 485
JMF criteria 76, 87–8, 91
joint aspiration 475
juice 209–11, 247, 557–8, 563, 632
junk foods 225, 247
juvenile absence epilepsy 384, 389
juvenile myoclonic epilepsy 384, 389, 391, 400

karyotyping 435–6, 449, 451

Kawasaki's disease
  diagnosis of 576
  early recognition of 582
  and fever 55
  investigations for 580
  management of 583–4, 588–9
  MCQs on 592
Kernig's sign 158, 580
ketogenic diet 392, 394, 398–9
ketone levels 540, 544–5
Kleine–Levin's syndrome 404
Klinefelter's syndrome 536
Koebner's phenomenon 598, 605
Koplik's spots 574
Krabbe's disease 431
Kussmaul's respiration 28, 538–9

LABA (long-acting beta agonist) 321, 329–30
lactase deficiency 204, 210, 218
Lactobacillus reuteri 110
lactose intolerance
  diagnosis of 208, 218
  and diarrhoea 204
  differential diagnosis for 137
  and excessive crying 98
  and feeding problems 119
  secondary 123
lactulose 202, 227, 229, 233–4
lamotrigine 384, 391, 396–7
language delays 65, 425–6, 428, 624
Laurence–Moon–Biedl's syndrome 525, 560
laxatives
  abuse of 205, 238
  and constipation 225, 277
lead poisoning 488
learning disabilities
  and ADHD 623
  and CHD 344, 348
  and developmental delay 437
left-to-right shunts 335–7, 342, 462
Legg–Calvé–Perthes disease 469, 480
Leigh's disease 432
Lennox–Gastaut's syndrome 385, 400
Lesch–Nyhan's syndrome 438
lethargy, and abdominal pain 190

leukaemia
  acute lymphoblastic 472
  and acute rash 578
  and anaemia 492, 498
  and IBT 582
leukotriene inhibitors 320–1
leuprolide 533
levetiracetam 384, 391
LGG (Lactobacillus GG) 196–7
lichen planus 598
limping
  causes of 467–72
  differential diagnosis of 474–5
  examination for 473–4
  history taking for 473
  investigations of 475
  management of 476–8
  MCQs for 484–5
  and obesity 558
  use of term 466
lipid profile 560
listening
  positive style of 13
  reflective 11
lithium 335, 340
liver function tests
  and abdominal pain 184
  and anaemia 493
  and FTT 244
  and obesity 560
  and puberty 529
long QT syndrome 388
loperamide 212–13
lorazepam 31, 40
LTRA (leukotriene-receptor antagonist) 329
lumbar puncture, contraindications to 31, 53, 73
lung hyperinflation 296, 316
Lyme disease 52, 472, 485
lymphadenopathy
  and acute rash 576, 580
  and anaemia 492
  generalised 45, 206, 474, 574
lymphopenia 82–3, 86, 90

macrocytic anaemia 486, 489, 493, 498, 505
macrolides 301
magnesium, and asthma 38–9
malabsorption
  and anaemia 499
  and iron deficiency 497
malaria 52, 491
malassezia yeast 599, 601

malnutrition 201, 203, 213, 254
malrotation
  and abdominal pain 177
  and bilious vomiting 156
  and excessive crying 99
  investigations for 183
  MCQs on 199
Mantoux test 299
Marfan's syndrome 335
mastitis 119–20, 123
McCune–Albright's syndrome 524, 530, 536
MCV (mean corpuscular volume) 487–8, 493, 495
mEASI (modified Eczema Area and Severity Index) 613–14
measles; *see also* MMR vaccine
  and acute rash 574, 579, 591
  prevention of 582
Meckel's diverticulum
  and abdominal pain 177–8
  diagnosis of 182
  management of 187
  MCQs on 199
meconium, delayed passage of 180–1, 223–4
medication, side effects of 629
medication adherence 319
melatonin 412–13, 418–19, 441, 447–8
menarche 242, 522–4, 526
meningism 50–1, 157, 387, 580
meningitis
  aseptic 61, 573, 576
  bacterial 28, 31, 53, 62
  and fever 43
  presentation of 49
  and seizures 386
  viral 53
meningococcal disease
  and acute rash 577, 582, 584, 587–8
  and limp 474
  MCQs on 73
  presentation of 49, 60
Menkes' kinky hair disease 431, 435
mental retardation 425, 525, 574, 623
Mentzer score 494
metabolic investigations 436–7
metabolism, inborn errors of 28, 385, 428–30, 441, 449

methotrexate 188, 477, 608

methylphenidate
  and ADHD 628–9, 635–6, 638
  and autism 441
  and giggle wetting 284
  and sleep problems 411

MI (motivational interviewing) 10–12
  and acute rash 582
  and obesity 564
  teaching 15

microalbuminuria 546, 553

microcytic anaemia 487–8, 493

midazolam 31–2, 40–1

migraine
  abdominal 178
  criteria for 362–3
  and diet 367, 369
  MCQs on 378–9
  paediatric 358–60, 362, 375
  prophylaxis of 375
  and seizures 388
  treatment for 368–9, 373–4
  and vomiting 157, 159

MMR vaccine 142–3, 441, 585–7

MMRV vaccine 143

MMS (multiple micronutrients supplement) 499–500

moist cough 20, 295–9, 301, 306, 310

molluscum dermatitis 597

montelukast 329

Moraxella catarrhalis 19, 46, 310

morning stiffness 476, 483

morphine 496–7, 500–1

Movicol 227, 229, 235

MRI (magnetic resonance imaging)
  and epilepsy 381, 392
  and limping 469, 475
  and seizures 389

mucopolysaccharidosis 434–5, 511

mumps; *see also* MMR vaccine
  and acute rash 573, 591

murmurs
  assessing 352–3
  and CHD 334
  and excessive crying 98
  explaining to parents 343–4, 348
  and FTT 243
  innocent 336, 347
  organic 344, 352, 356

myasthenia gravis 430

Mycoplasma pneumonia 316–17, 491

Mycoplasma pneumoniae 47, 79, 496

myelodysplastic syndromes 489

naevi 223, 263

NAI (non-accidental injury)
  and excessive crying 95–6, 102–4
  signs of 112

naproxen sodium 368, 376–7

naps, scheduling 411

narcolepsy 404
  and epilepsy 388
  investigations for 408
  MCQs on 420
  treatment of 411–12, 417–18

nasal discharge, purulent 301

nasal steroids 301, 308

nasogastric feeding 126, 322, 344

nasogastric tubes 162, 168, 186, 251, 255

NDFs (nutrient-dense formulas) 251–2

nebulisers 35, 320

neglect 98, 239, 248–9, 257

Neisseria meningitidis 79

neonates
  bilious vomiting in 156, 158, 164
  risk of infection 44

nephrolithiasis 155–6, 158–9, 179, 183, 189

neurocutaneous stigmata 387, 433–4

neurofibromatosis
  and ADHD 623–4, 626
  and developmental delay 427
  and enuresis 263
  and puberty disorders 523
  and short stature 511

neuroimaging, and headache 365, 367, 369–70, 379

neuronal ceroid lipofuscinosis 431

neuropathy, diabetic 546–7

neutropenia
  clinical features of 78
  cyclic 53
  incidental 56

Niemann–Pick's disease 429, 431, 435

night feeders 413

night terrors 405, 419

night-time awakening 403, 407, 411, 415–16, 539

night-time fears (NFs) 416–17

nightmares 375, 388, 405, 407, 419

Nikolsky's sign 576–7

nipples, cracked 119–20, 123

nitric oxide, fractional excretion of 318

NNH (number needed to harm) 5

NNT (number needed to treat) 5, 7

Nocardia 78

nocturia 278

nocturnal enuresis 259
  aetiology of 260–1
  behavioural interventions for 269
  and bladder capacity 268–9
  and diabetes mellitus 539–40
  differential diagnosis of 263
  examination for 262–3
  history taking for 261–2
  investigations for 263
  management of 264–8
  MCQs for 273–5
  treatment of 271–3

non-specific cough 294

Noonan's syndrome, and CHD 335, 343

normocytic anaemia 489, 491, 493

Norwood procedure 347

NPs (nurse practitioners) 605, 612–13

NSAIDs (non-steroidal anti-inflammatory drugs) 472–3, 477, 479

nutritional advice 560–1

obesity
  causes of 556–7
  drug therapy for 569
  and DS 458
  and enuresis 265
  examination for 559–60
  and exercise capacity 567
  and headache 361
  history taking for 558
  investigations for 560
  management of 560–4
  MCQs on 569–71
  models of care for 565
  and paediatricians 566
  and precocious puberty 523

and sleep disorders 406, 408, 413

social impact of 568

use of term 557

obstructive lesions 337

oestradiol 244, 528

olanzapine 256

oligohydramnios 468, 473

Omenn's syndrome 597

ondansetron 161–2, 164–6, 169, 174

ophthalmoplegic migraine 360

oral allergy syndrome 150

oral contraceptives 524, 526, 603

oral immunotherapy 139, 141, 148–9

orchitis 573

orlistat 562, 569

ORT (oral rehydration therapy) 163, 165–9, 173, 201, 209, 212–14

orthostatic syncope 23–4

Ortolani testing 453, 468

OSA (obstructive sleep apnoea) 406–7
  and Down's syndrome 451, 454, 456, 458–9, 464
  and enuresis 261, 265
  MCQs on 419
  treatment of 411–12

Osgood–Schlatter's disease 467, 470, 477, 485

osmotic diarrhoea 202, 212

osteochondritis dissecans 467, 470, 477–8

osteomyelitis 52
  acute haematogenous 482–3
  and excessive crying 99
  investigations for 475
  and limping 471, 479
  signs of 52
  treatment of 477, 482
  vertebral 468

otitis media
  acute, *see* AOM
  and adenoidectomy 66
  and DS 454
  and headache 359
  and measles 574
  persistent 57, 65
  risk factors for 72

otorrhoea 46, 52, 99

ovarian cyst 182, 524, 528, 530

over-the-counter medications
  and cough 299–300, 303, 307
  and rash 602

oxandrolone 534
oxybutynin 268, 284, 287, 290
oxycodone 192–3

PACCT (Paris Consensus on Childhood Constipation Terminology) 221
PACE programme 325–6
pacifiers 129–30
PACT (parent-mediated communication-focused treatment) 445–6
pain, and limp 466, 468
palivizumab 341, 344, 353–4, 457
pallor
  and anaemia 181, 206, 486–7, 492–4
  and coeliac disease 203
  and excessive crying 99
  investigations for 493
  and leukaemia 498
  and limping 474
  and migraine 178, 359
  and syncope 388
  and vomiting 155
palpitations 242, 335, 351, 388, 486
pancreatitis 156, 158, 173, 176–7, 573, 591
papilloedema
  and headache 367
  and hypertension 156, 361
  and intracranial pressure 387
  and puberty 527, 532
  and raised intracranial pressure 153
  and vomiting 158
papular purpuric gloves and socks syndrome 575
paracetamol
  and fever 60
  and limb pain 479
  and sickle-cell disease 496
  and vomiting 160
parasomnias 402, 405, 410–11, 413
parental anxiety 43, 54, 351, 588
parental beliefs 136, 185
parental response
  to abdominal pain 185, 195
  to crying 410–13
  to daytime wetting 282
  to diarrhoea 209
  to epilepsy 390
  to fever 54
  to nocturnal enuresis 264–5

  to soiling 225
  to vomiting 160
parenting styles 409, 626
parents
  coping skills of 410
  difficult encounters with 12–14
parvovirus B19 491, 572–3, 585, 590
patch testing 139
PBB (persistent bacterial bronchitis) 294, 306, 310
PDA (patent ductus arteriosus) 336–8, 343, 345, 356
peak flow meters 321
peanut allergy 134, 145–6, 149, 332
Pediatric Quality of Life Inventory 88
pelvic abscess 209
pelvic ultrasound 523, 527
Pendred's syndrome 425
penicillin
  and acute rash 582
  and sickle-cell disease 495–6
  and UTIs 58
perfusion, poor 44, 52, 95
peritonitis 99, 175, 177, 181–2, 185–6
permethrin 609–11, 616
persistent vomiting 27, 212–13, 363, 365, 367
Perthes disease 467, 469, 475, 477
pertussis 294, 297, 301, 305, 311
pet allergies 319–20
petechiae
  and acute rash 574–5, 577–8
  and fever 59
  and limping 474
  and pallor 492
Peyer's patches 176, 198
PFAPA syndrome 53
phagocytic defects 76, 78, 82
pharyngitis
  and abdominal pain 182
  complications of 45–6
  signs of 52
  treatment of 56–7
phenobarbitone 31–2
phenylketonuria, maternal 432, 434
phenytoin 31, 335, 391, 603
Philadelphia protocol 56, 61–3
photophobia 49, 155, 178, 363, 579–80

physiotherapy, and pneumonia 68–9
pica 491
PIDs (primary immunodeficiency disorders)
  clinical features of 77–8, 86
  evaluation for 87–8
  and immunoglobulin 82
  interpreting features of 79–80
  management of 84–5
  MCQs on 91
  and recurrent infections 75–6
  referral for 85
pityriasis rosea 598, 601
pityriasis versicolor 599, 601
plaque psoriasis 598, 601, 607, 611
Pneumocystis jirovecii 77, 79, 81
pneumonia
  and abdominal pain 182–3
  assessment of 47–8
  bacterial 52
  community-acquired 57, 59, 67
  and cough 297
  and diabetes mellitus 540
  MCQs on 73
  and measles 574
  and PIDs 80
  repeated 299
  treatment of 57, 68–9
  and varicella zoster 585
  viral 52
polycythaemia 455, 462
polydipsia
  and coma 28
  and daytime wetting 278
  and diabetes 539–40, 548
  and DKA 182
  and enuresis 261–3
polyethylene glycol (PEG) 227, 231–4
polymerase chain reaction tests 30–1
polysomnography 405, 408, 411, 420
polyuria
  and coma 28
  and daytime wetting 279, 281
  and diabetes 539, 548
  and DKA 182
  nocturnal 261–2
port wine stains 601–2

post-gastroenteritis syndrome 203
post-micturition dribble 278
post-viral cough 294, 297
Prader–Willi's syndrome
  and delayed puberty 525
  and developmental delay 427, 434
  MCQs on 535
  and obesity 559, 571
  and OSA 406
  and short stature 511, 514
PRAM (Preschool Respiratory Assessment Measure) 21, 102, 324
precocious puberty 523–4, 528–35
prednisolone
  and anaphylaxis 27
  and asthma 22, 36
  and Crohn's disease 187
  and Kawasaki's disease 589
  and wheeze 323–4
prednisone 187
pregnancy
  ectopic 182
  and vomiting 153
prematurity
  and cough 295
  and developmental delay 427
  and excessive crying 99
  and hearing loss 425
presyncope 22–4
probiotics
  and abdominal pain 187, 196–7
  and diarrhoea 213–14
progressive waiting 411
prolonged fever 52, 73
propranolol
  and CHD 345–6
  and haemangioma 609, 611, 615
  and migraine 373–4
  and syncope 24
proton pump inhibitors (PPIs) 162, 171–2, 301
pseudohypoparathyroidism 438, 511, 560
Pseudomonas species 299, 301
psoriasis
  and chronic rash 597–9
  and limping 473
  management of 610
  MCQs on 618
  treatment of 607–8
psychogenic non-epileptic seizures 388
psychosocial deprivation 425

pubertal development
examination for 527
history taking for 526
investigations for 527–9
management of 529–31
normal 521–2
parental reactions to 533
puberty, and chronic disease 529–30
PUJ (pelvi-ureteric junction) obstruction 155, 159, 162, 164
pulmonary flow murmur 336
pulmonary function tests 295, 314, 318, 333
pulmonary hypertension 345, 406, 408
pulmonary stenosis 335, 339–40, 343, 345
pulse oximetry 47, 342, 348–9
purpura fulminans 49, 73, 573, 577, 585
pyelonephritis 48, 58, 69–70, 73
pyeloplasty 162
pyloric stenosis
and failure to thrive 240
investigations in 159
management of 161
MCQs on 172
and vomiting 154, 164
pyogenic infections, recurrent 79–80
pyuria 70, 576, 592

quality of life (QoL)
and AEDs 394
and chronic infection 88–9, 93

radiological investigations
and developmental delay 436
and short stature 511
and UTIs 101
raised intracranial pressure
and excessive crying 99
and headache 361, 365
and obesity 563
and SBI 53
and seizures 387
and vomiting 153, 156
randomisation, correct 3–4
RAP (recurrent abdominal pain) 178, 189–90, 196–8; *see also* FAP
rash; *see also* acute rash; chronic rash

configuration of 596
describing 594
and diabetes mellitus 539
and fever 56
and food allergy 142
and limping 473
in meningococcal disease 49
morphology of 595
non-blanching 28, 58, 582, 587–8
scaly 618
RBC-7 device 303–4
RCTs (randomised controlled trials)
assessing quality of 6
and EBM 2–6
pitfall avoidance in 6–8
rebound headache 367, 369, 379
rectal biopsy 224
recurrent cough 294
recurrent fevers 43–4, 50, 53
recurrent headaches
examination for 364–5
history taking for 363–4
management of 365–7, 369
treatment of 367–8
types of 358–9
recurrent hypersomnia 404, 412
recurrent infections
causes of 75–6
differential diagnosis for 82
and DiGeorge's syndrome 428
and DS 457
examination for 81
and heart failure 335
history taking for 80–1
investigations of 82–3
management of 83–5
red flags in 92
recurrent otitis media 57, 65, 80, 317
recurrent pneumonias 91, 154, 306, 314, 332
recurrent UTIs 71–2, 280, 285, 289
recurrent vomiting
and anaphylaxis 26
causes of 159, 164, 173
and GERD 154
management of 160
red blood cell indices 486–7
red reflex 453
refeeding syndrome 248, 255

referred pain 176, 467, 476, 479
reflex-anoxic seizures 388, 400–1
Refsum's disease 435
relaxation, applied 372–3
renal failure, chronic 488, 511, 525
renal insufficiency, chronic 514
renal stones, *see* nephrolithiasis
respiratory burst assay 83
respiratory distress
and acute rash 580
and anaphylaxis 26–7
and bronchiolitis 313
and CHD 341–2
and cough 296
and DS 453
and excessive crying 99
and fever 51–2
and sickle-cell disease 496
and wheeze 315, 319
respiratory syncytial virus (RSV)
and acute rash 575
and bronchiolitis 314
and DS 454
and palivizumab 353
respite care 440
REST programme 109
reticulocyte count 487, 489, 491, 493, 495, 497
retinopathy
diabetic 546–7
pigmentary 429
Rett's syndrome 431, 438, 449
RH (retinal haemorrhage) 98–9, 101, 107, 492
rheumatic fever 46, 52, 574
rheumatoid arthritis 472, 483–4
rhinitis, allergic 134, 294–5, 596–7, 603
rhinorrhoea, purulent 317, 333
rhinosinusitis 457
rhythmic movement disorder 405
risperidone 441, 446–7, 558
Ritalin 635–6
Rochester criteria 56, 62–3
rolandic epilepsy 394
Rome II criteria 178, 195–6
rotavirus
and gastroenteritis 154, 203
tests for 208

vaccination against 209, 212, 216–17
RSI (rapid sequence intubation) 39–40
rubella 142, 441, 537, 573–4, 591
Russell–Silver's syndrome 245, 511, 514, 517

sacral dimple 223, 263
sacral lipoma 223, 263
salbutamol 22, 36–8, 327
saline
hypertonic, *see* HS
nebulised 33–5
salmon patch 602
salmonella
and diarrhoea 202, 212
and limping 471
and PIDs 79, 92
sample size, calculation of 3
Sandhoff's disease 431, 435
SBI (serious bacterial infection)
examples of 43
risk of 44, 56, 61–3
signs of 52
scabies 597, 609–11, 616
scalded skin syndrome 576, 583–4, 592
scalp treatment 607
scarlet fever 574, 582, 596
school
and daytime wetting 282
and epilepsy 390
SCID (severe combined immunodeficiency)
and FBC 82
frequency of 76–7
MCQs on 92–3
screening for 84, 89–90
signs of 78
SCIG (subcutaneous immunoglobulin) 90–1, 93
SCORAD (Scoring of Atopic Dermatitis) 611–13
secretory diarrhoea 202, 218
sedation 410, 413
seizures; *see also* epileptic seizures
categories of 381
differential diagnosis of 387–8
drug therapy of 40–1
and DS 454
examination for 387
febrile, *see* febrile convulsions
history taking for 386

investigations for 389
management of 389–93
MCQs on 399–401
nocturnal 410
and obesity 560
triggers for 390
self-care skills 455
self-hypnosis 302, 368, 373–4, 417
self-soothing 404, 413
sepsis
and diabetes mellitus 540
and fever 55
first response to 30
septic arthritis
differentiation from transient synovitis 479–80
and excessive crying 99
investigations for 475
and limping 470–1, 479
MCQs for 484
signs of 52
treatment of 477, 481–2
septicaemia
and acute rash 577, 580
and fever 43
meningococcal 31, 73
presentation of 49, 52
Serratia marcescens 78
serum tryptase 139, 143
sex steroid secreting tumours 524
sex steroids 523–5, 531
sexual abuse 239
SGA (small for gestational age) 513–15, 517–18
shock, first response to 29–30
short bowel syndrome 207
short stature
and brain tumours 361
and coeliac disease 203
and Crohn's disease 182
and delayed puberty 526, 529, 534
differential diagnosis of 511
and DiGeorge's syndrome 428
and DS 457–8, 465
examinations for 509–10
and GH treatment 514–15
history taking for 509
investigations in 511–12
MCQs on 519–20
and obesity 559
parent and child perceptions of 512–13, 516–17

and Prader–Willi's syndrome 427
use of term 507
shuddering attacks 387
shunt blockage 359, 362
siblings, and developmental delay 440
sick days, management of 545
sickle-cell disease
acute painful episodes in 495–6
and anaemia 490–1, 494–5
and enuresis 261–3
and excessive crying 104
information for parents 498
and limping 471
MCQs on 506
and pneumococcal disease 501–2
and recurrent infections 82
sickle-cell pain 500–1
sinopulmonary infections, recurrent 79–80
sinusitis 359, 361–2, 574
SJS (Stevens–Johnson syndrome) 391, 576–7, 583, 585
skin infections 79, 85, 577, 583, 602
sleep, MCQs on 419–20
sleep apnoea 262, 563; see also OSA
sleep deprivation
and cough 300, 303
and epilepsy 383–4, 386
and migraine 360
parental 409
sleep-deprived EEG 389
sleep-disordered breathing 402, 406, 408
sleep disorders 403–5
examination for 407–8
management of 410
and seizures 388
sleep disturbance
and autism 441, 447–8
behavioural 412
and cough 297
and GERD 154
natural history of 414
negative effects of 402
sleep hygiene 409, 411–13
sleep logs 413
sleep patterns
assessing 410
normal 367, 403, 406, 409
sleepwalking 405, 407, 419

SLIT (sublingual immunotherapy) 309
Smith–Lemli–Opitz's syndrome 434, 438
smoking
and cough 300, 302
and eczema 597
and otitis media 57
and recurrent infections 87
and retinopathy 546
and wheeze 314–15, 320–2
social class 87, 414
sodium oxybate 411, 417–18
sodium valproate
and obesity 558
and seizures 384, 391
soiling 220–2, 225–6, 228–9, 235–6
somatic pain 176
soothers 122, 132
spacer devices 301, 316, 320, 326–8
speech
acquisition of 422–4
and seizures 383
speech delay 425, 436, 440, 622
spherocytosis, hereditary 490, 493, 497, 499, 505–6
spinal abnormalities 223, 263
spinal dysraphism 261
spirometry 299, 329, 333, 496–7
'spitting up' 119, 125; see also infant regurgitation
splenectomy 490, 497, 504
splenic infarction 183
splenic sequestration 491, 498
SPT (skin prick testing)
errors in 138
and food allergy 133–4, 143
MCQs on 150
spurious diarrhoea 209, 211
sputum cultures 295, 299, 301
Staphylococcus aureus
and cough 299, 301
and eczema 606
and granulomatous disease 78
and mastitis 120
and PIDs 79
and septic arthritis 471
and toxic shock 576
and tracheitis 19
status epilepticus 28, 31–2, 39–40, 389
steatorrhoea 202, 206, 242

'steeple sign' 18
steroids
anabolic 524
and asthma 36, 320–2, 329
and croup 33
and diabetes mellitus 539
and eczema 605–6, 610–11
and IBD 187–8
and Kawasaki's disease 583, 588–9
and septic arthritis 477
and short stature 509
and wheeze 315, 319, 323–4, 328
Still's murmur 336, 355
stool avoidance 225
stool culture 62, 183–4, 208, 214
stool pattern, normal 205, 220–1
stools
hard 221–2, 228, 230–2
occult blood tests for 224
straining 98, 277–8
strep throat 59, 72
Streptococcus
group A 596
group B 471, 606–7
Streptococcus pneumoniae 19, 46–7, 310
stress
and headaches 360, 370
on parents 103
stress incontinence 280
stridor
acute 16, 34
and anaphylaxis 27
and cough 296
and haemangioma 601
stroke 28, 491, 498, 573, 581
Sturge–Weber's syndrome 602
sudden infant death syndrome 432
SUFE (slipped upper femoral epiphysis) 467, 470, 476–7, 479
suicidal ideation 242, 629
sulfamethoxazole 71, 85
sulfasalazine 188
sumatriptan 162, 368, 376–7
suppositories 225
sweat test 299
sweating, and puberty 530
syncope
acute 22–4
of cardiac origin 388
and sleep disorders 407

synovitis, transient 467, 469, 475–81, 484
systemic lupus erythematosus 52, 223, 525

T-cell deficiency 78, 92
T-cell function, tests of 83
T-cell lymphopenia (TCL) 89–90, 92
T-cell-mediated deficiencies 80
T-lymphocyte deficiency 79
tachycardia, supraventricular 23–4, 100, 158, 340, 351
tachypnoea
    and diabetes mellitus 539–40
    and DS 453
    and fever 47, 49
    and hypovolaemia 202
    and wheeze 20
tacrolimus 606, 611, 613–14
TAPVD (total anomalous pulmonary venous drainage) 340, 346
Tay–Sachs's disease 429, 431, 434–5
temporal lobe seizures 394
TEN (toxic epidermal necrolysis) 576–7
tension headaches
    criteria for 360, 363
    and distraction 367
    recurrent 358
testes, undescended 509
testicular torsion 176, 182, 184, 186, 199, 467
testosterone 521, 523–4, 528, 531–2, 604
testotoxicosis 524, 530
tetralogy of Fallot 335, 339, 342–3, 346, 350, 355–6
TGA (transposition of the great arteries) 335, 339–40, 346, 354–6
thalassaemia
    assessing 494
    ethnic risk for 487
    and HU 503–4
    and iron overload 502
    management of 497–8
    types of 488
thalassaemia intermedia 497
thelarche, premature 522–4, 529, 532, 535
thrombocytopenia 78, 82, 472, 574, 580

thyroid function tests
    and DS 455
    and obesity 560
Tinea infections
    and chronic rash 597–8
    differential diagnosis of 601
    investigations into 604
    MCQs on 618
    treatment of 608–9
    varieties of 600
TIPS AEIOU 27
toddler's diarrhoea 202, 204, 212, 218
toddler's fracture 467–8, 475, 485
tolterodine 273, 290
tonic-clonic seizures 382, 384, 388, 390–1
tonic seizures 385, 388
topiramate 368, 375, 391
toxic shock syndrome 576, 584, 592
tracheitis, bacterial 19
transformation migraine 360
trauma, and limp 468
Treacher Collins syndrome 425
TREC (T-cell receptor excision circle) 89–90, 92
Trendelenburg gait 466, 468–9
Trichophyton 598, 600, 609
tricuspid atresia 339–40, 343, 347
trimethoprim 71, 85
triple X syndrome 525
tripping 262, 279–81, 285
triptans 368, 376
truncus arteriosus 335, 339–40, 346
tuberculosis
    and anaemia 488
    and cough 295, 298
    and failure to thrive 240
    and fever 52
tuberous sclerosis
    and developmental delay 427
    and seizures 385, 391
Turner's syndrome
    and CHD 335
    and delayed puberty 525
    MCQs on 536
    and short stature 511, 514–17, 520
tympanostomy tubes 66

ulcerative colitis 179, 184, 188

upper airway cough syndrome
    and dark circles under eyes 142
    MCQs on 311–12
    treatment of 301
urge incontinence 280
urgency, use of term 278
urinalysis
    and abdominal pain 183
    and constipation 224
    and daytime wetting 281
    and excessive crying 101, 104
    and fever 54
urine culture
    and daytime wetting 281
    and UTIs 54, 57, 59
urine dipstick 54, 263
urodynamic studies 260, 281, 288–9
urotherapy 281, 283–5, 288
urticaria
    and acute rash 578–9
    and food allergy 135–6, 138, 142
    management of 583–4
URTIs (upper respiratory tract infections)
    and AOMs 46
    and cough 294–5, 297, 300–1
    and intussusception 176
    MCQs on 312
    treatment of 307
    and wheeze 315, 317
UTIs (urinary tract infections)
    assessment of 48, 54
    and constipation 224
    and daytime wetting 276–7, 279, 282, 284, 291
    and excessive crying 101
    and fever 43
    MCQs on 73
    and nocturnal enuresis 262–3
    prevention of 70–2
    signs of 52
    treatment of 57–8

vaccinations, complications with 86
vagal nerve stimulation 393
vaginal reflux 280, 284
valproic acid 396–7

varicella zoster
    and acute rash 573
    complications of 585
    immunisation from 582
    MCQs on 591
    and PIDs 79, 84, 86
vasodepressor syncope 24
vasopressin 261
venous hum 336, 348, 355
venous sinus thrombosis 46, 359
ventricular hypertrophy 339, 343, 462
vertigo 23, 152, 360, 364
video games
    and epilepsy 393
    and sleep disorders 409
vigabatrin 384–5, 391, 397–8
VIPomas 202, 207
visceral pain 110, 175–6
visual field defects 361, 373, 382
visual impairment 418, 436, 439
vital signs, normal 45
vitamin A 361
vitamin B$_{12}$ deficiency 244
vitamin C 487
vitamin D 607, 611
vitamin K 490
vitamins, and immune system 85
voiding, timed 281, 283, 287–8
voiding diaries 277, 282–3, 285–6, 291
voiding dysfunction 224, 283, 286, 289
voiding postponement 280, 291
voiding problems, terminology of 259–60
volvulus
    and abdominal pain 177
    and bilious vomiting 156
    and excessive crying 99
    management of 186
vomiting; see also bilious vomiting; recurrent vomiting
    and acute rash 576, 578–9
    causes of 154–6
    central stimuli of 152–3
    and diabetes 539
    examination for 157–8
    and failure to thrive 242, 245
    and FTT 245, 257
    and headache 370
    history taking for 157

management of 160–1, 163
MCQs on 172–3
pharmacological reduction of 165–6
self-induced 238
VSDs (ventricular septal defects) 336
  and cyanotic CHDs 339–40
  in Down's syndrome 335
  management of 345
  MCQs on 355
  and murmurs 348
VTs (ventilation tubes) 57, 65, 457, 463
VUR (vesicoureteric reflex)
  and daytime wetting 276–7

radiological investigations for 101
  and UTIs 48, 52, 58, 71

WAAPs (written asthma action plan) 325–6
Waardenburg's syndrome 425
wakening, anticipatory 411
watchful waiting (WW) 57, 59, 65, 300, 601
weaning
  early 129
  process of 115, 117–18, 122
weight gain, medications causing 570
weight loss
  and cough 302
  and diabetes 538, 548

and FTT 241–3
  and sleep disorders 412
weight maintenance 254, 561–4
West's syndrome 384–5
wet wraps 606
wheeze; see also asthma
  acute, see acute wheeze
  and allergenic food 144–5
  differential diagnosis of 317
  episodic 317
  examination for 316
  history taking for 315–16
  investigations for 318
  management of 318–19
  MCQs on 331–3
  nocturnal 322

white cell scanning 184
white matter disease 431
Williams's syndrome 335, 427–8, 438, 449, 623–4
Wilson's disease 435
Wiskott–Aldrich's syndrome (WAS) 78–80, 82, 91, 597
WLSPT (water load symptom provocation test) 194–5
Wolff–Parkinson–White's syndrome 23–4

XLA (X-linked agammaglobulinaemia) 76–7, 88–90, 92–3

zinc deficiency 597
zolmitriptan 376

T - #0954 - 101024 - C0 - 246/174/29 - PB - 9781908911902 - Gloss Lamination